American Medical Association
Physicians dedicated to the health of America

The Family Practice Desk Reference

Driscoll • Bope

Edited by

Charles E. Driscoll, MD
Lynchburg Family Practice Residency
Lynchburg, Virginia

Edward T. Bope, MD
Riverside Methodist Hospital
Columbus, Ohio

FOURTH EDITION

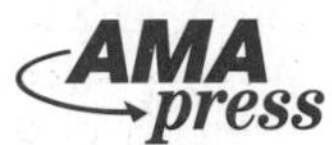

The Family Practice Desk Reference
Fourth Edition

AMA Press
Vice President, Business Products: Anthony J. Frankos
Publisher: Michael Desposito
Editorial Director: Mary Lou White
Director, Production and Manufacturing: Jean Roberts
Senior Acquisitions Editor: Eileen Lynch
Developmental Editor: Katharine Dvorak
Director, Marketing: J. D. Kinney
Marketing Manager: Reg Schmidt
Senior Production Coordinator: Rosalyn Carlton
Senior Print Coordinator: Ronnie Summers
Proofreader: Nicole Netter

Internet address: www.ama-assn.org

Additional copies of this book may be ordered by calling 800 621-8335 or visiting www.amapress.com. Mention product number OP830102.

ISBN 1–57947–190–0

Library of Congress Cataloging-in-Publication Data

The family practice desk reference / edited by Charles E. Driscoll,
Edward T. Bope.—4th ed.
p. ; cm.
Includes bibliographical references and index.
ISBN 1-57947-190-0
1. Family medicine—Handbooks, manuals, etc.
[DNLM: 1. Family Practice—Handbooks. WB 39 F198 2002] I. Driscoll,
Charles E. II. Bope, Edward T.
RC55 .F22 2002
610—dc21 2002074646

BP57:02–P–045:010/02

We dedicate this book to Jackie Driscoll, who has inspired, supported, and loved us through this book and previous editions, and to Charles E. Bope, MD, who is a role model for the family doctor that everyone needs and an inspiration to both of us.

CONTENTS

PREFACE

Medical information for physicians is now available in many electronic formats. In this era of handheld computers and the Internet, there are many ways to get quick, up-to-date answers to questions about patient care. Why then would we want to continue to do a book form of *The Family Practice Desk Reference*? The simpler of several answers is that there is still need to have a good clinical resource in a print format. Internet access can be slowed by sign-on and sign-off times, and often physicians must leave the patient care area to get to a computer. And unless a dedicated line is kept open for Internet use during patient care, the computer may be in use for another task. A book, however, can go wherever needed and does not depend on an Internet connection or batteries!

As with our previous editions, the fourth edition of *The Family Practice Desk Reference* contains the necessary nuggets of information about the most common conditions encountered by family physicians. We set out to provide a quick reference to the most important aspects of health and illness management, rather than an exhaustive discourse. We organized the book using the life-cycle approach (care of children, maternity care, etc) and by body system (cardiovascular, lung, etc), rather than by discipline, and each chapter is written by practicing family physicians, residency faculty, or senior family practice residents. In addition, each chapter contains a list of references for more in-depth study.

We are indebted to Eileen Lynch, our editor at AMA Press, who has encouraged us and kept us on schedule along the way. We would also like to thank our secretaries, Teresa Henderson, Deborah Donnigan, and Nakisha Pannell, for their assistance in preparing the manuscript, and Andrew Wilds for his photographic work.

Charles E. Driscoll, MD
Edward T. Bope, MD

CONTRIBUTORS

Ann M. Aring, MD
Riverside Family Practice Residency
Riverside Methodist Hospital
Columbus, Ohio

Michael R. Cook, MD
Lynchburg Family Practice Residency
Lynchburg, Virginia

William C. Crow, Jr, MD
Lynchburg Family Practice Residency
Lynchburg, Virginia

Jacquelyn S. Driscoll, RN
Lynchburg, Virginia

Robert I. Elliott, MD, FAAFP
Lynchburg Family Practice Residency
Lynchburg, Virginia

Dean G. Gianakos, MD
Lynchburg Family Practice Residency
Lynchburg, Virginia

Curtis L. Gingrich, MD
Riverside Family Practice Residency
Riverside Methodist Hospital
Columbus, Ohio

David S. Gregory, MD
Lynchburg Family Practice Residency
Lynchburg, Virginia

John W. Hedrick, MD
Louisiana State University Family Practice Residency
Alexandria, Louisiana

J. Dan Johnson, DO
Lynchburg Family Practice Residency
Lynchburg, Virginia

Anitha Lokesh, MD
Lynchburg Family Practice Residency
Lynchburg, Virginia

Michael L. Madden, MD
Louisiana State University Family Practice Residency
Alexandria, Louisiana

Stephen E. Markovich, MD
Riverside Family Practice Residency
Riverside Methodist Hospital
Columbus, Ohio

Dawn Mattern, MD
Riverside Family Practice Residency
Riverside Methodist Hospital
Columbus, Ohio

H. Dale Meade, MD
Louisiana State University Family Practice Residency
Alexandria, Louisiana

Dana Nottingham, MD
Riverside Family Practice Residency
Riverside Methodist Hospital
Columbus, Ohio

Patricia A. Pletke, MD
Lynchburg Family Practice Residency
Lynchburg, Virginia

Mrunal Shah, MD
Riverside Family Practice Residency
Riverside Methodist Hospital
Columbus, Ohio

Brenda L. Stokes, MD
Lynchburg Family Practice Residency
Lynchburg, Virginia

John A. Vaughn, MD
Riverside Family Practice Residency
Riverside Methodist Hospital
Columbus, Ohio

Alex Wilgus, MD
Lynchburg Family Practice Residency
Lynchburg, Virginia

George C. Wortley, MD
Lynchburg Family Practice Residency
Lynchburg, Virginia

chapter 1

Family-Centered Care

Charles E. Driscoll, MD

IN THIS CHAPTER

- Facts about family medicine
- Recommendations for periodic health examinations
- Negative recommendations for periodic health examinations
- Office follow-up of asymptomatic chronic conditions
- Disqualifying conditions for Department of Transportation examinations
- Health teaching for patients
- Strategies for health promotion
- Techniques to improve patient adherence
- Developmental stages of family
- Assessing family function coping
- Counseling for prevention of domestic violence
- Family genograms
- Guidelines for involving the family in a patient's care
- Helping families cope with chronic illness
- Home visits
- Acquiring information to support clinical practice

BOOKSHELF RECOMMENDATIONS

- *American Family Physician*. A peer-reviewed journal of the American Academy of Family Physicians. Leawood, KS: American Academy of Family Physicians. Published 24 times per year.

TABLE 1.1A

Defining Family Medicine

Family practice is the medical specialty that provides continuing and comprehensive health care for the individual and family. It is the specialty in breadth that integrates the biological, clinical, and behavioral sciences. The scope of family practice encompasses all ages, both sexes, each organ system, and every disease entity. (From American Academy of Family Physicians Official Definitions of "Family Practice," located at www.aafp.org/about/300_c.html.)

Of all office visits to physicians, General and Family Practice physicians see the largest share—22.5%. This is followed by Internal Medicine (17.9%) and Pediatrics (9.8%).

Reason for Visit to Family Physician	Percentage of Total Office Visits
Acute problem	49.5
Chronic problem, routine	23.0
Chronic problem, flare-up	7.6
Pre/post surgery or injury follow-up	3.0
Non-illness care	15.0
Unknown or not reported	1.9

TABLE 1.1B

Top 10 Diagnoses by Age Group for Visits to Family Physicians

	All Ages	Under 3 Years	3–17 Years	18–24 Years	25–44 Years	45–64 Years	65–74 Years	75+
1	General exam	Well-child exam	Throat symptoms	Throat symptoms	General exam	General exam	General exam	General exam
2	Cough	Cough	Cough	Abdominal pain	Throat symptoms	Hypertension	Hypertension	Hypertension
3	Throat symptoms	Fever	School/work physical	Cough	Cough	Cough	Progress visit	Leg symptoms
4	Progress visit	Ear symptoms	General exam	Prenatal exam	Back symptoms	Progress visit	Diabetes mellitus	Medications
5	Hypertension	Nasal congestion	Prophylactic inoculation	Head cold	Headache	Check blood pressure	Medications	Check blood pressure
6	Back symptoms	Prophylactic inoculation	Skin rash	General exam	Prenatal exam	Back symptoms	Abdominal pain	Cough
7	Abdominal pain	Skin rash	Head cold	Depression	Progress visit	Diabetes mellitus	Check blood pressure	Progress visit
8	Headache	Diarrhea	Earache or infection	Back symptoms	Sinus problems	Sinus problems	Cough	Abdominal pain
9	Medications	Sinus problems	Medications	Skin irritations	Skin rash	Medications	Back problems	Shortness of breath
10	Sinus problems	Head cold	Fever	Painful urination	Low-back symptoms	Headache	Skin lesion	Skin rash

Source: US Department of Health and Human Services, Public Health Service, Centers for Disease Control, National Center for Health Statistics, 1999. Available online at www.aafp.org/facts/FactsIndex.xml.

TABLE 1.2

Recommendations for Periodic Health Examinations

The recommendations for periodic heath examinations are adapted from the clinical policies of the American Academy of Family Physicians (AAFP). Every effort has been taken by the AAFP Commission on Clinical Policy and Research to make the recommendations consistent with evidence-based medical practice. For updates to these recommendations or for the complete policy for a number of periodic health interventions for the general and specific populations, refer to www.aafp.org/exam.

Strongly Recommended* and Recommended** Interventions for Periodic Health Exam in Asymptomatic Persons of the General Population

Patient Population	Target Disease	Screenings
Neonates and Infants	PKU, Thyroid function, Hemoglobinopathies	Order these tests for all
	Accidental injury	Advise child safety seat
	Lead poisoning where prevalent in community	Determine lead levels
	Otitis media	Counsel parents re smoke-free environment and promote breastfeeding
	Hip dysplasia, trauma, retinoblastoma, heart and other congenital abnormalities	Initial physical exam in the newborn period
	Diphtheria, pertussis, tetanus, polio, mumps, measles, rubella, Haemophilus influenzae B, pneumococcal disease, hepatitis B, varicella	Instruct parents on proper number and timing of immunizations and begin in hospital or on first well-child visit
Children 2–5 Years	Visual difficulties	Screen for amblyopia and strabismus
	Obesity	Measure height and weight periodically
	Accidental injury	Advise re injury prevention; child safety seats, helmets, seat belt use, smoke detectors, poison control center numbers, bike safety
	Coronary artery disease, hypertension, obesity, and diabetes	Advise to engage in regular physical activity

Patient Population	Target Disease	Screenings
Children 6–12 Years	Obesity	Measure height and weight and encourage physical activity and proper diet
	Tobacco use	Discourage use of tobacco and, if started, encourage discontinuation; counsel parents about effects of smoking on child's health
Adolescents	Obesity	Measure height and weight and, encourage physical activity and proper diet
	Tobacco use	Discourage use of tobacco and, if already started, encourage discontinuation
	Congenital rubella	Ensure rubella immunity
	Osteoporosis	Counsel for adequate calcium intake
	Sexually transmitted diseases and unwanted pregnancy	Counsel on risks of sexually transmitted diseases and pregnancy prevention
All Men and Women	Hypertension	Measure blood pressure
	Obesity	Measure height and weight and encourage physical activity and proper diet
	Lipid disorders	Fasting lipid profile if ≥45 years in females and ≥35 years in males
	Tobacco use	Discourage use or encourage discontinuation of tobacco
	Tetanus, diphtheria, influenza, hepatitis B	Immunize those who need it with booster or start series
	Accidental injury	Counsel re injury prevention
	Automobile accidents	Advise against driving while intoxicated
Women	Breast cancer	Clinical exam and mammogram every 1–2 years if 50–69 years of age
	Colorectal cancer	Screening annually with fecal occult blood test and endoscopy after age 50; start earlier if family history of early cancer

Continued

TABLE 1.2

Recommendations for Periodic Health Examinations, cont'd

Patient Population	Target Disease	Screenings
	Cervical cancer	Pap smear every 3 years if ever had sex and have a cervix
	Chlamydia	Screen in women aged 25 or younger and sexually active
	Osteoporosis	Counsel for adequate calcium intake
	Neural tube defects	0.4 mg of folate daily supplementation for those planning pregnancy
Men	Colorectal cancer	Screening annually with fecal occult blood test and endoscopy after age 50; start earlier if family history of early cancer
	Coronary artery disease	Advise of risk and benefits for aspirin prophylaxis if risk factors present
	Prostate cancer	Counsel re known risks and uncertain benefits of prostate cancer screening; begin in 40s for blacks and 50s for whites
Elderly Patients	Pneumococcal disease	Immunize those ≥65 years old
	Visual difficulties	Snellen acuity testing
	Hearing difficulties	Question about hearing impairment; refer if needed
	Osteoporosis	All perimenopausal and postmenopausal patients advised of risk and benefits of hormone replacement therapy

Adapted from AAFP Policy Action, November 1996, Revision 5.0, August 2001, No. 962, Reprint No. 510, American Academy of Family Physicians.

* *Strongly recommended:* Good-quality evidence exists that demonstrates substantial net benefits over harm, is cost-effective, and is acceptable to nearly all patients.

** *Recommended*: Evidence exists that demonstrates net benefit, but either the benefit is moderate in magnitude or evidence is only rated as "fair," cost-effective, and acceptable to nearly all patients.

TABLE 1.3

Periodic Health Examination: Negative Recommendations

The following are negative recommendations and should *not* be a routine part of the periodic health exam. The recommendation is with good to fair evidence that shows no net benefit over harm.

Patient Population	Target Disease	Interventions *Not* Recommended
Asymptomatic persons	Pancreatic cancer	Use of ultrasound and/or serological markers
Asymptomatic persons	Bladder cancer	Use of urinalysis (microscopic or dipstick)
Asymptomatic persons	Peripheral arterial disease	Use of Doppler or duplex ultrasound or other vascular laboratory tests
Asymptomatic persons	Lung cancer	Use of chest x-ray and/or sputum cytology
Asymptomatic persons	Thyroid cancer	Use of ultrasound screening
Asymptomatic persons	Insulin-dependent diabetes mellitus	Use of immune marker screening
Asymptomatic persons	Genital herpes simplex virus infection	Screening with culture, serology, or other tests
Asymptomatic children and adults	Cardiac disease	Use of routine ECG as part of a periodic health or preparticipation physical exam
All children	Poisoning	Mr Yuk stickers
Patients less than 60 years old and not neonates	Thyroid disease	Use of thyroid function test
Males	Asymptomatic bacteriuria	Use of urinalysis (microscopic or dipstick)
Females, except for two groups, those who are non-institutionalized elderly and those who have diabetes, for whom there is insufficient evidence to recommend for or against routine screening	Asymptomatic bacteriuria	Use of urinalysis (microscopic or dipstick)
Women who have had hysterectomies for reasons other than cancer	Vaginal cancer	Use of Pap smears

Continued

TABLE 1.3

Periodic Health Examination: Negative Recommendations, cont'd

Patient Population	Target Disease	Interventions *Not* Recommended
Women without a family history of frequent ovarian cancer. For this latter group, there is insufficient evidence to recommend for or against routine screening	Ovarian cancer	Use of ultrasound of the pelvis, and/or serum tumor markers

Adapted from AAFP Policy Action, November 1996, Revision 5.0, August 2001, No. 962, Reprint No. 510, American Academy of Family Physicians.

TABLE 1.4

Office Follow-up Recommendations for Stable, Asymptomatic Chronic Conditions

Diagnoses	Every 2 to 4 Months	Every 6 Months to Annually	Becomes Symptomatic
Hypertension	HX-end organ changes; MR; PX-BP, lung, heart, edema, peripheral pulses; PE-all visits	LAB-glucose, electrolytes, uric acid, lipids, BUN, creatinine; PX-retinas	ECG, chest X-ray, echocardiogram, EST, peripheral vascular studies
Type II diabetes	HX-end organ changes, sugars too high or too low, diet, psyche, exercise, home monitoring; MR; PX-feet, lung, heart, vascular, neurological, BP, weight; PE-all visits	LAB-hemoglobin A_{1C}, BUN, creatinine, urinalysis, micro albumin/creatinine ratio of urine; PX-complete dilated eye exam	ECG, arterial doppler studies, EST, blood sugar, creatinine clearance, urinalysis
Coronary artery disease	HX-functional status, angina, dysrhythmias; diet, exercise, smoking; MR; PX-retinas, lung, heart, edema, BP, pulse, weight; LAB-Protime and INR if anticoagulated; PE-all visits	LAB-lipids, digoxin level if indicated, serum glucose and potassium, serum magnesium, drug levels of antiarrhythmics; ECG	EST, radio nuclide scan, chest X-ray, echocardiogram, troponin, coronary angiography
CHF	HX-salt intake, fluid balance, weight changes, functional status, sleep, orthopnea, PND; MR; PX-feet, lung, heart, vascular,	LAB-lipids, digoxin level if indicated, serum glucose, calcium, serum BUN, creatinine and electrolytes, serum magnesium, ECG; chest x-ray	EST, chest x-ray, echocardiogram, radionuclide scan, sleep study for apnea, pulse oximetry, or blood gases

Continued

TABLE 1.4

Office Follow-up Recommendations for Stable, Asymptomatic Chronic Conditions, cont'd

Diagnoses	Every 2 to 4 Months	Every 6 Months to Annually	Becomes Symptomatic
	BP, weight, pulse, neck veins, liver size, cyanosis; PE-all visits		
Asthma/COPD	IHX-functional status, home monitoring with peak flows, sputum, cough, sleep, infections, allergic symptoms; MR; PX-BP, lung, heart, pulse, oximetry, ear-nose-throat exam; PE-all visits	LAB-spirometry or pulmonary function tests, drug levels of therapeutic agents if applicable; IHX-immunization review	Pulse oximetry or arterial blood gases, chest X-ray, pulmonary function tests, VQ scan, EST monitoring oxygen status with exercise
TIA/Stroke	IHX-neurological deficits, smoking, headaches, balance, swallowing, strength, sensory changes; MR; PX-focused neurological exam, lung, heart, carotid auscultation; PE-all visits	PX-full neurological exam, retinas, mental status; LAB-lipids, serum electrolytes if on diuretic, glucose, drug levels of therapeutic agents if applicable	EEG, ECG, carotid duplex studies, echocardiogram, computed tomography scan of the head

BP indicates blood pressure; BUN, blood urea nitrogen; CHF, congestive heart failure; COPD, chronic obstructive pulmonary disease; ECG, electrocardiogram; EEG, electroencephalogram; EST, exercise stress test; IHX, interval history; INR, international normalized ratio; LAB, laboratory and other studies; MR, medication review (dose, interval, compliance, side effects, cost); PE, patient education; PND, paroxysmal nocturnal dyspnea; PX, physician exam; TIA, transient ischemic attack; VQ, ventilation-perfusion.

TABLE 1.5

Disqualifying Conditions for Department of Transportation Physical Examinations

1	Loss of foot, leg, hand or arm	Disqualify; waiver may be available from regional director of motor carriers
2	Significant hand or lower extremity impairment (eg, fused hip or partial paralysis)	Disqualify; waiver may be available from regional director of motor carriers
3	Insulin used for diabetic control	Disqualify; oral agents acceptable
4	Cardiovascular disease	Disqualify; refer to cardiologist if patient insists on trying to qualify
5	Respiratory dysfunction with PaO_2 >65 mm Hg or $PaCO_2$ >45 mm Hg	Disqualify
6	Uncontrolled hypertension	Disqualify if blood pressure >181/105 mm Hg
7	Muscular, neurological, or vascular disease	Disqualify if condition significantly impairs ability to control steering wheel or pedals of vehicle or impairs reaction times
8	Epilepsy	Disqualify if recurrent seizures; if an isolated seizure patient should be off medication and seizure free for 5 years to qualify
9	Mental or nervous condition	Disqualify if judgment or reaction time is impaired
10	Vision < 20/40 in each eye with correction	Disqualify
11	Hearing loss of > than average of 40 dB in best ear	Hearing aid may be worn for the test; disqualify if unable to pass
12	Schedule I or consciousness-altering drugs	Disqualify
13	Current diagnosis of alcoholism	Disqualify and refer for treatment

TABLE 1.6

Health Teaching for All Patients

Nutrition

- Eat foods from each of the four basic food groups in amounts recommended by the food pyramid.
- Decrease red meats in the diet, particularly those marbled with fat.
- Eat more fish and poultry; remove the skins and boil or broil.
- Increase soluble fiber content in the diet such as oat bran, dry beans, and peas; eat high-fiber vegetables.
- Seek calcium and potassium and avoid sodium and phosphate.
- Drink three or more glasses of water daily.
- Eat one main meal of the day (prior to a period of activity and not before being sedentary) and two smaller ones.
- Read food labels and avoid high fat, cholesterol, sodium, and sugar intakes.
- Nutritional supplements that may be beneficial if taken daily include vitamin E (400 IU) and folic acid (1 mg). Calcium may be added to bring daily total to 1200–1500 mg.

Activity

- Maintain ideal body weight for height $\pm$10% or ideal BMI (body mass index = wt in kg/ht in m^2).
- Be physically active five to six times per week for 30 minutes at your target pulse rate (target pulse = [220−age] $\times$ 0.8).
- Vary exercise between endurance and strengthening activities.

Safety

- Use no form of tobacco.
- Avoid excess alcohol intake; one glass of wine daily may be helpful.
- Always wear seat belts.
- Do not keep firearms in the house unless unloaded and locked in a gun safe with trigger locks.
- Understand *and* practice the concepts of "safer sex."
- Have a written medical power of attorney and advanced directives.
- Use protective equipment for work (hearing and vision protection, respirators, or masks) and for play (helmets, knee and wrist protectors).
- Get help for depression, anger management, and domestic violence.

Risk Adjustment

- Know your numbers and keep cholesterol $<$200 mg/dL, HDL $>$35 mg/dL, fasting glucose $\leq$110 mg/dL. Systolic blood pressure should be $\leq$130 mm Hg and diastolic $\leq$80 mm Hg.
- Keep immunizations current.
- Know your family history risk factors, especially for cancer, heart disease, and diabetes.
- After age 40, prophylactic use of 81 mg of aspirin daily may be helpful for cardiovascular and malignancy prevention.

TABLE 1.7

Strategies for Success in Health Promotion

- Keep health promotion activities patient centered.
- Share decision making with the patient and his or her family.
- Obtain informed consent after education about the purpose and expected effects of all interventions.
- Encourage patients to take responsibility for their own decisions/actions.
- Use every patient encounter to look for opportunities to address modifiable risk factors.
- Observe current health behaviors and adapt health promotion interventions to fit the individual's lifestyle.
- Make smaller, incremental changes rather than one big one—keep goals realistic and achievable.
- Make a list of specific recommendations into a prescription for change.
- Acknowledge that change is difficult and it may be easier to add new behaviors than to change old ones.
- Obtain a firm commitment from the patient to make an intervention or change.
- Use follow-up visits to monitor progress toward mutually agreed upon goals.
- Involve office staff in supportive encouragement for change and monitoring.

TABLE 1.8

Techniques to Improve Patient Adherence

Techniques	Rationale
Tell patients what their "numbers" are at each visit (eg, blood pressure, weight, cholesterol, blood sugar, etc). Give patients a framework to interpret their tests.	Encourages ownership; reinforces reality, particularly in asymptomatic conditions. Leads to an active rather than passive approach.
Use home monitoring devices such as glucose meters and blood pressure cuffs.	Establishes validity of patient's self-care and provides ongoing motivation.
Use simple language and assess for understanding.	Patients must understand what's wrong and what to do before they will act.
Set realistic goals for diet, exercise, and medication taking; make recommendations compatible with patient's lifestyle.	Success at smaller goals (eg, 5 lb of weight loss) leads to fulfillment and more effort.
Recommend support groups or national disease entities such as National Arthritis Foundation, Weight Watchers, American Heart Association, etc.	Additional learning and motivation from others with similar conditions; encourage patients to tell you what they have learned to ensure no harmful practices.
Be supportive of patient-selected therapies if they can cause no harm.	Reinforces your wish that the patient take an active role in his or her care.
Provide written material for patient education; best to personalize for the individual patient needs.	Reinforces the main points and underscores patients' need to know more about themselves. Discourages dependence on the physician.
Encourage use of the Internet; use information from www.familydoctor.org as a starting point.	Patient information from Internet stimulates questions and patient may use email to doctor to check in with progress.
Ask patients to tell in their own words how they have complied with recommendations/goals.	Avoids assumptions about how patients take their medications.
At each follow-up, give objective feedback on progress toward goal.	Shows patient relationship between behavior and change; shows you care about how they are doing.
At each follow-up, be sure to go "heavy" on the praise and "light" on admonishment.	A sense of failure may lead to hopelessness, helplessness, and resistance to change.
At the end of visit, provide a "prescription" on a piece of paper. This can be brief instructions, a diagram, a copy of their flowsheet, etc.	Patients expect some tangible result of their visit. Medication prescriptions are not appropriate for all visits.

TABLE 1.9

Developmental Stages of the Family

Major Stages of the Family	Average Length	Definition	Tasks
Newly married	2 years	Union of couple; no children	Disengage from family of origin; adjust to each others' personality; meet social, economic, and sexual needs; establish effective methods of communication
Birth of first child	2.5 years	Oldest child age 0–30 months	Assume parental role while maintaining marital role; institute new schedule; deal with fatigue, financial stress, home confinement, and decreased leisure activity
With preschool children	3.5 years	Oldest child age 30-months to 6 years	Socialization of the children; child learns to relate emotionally to others, undergoes early individuation and sexual identity
With children in school	7 years	Oldest child age 6–13 years	First official separation from home; parents' social activities widen to include school activities; child develops physically, socially, emotionally, and intellectually
Families with teenagers	7 years	Oldest child age 13–20 years	Stressful stage; family must maintain closeness and cohesiveness while simultaneously encouraging child's development of independence; child begins disengagement process; adolescent sexual feelings conflict with social restriction
Launching years	8 years	First child leaves home to last child gone	Parent-child relationship change to adult-adult type; parents face prospect of time alone

Continued

TABLE 1.9

Developmental Stages of the Family, cont'd

Major Stages of the Family	Average Length	Definition	Tasks
			and need to reinvest in each other instead of children
Parents alone in middle years	15 years	Last child leaves; empty nest	Reappraisal of lifetime goals, realignment of priorities; couples who have remained together for sake of children divorce; most difficult time for women, causing emotional crises; adaptation to grandparent role
Retirement and later years	10-15 years	Retirement; death of both spouses	Coping with aging process; loss of occupation; societal disengagement; depression may arise

Adapted from Duvall EM. *Family Development*. 4th ed. Philadelphia: JB Lippincott; 1971.

TABLE 1.10

Types of Family Crises

Family development is usually consistent and predictable, though occasionally crises will occur that disrupt the emotional well-being of the family unit. Assessment of family function and coping abilities helps to successfully navigate individuals and their family through the health care system.

Assess for family strength, coping skills, and crises:

- When family first enters your practice
- When family members become caregivers for others in the family
- When psychosomatic illness is diagnosed
- When stress is present in the patient-physician relationship

Dismemberment
Hospitalization
Loss of child
Loss of spouse
Prolonged separation (military service, work)
Demoralization
Disgrace (alcoholism, crime, delinquency, drug addition)
Infidelity
Prolonged unemployment
Sudden impoverishment
Progressive dissension
Accession
Adoption
Relative moves in
Stepmother/stepfather marries in
Demoralization Plus Dismemberment or Accession
Desertion
Divorce
Illegitimacy
Imprisonment
Institutionalization
Runaway
Suicide or homicide

Adapted from Rakel RE. *Principles of Family Medicine*. Philadelphia: WB Saunders; 1977:351.

TABLE 1.11A

Using the Family APGAR to Assess Family Function

Five Components of Family Function (Family APGAR)

The Family APGAR is a five-item family function screening questionnaire in which the patient is asked to describe how family members communicate, eat, sleep, and carry out home, school, and job responsibilities.

1. **Adaptation.** The utilization of intrafamilial and extrafamilial resources for problem solving in times of crisis.
2. **Partnership.** The sharing of decision-making and nurturing responsibilities by family members.
3. **Growth.** The physical and emotional maturation and self-fulfillment that are achieved by family members through mutual support and guidance.
4. **Affection.** The caring or loving relationship that exists among family members.
5. **Resolve.** The commitment to devote time to other members of the family for physical and emotional nurturing, involving a decision to share wealth and space.

Adapted from Rosen GM, Geyman JP, Layton RH. *Behavioral Science in Family Practice*. New York: Appleton-Century-Crofts; 1980:145, and Smilkstein G. The family APGAR: a proposal for a family function test and its use by physicians. *J Fam Pract*. 1978;6:1231.

TABLE 1.11B

Family APGAR Questionnaire

Scoring: The patient checks one of the three choices, which are scored as follows: "Almost Always" (2 points), "Some of the Time" (1 point), or "Hardly Ever" (0 points). The scores for each of the five questions are then totaled. A score of 7 to 10 suggests a highly functional family. A score of 4 to 6 suggests a moderately dysfunctional family. A score of 0 to 3 suggests a severely dysfunctional family.

	Almost Always	Some of the Time	Hardly Ever
I am satisfied that I can turn to my family when something is troubling me.			
I am satisfied with the way my family talks things over with me and shares problems with me.			
I am satisfied that my family accepts and supports my wishes to take on new activities or directions.			
I am satisfied with the way my family expresses affection and responds to my emotions, such as anger, sorrow, and love.			
I am satisfied with the way my family and I share time together.			

Adapted from Rosen GM, Geyman JP, Layton RH. *Behavioral Science in Family Practice*. New York: Appleton-Century-Crofts; 1980:147, and Smilkstein G. The family APGAR: a proposal for a family function test and its use by physicians. *J Fam Pract*. 1978;6:1231.

TABLE 1.12

Action Plan for Victims of Abuse and Domestic Violence

Magnitude of the Problem

- Approximately 95% of victims are women.
- 4,000,000 women a year are assaulted by their partners—one every 9 seconds.
- Every day four women are murdered by boyfriends or husbands.
- 93% of women who kill their mates have been battered.
- 25% of all crime is wife abuse.
- 70% of men who batter their partners, also sexually or physically abuse their children.
- Domestic violence costs the United States $67 billion annually.

Natural History of the Problem

- There are three types of abuse: physical, emotional, and sexual.
- There are three phases of domestic violence:
    1. **Tension Phase:** May last weeks to months; stress builds; communication breaks down; victim can sense danger is imminent; "minor" incident occurs and then escalation.
    2. **Crisis Phase:** May last 1 to 3 days; anxiety peaks; major uncontrolled violence occurs; serious injury or death possible; abuser blames victim; victim accommodates in order to survive; believes escape impossible; victim may escape, but returns.
    3. **Calm Phase:** May last for days or weeks; whole family in shock; abuser remorseful and seeks forgiveness; everyone relieved violence is passed and victim accepts promises; wants to believe violence won't recur; survival via denial and negotiation.

Action Plan

- Make and hide extra keys for your car and home.
- Have a deadbolt lock on at least one interior door in your home in a room with an escape route.
- Keep important documents such as birth certificate and social security card in a safe and accessible place.
- Make a neighbor or friend aware of your situation.
- Keep a small suitcase packed and ready if it becomes necessary to flee.
- If leaving, do not go without your children.
- Establish a business relationship with an attorney.
- If you take legal action, be prepared to follow through.
- Keep emergency money aside and hidden.
- Memorize the National Domestic Violence Hotline (1-800-799-SAFE).
- Locate the nearest domestic violence shelter.
- In an emergency, call 911 and tell police you are in danger.
- Keep a diary of what happens to you hidden in a safe place.

FIGURE 1.1

Using the Family Genogram

Family genograms provide a "snapshot" of family structure and help to identify, in shorthand format, areas of concern for the patient's medical care. Standardized symbols are used to indicate gender, the family relationships, medical conditions that may be inherited, and areas of conflict within the family. Completion of the genogram often supplies the "missing link" for diagnosis and treatment.

Genograms help to:

- Record data on repetitive conditions (eg, bipolar illness, Down syndrome)
- Understand family interactions and relationships (eg, enmeshment, conflict)
- Establish a plan for follow-up and screening (eg, familial polyposis coli)
- Identify influential decision makers or significant others

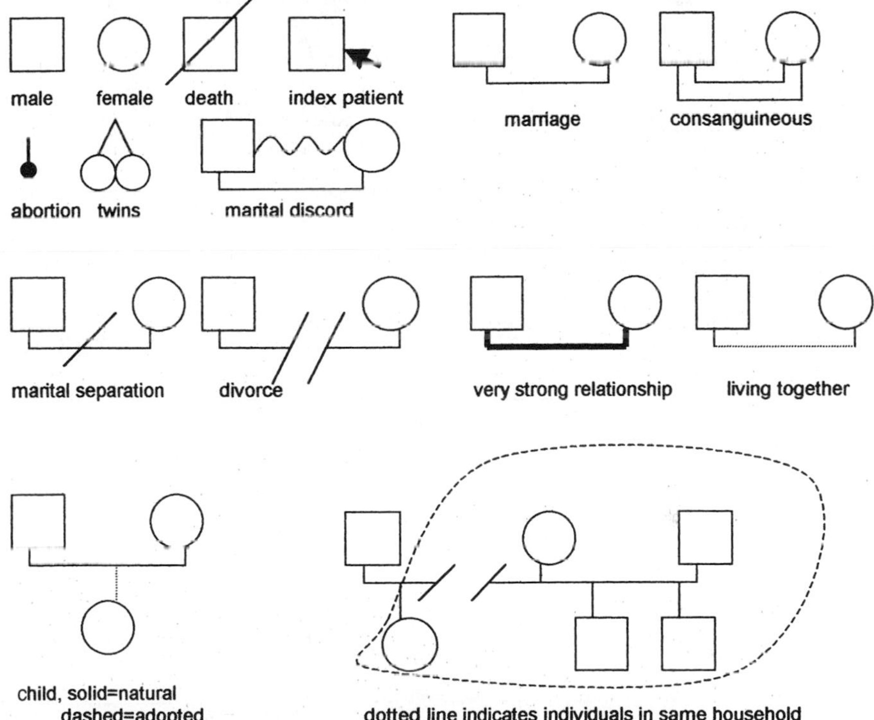

TABLE 1.13

Guidelines for Involving Family in Patient's Care

See Patient Only

- Minor and acute problems (eg, upper respiratory infection, urinary tract infection)
- Self-limited problems with consistent history (eg, back pain, minor trauma)
- Routine preventive/wellness care in patient who has own decision-making capacity

Family Conference Desirable

- Treatment failure or repeated occurrences of illness
- Routine preventive/wellness care in dependent patients (eg, child, senior patient with dementia, mental retardation)
- Care that has already involved others (eg, premarital exam, prenatal exam, and follow-up care)

Family Involvement Essential

- Continuing care for chronic illness (eg, cancer, diabetes, congestive heart failure)
- Serious acute trauma or major illness (eg, motor vehicle accident, myocardial infarction)
- Social problems (eg, substance abuse, trouble with school, trouble with the law, in questions of violence or abuse)
- Psychiatric illness (eg, bipolar disorder, depression, anxiety, dementia)
- Difficult-to-manage patients (eg, aggressive, combative, noncompliant)
- Diagnostic or treatment dilemmas
- Ethical issues of concern (eg, assessing driving capability, decision-making capacity)
- Admission to special intensive care units
- Death

TABLE 1.14

Strategies for Helping Families Cope with Chronic Illness

1. Provide regular physician contact for empathic guidance; explain the diagnosis and management (carefully, clearly, slowly, and repeatedly).
2. Have a family meeting and involve all members in decisions and care.
3. Involve competent assistants in the family's care (social worker, visiting nurse, clergy member).
4. Assist family in recognizing financial and legal issues.
5. Suggest resources that can provide respite for the caregivers (hospice, church groups) and places available for placement if it should eventually be needed.
6. Focus on the needs of the entire family, not just the patient. Have family develop a "coping notebook" with names and phone numbers of doctors, friends, agencies, self-help support groups, and emergency care services.
7. Strive to maintain patient's general health, mental status, and skills for independent activities.
8. Ensure patient safety. Reduce objects that may cause falls; install tub/toilet rail; reduce bathwater temperature; wear ID bracelet; install intercom or call bell system; use lifeline system (automatic dialing of emergency number by single button push).
9. Provide names of other families who have successfully dealt with a similar medical problem.
10. Provide periodic written summary of patient's course and your assessment and plans to family caregivers and any other physicians or professionals involved in the patient's care.

TABLE 1.15

Home Visits

Initial assessment/management of an acute illness when:

- Patient is too elderly to come to office (no transportation capabilities)
- Patient is too ill (acute back injury, severe influenza)
- Pain is exacerbated by movement (febrile hospice patient with malignancy)
- Ambulation is impaired (elderly person with casted leg)
- Patient would be infectious to other patients (chickenpox)
- Patient's problem needs treatment before transport to hospital can be effected (acute asthma in elderly single patient, CPR, relief of pain)
- Need to assess indications for admission to hospital

When patient needs follow-up after release from the hospital:

- Assess rehabilitation progress and adaptation to illness
- Assess coping abilities of family members to deal with chronic disease
- Help patients who need more time to recover from disfiguring trauma or surgery

Patients with chronic diseases:

- Patients confined to the home (severe arthritis, multiple sclerosis, chronic obstructive pulmonary disease, congestive heart failure)
- Patients with a dementing illness or problems with toileting control
- Patients with a terminal illness

When disturbed home situation or family dysfunction is suspected:

- Assess financial capabilities, hygiene, family's ability to care for patient
- Recommend family counseling to include members who won't come to office

Further information about house calls and a form for proper documentation may be found online at www.aafp.org/fpm/20000600/49hous.html.

TABLE 1.16

Information to Be Learned from Home Visits

O—Outside
Type of neighborhood
Type of house
Play area for children
Condition of patient's home and other homes in area
Environmental hazards

B—Behavior of family members
How do they relate to one another? (Degree of love and intimacy; strength; nature of nurturing process; character of communication; exchange of looks; verbal exchange; nature of physical contact [warm and supportive; quarrelsome and rejecting]; if different ethnic group, don't misinterpret signs)
How do they relate to the children?
How do they relate to the physician? Is the TV on?
Is there a caretaker (hidden patient)? How is the caretaker coping?
Cultural or ethnic activities?

S—Safety
High rate of accidents in home?
Is there much clutter around?
Are there exposed wires, fans, hot water vaporizers, poor lighting, flaking paint, smoke detectors?
Is it poison proof? Presence of ipecac?
Medicines?

E—Eating area: habits and patterns
Where does the family eat? (Kitchen, dining room; in front of TV; at round table or long, narrow one?)
Sanitation of the kitchen?
Is garbage disposed of properly?
What about cooking and storage facilities?
What food is available?

R—Relationships and support groups in wider community
Is extended family nearby?
Do they know neighbors? Are they supportive? Hostile? Indifferent?
Do they have friends they can contact in an emergency?
Do they belong to a church or civic organization?
Do family members work nearby? Who works? Economic background?
When do they shop?

Continued

TABLE 1.16

Information to Be Learned from Home Visits, cont'd

V—Variations
Had you expected the home to be different? More adequately furnished? Less? Does the inside look different from the outside?
Family member or friend present who was not previously mentioned?
Evidence of children's toys, etc?

E—Environment
Furnishings, etc?
Housekeeping?
Bathroom sanitation?
Homey? (Family pictures, mementos, religious artifacts, hobbies, etc)
Study area? Play area for children?
Family space? Private space? Where does the family congregate? (What people do in a physical setting turns a space into a place. For example, the bathroom may be the library, a think tank, an escape from the family, or a haven for suicides.)
Sleeping arrangements? (The stage of the family in its life cycle; use of space; communal versus private space within the home)

S—Sickness
Medications?
Provisions for ill persons? (Bed-bound patient locations; dust-proofing for asthmatics; handrails for cardiac patients) How does the family perceive the illness?

Courtesy Antonnette V. Graham, RN, LISW, Assistant Professor of Family Medicine, Case Western Reserve University, Cleveland, Ohio.

TABLE 1.17

Acquiring Information to Support Clinical Practice

The National Library of Medicine (www.nlm.nih.gov) can be accessed via the Internet. A brochure outlining the basics of how to get information via PubMed is available for free reproduction at http://nnlm.gov/nnlm/online/pubmed/pmtri.pdf. PubMed is available free on the Internet at http://www.ncbi.nih.gov/entrez/query.fcgi. PubMed provides:

- Free access to MEDLINE
- Sets of related articles pre-computed for each article cited in MEDLINE
- Clinical Queries form with built-in search filters for therapy, diagnosis, etiology, and prognosis
- Links to sources of full text journal articles (fees may be required)
- Link to Clinical Alerts for findings on NIH-funded clinical trials that significantly affect morbidity and mortality
- Links to www.clinicaltrials.gov, Consumer Health Information (MEDLINEplus), and the NLM Gateway

Practice guidelines can be accessed from The National Guideline Clearing House at www.guideline.gov. At this site you can browse for evidence-based guidelines and if more than one has been published, they can be compared in a side-by-side view.

Treatment guidelines can be located at www.medexact.com.

Information regarding various topics can be accessed at www.cdc.gov. This is a useful site for obtaining immunization requirements and advice for travelers, infectious disease recommendations, and guidance on management of bioterrorism. The *Morbidity and Mortality Weekly Report* (*MMWR*) is also available.

At www.uib.no/isf/guide/family.htm, you will find the Primary Care Internet Guide. After arriving at this site, click on one of the more than 220 links to get to family practice, family medicine, and general practice sites. The links are grouped as: News groups and mailing lists; Societies and organizations; Documents, textbooks and CME; University Family Practice Departments (USA); University Departments (Non US); and other sites.

Web links to health agencies, professional health societies, and non-profit consumer health organizations can be located at www.vh.org/Beyond/MedicalSocieties.html.

chapter 2

Care of Children

Brenda L. Stokes, MD

IN THIS CHAPTER

- Apgar scoring of the newborn
- Conditions of high risk for the newborn
- Maturity rating of the newborn
- Classification of the newborn
- Neonatal resuscitation
- Newborn problems: jaundice, hepatitis B prophylaxis, ambiguous genitalia, gynecologic conditions, formulas
- Immunization schedule
- Developmental evaluation
- Dental development
- Timing of appearance of sexual characteristics and Tanner staging
- Pediatric vulvovaginitis
- Common infectious diseases
- Common respiratory diseases
- Otitis media
- Parasitic infections
- Rabies prophylaxis
- Febrile seizures
- Meningitis
- Stooling disorders
- Attention deficit hyperactivity disorder (ADHD)
- Rheumatic fever
- Pediatric sedation
- Anemia
- Lead poisoning

BOOKSHELF RECOMMENDATIONS

- American Academy of Pediatrics. Pickering LK, ed. *Red Book 2000, Report of the Committee on Infectious Diseases*. 25th ed. Elk Grove Village, IL: American Academy of Pediatrics; 2000.
- Schwartz MW, ed. *The 5-Minute Pediatric Consult*. Baltimore, MD: Williams and Wilkins; 1997.
- Siberry GK, Iannone R, eds. *The Harriet Lane Handbook: A Handbook for Pediatric House Officers*. 15th ed. St Louis, MO: Mosby Inc; 2000.

TABLE 2.1

Apgar Scoring of the Newborn

Condition	Apgar Score at 5 Minutes
Best	8–10
Moderately depressed	5–7
Severely depressed	4 or less

Using the Apgar Score: The newborn is examined at 1 and 5 minutes after birth. Points are given based on the criteria in Table 2.2 and added for a total score. The score at 5 minutes is the most predictive of long-term prognosis.

TABLE 2.2

Apgar Score

Aspect	0	1	2
Heart rate	Absent	Slow (<100)	Normal (>100)
Respiratory effort	Absent, irregular	Slow, crying	Good
Muscle tone	Limp	Some flexion of extremities	Active motion
Reflex irritability (response to catheter in nostril)	No response	Grimace	Cough or sneeze
Color	Blue or pale	Body pink, extremities blue	Completely pink

TABLE 2.3

Conditions of High Risk for the Newborn

Antenatal	Natal	Postnatal
Maternal age <16 or >35	Abnormal fetal heart rate	Birth asphyxia
Maternal diabetes	Abnormal presentation, such as breech or face	Fetal malformations
Maternal hypertension	Cesarean section	HIV infection
Maternal hemorrhage	Chorioamnionitis	Hypothermia
Maternal hypoxia	Heavy sedation of mother	Macrosomia
Maternal infection	Maternal hypotension	Meconium staining
Maternal drug therapy Reserpine Lithium carbonate Magnesium Alcohol Adrenergic blocking drugs	Maternal infection Herpes HIV Group B streptococcus	Preterm infant
Maternal substance abuse Cocaine Heroin, alcohol Methadone	Meconium-stained fluid	Respiratory distress
Maternal anemia or isoimmunization	Mid- or high-forceps delivery	Small-for-dates infant
Smoking	Multiple births	
	Polyhydramnios	
	Precipitus delivery	
	Premature delivery	
	Prolapsed chord	
	Prolonged labor	
	Prolonged rupture of membranes	
	Shoulder dystocia	

FIGURE 2.1

The New Ballard Score: Maturational Assessment of Gestational Age

UROMUSCULAR MATURITY

NEUROMUSCULAR MATURITY SIGN	SCORE -1	SCORE 0	SCORE 1	SCORE 2	SCORE 3	SCORE 4	SCORE 5	RECORD SCORE HERE
[illegible]								
SQUARE WINDOW (Wrist)	>90°	90°	60°	45°	30°	0°		
ARM RECOIL		180°	140°-180°	110°-140°	90°-110°	<90°		
POPLITEAL ANGLE	180°	160°	140°	120°	100°	90°	<90°	
SCARF SIGN								
HEEL TO EAR								
							TOTAL NEUROMUSCULAR MATURITY SCORE	

IYSICAL MATURITY

PHYSICAL MATURITY SIGN	SCORE -1	SCORE 0	SCORE 1	SCORE 2	SCORE 3	SCORE 4	SCORE 5	RECORD SCORE HERE
SKIN	sticky friable transparent	gelatinous red translucent	smooth pink visible veins	superficial peeling &/or rash, few veins	cracking pale areas rare veins	parchment deep cracking no vessels	leathery cracked wrinkled	
LANUGO	none	sparse	abundant	thinning	bald areas	mostly bald		
PLANTAR SURFACE	heel-toe 40-50 mm:-1 <40 mm:-2	>50 mm no crease	faint red marks	anterior transverse crease only	creases ant. 2/3	creases over entire sole		
BREAST	imperceptible	barely perceptible	flat areola no bud	stippled areola 1-2 mm bud	raised areola 3-4 mm bud	full areola 5-10 mm bud		
EYE/EAR	lids fused loosely: -1 tightly: -2	lids open pinna flat stays folded	sl. curved pinna; soft; slow recoil	well-curved pinna; soft but ready recoil	formed & firm instant recoil	thick cartilage ear stiff		
GENITALS (Male)	scrotum flat, smooth	scrotum empty faint rugae	testes in upper canal rare rugae	testes descending few rugae	testes down good rugae	testes pendulous deep rugae		
GENITALS (Female)	clitoris prominent & labia flat	prominent clitoris & small labia minora	prominent clitoris & enlarging minora	majora & minora equally prominent	majora large minora small	majora cover clitoris & minora		
							TOTAL PHYSICAL MATURITY SCORE	

SCORE

Neuromuscular_________

Physical_________

Total_________

[illegible]

score	weeks
-10	20
-5	22
0	24
5	26
10	28
15	30
20	32
25	34
30	36
35	38
40	40
45	42
50	44

GESTATIONAL AGE (weeks)

By dates_________

By ultrasound_________

By exam_________

Reproduced with permission from Mosby, Inc. (Ballard JL, Khoury JC, Wedig K, et al. New Ballard Score, expanded to include extremely premature infants. *J. Pediatr.* 1991, 119:417–423.)

FIGURE 2.2

Classification of Newborns by Intrauterine Growth and Gestational Age

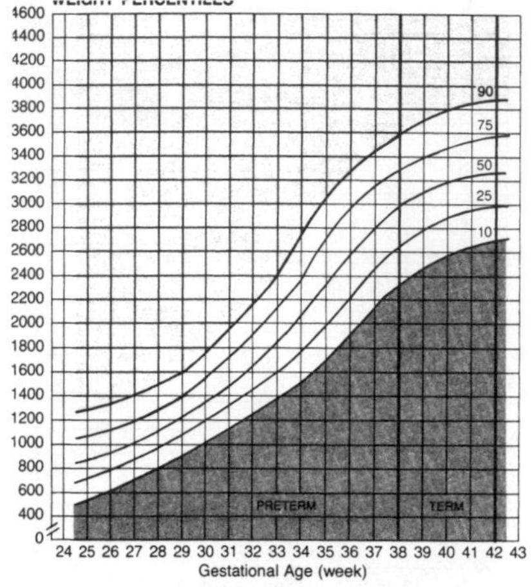

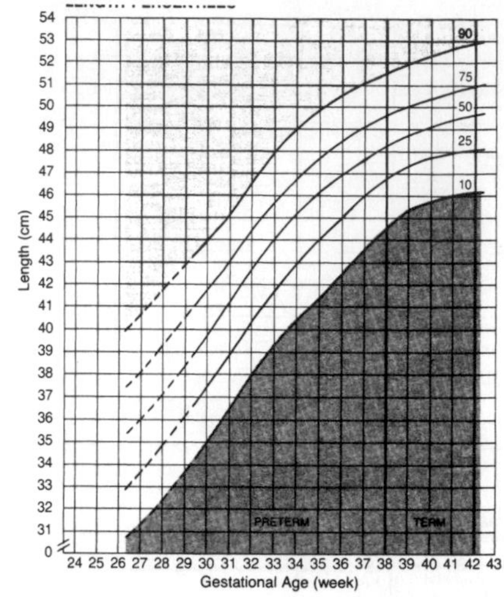

HEAD CIRCUMFERENCE PERCENTILES

38 37 36 35 34 33 32 31 30 29 28 27 26 25 24 23 22 0

90 75 50 25 10

PRETERM TERM

24 25 26 27 28 29 30 31 32 33 34 35 36 37 38 39 40 41 42 43

Gestational Age (week)

CLASSIFICATION OF INFANT*	Weight	Length	Head Circ.
Large for Gestational Age (LGA) (>90th percentile)			
Appropriate for Gestational Age (AGA) (10th to 90th percentile)			
Small for Gestational Age (SGA) (<10th percentile)			

*Place an "X" in the appropriate box (LGA, AGA or SGA) for weight, for length and for head circumference.

Reproduced with permission from the American Academy of Pediatrics and Mosby, Inc. (Lubchenco LO, Hansman C, Boyd E. Intrauterine growth in length and head circumference as estimated from live births at gestational ages from 26 to 42 weeks. *Pediatrics.* 1966, 37:403–408; Buttaglia FC, Lubchenco LO. A practical classification of newborn infants by weight and gestational age. *J. Pediatr.* 1967,71:159–163.)

FIGURE 2.3

Neonatal Resuscitation: Actions

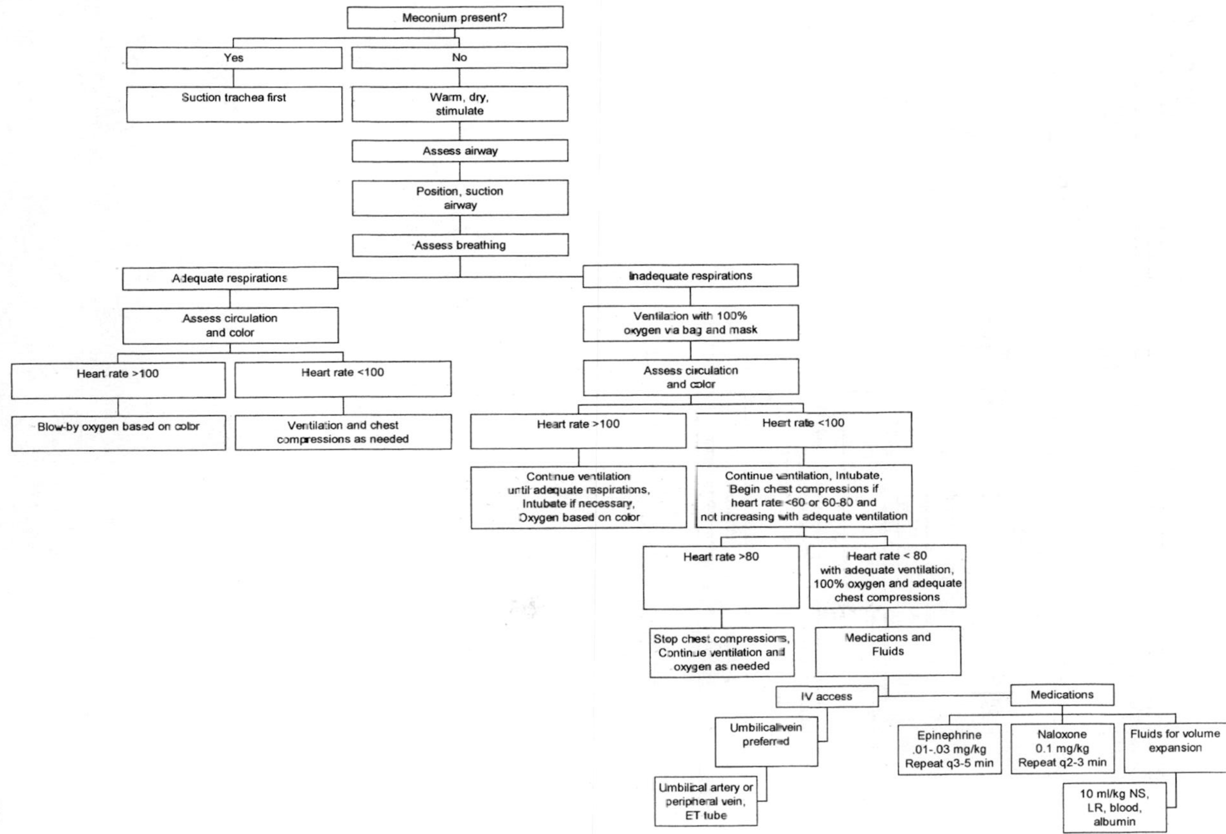

FIGURE 2.4

Neonatal Resuscitation: Medications

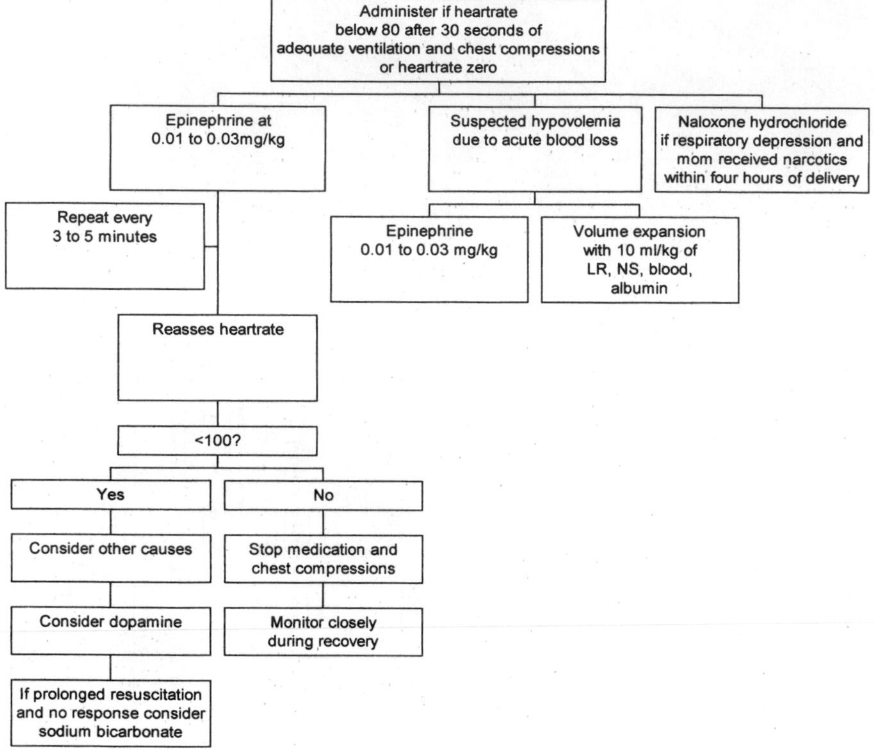

TABLE 2.4A

Drugs Used in Pediatric Advanced Life Support

Drug	Dosage	Remarks
Adenosine	0.1–0.2 mg/kg Maximum single dose: 12 mg	Rapid IV bolus
Atropine sulfate*	0.02 mg/kg	Minimum dose: 0.1 mg Maximum single dose: 0.5 mg in child, 1.0 in adolescent
Bretylium	5 mg/kg; may be increased to 10 mg/kg	Rapid IV
Calcium chloride 10%	20 mg/kg	Give slowly
Dopamine hydrochloride	2–20 μg/kg per min	α-Adrenergic action dominates at ≥15–20 μg/kg per min
Dobutamine hydrochloride	2–20 μg/kg per min	Titrate to desired effect
Epinephrine for bradycardia*	IV/IO: 0.01 mg/kg (1:10 000, 0.1 mL/kg) ET: 0.1 mg/kg (1:1000, 0.1 mL/kg)	
Epinephrine for asystolic or pulseless arrest*	**First dose:** IV/IO: 0.01 mg/kg (1:10 000, 0.1 mL/kg) ET: 0.1 mg/kg (1:1000, 0.1 mL/kg) IV/IO doses as high as 0.2 mg/kg of 1:1000 may be effective	
	Subsequent doses: IV/IO/ET: 0.1 mg/kg (1:1000, 0.1 mL/kg) IV/IO doses as high as 0.2 mg/kg of 1:1000 may be effective	Repeat every 3–5 minutes
Epinephrine Infusion	Initial at 0.1 μg/kg per min	Titrate to desired effect (0.1–1.0 μg/kg per min) Higher infusion dose used if asystole present
Lidocaine*	1 mg/kg	

Continued

TABLE 2.4A

Drugs Used in Pediatric Advanced Life Support, cont'd

Drug	Dosage	Remarks
Lidocaine infusion	20–50 μg/kg per min	
Naloxone*	If ≤5 years old or ≤20 kg: 0.1 mg/kg If >5 years old or >20 kg: 2.0 mg	Titrate to desired effect
Prostaglandin E_1	0.05–0.1 μg/kg per min	Monitor for apnea, hypotension, hypoglycemia
Sodium bicarbonate	1 mEq/kg per dose or 0.3 × kg × base deficit	Infuse slowly and only if ventilation is adequate

Adapted from Chameides L, Hazinski MF, eds. *Pediatric Advanced Life Support*. Dallas: American Heart Association; 1997.

*For ET administration, dilute medication with normal saline to a volume of 3 to 5 mL and follow with several positive-pressure ventilations.

TABLE 2.4B

Preparation of Catecholamine Infusions in Infants and Children*

Medication	Dilution*	Delivery Rate
Isoproterenol Epinephrine	0.6 × body weight (kg) is the mg dose added to sufficient diluent to create a total volume of 100 mL†	1 mL/h delivers 0.1 μg/kg/min
Dopamine Dobutamine	6 × body weight (kg) is the mg dose added to sufficient diluent to create a total volume of 100 mL†	1 mL/h delivers 1 μg/kg/min

Adapted from Chameides L, Hazinski MF, eds. *Pediatric Advanced Life Support*. Dallas: American Heart Association; 1997.

*This provides an initial concentration only. Drug concentration can be adjusted based on the patient's fluid requirements or limitations.

†In large patients the amount of drug used to create 100 mL of the drug infusion may deplete the available supply of the drug. To reduce the volume of drug needed to prepare the infusion, decrease the drug concentration by a factor of 10 and increase the hourly infusion rate by a factor of 10. For example, according to the formula above, a 20-kg child would require 12 mg (20 × 0.6) or 60 mL (0.2 mg/mL) of isoproterenol per 100 mL. Instead, dilute 1.2 mg (6 mL) in a solution totaling 100 mL and infuse the final solution at 10 mL/h (instead of 1 mL/h). If high doses of the drug are required (eg, greater than or equal to 10 μg/kg per minute), the resulting amount of fluid delivered may be excessive for small infants or children. Under these conditions, the concentration of the drug may be *increased* by a factor of 3, 5, or 10 and the rate of infusion *decreased* by the same factor.

PROBLEMS OF THE NEWBORN

TABLE 2.5

Hyperbilirubinemia: Common Causes of Jaundice in the First Week of Life

Diagnosis	Clinical and Laboratory Data
Physiological jaundice	Observed on day 2–4 after birth. Transient. Elevated indirect bilirubin. Peak usually <12.9 mg/dL on day 3–4 in term infants and <15 mg/dL on day 5–7 in preterm infants.
ABO incompatibility	Jaundice within 24 hours of birth. May have mild anemia and hepatosplenomegaly. Mother's blood type is O and infant either A or B. More severe if infant's blood type is B. Coombs' test positive. Reticulocyte count is elevated.
Hemolytic disease, Rh incompatibility	Jaundice within 24 hours of birth. Mother is Rh negative and infant is Rh positive. Hepatosplenomegaly and petechiae. Coombs' test positive, anemia, reticulocytosis, elevated indirect bilirubin. Worse with each subsequent pregnancy.
Congenital spherocytosis	Anemia and splenomegaly. Coombs' test negative, elevated indirect bilirubin. Peripheral smear with spherocytes.
Breastfeeding jaundice	Jaundice appears between days 4 and 14. Bilirubin elevated up to 12–20 mg/dL. Disappears rapidly when formula is substituted.

TABLE 2.6

Management of Hyperbilirubinemia in the Healthy Term Neonate

	TSB* Level, mg/dL (μmol/L)			
Age, hours	**Consider Phototherapy****	**Phototherapy**	**Exchange Transfusion if Intensive Phototherapy Fails********	**Exchange Transfusion and Intensive Phototherapy**
<24	***	***	***	***
25–48	>12 (170)	>15 (260)	>20 (340)	>25 (430)
49–72	>15 (260)	>18 (310)	>25 (430)	>30 (510)
>72	>17 (290)	>20 (340)	>25 (430)	>30 (510)

Adapted from Practice parameter: management of hyperbilirubinemia in the healthy term newborn. American Academy of Pediatrics. Provisional Committee for Quality Improvement and Subcommittee on Hyperbilirubinemia. *Pediatrics.* 1994;94(4):558–565.

* TSB, Total Serum Bilirubin

** Phototherapy at these TSB levels is a clinical option.

*** Term infants who are clinically jaundiced at <24 hours old are not considered healthy and require further evaluation.

**** Intensive phototherapy should produce a decline of TSB of 1–2 mg/dl within 4 to 6 hours, and the TSB level should continue to fall and remain below the threshold level for exchange transfusion. If this does not occur, it is considered a failure of phototherapy.

TABLE 2.7

Ruling Out Physiological Jaundice

Criteria that Rule Out the Diagnosis of Physical Jaundice*

1. Clinical jaundice in the first 24 hours of life.
2. Total serum bilirubin concentrations increasing by more than 5 mg/dL (85 μmol/L) per day.
3. Total serum bilirubin concentration exceeding 12.9 mg/dL (221 μmol/L) in a full-term infant on day 3–4, or 15 mg/dL (257 μmol/L) in a premature infant on day 5–7.
4. Direct serum bilirubin concentration exceeding 2 mg/dL (34 μmol/L).
5. Clinical jaundice persisting for >1 week in a full-term infant or 2 weeks in a premature infant.

* The absence of these criteria does not imply that the jaundice *is* physiological. In the presence of any of these criteria, the jaundice must be investigated.

TABLE 2.8
Neonatal Hepatitis B Prophylaxis

	Maternal Hepatitis B Status		
	HBsAg Negative	**HBsAg Positive**	**HBsAg Unknown**
HBIG	Not needed	Administer within 12 hours of birth	Test mom. If positive, give as soon as possible but no later than 7 days after birth
Vaccine	Give as routinely scheduled	Give first dose within 12 hours of birth, second dose at 1–2 months, and third dose at 6 months of age	Give first dose within 12 hours of birth, second dose at 1–2 months, and third dose at 6 months of age

HBIG indicates hepatitis B immune globulin; HbsAg, hepatitis B surface antigen.

TABLE 2.9
Ambiguous Genitalia

Fetal Development

Genital structures arise as follows:	Internal gonad from genital ridge differentiates at 6–7 weeks External gonad from genital tubercle at 10–12 weeks

Evaluation

Carefully examine before informing of child's sex

Unclear sex from exam needs further testing

Chromosomes sent for analysis prior to assigning sex to the neonate

Support for parents while waiting results

TABLE 2.10

Gynecological Conditions of the Infant

Condition	Etiology	Diagnosis	Treatment	Prognosis
Vaginal atresia	Dysplasia or aplasia of müllerian ducts	Absent uterus on palpation, no vaginal orifice, may have associated urinary tract anomaly	Emergency urinary drainage, surgical vaginal construction	Sterile
Gonadal agenesis	21 Different abnormal chromosome complements associated (1/2500 births)	Edema of hands and feet of newborn; somatic anomalies (low hairline, low-set ears, cubitus valgus, growth failure, high palate); abnormal karyotype	Surgical removal of ovarian streaks if Y chromosome is present to prevent malignancy; estrogens to develop secondary sex characteristics	Sterile
Testicular feminization	Congenital insensitivity to androgens, familial tendency	Girl with inguinal "hernias," blind vaginal pouch, absent uterus; buccal chromatin-negative; 46 XY; primary amenorrhea	Surgical removal of testes, hormone therapy with estrogens, female sex assigned	Sterile
True hermaphroditism	Ovotestis develops often in absence of Y chromosome (rare)	Hypospadic, small phallus; small vagina; gonads may be palpable in labial or scrotal folds; buccal chromatin-positive	Gonads excised to prevent dysgerminoma, surgical sex assignment carried out, hormones for secondary sex characteristics	Sterile
Labial agglutination	Congenital or inflammatory process with adhesions	Visible adhesion of labia, thin livid line; vaginal orifice, usually partially patent	Topical estrogen cream twice daily for 7–14 days	Normal, may recur

Condition	Etiology	Diagnosis	Treatment	Prognosis
Vaginal bleeding age 3–5 days	Withdrawal of placental estrogens	Normal examination; bleeding stops spontaneously	None; reassurance	Normal
Urethral prolapse	?	Painful, friable mass at vaginal orifice; cathether inserted in center of mass enters bladder	Topically applied estrogen and antibiotic creams; surgical excision if medical therapy fails	Fertile
Adrenal virilization (pseudoherm-aphroditism)	Inborn error of cortisol metabolism (1/15,000 births)	Labial fusion, clitoral enlargement, uterus palpable; buccal chromatin-positive; elevated urinary 17-ketosteroids and pregnanetriol; check electrolytes	Cortisone; surgical excision of large clitoris, reconstruct vagina, estrogens at puberty	Sterile
Nonadrenal virilization	Maternal progestins taken before 12 weeks and up to 16 weeks	Labial fusion, clitoral enlargement, uterus palpable, buccal chromatin-positive; normal urinary 17-ketosteroids and pregnanetriol, history of progestins to mother	Reassurance, surgical correction of fused labia and clitoral enlargement before age 3; no hormone therapy	Fertile

TABLE 2.11

Formulas for Specific Feeding Problems

Problem	Formula
Lactose intolerance	Lactofree, Similac lactose free
Cow protein allergy/intolerance	ProSobee, Isomil, Alsoy
Protein intolerance	Nutramigen, Alimentum
Prematurity	Premature Enfamil, Premie SMA
Inborn errors of metabolism:	
Amino acid	Lofenalac (low phenylalanine content)
Galactosemia	Soy formulas, Nutramigen (galactose free)
Fructose	Similac, Enfamil, SMA (fructose free)
Reflux	Enfamil AR (thickened formula)
Acute diarrhea	Isomil DF, lactose-free formulas

TABLE 2.12

Immunization Schedule*

Immunization	Routine Schedule	Minimum Interval Between Doses
Hepatitis B	Birth-2 mos, 1 mo–4 mos, 6 mos–18 mos	4 weeks between doses 1–2 and 8 weeks between doses 2–3
Hib	2 mos, 4 mos, 6 mos, 12–15 mos	4 weeks
Hib-hepatitis B	2 mos, 4 mos, 12–15 mos	2 months for doses one and two, at least 8 months for doses 2 and 3.
IPV	2 mos, 4 mos, 6–18 mos, 4–6 yrs	4 weeks
Pneumococcal conjugate	2 mos, 4 mos, 6 mos, 12–15 mos	4 weeks
DTaP	2 mos, 4 mos, 6 mos, 15–18 mos	4 weeks for first 3 doses, 6 months between doses 3 and 4
MMR	12–15 mos, 4–6 yrs	4 weeks
Varicella	12–18 mos	4 weeks
Hepatitis A	Only in selected areas after 24 mos	6 months
dT	11–18 yrs	

Hib indicates *Haemophilus influenzae* type b; IPV, inactivated poliovirus vaccine; DTaP, diphtheria and tetanus toxoids with acellular pertussis vaccine; MMR, measles, mumps, and rubella; dT, tetanus-diphtheria toxoids (adult type).

*These recommendations are updated annually. See www.aafp.org for most recent update.

TABLE 2.13

Contraindications to Vaccine Administration

- Very few absolute contraindications
- Anaphylactic reactions to previous vaccine doses or any vaccine components
  - —Egg allergy with influenza and yellow fever vaccines
  - —Mercury sensitivity; need to check individual vaccines for thimerosal as a preservative
  - —Antibiotic allergies to streptomycin, neomycin, and polymyxin B with IPV and to neomycin with varicella, MMR, or individual measles, mumps, or rubella
  - —Baker's yeast reaction with hepatitis B
  - —Gelatin allergy with varicella vaccine
- Pregnancy with MMR or varicella vaccine
- Immunodeficiency with MMR or varicella
- HIV infection with varicella (MMR if advanced HIV infection)
- DTaP if development of encephalopathy within 7 days of previous vaccination
- Precautions include the following:
  - —Moderate or severe current illness
  - —High fever (>104.8°F), collapse or shock, inconsolable crying over 3 hours within 48 hours, seizures within 3 days, or Guillain-Barre syndrome within 6 weeks after a previous DTaP vaccination
  - —Pregnancy with IPV
  - —Recent administration of immune globulin

IPV indicates inactivated poliovirus vaccine; MMR, measles, mumps, and rubella; HIV, human immunodeficiency virus; DTaP, diphtheria and tetanas toxoids with acellular pertussis vaccine.

TABLE 2.14

Immunization Schedule for Children Who Start After 12 Months of Age

Ages 12 months to 7 years

Time Line	Immunizations	Guidelines
First visit	MMR, Hib, HBV, DTaP, PCV7	Hib is not given if over 5 years old and PCV7 is not given if over 2 years old, except in certain higher-risk patients.
4 weeks later	HBV, DTaP, IPV, varicella	
8 weeks after first visit	Hib, DTaP, IPV, PCV7	Second Hib given only if first dose was given under 15 months old. Second PCV7 given if first dose was given under 24 months, unless patient is high risk.
8 months or more after first visit	HBV, DTaP, IPV	
At 4–6 years old	MMR, DTaP, IPV	Fourth dose of IPV and fifth dose of DTaP not needed if previous doses were given after 4 years old.

Ages 7–12 years

Time Line	Immunizations	Guidelines
First visit	MMR, HBV, IPV, dT	
8 weeks after first visit	MMR, HBV, IPV, dT, varicella	Second IPV can be given 4 weeks after first dose if necessary.
8 months after first visit	HBV, IPV, dT	

Over 13 years

Immunization	Schedule	Guidelines
Hepatitis B	First visit, 4 weeks later, 6 months later	Start at any age
Varicella	First visit, 4 weeks later	Give two doses after 13 years old
dT	First visit, 4 weeks later, 6–12 months later	Booster doses every 10 years
MMR	First visit, 4 weeks later	Caution in postmenarchal females, document not

Continued

TABLE 2.14

Immunization Schedule for Children Who Start After 12 Months of Age, cont'd

Immunization	Schedule	Guidelines
		pregnant and prevent pregnancy for 3 months after administration.
IPV	3 doses at least 28 days apart	No definite recommendations, give if high risk of exposure.

TABLE 2.15

Developmental Evaluation

Age	Gross Motor	Fine Motor	Cognitive	Language	Social	Anticipatory Guidance
1 month	Lifts chin up when prone	Tight grasp	Regards face	Responds to noise	Social smile	Car seat, signs of illness, back to sleep, tummy time while awake, colic, smoke-free environment
2 months	Lifts chest up when prone, some head control	Loses tight grasp	Follows object past midline	Coos, smiles in response to stimulation	Recognizes parent	Safety with small objects in mouth and rolling over, talk to baby, babysitters
3 months	Supports self on elbows when prone, holds head steady	Holds hand open >50%, hands together at midline	Follows circular pattern, responds to visual threat			Lower water temperature <120 °
4 months	Extends elbows when prone, rolls prone to supine, no head lag when pulled to sitting position	Grasps rattle	Reaches for and bats object with both hands	Orients to voice, vocalizes responsively, laughs, squeals, razzes	Regards own hands and reflection in mirror	Childproof home, nutrition, introduce solid foods, no baby walkers, no bottles in bed

Continued

TABLE 2.15

Developmental Evaluation, cont'd

Age	Gross Motor	Fine Motor	Cognitive	Language	Social	Anticipatory Guidance
5 months	Rolls supine to prone, sits well when propped	Transfers object, unfisted 100%, ulnar rake	Grasps 1 block	Says "ah-goo," orients laterally to sound		Teething
6 months	Sits well with support	Radial rake, grasps feet when supine	Reaches for objects with either hand, looks for dropped toy	Babbles	Recognizes strangers	Safety, brush teeth, supervise eating, stranger anxiety, allow exploration
7 months	Sits unsupported, belly crawl			Echolalia, orients to sound in 2 planes		Childproof home, syrup of ipecac
8 months	Creeps, pulls to stand		Inspects objects, works for toy	Nonspecific "mama" and "dada," responds to name, understands "no"	Stranger/separation anxiety	Stranger anxiety, gun safety
9 months	Cruises	Finger feeds self	Search for hidden object, combine blocks	Imitates sounds, plays peek-a-boo or pat-a-cake	Reaches to be taken, explores environment	Avoid choke foods, no baby walkers, interact with reading, singing, games
10 months	Walks with 2 hands held	Immature pincer grasp		Specific "mama" and "dada"		Limit rules and enforce consistently

Age	Gross Motor	Fine Motor	Cognitive	Language	Social	Anticipatory Guidance
11 months	Walks with 1 hand held, stands alone	Mature pincer grasp		First word, orients to 3 planes		Supervise closely
12 months	Takes a few steps, creeps up steps	Release object, drinks from cup	Looks for dropped or hidden objects, functional use of objects	2-4 words, follows command with gesture, indicates needs by pointing	Waves "bye-bye"	Offer healthy food choices, change to whole milk, establish routines, lower crib mattress
15 months	Walks well, stands without pulling up, stoops and recovers, climbs onto furniture	Uses spoon to feed, drinks from open cup	Tower of 3 blocks, imitates scribble	4–6 words, 1 body part, immature jargon (13 months), follows 1-step command without gesture	Solitary play	Self-feeding, family meals, temper tantrums, discipline: set limits, positive reinforcement
18 months	Walks up stairs with help, runs	Turns 2–3 pages at a time	Scribbles spontaneously, tower of 4 blocks	10–25 words, mature jargon, 3 body parts		Supervise play, bedtime routine, toilet training, read books
22 months	Walks down stairs with help, throws ball overhand	Unzips	Tower of 6 blocks, 3–4 block train	50+ words, 2 word phrases, uses me and mine, names 1 picture		

Continued

TABLE 2.15

Developmental Evaluation, cont'd

Age	Gross Motor	Fine Motor	Cognitive	Language	Social	Anticipatory Guidance
24 months	Kicks ball, walks up and down steps without help	Turns pages one at a time, removes some clothes		Names 6 objects in a picture, repeats 2 digits, follows 2-step commands	Parallel play, imitates adults	Safety, airbag safety, supervise closely, picky eater, nutritious snacks, discipline
30 months	Walks up stairs, alternating feet using the rail, jumps in place	String beads, fold paper	Tower 10 cubes	Understands the concept of "I", no echolalia, functional use of objects	Washes hands, tells first and last name	
3 years	Walks up stairs, alternating feet without using the rail, pedals tricycle, balance on 1 foot, heel to toe walk	Cut with scissors, dresses self with help	Draws circle and cross, adds 2 parts to drawing of incomplete person	Knows age, name, and sex, 3-word phrases, uses plurals correctly	Plays well with others, shares, takes turns, independent with eating, toilet trained	Dentist, review car, water, and bike safety, limit TV, good, balanced diet, sexual curiosity
4 years	Walks down stairs alternating feet, hops on 1 foot, skips	Catches ball	Copies square, distinguishes between fantasy and reality, draws a person with 3 parts	Knows all colors, sings a song, asks questions, gives first and last name		Firm rules and reinforce limits, stranger safety

Age	Gross Motor	Fine Motor	Cognitive	Language	Social	Anticipatory Guidance
5 years	Jumps over low obstacles, catches ball, heel to toe walking	Dresses self without help, ties shoe, buttons clothes	Copies triangle, counts on fingers, draws stick figure (6 parts), picks longer line, knows some opposites	Prints first name, asks for word meanings, learns address and phone number	Separates easily	School readiness, respect for authority, family rules, review safety on playground, street, and water

TABLE 2.16

Dental Development

	DECIDUOUS TEETH				PERMANENT TEETH	
	Eruption		Shedding		Eruption	
	Maxillary	**Mandibular**	**Maxillary**	**Mandibular**	**Maxillary***	**Mandibular***
Central incisors	6–10 months	5–8 months	7–8 years	6–7 years	7–8 years (4)	6–7 years (3)
Lateral incisors	8–12 months	7–10 months	8–9 years	7–8 years	8–9 years (6)	7–8 years (5)
Cuspids	16–20 months	16–20 months	11–12 years	9–11 years	11–12 years (12)	9–11 years (7)
First premolar	—	—	—	—	10–11 years (8)	10–12 years (9)
Second premolar	—	—	—	—	10–12 years (10)	11–13 years (11)
First molars	10–18 months	10–18 months	9–11 years	9–12 years	6–7 years (1)	6–7 years (2)
Second molars	20–30 months	20–30 months	10–12 years	11–13 years	12–14 years (13)	12–13 years (14)
Third molars	—	—	—	—	17–30 (15)	17–30 (16)

Note: Sexes are combined, although girls tend to be slightly advanced over boys. Averages are approximate values derived from various studies.

*Numbers in parenthesis give order of eruption.

TABLE 2.17

Time of Appearance of Sexual Characteristics: American Girls

Aspect	Comments	Age
Puberty	Age at onset is earlier now but has leveled off in developed countries	Onset at 8–13 years
Breasts	Budding is usually the first sign of puberty	10–11 years
Pubic hair	Sparse hair is first seen	6–12 months after breast buds appear
Menarche	Usually anovulatory at onset	2–2.5 years after breast buds, can be up to 6 years later

TABLE 2.18

Time of Appearance of Sexual Characteristics: American Boys

Aspect	Comments	Age
Puberty	Age at onset; first signs are growth of testes and thinning of the scrotum	Onset at 8.5–13.5 years
Genitals	Pigmentation and growth of the scrotum and growth of the penis	
Pubic hair	Gradually darkens and becomes coarse and thicker	
Axillary hair	Appears at midpuberty	

FIGURE 2.5

Tanner Staging: Female Pubic Hair Development

Tanner Stage	Comment
I	Prepuberty; no pubic hair
II	Sparse, straight hair on the labia
III	Thicker, darker hair; present in typical female triangle
IV	Thicker, curled hair in adult distribution, but not as abundant
V	Adult pattern; may extend to the medial thighs

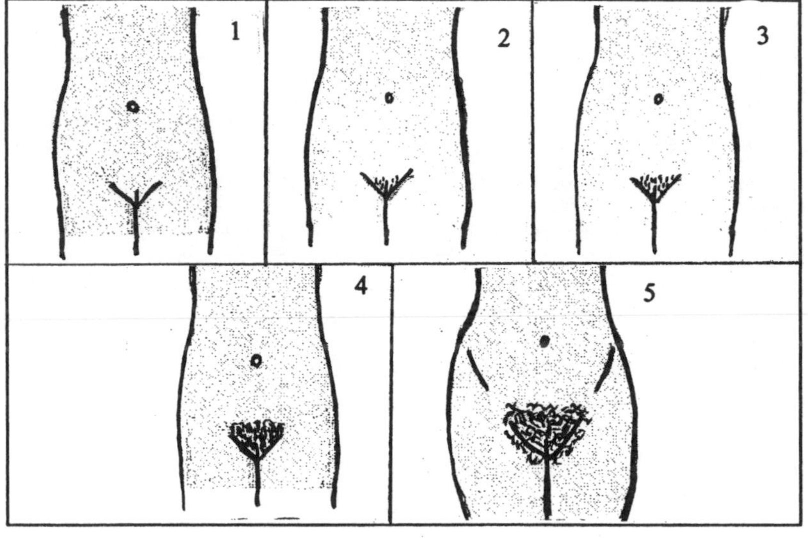

FIGURE 2.6

Tanner Staging: Female Breast Development

Tanner Stage	Comments
I	Prepuberty; elevations of papilla only
II	Breast buds appear; areola in mound and wider
III	Enlargement of the entire breast with no protrusion of the papilla or nipple
IV	Enlargement of the breast with protrusion of areola and papilla as a separate mound
V	Adult breast with projection of the nipple only

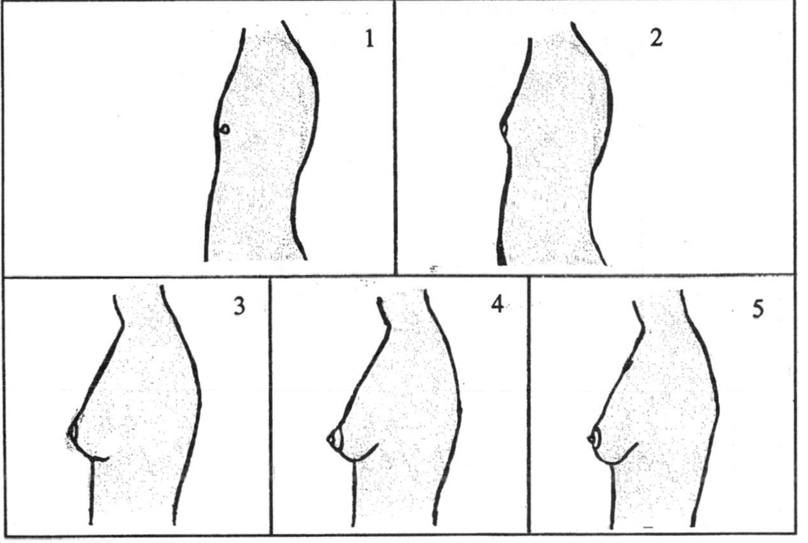

FIGURE 2.7

Tanner Staging: Male Genital and Pubic Hair Development

Tanner Stage	Comments
I	Prepuberty; no pubic hair and childhood genitalia
II	Testes and penis slightly enlarge; skin on scrotum becomes more textured; light, thin hair develops laterally and darkens
III	Testes, scrotum, and penis further enlarge; pubic hair extends across the pubis
IV	Genitalia resembles adult; scrotum is darker; glans is broader and larger; pubic hair curls and thickens
V	Genitalia is adult size; pubic hair is thicker and extends onto medial thighs

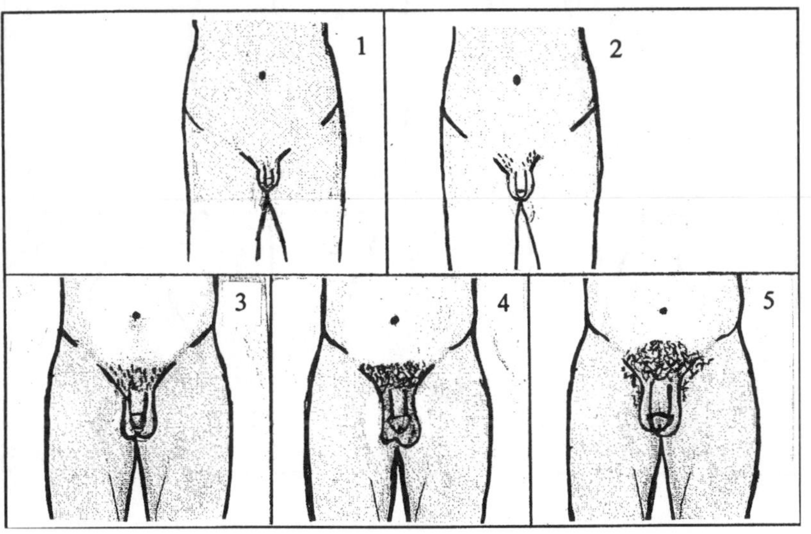

TABLE 2.19

Pediatric Vulvovaginitis

Signs and Symptoms
Vaginal discharge
Erythema
Pruritus
Dysuria

Common Etiology
Poor perineal hygiene
Candida infection
Foreign body
Other infections such as pinworms, *Gardnerella vaginalis*, streptococcal, staphylococcal, enterococci, anaerobic bacteria, Trichomonas; if *Trichomonas* is present, think of gonorrhea and chlamydia and suspect abuse

Exam and Labs
External genitalia
Vaginoscopy may be indicated
Vaginal pH (normal is 7–8 in prepuberty and 5–5.5 after puberty)
Microscopic exam of vaginal discharge
Urinalysis
Cultures

Treatment
Teach perineal hygiene, wiping from front to back
Treat specific infection with appropriate antimicrobial agent
Topical estrogen cream or polysporin ointment can be used to speed resolution

TABLE 2.20

Common Infectious Diseases

Disease	Incubation	Prodrome	Signs and Symptoms	Isolation	Treatment
Chickenpox (varicella)	10–21 days	Minimal URI symptoms	Rash with macules, papules, and vesicles. Spreads from trunk to extremities for 5–20 days.	Until all lesions are crusted. Infectious prior to rash.	If over 12 years old, immunocompromised, or severe infection, treat with oral or IV acyclovir, famciclovir, or valacyclovir and foscarnet. Symptomatic with bed rest, antipyretics, and topical antipruritics.
Diphtheria	2–7 days	Rapid onset	Moderate fever, malaise, sore throat. Gray, tenacious membrane in throat. Respiratory distress.	Until two negative nose and throat cultures 24 hours apart.	Antitoxin and erythromycin or pencillin G for 14 days. Supportive treatment as needed.
Fifth disease (erythema infectiosum, parvovirus B19)	4–21 days	Mild, nonspecific symptoms of fever, myalgias, malaise, and headache	Maculopapular rash on face with circumoral pallor (slapped cheek) appears 7–10 days after mild symptoms start. Spreads to extremities, lasts a few days to a few weeks and brought out by warmth.	None. Not infectious after rash appears.	Symptomatic.

Disease	Incubation	Prodrome	Signs and Symptoms	Isolation	Treatment
Hepatitis A	15–50 days	Rapid onset	Fever, anorexia, headache, abdominal pain, jaundice, and liver enzyme elevation, usually mild symptoms in children.	Stool, urine, and blood for one month.	Supportive, bed rest, fluids, serum gamma-globulin to contacts.
Hepatitis B	6 weeks to 6 months	Insidious onset	Wide spectrum from asymptomatic to fulminant hepatitis.	Body secretions until surface antigen negative.	Supportive, bed rest, fluids, hepatitis B immune globulin and vaccine to intimate contacts and vaccine to other contacts.
Hand-foot-and-mouth disease (coxsackie-virus A16)	4–6 days	None	Ulcers on buccal mucosa, tongue, and gums. Vesicular rash on hands, feet, and occasionally buttocks.	None	Symptomatic
Herpangina (coxsackie-virus group A)	3–6 days	None	High fever, vomiting, sore throat, and ulcers of oral mucosa for 5–6 days.	2–6 days	Symptomatic
Menigococcal meningitis	1–10 days	URI, fever, headache, diarrhea	Meningeal signs, purpuric or petechial rash, septic arthritis. CSF shows signs of infection.	24 hours after first dose of antibiotics	Supportive and antibiotics with cefotaxime or ceftriaxone or meropenem and dexamethasone and vancomycin or chloramphenicol and TMP/SMX and vancomycin.

Continued

TABLE 2.20

Common Infectious Diseases, cont'd

Disease	Incubation	Prodrome	Signs and Symptoms	Isolation	Treatment
Mononucleosis (Ebstein-Barr virus)	2–8 weeks	None	Fatigue, anorexia, exudative tonsillitis, lymphadenopathy, splenomegaly, maculopapular rash, and atypical lymphocytosis.	Avoid saliva contact for 3 months	Symptomatic
Mumps	12–25 days	None	Swelling and pain in salivary glands and fever; 30–40% are asymptomatic.	Until salivary swelling has resolved	Symptomatic, bed rest, analgesics, fluids.
Poliomyelitis	7–21 days	Usually none, mild fever and sore throat	Asymmetric flaccid paralysis with nuchal rigidity and back stiffness, pain and tenderness in affected muscles.	Secretions for 1 week and stool for 6 weeks	Supportive, bed rest, physical therapy when pain subsides
Roseola	5–15 days	3–5 days of sustained high fever	Fine pink rash on neck and trunk begins at defervescence and lasts 2 days. Usually seen at 6 months to 2 years old.	Unknown	Supportive, antipyretics.

Disease	Incubation	Prodrome	Signs and Symptoms	Isolation	Treatment
Rubella (German measles or 3-day measles)	14–23 days	Lymphadenopathy, fever, headache, malaise	Erythematous, maculopapular rash appears on face and spreads to trunk and proximal extremities, lasting 1–3 days. Postauricular, suboccipital, and cervical lymphadenopathy.	Infectious from 5 days before to 7 days after the rash appears	Symptomatic
Measles (rubeola)	8–12 days	High fever, coryza, cough, and conjunctivitis for 3–4 days	Koplik's spots appear 1–2 days before maculopapular rash. Rash is confluent and spreads from hairline to face to body then feet and lasts 4–5 days.	5 days after onset of rash	Symptomatic
Whooping cough (pertussis)	5–20 days	1–3 weeks of cough, coryza, and occasional emesis (catarrhal stage)	Short paroxysmal cough ending with inspiratory "whoop" (paroxysmal stage)	5 days on treatment or 3 weeks after onset of paroxysmal cough if no therapy	Supportive, erythromycin for 14 days, corticosteroids and albuterol may reduce cough

CSF indicates cerebrospinal fluid IV, intravenous; TMP/SMX, trimethoprim-sulfamethoxazole; URI, upper respiratory infection.

TABLE 2.21
Common Respiratory Diseases

	Bronchiolitis	**Asthma**	**Pneumonia**	**Epiglottitis**	**Croup**
Onset	3 months to 3 years	All ages	All ages	2–7 years	Under 3 years
Previous History	Negative	Usually positive	Negative	Negative	Cough and rhinorrhea
Seasonal Incidence	Winter	All seasons	Winter	Any season	Late fall and winter
Fever	None or low grade	None	Present	High fever	High fever
Lung Exam	Prolonged expiration, wheezes, rales, or rhonchi	Prolonged expiration, wheezes	Normal expiration, rales	Normal expiration	Normal expiration
Percussion	Hyperresonant	Hyperresonant	Hyperresonant	Normal	Normal
Airway Compromise	Inspiratory and expiratory obstruction	Expiratory obstruction	Usually no obstruction	Inspiratory stridor	Inspiratory obstruction, barking cough
Respiratory Distress	Mild to severe	Mild to severe	Mild to severe	Severe	Mild to severe
WBC	Lymphocytosis	Normal to eosinophilia	Lymphocytosis to leukocytosis	Marked leukocytosis	Normal
Chest X-Ray	Hyperaeration	Hyperaeration	Lobar infiltrate	Normal, neck x-ray with "steeple sign"	Normal
Treatment	Oxygen, bronchodilators if wheezes present	Oxygen, bronchodilators, systemic corticosteroids	Appropriate antibiotics, oxygen	Cefuroxime, cefotaxime, or ceftriaxone	Cool mist if mild, racemic epinephrine, dexamethasone, nebulized steroids if severe

TABLE 2.22

Otitis Media

Diagnosis

Differentiate between acute otitis media and otitis media with effusion. Hyperemic, buldging, opacified, immobile tympanic membrane with both. Effusion with signs and symptoms of acute, local, or systemic illness consistent with acute otitis media.

Etiology

Viral (40%–50%)
Streptococcus pneumoniae (40%–50%)
Haemophilus influenzae (20%–25%)
Moraxella catarrhalis (10%–15%)

Treatment

Otitis media with effusion:

- No treatment unless present over 3 months
- If persistent after treatment, do not retreat

Acute otitis media:

- 80% will resolve in 3 days without treatment
- Length of treatment depends on age and underlying medical conditions
- 5–7 days if over 2 years old in selected patients; 10 days if 2 years old or younger and with certain underlying medical conditions

Antibiotics:

- Amoxicillin at usual dose of 40–45 mg/kg/day or high dose of 80–90 mg/kg/day divided bid or tid
- If allergic to amoxicillin, TMP/SMX 8 mg/kg/day divided bid or clarithromycin 15 mg/kg/day divided bid or azithromycin 10 mg/kg for 1 day then 5 mg/kg for 4 more days
- If treatment failure or used antibiotics in the past month, high dose amoxicillin or high-dose amoxicillin/clavulanate 80–90 mg/kg/day of amoxicillin component and keep clavulanate at 10 mg/kg/day or use cefdinir, cefpodoxime, or cefuroxime axetil

TABLE 2.23

Parasitic Infections

Parasite	Diagnosis	Treatment	Dose (oral)
Pinworm (*Enterobius vermicularis*)	Microscopic visualization of ova on tape sample from anus or direct visualization of pinworm	Mebendazole	100 mg in one dose, repeat in 2 weeks
		Pyrantel pamoate	11 mg/kg in one dose (maximum 1 gram), repeat in 2 weeks then in 4 weeks
Giardiasis (*Giardia lamblia*)	Microscopic visualization of trophozoites or cysts from stool sample or detection of giardia-specific antigen in stool	Metronidazole	5 mg/kg tid for 5 days (max 250 mg/dose)
		Quinacrine	7 mg/kg/day divided tid for 5 days (max 300 mg/day)
Roundworm (*Ascaris lumbricoides*)	Adult worm in emesis or stool or ova in stool	Mebendazole	100 mg bid for 3 days
		Pyrantel pamoate	11 mg/kg in one dose (max 1 gram)
Visceral larva migrans, toxocariasis (*Toxocara canis, T cati*)	History of exposure to cats or dogs, hypereosinophilia, hypergammaglobulinemia, may be anemic, fever, hepatomegaly	Symptomatic treatment, self-limited disease;	
		Mebenazole	100–200 mg bid for 5 days
Tapeworm (*Taenia saginata* [beef], *T. solium* [pork])	Worm segments or ova in stool	Praziquantel	10 mg/kg for one dose

TABLE 2.24

Guidelines for Postexposure Rabies Prophylaxis

Animal Species	Condition of Animal at Time of Attack	Treatment
Domestic dog or cat	Healthy and available for 10 days of observation	None, unless animal develops rabies
	Suspicious	HRIG and HDCV or RVA; discontinue after 5 days if animal is healthy
	Rabid	HRIG and HDCV or RVA
	Unknown	Consult public health officials; if treatment is indicated, give HRIG and HDCV or RVA
Wild animals: skunk, bat, fox, coyote, raccoon, bobcat, and other carnivores	Regard as rabid unless proven negative by laboratory test	HRIG and HDCV or RVA
Other animals: livestock, rodents, rabbits, and hares	Consider individually. Bites of provoked squirrels, hamsters, guinea pigs, gerbils, chipmunks, rats, mice, other rodents, rabbits, and hares almost never call for antirabies prophylaxis	Local or state public health officials should be consulted concerning questions that arise about the need for rabies prophylaxis

HRIG indicates human rabies immune globulin; HDCV, human diploid cell vaccine; RVA, rabies vaccine absorbed.

Regimen is: Day 0 HRIG + HDCV or RVA. Day 3, 7, 14, and 28 HDCV or RVA alone. HRIG dosage is 20 mg/kg half dose intramuscularly and half dose in wound edge. HDCV and RVA dose is 1.0 mL intramuscularly (deltoid).

TABLE 2.25
Febrile Seizures

Definition
Simple, tonic-clonic seizure lasting less than 15 minutes
Usually occurs at the onset of illness
Occurs in children aged 6 months to 5 years
Fever present
No evidence of meningitis or encephalitis
No neurologic signs or symptoms

Risk Factors
Family history
Abnormal neurodevelopmental history
Atypical seizure (lasting more than 15 minutes, repetitive, abnormal neurologic exam, abnormal electroencephalogram)
Past history of febrile seizures
Risk of recurrence is 30% for second, 17% for third, and 9% for more than three

Treatment
Temperature control with each subsequent illness
Anticonvulsant therapy is not routinely recommended
(risk of epilepsy is 2%)

TABLE 2.26
Meningitis

Signs and Symptoms

Fever	Irritability	Altered mental status
Headache	Nausea	
Nuchal rigidity	Vomiting	

Diagnosis
Cerebrospinal fluid sent for analysis: protein, glucose, cell counts, gram stain, cultures, and specific antigen or antibody tests

Treatment
Do not wait for cerebrospinal fluid results to initiate. Antibiotics based on age, see Table 2.28.

TABLE 2.27

CSF Characteristics

CSF	Normal	Bacterial Meningitis	Aseptic Meningitis
Opening pressure	70–180 mm H_2O	Normal to increased	Usually normal
Protein	15–45 mg/dL	Increased	Normal to increased
Glucose	45–80 mg/dL	Decreased	Normal to decreased
WBC count	0 to 10	25 to 10 × 10^3	5 to 2 × 10^3
Predominant cells	Mononuclear	Polymorphonuclear	Lymphocytes
Gram stain	Negative	May be positive	Negative

TABLE 2.28

Presumptive Therapy for Bacterial Meningitis

Age	Therapy	Pathogens
Under 1 month	Ampicillin and cefotaxime or ampicillin and gentamicin	Group B streptococci (45%) *E. coli* (18%) Gram-negative bacteria (10%) Gram-positive bacteria (10%) *Listeria monocytogenes* (7%)
1 month to adult	Cefotaxime 50 mg/kg IV/IM q6 hours (max 3 g/dose) or ceftriaxone 50 mg/kg IV/IM q12 hrs (max 2 g/dose) and vancomycin 15 mg/kg q6 hours (max 1 g/dose) and dexamethasone 0.4 mg/kg q12 hours for 2 days given with or just prior to first dose of antibiotics	*S. pneumoniae* *N. meningitidis* *H. influenzae* (rare)

IV indicates intravenous, IM, intramuscular; of 6 h, every 6 hours; of 12 h, every 12 hours.

TABLE 2.29
Stooling Disorders with Diarrhea

Condition	First-Stage Screening	Second-Stage Screening	Specific Diagnostic Studies
Hirschsprung's disease (1)*	Abdominal radiograph	Barium enema	Rectal biopsy
Stenosis of the bowel (1)	Abdominal radiograph	Gastrointestinal series	Exploratory laparotomy
Milk protein sensitivity (1)	Cow's milk elimination	Rechallenge with cow's milk	Consistent response to cow's milk protein
Agammaglobulinemia (Swiss type) (1)	Peripheral blood smear (lymphocytes)	Serum protein electrophoresis	Biopsy of lymph nodes
Disaccharide intolerance (1, 2)	Stool pH test for reducing substances	Tolerance test for sugars	Trial carbohydrate elimination; may use fructose
Cystic fibrosis (1, 2)	Sweat test	—	Repeat sweat test
Celiac disease (2, 3)	History	Trial of gluten-free diet	Intestinal biopsy
Ulcerative colitis (3)	Stool guaiac	Sigmoidoscopy, barium enema	Intestinal biopsy
Ova and parasites (1, 2, 3)	Stool cultures	Repeat stool cultures	
Antibiotic-associated toxin (1, 2, 3)	Culture for *C difficile*	Sigmoidoscopy	Culture

*Age at onset: (1), infant; (2), toddler; (3), toddler or older child.

TABLE 2.30

Constipation

Etiology
Dietary
Resistance to toilet training
Rashes/fissures
Hirschsprung's disease
Hypothyroidism
Medications (antidepressants)

Treatment
Increase dietary fiber
Stool softeners
Enema

TABLE 2.31

Stooling Disorders with Constipation

Clinical	Hirschsprung's Disease	Encopresis
Age	Birth or soon after; male > female	After age 4
Toilet training	Usually successful	Usually successful initially
Constipation	Yes	Yes
Toilet use	Usually	Infrequent
Soiling	Rarely	Constant
Rectum	Usually empty	Stool present
Stool	Pellet or ribbonlike; offensive odor	Very large. Some retain and others deposit in inappropriate places
Evaluation	Plain x-ray examination and barium enema; rectal biopsy	Psychiatric since many will have retardation or serious psychopathology
Resolution	Surgery	Psychotherapy, behavior modification

TABLE 2.32

Attention Deficit Hyperactivity Disorder (ADHD)

Diagnosis

Observe child's behavior (attention difficulties, hyperactivity, impulsivity)
History from parents and teachers
Evaluate for any comorbid conditions (learning disabilities, conduct disorder, oppositional defiant disorder, mood disorders, anxiety disorders, substance abuse [adolescents])

Assessment Tools

Screening questionnaires for parents and teachers (ACTERs, Connors, etc)
Neurologic exam
Psychometric testing

Treatment

Behavior management at home and school with structured schedule, simple rules, firm rewards and punishment
Special education
Psychotherapy
Pharmacotherapy

TABLE 2.33

Drug Therapy for Attention Deficit Hyperactivity Disorder (ADHD)

Drug	Age (years)	Initial Dose	Subsequent Dose	Maximum Dose (per day)
Methylphenidate (Ritalin)	6–8 9–12	5 mg in AM 10 mg in AM	Increase by 5 mg a week divided up to tid until desired effect	60 mg
Ritalin SR		20 mg in AM		60 mg
Concerta		18–36 mg in AM		54 mg
Magnesium Pemoline (Cylert)	6	37.5 mg in AM	Increase by 18.75 mg a week divided up to tid	112.5 mg
Dextroamphetamine (Dexedrine)	3–5 6–7	2.5 mg qd 5 mg qd	Increase by 5 mg a week	40 mg
Adderall (dextroamphetamine and racemic amphetamine)	3–5 >6	2.5 mg qd-bid 5 mg qd-bid	Increase by 2.5 to 5 mg a week	40 mg
Imipramine (Tofranil)	6 7–8	10 mg in AM 25 mg in AM	Increase by 10 mg a week, divide dose tid	75 mg
Clonidine (or guanfacine hydrochloride [Tenex])	Use as add on med			

TABLE 2.34

Rheumatic Fever: Diagnosis

Use Jones criteria (see Table 2.35); need two major criteria or one major and two minor criteria. Evidence of recent group A streptococcal infection (scarlet fever, positive throat culture, or increased antistreptolysin titer).

TABLE 2.35

Diagnosis of Rheumatic Fever: Jones Criteria Revised

Major Criteria	Minor Criteria
Carditis	Arthralgia
Chorea	Fever
Erythema marginatum	Previous rheumatic fever or rheumatic heart disease
Polyarthritis	Prolonged PR interval
Subcutaneous nodules	Elevated sedimentation rate, C-reactive protein, or leukocytosis

TABLE 2.36

Differential Diagnosis of Rheumatoid Diseases

Aspect	Rheumatic Fever	Juvenile Rheumatoid Arthritis	Systemic Lupus Erythematosus
Age trend	6–16 years	5 years	0–15 years
Sex ratio	Equal	Girls 1.5:1	Girls 8:1
Joint findings			
Pain	Severe	Moderate	—
Swelling	Nonspecific	Nonspecific	Nonspecific
Tenderness	Severe	Moderate	—
Bone x-ray	None	Frequent	Occasional
Morning stiffness	Yes	Yes	Yes
Rash	Erythema marginatum	Rheumatoid arthritis rash	Malar flush
Chorea	Yes	No	Rarely
Clinical carditis	Possible	Rare	Late
Laboratory tests			
WBC	Normal to high	Normal to high	Decreased to normal
Latex	Negative	+ (15%)	+ Occasionally
Sheep cell agglutination	Negative	+ (10%)	—
LE cell prep	Negative	+ (5%)	+ Always
Biopsy			
Skin rash	Nonspecific	Nonspecific	Diagnostic
Nodules	Nonspecific	Nonspecific	Nonspecific
Response to salicylates	Rapid	Slow, usually	Slow or none
Fever	Low grade	Low grade	Possible

LE indicate lupus erythematosus; WBC, white blood cell count.

TABLE 2.37

Pediatric Sedation

Medication	Oral Dose (mg/kg/dose)	IV Dose (mg/kg/dose)	IM Dose (mg/kg/dose)	PR Dose (mg/kg/dose)	Maximum Dose (mg)
Diazepam	0.2–0.3	0.1–0.2	Painful	0.2–0.3	
Lorazepam	0.05	0.05	0.05	0.05	2 mg IV, 4 mg IM/PO/PR
Midazolam*	0.5–0.75	0.05	0.1–0.2	0.3–1.0	20 mg PO/PR, 10 mg IV/IM
Pentobarbital	2–6	0.5–1.0		2–6	200 mg PO/PR, 150 mg IV/IM
Chloral hydrate	25–100	—	—	25–100	2000 mg
Ketamine	4–6	Induction of anesthesia only	2–3	4–6	—

IM indicates intramuscular; IV, intravenous; PO, oral; PR, rectal.

*Can be given intranasally at 0.2–0.3 mg/kg/dose up to 7.5 mg.

TABLE 2.38

Common Causes of Microcytic Anemia

	Chronic Inflammation	Iron Deficiency	β-Thalassemia Trait
ESR	↑	Normal	Normal
Ferritin	Normal to ↑	↓	Normal to ↑
Iron	↓	↓	Normal
TIBC	↓	↑	Normal
RDW	Normal	↑	↓
FEP	↑	↑	Normal
Reticulocyte count	Normal	↓	Normal to ↑
Peripheral smear	Variable	Microcytic, hypochromic, target cells, fine basophilic stippling	Microcytic, normochromic, coarse basophilic stippling
Hemoglobin electrophoresis	Normal	Normal	↑ Hemoglobin A2

Adapted from Siberry GK, Iannone R, eds. *The Harriet Lane Handbook: A Handbook for Pediatric House Officers*. 15th ed. St. Louis: Mosby, Inc; 2000.

ESR indicates erythrocyte sedimentation rate; TIBC, total iron-binding capacity; RDW, red cell distribution width; FEP, free erythrocye protoporphyrin.

TABLE 2.39

Age-Specific Blood Cell Indices

Age	Hb (g%)[a]	Hct (%)[a]	MCV (fL)[a]	MCHC (g/% RBC)[a]	Reticulocytes	WBCs (X 10,000/mm^3)[b]	Platelets (10,000/mm^3)[b]
26–30 wk gestation[c]	13.4 (11)	41.5 (34.9)	118.2 (106.7)	37.9 (30.6)	—	4.4 (2.7)	254 (180–327)
28 wk	14.5	45	120	31.0	5–10	—	275
32 wk	15.0	47	118	32.0	3–10	—	290
Term[d] (cord)	16.5 (13.5)	51 (42)	108 (98)	33.0 (30.0)	3–7	18.1 (9–30)[e]	290
1–3 days	18.5 (14.5)	56 (45)	108 (95)	33.0 (29.0)	1.8–4.6	18.9 (9.4–34)	192
2 weeks	16.6 (13.4)	53 (41)	105 (88)	31.4 (28.1)		11.4 (5–20)	252
1 month	13.9 (10.7)	44 (33)	101 (91)	31.8 (28.1)	0.1–1.7	10.8 (4–19.5)	
2 months	11.2 (9.4)	35 (28)	95 (84)	31.8 (28.3)			
6 months	12.6 (11.1)	36 (31)	76 (68)	35.0 (32.7)	0.7–2.3	11.9 (6–17.5)	
6 mo-2 years	12.0 (10.5)	36 (33)	78 (70)	33.0 (30.0)		10.6 (6–17)	150–350
2–6 years	12.5 (11.5)	37 (34)	81 (75)	34.0 (31.0)	0.5–1.0	8.5 (5–15.5)	150–350
6–12 years	13.5 (11.5)	40 (35)	86 (77)	34.0 (31.0)	0.5–1.0	8.1 (4.5–13.5)	150–350
12–18 yr male	14.5 (13)	43 (36)	88 (78)	34.0 (31.0)	0.5–1.0	7.8 (4.5–13.5)	150–350

Age	Hb (g%)[a]	Hct (%)[a]	MCV (fL)[a]	MCHC (g/% RBC)[a]	Reticulocytes	WBCs (X 10,000/mm^3)[b]	Platelets (10,000/mm^3)[b]
12–18 yr female	14.0 (12)	41 (37)	90 (78)	34.0 (31.0)	0.5–1.0	7.8 (4.5–13.5)	150–350
Adult male	15.5 (13.5)	47 (41)	90 (80)	34.0 (31.0)	0.8–2.5	7.4 (4.5–11)	150–350
Adult female	14.0 (12)	41 (36)	90 (80)	34.0 (31.0)	0.8–4.1	7.4 (4.5–11)	150–350

Adapted from Siberry GK, Iannone R, eds. *The Harriet Lane Handbook. A Handbook for Pediatric House Officers.* 15th ed St. Louis: Mosby Inc; 2000.

Hb indicates hemoglobin; Hct, hematocrit; MCV, mean corpuscular volume; MCHC, mean corpuscular hemoglobin concentration; RBC, red blood cell count; WBC, white blood cell count.

[a]Data are mean (−2 SD).

[b]Data are mean (+2 SD).

[c]Values are from fetal samplings.

[d]<1 month, capillary hemoglobin exceeds venous: 1 hour −3.6 g difference; 5 days −2.2 g difference; 3 weeks −1.1 g difference.

[e]Mean (95% confidence interval).

TABLE 2.40

Interventions in Lead Poisoning

Class	Blood Lead Level (μg/dL)	Intervention
I	≤9	Rescreen annually, unless high risk.
IIA	10–14	If large number of children in community in this range, community-wide prevention should be started. Individual children in this range should be tested every 3–4 months, until two consecutive measurements are <10 μg/dL; then retest in 1 year.
IIB	15–19	Education on environment, cleaning, and nutrition should be started; Health Department should be notified. Patient should be tested for iron deficiency. Rescreen every 3–4 months until two consecutive levels <10 μg/dL. Consider abatement.
III	20–44	Conduct a complete medical evaluation. Identify and eliminate environmental sources of lead. These children require close follow-up. Chelation may be considered in selected children.
IV	45–69	Begin both medical and environmental intervention. Chelation treatment (either oral or intravenous/intramuscular) should begin within 48 hours with close follow-up.
V	≥70	This is a medical emergency requiring immediate intervention, which includes hospitalization. In addition, environmental remediation should be started.

Adapted from Siberry GK, Iannone R, eds. *The Harriet Lane Handbook: A Handbook for Pediatric House Officers*. 15th ed. St. Louis: Mosby, Inc; 2000.

chapter 3

Sexuality and Reproductive Medicine

Charles E. Driscoll, MD
Jacquelyn S. Driscoll, RN

IN THIS CHAPTER

- Taking an initial sexual history
- Sexological exam for patients with sexual complaints
- Sex education throughout the life cycle
- Drug effects on sexuality
- Internet resources for patients and physicians
- Sexual assault
- Sexual therapy using the PLISSIT model
- Kegel exercises
- Guidelines for use of sildenafil
- Care for homosexual patients
- Care for common sexual concerns
- Aging effects on sexuality
- Effects of illness on sexuality
- Infertility evaluation

BOOKSHELF RECOMMENDATIONS

- Berman J, Berman L. *For Women Only: A Revolutionary Guide To Reclaiming Your Sex Life*. New York: Owl Books; 2001.
- Butler RN, Lewis MI. *The New Love and Sex After 60*. New York: Ballantine Books; 2002.
- Comfort A. *Sexual Consequences of Disability*. Philadelphia: Stickley; 1978.

- Nusbaum MRH. *Monograph 267 Sexual Health*. Leawood, KS: AAFP Home Study Self-Assessment; 2001.
- Zilbergeld B. *The New Male Sexuality*. Rev ed. New York: Doubleday; 1999.

TABLE 3.1

Taking an Initial Sexual History

Taking a sexual history can be uncomfortable for both the physician and the patient. The physician must create an atmosphere of confidentiality and permissibility for honest answers to be forthcoming from the patient. Intensity of the questions should progress from general to specific, and from less intrusive to very personal.

Permissive, Confidential Atmosphere

- Let the patient know this is a routine part of history taking.
- Assure confidentiality; do not take notes in front of the patient.
- Make patient information handouts about sexuality topics available in office.
- A textbook or journal may convey the message that sex is an "OK" topic.
- Convey a feeling of comfort in talking about sexuality issues.
- Your body language and facial expression should be congruent with a message of permissibility.

Opener

- "To take better care of you, I need to ask some things about your life style. These questions will include information about your use of tobacco, alcohol, seatbelts, your exercise habits, and sexual activity."

First-Level Questions Asked of Everyone

- "How satisfactory is your sexual functioning?"
- "Do you have any concerns (questions) about sex?"
- "What is your understanding of the term 'safer sex'?"

Second-Level Questions (when patient is determined to be sexually active and comfortable with questioning)

- "How many different sexual partners have you had?"
- "Do you have sex with men, women, or both?"
- "Do you or all of your sexual partners use condoms?"
- "Which behaviors have you engaged in that might have increased your personal risk for a sexually transmitted disease?"

Continued

TABLE 3.1

Taking an Initial Sexual History, cont'd

Diagnostic-Level Questions (when a sexual problem is presented by the patient)

- "How has sex changed for you? For your partner?"
- "What happens [explained in reference to sexual response cycle] when you have this problem?"
- "How do you feel when you have this problem?"
- "What does your partner [say/do/feel] when you have this problem?"
- "How would you (and your partner) like it to be different?"
- "What is your explanation for the problem?"
- "Has anything sexual ever been done to make you feel uncomfortable?"

TABLE 3.2

Physical Examination for Sexual Complaints

General Physical Examination
■ Chronic illnesses (eg, diabetes, cancer)
■ Neurological system alterations, especially spinal nerves
■ Peripheral vascular and cardiovascular systems
■ Thyroid
■ Mental status and mood disorders
Breast Examination
■ Check for nipple erection response
■ Galactorrhea
■ Pain, mass
Genital Examination
■ Lesions on external genitalia; pubic hair amount and distribution
■ Clitoral hood retracts painlessly, no adhesions
■ Bulbocavernosis reflex—anal wink with pressure on glans penis or clitoris (present in 70% of normal subjects with intact sacral nerves)
■ Absence of the abnormal bulbocavernosis muscle spasm of vaginismus
■ Normal vaginal speculum exam, wet mount, single finger, and then bimanual exam (no evidence of trauma, pain, relaxation, infection)
■ No pain or discharge on urethral palpation
■ Test vaginal muscle tone by asking patient to squeeze vaginal examining finger
■ Consider colposcopy if patient has chronic burning pain of vulva or penis (occult human papillomavirus)
■ Penis without deformity, no palpable plaques
■ If uncircumcised, check to see if patient can retract foreskin painlessly and no evidence of infection or lesion underneath
■ Testes normal size and not tender
■ Prostate normal
■ Normal cremaster reflex
■ Palpate perineal body and perianal tissues for abnormality
■ If patient complains of crooked penis with erection, have him take picture at home and bring into office
Consider Special Studies (not indicated in all patients)
■ Pelvic ultrasound if dyspareunia
■ Cultures for infection from urethra and/or cervix
■ Serum glucose, creatinine, thyrotropin, prolactin level (if galactorrhea), complete blood cell count, testosterone (AM specimen), follicle-stimulating hormone

TABLE 3.3

Anticipatory Guidance/Sexual Education in the Life Cycle

Life Cycle Stage	Issues That May Be Considered for Education
Childhood	*For Parents* ■ Babies respond sexually to touch with arousal ■ Nursing may cause normal sexual arousal in mom ■ Normal children touch their own genitals in self-exploration; do not punish ■ Begin sex education when child shows curiosity ■ By school age, normally modesty increases and overt sex play decreases ■ Boys and girls differ in age and understanding *For the Child* ■ Body changes are progressing in a normal way ■ What understanding do they have about sexual issues seen in movies, television, etc? ■ Sexual behavior has consequences (eg, pregnancy, sexually transmitted diseases) ■ Appropriate and inappropriate touching, nudity, and sexual abuse prevention *Reference Recommendation* ■ Mayle P, Robins A. *Where Did I Come From? The Facts of Life Without Any Nonsense and With Illustrations.* Secaucus, NJ: Carol Publishing; 1999.
Adolescence	*For Parents* ■ Normal stages of sexual maturation of their teen ■ Teen needs open, honest talk about sexuality ■ Teens are generally unwilling to ask questions, but want information *For Teens* ■ Sexual arousal and "wet dreams" may occur naturally, even when unwanted ■ Responsibilities of initiating sexual activity include prevention of pregnancy and sexually transmitted diseases ■ Dating, avoidance of alcohol or drugs that lower inhibitions, prevention of rape or sexual abuse ■ What are sources of sexual information and how accurate are they? ■ Isolated same-sex encounters may occur normally and do not imply homosexuality

Life Cycle Stage	Issues That May Be Considered for Education
	Reference Recommendation ■ Madaras L, Madaras A. *My Body, My Self* (there are 2 editions, one for boys and one for girls). New York: Newmarket Press; 2000.
Adults Young to midlife	*For All Patients* ■ Sexuality is a part of health and an "OK" subject for discussion in the doctor's office ■ Sexual attraction/activity with another involves letting go of shyness and building self-esteem ■ Good sex is 90% mental and only 10% physical ■ Responsible sexuality requires attention to "safer sex" rules and prevention of unwanted pregnancy ■ Sex is not for bartering in solving relationship conflicts ■ If sexually naive, recommend accurate resources for education ■ How to get help for a sexual problem ■ Sexual patterns and enjoyment change with aging, illness, energy, stress, and children ■ Over 50% of couples will experience a sexual concern during marriage; this is normal ■ Keeping the romance and good communication are essential to keeping sexual health *Reference Recommendations* ■ Berman J, Berman L. *For Women Only: A Revolutionary Guide to Reclaiming Your Sex Life.* New York: Owl Books; 2001. ■ Zilbergeld B. *The New Male Sexuality.* Rev ed. New York: Doubleday; 1999.
Seniors	*For All Patients* ■ Sexual life and intimacy are still important ■ Normal changes of aging alter the sexual pattern, but do not ordinarily interrupt it ■ Sexual performance failures are not a normal part of aging ■ A continued risk for STDs exists ■ Illness and medications will all have a potential impact on sexual functioning ■ Menopause has an impact on sexual functioning ■ Loss of a partner has significant consequences *Reference Recommendation* ■ Butler RN, Lewis MI. *The New Love and Sex After 60.* New York: Ballantine Books; 2002.

TABLE 3.4

Drug-Induced Sexual Dysfunction

Adverse Effect	Drugs Known to Cause Effect
Decreased Libido	Antidepressants (tricyclics and SSRIs), amiodarone, benzodiazepines, ACEIs, antihistamines, most antihypertensives (including diuretics), barbiturates, benzepril, beta-blockers, antipsychotics, cimetidine, digoxin, finasteride, gemfibrozil, hydroxyzine, ketoconazole, medroxyprogesterone, narcotics, metoclopramide, metronidazole, niacin, ranitidine, weight loss medications
Increased Libido	Amphetamines, danazol, ethosuximide, levodopa, pergolide, physostigmine, propofol, trazodone, testosterone
Delayed/Inhibited Orgasm	Alcohol, benzodiazepines, amoxapine, amphetamines, anorexiants, clomipramine, clonidine, SSRIs, fluvoxamine, imipramine, isocarboxazid, MAOIs, methadone, methyldopa, nefazodone, phenothiazines, sedative-hypnotics, trazodone
Improved Erection	Nifedipine, sildenafil
Improved Orgasm	Nifedipine
Erectile Dysfunction	Alcohol, amiodarone, antidepressants (tricyclics and SSRIs), amphetamines, anticholinergics, antihistamines, beta-blockers, baclofen, barbiturates, ACEIs, benztropine, bromocriptine, buspirone, anticonvulsants, benzodiazepines, antipsychotics, cimetidine, clofibrate, cocaine, cyclobenzaprine, dicyclomine, digoxin, diltiazem, disulfiram, estrogens, famotidine, finasteride, fluvastatin, hydralazine, hydroxyzine, thiazide diuretics, indomethacin, indapamide, itraconazole, ketoconazole, leuprolide, lithium, losartan, MAOIs, meclizine, progesterones, meprobamate, methadone, methyldopa, methysergide, metoclopramide, narcotics, naproxen, nitrites, nizatidine, omeprazole, orphenadrine, phenytoin, prazosin, ranitidine, reserpine, risperidone, scopolamine, sulfasalazine, terazosin, verapamil
Ejaculation Dysfunction, Delayed or Retrograde Ejaculation	Aminocaproic acid, amitriptyline, amoxapine, amphetamines, anorexiants, antihistamines, baclofen, barbiturates, buspirone, chlordiazepoxide, clomipramine, cocaine, desipramine, diazepam, doxepin, finasteride, fluoxetine and SSRIs, fluphenazine, fluvoxamine, guanadrel, guanethidine, phenothiazines, haloperidol,

Adverse Effect	Drugs Known to Cause Effect
	isocarboxazid, isotretinoin, labetalol, MAOIs, mazindol, methadone, methotrexate, methyldopa, metyrosine, naltrexone, naproxen, nefazodone, neuroleptics, olanzapine, narcotics, pargyline, pimozide, prazosin, reserpine, risperidone, sedative-hypnotics, tamsulosin, trazodone, trimipramine, tricyclic antidepressants
Priapism	Buspirone, chlorpromazine, clozapine, fat emulsions, fluvoxamine, heparin, labetalol, mesoridazine, molindone, nefazodone, omeprazole, papaverine, pergolide, perphenazine, phenothiazines, phenytoin, risperidone, tamoxifen, testosterone, trazodone
Painful Clitoral Swelling	Bromocriptine
Gynecomastia	Cimetidine, cyclobenzaprine, digoxin, spironolactone
Testicular Swelling/Pain	Cyclobenzaprine, mazindol
Decreased Male Fertility	Gemfibrozil, antineoplastics, glucocorticoids, sulfasalazine
Peyronie's Disease	Phenytoin
Painful Orgasm	Desipramine, protriptyline

ACEIs indicate angiotensin-converting enzyme inhibitors; MAOIs, monoamine oxidase inhibitors; SSRIs, selective serotonin reuptake inhibitors.

TABLE 3.5

Effects of Psychotropic Medications on Sexuality

Assessment for drug-induced sexual dysfunction:

- Problem began *after* drug therapy initiated
- Problem not partner- or situation-specific
- Not a life-long or recurrent problem
- No other obvious precipitating event (eg, alcohol use, relationship problem)
- Problem clears when medication is stopped
- Problems by self-report will be 2–10%, but if questioned increase to 40–50%

Drug (% of patients with side effects)	Side Effect/ Men	Side Effect/ Women	Treatment Strategy
Antidepressant, SSRI-type (50–60%)	Erectile dysfunction, low libido, poor-quality orgasm, delay ejaculation; may have a positive effect upon premature ejaculation	Orgasmic delay or absence, decreased lubrication, poor-quality orgasm, low libido	Wait for remission of symptoms; drug holiday; reduce to minimal effective dose; switch to another antidepressant (bupropion or tricyclic); cyproheptadine 4 mg 1–2 h before sexual activity; yohimbine or ginkgo biloba
Antidepressant, Tricyclic-type	Erectile dysfunction, prostatism, low libido	Decreased lubrication, delayed orgasm, low libido	Vaginal lubricants; change antidepressants
Antidepressant, Bupropion	Increase libido	Increase libido	No other reported sexual side effects, therefore may be good alternative to others causing problems
Antidepressant, Trazodone	Increase libido; may rarely cause priapism	Increase libido	Use more cautiously with males; sedation limits its usefulness as an alternative antidepressant, but may help with sleeplessness

Drug (% of patients with side effects)	Side Effect/ Men	Side Effect/ Women	Treatment Strategy
Antipsychotic (35–45%)	Priapism, erectile dysfunction, and retrograde ejaculation or ejaculatory pain	Orgasmic failure; libido may improve	Imipramine 25–50 mg/d for retrograde ejaculation; check for elevated prolactin levels; lower the drug dose
Antianxiety (20–30%)	Ejaculatory delay; may help premature ejaculation	Orgasmic delay	Substitute buspirone to control anxiety; try a different anxiolytic, use dose reduction
Lithium (worse if combined with benzodiazepine)	Decreased libido, erectile dysfunction	Decreased libido	Lower the lithium dose; discontinue benzodiazepine; substitute valproic acid or carbamazepine for lithium

SSRIs indicates selective serotonin reuptake inhibitors.

FIGURE 3.1

Management of Antidepressant Sexual Dysfunction

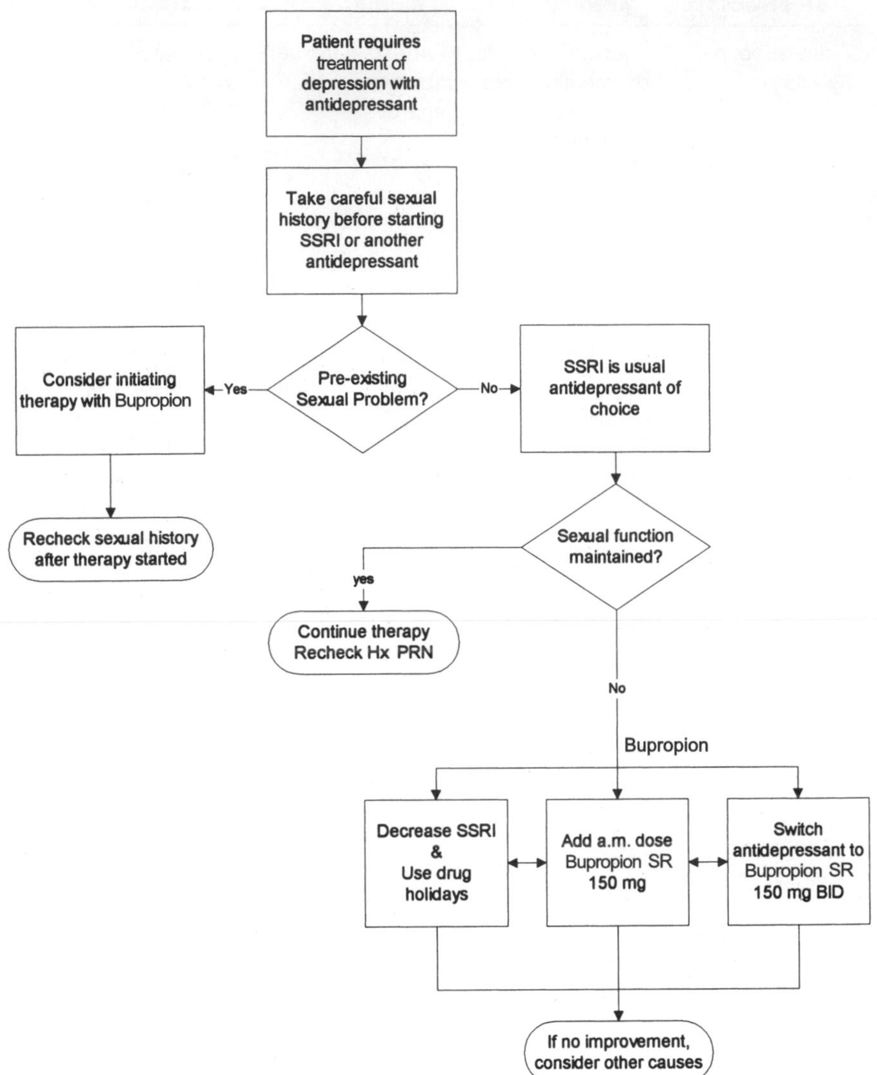

TABLE 3.6

Herbal Therapies for Sexual Dysfunction*

Name of Herb	Proposed Effect	Notes/Precautions
Yohimbine (Pausinystalia yohimbe)	Aphrodisiac, relieve erectile failure	Anxiety, restlessness, may provoke panic attack, drug-herb interactions; hypertensive crisis when given with sympathomimetics or tyramine
Avena Sativa	Relieve erectile failure, increase libido	May be obtained from homeopathic doctors, used for men; no adverse effects determined as yet
Ching Chun Bao (ginseng and other Chinese herbs)	Reduce fatigue, improve libido	Use by licensed Chinese herbalists, women may experience post-menopausal bleeding
DHEA (dehydroepi-androsterone)	Increase libido and improve sexual function	Elevates testosterone, may virilize females, men need PSA before use
Ginkgo Biloba	Restore erectile function, used to counteract effects on sexuality by antidepressant	Uncommon side effects (H/A, GI upset, may interact with anticoagulants)
Ginseng (also in varieties of Siberian and Red)	Improves sexual dysfunctions in men and women	May elevate corticosteroid levels, causes insomnia, may cause excessive stimulation, caution with hypertension, MAOIs; contra-indicated in asthma and renal failure
Men's Treasure, Men's Vital Force, Restorative Tablets for women, Women's Vital Force, and others	Mixtures of Chinese herbs, usually including ginseng in the formula, but may have some unknown ingredients	Caution in use, supervision by licensed Chinese herbalist is safest, may cause overstimulation, see precautions with ginseng
Vitamin E	Promote better erectile function	Antioxidant, antiplatelet and may interact with coumadin

PSA indicates prostate-specific antigen; GI, gastrointestinal; and MAOIs, monoamine oxidase inhibitors

*Avoid herbal remedies in pregnancy and breastfeeding.

TABLE 3.7

Internet Resources for Patient and Physician Use

Web URL	Resources at This Site
www.medicalsexuality.org	*Medical Aspects of Human Sexuality*, a free journal and links available for physicians
www.familydoctor.org	Patient education items on sexuality subjects
www.aasect.org	American Association of Sex Educators, Counselors and Teachers; find certified sex therapists
www.glma.org	Gay and Lesbian Medical Association; health issues and counseling
www.hivatis.org	HIV/AIDS Treatment Information Service; prevention counseling
www.indiana.edu/~kinsey/	The Kinsey Institute; links to sexology resources and journals
www.hisandherhealth.com/ index.html	Medical/Sexual Health Views; numerous links
www.siecus.org	Sexuality Information and Education Council of the US
www.sexuality.org	Society for Human Sexuality; review before recommending
www.umkc.edu/sites/hsw/ index.html	University of Missouri site; sex education and issues
www.newshe.com	Drs Laura and Jennifer Berman provide women's information
www.sexualhealth.com	Sexuality information for persons with disability/illness

TABLE 3.8

Caring for Victims of Sexual Assault

Definition

Rape is a crime of violence in which sex is utilized as one of the weapons of assault.

Types of Sexual Assault

Stranger rape, acquaintance rape, date rape, intimate or partner rape, aggravated assault (excess force/injury), incest, statutory rape (victim a minor)

Epidemiology

Victims are usually female, but may be male. Males are more reluctant to report than females; the true incidence is unknown as many cases go unreported. The prevalence has been increasing. Estimation suggests one in four adolescent girls are victims of forced sex or incest. Children <14 may account for up to 60% of all rape victims.

Predisposing Risk Factors

Risk-taking behavior; feeling a need for independence and exploration
Use of alcohol or drugs
Volunteering to go into a house alone with a new, older male acquaintance
The victim knows perpetrator more often than not
Past victimization and acceptance of interpersonal violence as the norm
Physical, emotional, or intellectual limitations

Psychological Sequelae of Rape

Immediate relief in escaping alive
Self-blaming and preoccupation with the event follow
Sense of loss of control of own life
"Rape Trauma Syndrome" most severe 6 weeks to 3 months or more after attack
Depression very common and suicide attempts are fairly frequent
Somatic complaints and sexual problems are common and may surface later
Anything resembling the rape situation may trigger posttraumatic stress
Reintegration and recovery with increased feeling of safety may take 1 year or longer

Continued

TABLE 3.8

Caring for Victims of Sexual Assault, cont'd

Steps to Assist Victims

- Communicate to patient she is a normal, healthy individual who escaped a serious life crisis.
- Convey to patient that it was not her fault and that recovery is possible though will take counseling and time; withhold judgmental statements.
- Two members of the health care team, a rape victim advocate/counselor and the physician, should stay with the patient at all times when in the examination phase.
- Assure confidentiality; health issues come first; encourage police reporting later and after securing the patient's permission.
- Assist the victim to maintain control of her body by explaining evidence collection techniques completely and proceeding only when the victim is ready to do so.
- Show empathy and support continuously; be gentle in voice and touch.
- Direct the focus toward safety of the victim from this point on.
- Provide preventive treatment for STDs and unwanted pregnancy.
- Be willing to listen as she often will want to tell her story over and over; reassure that feelings such as anger, revenge, helplessness are normal.
- Arrange for follow-up visits after the acute situation is handled.

Evidence Collection Steps

1. Complete history
   a. Time, place, and circumstances of the rape
   b. Identity of assailant recorded and witnesses if any
   c. Details of physical injury other than the sexual assault and whether weapon used
   d. Details of the type, location on the body, penetration, and amount of sexual activity
   e. Type and degree of resistance by the victim recorded
   f. Circumstances after rape and before exam (eg, bathing, douching)
   g. Last menstrual period, last consensual sexual contact, contraception used
   h. Past medical history, use of alcohol or medications, allergies to medications

2. Complete examination
   a. General physical exam; assess for trauma or injury; take photographs for documentation
   b. Inspect clothing and skin with Woods ultraviolet light for bright green fluorescence indication presence of semen
   c. Genital exam for presence of injury, condition of hymen
   d. Use rape evidence kit available in emergency department
   e. Swab any secretions and examine for presence of sperm under microscope; careful attention to chain of evidence and labeling/sealing
   f. Comb pubic hair into a plain white envelope; enclose the comb and seal it
   g. Pluck pubic hair from the patient and seal in a separate envelope
   h. Fingernail scrapings labeled for each finger in separate containers
   i. Cultures taken for STDs
   j. Smear from vagina, cervix, and anus for sperm, prostatic acid phosphatase and then wash cervix with 10 mL of sterile saline and aspirate the vaginal pool
   k. Test urine specimen for presence of sperm and pregnancy
   l. Obtain blood for serology
   m. All specimens transferred to clinical laboratory with signed receipts
   n. Bimanual examination for uterine size and tenderness or preexistent pelvic pathology
   o. Collect clothing and seal in paper bag and send to lab
3. Treatments offered
   a. Gonorrhea occurs in 3–4% of victims and syphilis in 0.1%—give ceftriaxone sodium, 250 mg IM
   b. Oral doxycycline 100 mg p.o. BID for 1 week for chlamydia
   c. Repeat STD testing in 4–6 weeks for proof of cure
   d. Pregnancy prevention with ethinyl estradiol 5 mg daily for 5 days or Ovral, 2 tabs stat and 2 again in 12 hours
   e. Tetanus booster if injured

BID indicates twice daily; IM, intramuscularly; po, orally; STDs, sexually transmitted diseases.

FIGURE 3.2

Treating Patients with Sexual Concerns—Incorporating the PLISSIT Model

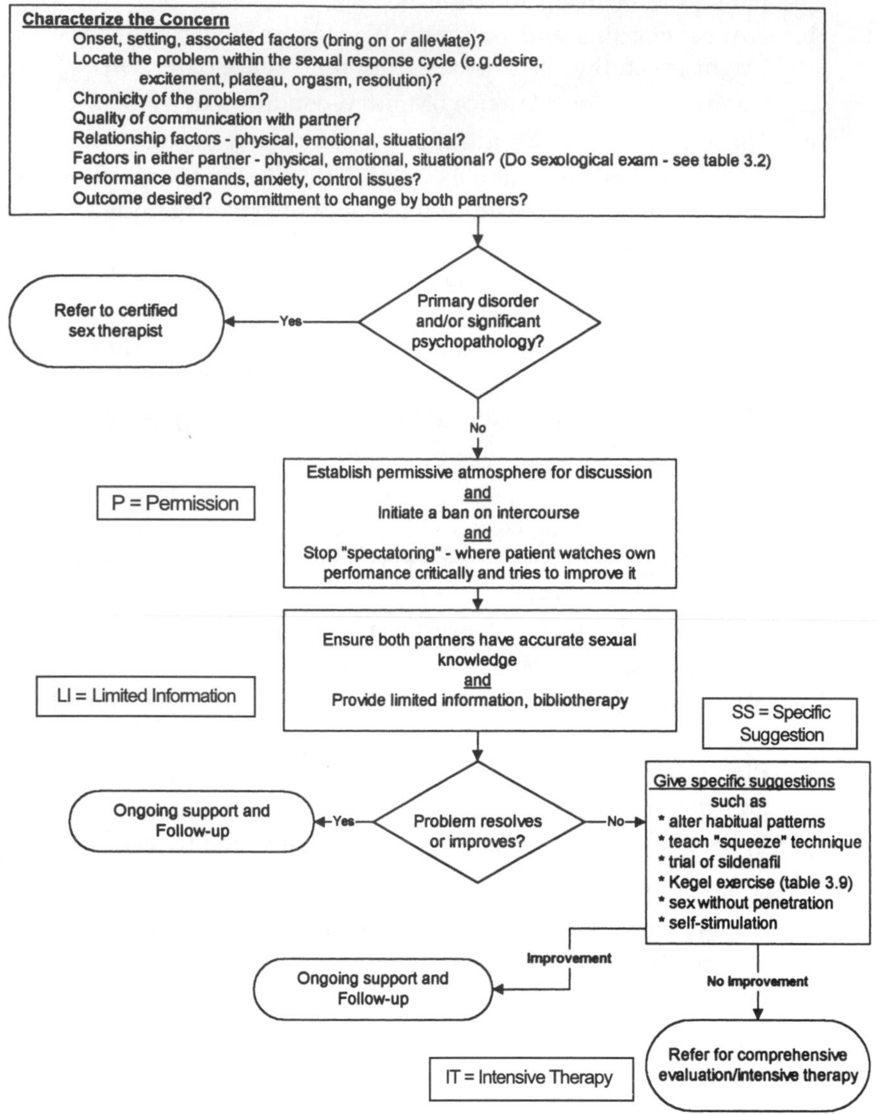

TABLE 3.9

Kegel Exercises for Improvement of Sexual Function

The exercises are intended to strengthen the pubococcygeus (PC) muscle in the pelvic floor. This allows the vagina to "grasp" the penis better and results in heightened arousal for both partners. Benefits include more intense orgasms and better bladder control. There are no contraindications to performing the exercises.

1. Learn how to control the muscle by sitting on the toilet with legs apart and stopping urination by clenching the muscle surrounding the vaginal opening. Start and stop the flow until you can identify and control contraction of the muscle.
2. Once learned, the exercise can be done anytime or anywhere, lying, sitting, or standing, and no one will know it is being done.
3. Contract and hold the PC muscle for 3 seconds, then relax. Repeat 10 times as a set of exercise and do this 4–5 times in a day. As the muscle strength improves, lengthen the contraction time to 8–10 seconds.
4. In addition to using prolonged contraction of the PC muscle, perform a set of exercise use a short "flicking" contraction of the muscle and do a set of 10 of them in rapid succession.
5. Another variation of the Kegel is to inhale deeply and imagine that air is being drawn in through the vagina in combination with the PC muscle contraction. This produces an elevation of the entire pelvic floor. Exhale during relaxation of the muscle.
6. Advise patience as it takes 6–8 weeks of daily exercise before changes are noticed.

TABLE 3.10

Guidelines for the Use of Sildenafil (Viagra)

Beneficial Effects

- Makes more nitric oxide available at nerve endings in the penis to allow tumescence to occur

Contraindications to Use

- Not for use in patients who require nitrate therapy, either chronically or intermittently
- Known allergic reaction to sildenafil

Safe Administration of Nitrates After Use of Sildenafil

- Nitrates can be safely administered in 24 hours after use of sildenafil; sildenafil plasma levels approximate 2 ng/mL compared to 440 ng/mL at peak

Drug-Drug Interactions

- Sildenafil is metabolized by the cytochrome P450 system via the liver; therefore, inhibitors of these isoenzymes will reduce clearance and elevate the sildenafil levels to 3–8 times normal. Drugs to avoid in combination are:

  —Erythromycin (a CYP3A4 inhibitor)

  —Cimetidine

  —Saquinavir and other protease inhibitors

  —Ketoconazole, itraconozole

- Rifampin, a drug that is a CYP3A4 inducer, significantly decreases plasma levels of sildenafil.
- Sildenafil does not interact with alcohol.
- Sildenafil is highly protein bound and renal dialysis does not hasten removal from the system.

Side Effects of Note

- Headache 16%, flushing 10%, dyspepsia 7%, blue-green color tinge to vision 3%. *Severe hypotension may result if combined with nitrates.*

Dosing

- For frail elderly, patients with hepatic or renal impairment, hypotension, coronary artery disease, and congestive heart failure—proceed with caution. Start at 25 mg dose and titrate up.
- For all other patients, start at 50 mg dose and titrate.
- Maximum of one dose per 24 hours

TABLE 3.11

Care for Homosexual Patients

Between 5–10% of the patients in a typical family practice are homosexual. Sensitive care for homosexual patients includes respect, confidentiality, candid communication, an inclusive environment for care, nonjudgmental atmosphere, and awareness of resources available. Eliminate bias from history taking. Take disclosure in stride and recognize the partner.

Risk Factors for Health in Homosexual Patients

- Lack of regular, routine medical care with screening (eg, Pap, mammography, PSA) due to avoidance of the medical system
- Failure to self-disclose sexual orientation may mislead diagnoses
- Extreme stress experienced, often in isolation, during "coming out"
- High prevalence of overuse of alcohol and tobacco
- High prevalence of domestic violence, sexual abuse, exploitation
- Gay men are at higher risk of traumatic injury with intercourse than their heterosexual counterparts
- Depression is more common
- Potential for suicide higher in homosexual teenagers
- Romantic and relationship failures are covert causes for stress-related illness
- Eating disorders due to subcultural attitudes toward beauty and thinness
- Desire for parenting is often unmet
- More likely to have had multiple sexual partners
- Anal intercourse in homosexual men favors transmission of HIV, gastrointestinal infections, hepatitis B virus, and other STDs
- Homosexual men are more likely to have an STD than their heterosexual counterparts, while lesbians are less likely to have an STD than heterosexual women.

Resources for Assisting in the Care of Homosexuals

- Gay and Lesbian Medical Association (www.glma.org)
- Family Pride Coalition (for families of homosexuals) (http://familypride.org)
- Gay and Lesbian Parents' Coalition (www.qrd/org/qrd/orgs/GLPCI)
- Children of Lesbians and Gays Everywhere (http://colage.org)
- Parents, Families and Friends of Lesbians and Gays (http://pflag.org)

HIV indicates human immunodeficiency virus; PSA, prostate-specific antigen; STDs sexually transmitted diseases.

TABLE 3.12

Managing Erectile Dysfunction

Definition

- Inability to develop and sustain an erection adequate for intercourse on at least 50% of attempts.

Modifiable Factors

- Tobacco addiction, diabetes mellitus, hyperlipidemia, drug effects, depression, anxiety, alcoholism, hypothyroidism, testosterone deficiency, renal or hepatic disease

History and Physical

- Have patient explain the problem in his terms; look for sexual abuse, trauma, pelvic "steal" syndrome, deviation of penis when erect, situational factors, role of the partner, unrealistic expectations, and coexistent sexual pathology (eg, premature ejaculation)
- Check testicular size (>3.5 cm is normal), penis for plaque or fibrosis, breast for galactorrhea, prostate for mass or enlargement, pulmonary and cardiovascular systems, thinning or loss of body hair, and neck for thyroid size

Laboratory Tests

- Serum glucose, TSH, liver function tests, cholesterol, prolactin (if galactorrhea), creatinine and BUN, AM testosterone

Sleep Test for Nocturnal Erection

- Snap-Gauge (Dacomed, Inc) or postage stamp test

Modes of Therapy

- Counseling to restart sexual intimacy via methods of sex without penetration
- Sildenafil—see Table 3.10 (~$8.50/tablet)
- Stop unnecessary medications and choose alternatives to offending ones
- Use of vacuum device with constriction ring (ErecAid by Osbon) (~$600)
- Prostaglandin E_1 (PGE_1) intra-cavernosal injection (~$8–35, depends on dose)
- Alprostadil intraurethral pellet (~$19–23 per pellet, depends on dose)
- Testosterone replacement therapy only if deficiency confirmed by 2 separate AM measurements—by IM self-injection every 2–4 weeks (~$10–20/mo)
- Yohimbine—limited effectiveness (~$24/month at TID dosing)
- Implantable penile prosthesis (~$6000–15,000)
- Rejoyn penile support sleeve with lubricated cover (~$6.50/single use)

Indications for Referral

- Presence of significant psychiatric pathology or when surgical therapy is indicated or for couples therapy and counseling by a certified sex therapist.

BUN indicates blood urea nitrogen; IM, intramuscular; TSH, thyrotropin; TID, three times daily.

TABLE 3.13

Managing Orgasmic Dysfunction in Women

Definition

- A difficulty or inability to reach orgasm after sufficient sexual stimulation and arousal

Modifiable Factors

- Medication or illicit drug use, hormonal problems, depression, inadequate sexual knowledge or experience, restrictive or "puritanical" attitudes, "spectatoring" during sexual activity, situational factors (no lock on the bedroom door), partner factors

History and Physical

- Have patient explain problem in her terms; check for sexual abuse; determine if problem is primary or acquired; ability to reach orgasm with self-stimulation; surgical history; sexual desire and fantasies are normal; unrealistic expectations
- Examine clitoris for adhesions of hood; tender areas at introitus or intravaginally; normal vaginal and bimanual exam; galactorrhea; thyroid normal; estrogenization normal

Laboratory Tests

- Serum glucose, thyrotropin, prolactin (if galactorrhea), total and free testosterone

Modes of Therapy

- Educate patient about her body and sexual response cycle
- Use of vibrator and self-stimulation to learn how to be orgasmic
- Use of fantasy or erotic literature as a focusing aid
- Coach patient how to teach her partner what she has learned about the kind of stimulation she needs to reach orgasm
- Sensate focus therapy by certified sex therapist
- Postmenopausal hormone replacement therapy (~$30/mo)
- Methyltestosterone (Estratest) one to three times weekly (~$12–15/mo) if deficiency state
- The Eros-CTD (clitoral therapy device) enhances blood flow to clitoris
- Trial of bupropion therapy (~$21/mo)

Indications for Referral

- Presence of significant psychopathology *or* when couple therapy or other intensive therapy by sex therapist required *or* when patient requests referral

TABLE 3.14

Diagnosis and Management of Psychosexual Disorders

Psychosexual Disorder	Definition	Diagnostic Search Keys	Management Modalities
Hypoactive Desire	Lack of sexual fantasies; desire for activity absent	Primary or acquired; partner specific; hormonal; sexual abuse history; drug use	Behavioral psychotherapy, self-pleasuring, treat with HRT if menopausal
Sexual Aversion Disorder	Extreme aversion and avoidance of all genital contact with sex partner	Panic disorder; sexual abuse history; foreign bodies in vagina	Behavioral psychotherapy; some women respond to MAOIs
Female Arousal Disorder	Inability to maintain state of arousal until completion of the sex act	Associated desire disorder; atrophic vaginitis; foreplay inadequate; drug-induced	Postmenopausal HRT, lubrication, behavioral therapy
Male Erectile Disorder	Inability to attain or maintain an erection until completion of the sex act	Primary or acquired; leg claudication; erect with self-stimulation; morning erections; drug-induced	Trial of sildenafil, PGE_1 intracavernosal injection, stop offending drugs, use of vacuum device
Female Orgasmic Disorder	Delay or absence of orgasm following normal arousal	Primary or acquired; surgery; discord; restrictive attitudes	Self-stimulation program, stop alcohol use, couple or relationship therapy
Male Orgasmic Disorder	Delay or absence of orgasm following normal arousal	Usually acquired; drugs; prostatectomy	Stop offending drugs, nerve-sparing prostate surgery
Premature Ejaculation	Ejaculation before or shortly after penetration and before the person wishes	Rarely organic; possible to be drug-induced; usually life-long	Behavioral therapy, may respond to SSRI or clomipramine
Dyspareunia (male or female)	Recurrent genital pain associated with sex	Rule out treatable medical disorder; drug-induced	Adequate lubrication, treat endometriosis, change medications

Continued

TABLE 3.14

Diagnosis and Management of Psychosexual Disorders, cont'd

Psychosexual Disorder	Definition	Diagnostic Search Keys	Management Modalities
Vaginismus	Involuntary spasm of muscles around vagina that interferes with sex	Primary or acquired; earlier sexual trauma; marriage is unconsummated	Adequate lubrication, treat endometriosis, progressive dilation therapy
Sexual Dysfunction of Illness	Disorder fully explained by the direct effects of a medical condition	Underlying medical condition; emotional stress	Provide alternatives to usual sexual repertoire, treat medical condition
Drug-induced Sexual Disorder	Disorder fully explained by drug use or side effects	Prescribed and illicit drug use	Provide alternative medications, stop drug use

HRT indicates hormone replacement therapy; MAOIs, monoamine oxidase inhibitors; PGE_1, prostaglandin E_1; SSRIs, selective serotonin reuptake inhibitors.

TABLE 3.15

Aging and Sexual Functioning

Common Changes of Aging Affecting Female Sexual Response

- Lack of available partner and privacy
- Lessening of desire for sex, but more need for intimacy
- Less engorgement of genital tissues during arousal
- Thinner vaginal mucosa; atrophic vaginitis
- Lessening of skin flush and breast enlargement
- Lubrication occurs more slowly and in reduced amount
- Lengthening of plateau phase and slower approach to orgasm
- Orgasm may be less intense (sometimes painful, tetanic uterine contractions can occur during orgasm)
- Joint and other discomforts blunt arousal effect

Common Changes of Aging Affecting Male Sexual Response

- Increased time and intensity of stimulation required to achieve erection
- Lessening of desire for sex, but more need for intimacy
- Decrease in seminal fluid secretion and lubrication
- Loss of elasticity in penis with drooping of erection
- Decreased turgor of erection
- Decrease in penis size (length and circumference)
- Longer refractory period between sexual response cycles
- Lessening of intensity in orgasm
- Arousal more easily interrupted by distractions

TABLE 3.16A

Modulating Effects of Illness on Sexuality

Sexuality may be *enhanced* (partners drawn more close to each other) or *inhibited* (fear triggers withdrawal and discord). All patients deserve inquiry regarding how their sexuality is affected and what, if anything, do they wish to do about it.

Adverse Effects

- *Somatic:* Pain, immobility, disfigurement, altered physiology
- *Psychological:* Fear, anxiety, depression, defensive behavior, anger
- *Combined:* Partial sexual dysfunction triggers exaggerated emotional response

Motivation for Sex Can Change

- Affirm masculinity or femininity
- Receive nurturing and secondary gain
- Need to be dependent or independent
- Need to protect and parent

Basic Rules in Assisting Couples Facing Illness to Improve Sexuality

1. All patients deserve a sexual history, but not all require counseling or therapy.
2. Give anticipatory guidance to prevent dysfunction (eg, before prostate surgery) and warn of predictable problems.
3. Learn from other patients what works for them and pass ideas on to others.
4. Increase the sexual repertoire and widen the sexual possibilities by specific suggestions for working around the disability.
5. Perform a careful history of problems, do a sexological examination and set realistic expectations.
6. Recognize limitations and seek consultation from a sex therapist when necessary.

Elements to Be Included in Sexual History of Patients with Illness

- Preillness level of functioning
- Present level of functioning
- Medication history
- Effects of illness on self-image
- Which part of the sexual response cycle is affected?
- Attitudes, fears, and ability of the couple to communicate
- Outcome desired after intervention

TABLE 3.16B

Approach to Specific Problems

Disability	Specific Suggestions to Improve Sexuality
Arthritis	■ Share hot bath and limbering up exercise before sex
	■ Warm bed (water bed) and warm room reduce discomfort and lessen work needed for coitus
	■ Use pillows to cushion joints
	■ If no reduction in sexual sensitivity, take pain medications before sexual activity
	■ Have sex when rested, perhaps at mid-day
	■ Reduced weight bearing by changing coital position to side-to-side or rear entry
	■ Vaginal lubrication if Sjogren's syndrome present
	■ Surgery (eg, hip replacement) may be needed
Diabetes	■ Counteract vaginal dryness with lubrication
	■ Restore vaginal epithelium with HRT if needed
	■ Advise against coitus if penile or vaginal infection
	■ Educate about retrograde ejaculation
	■ Correct zinc depletion
	■ Supply variety of ways to improve erections (eg, sildenafil, ErecAid, intracavernous penile injection)
Heart Disease	■ Assess for and treat depression, common post-MI
	■ Educate and reassure regarding safety of sexual intercourse
	■ Submaximal exercise testing and rehabilitation
	■ Resume intimacy first, then sexual activity slowly and only with regular sexual partner
	■ Comfortable temperature in bedroom
	■ Use of long-acting nitrates if angina (avoid sildenafil)
	■ Avoid sex in context of oxygen-robbing situations (eg, smoking, eating, alcohol, or arguments)
	■ Healthy partner on top or sitting position may reduce oxygen demand
	■ Stop sexual activity if angina persists
	■ Coronary bypass surgery may be considered
Cancer	■ Elicit feelings of both partners for discussion
	■ Introduce discussion of sex before therapies begin
	■ Resume intimate touch and affection as soon as possible after surgery
	■ Discuss alternatives to intercourse
	■ Plan for alleviation of pain if anticipated

Continued

TABLE 3.16B

Approach to Specific Problems, cont'd

Disability	Specific Suggestions to Improve Sexuality
	■ Suggest water-soluble lubricants and perhaps condoms as semen may irritate vaginal mucosa, especially after radiation therapy ■ Try different coital positions to relieve pressure on incisions ■ Recommend cancer support groups for sharing
COPD and Other Lung Disease	■ Avoid sex in context of oxygen-robbing situations (eg, smoking, eating, alcohol, or arguments) ■ Assist with smoking cessation program ■ Change coital position to alleviate pressure on the chest and reduce work (eg, sitting, side-to-side, rear entry) ■ Supply additional oxygen with nasal prongs ■ Pretreat with inhaler before sex ■ Pulmonary rehabilitation program improves endurance ■ Women with decreased vaginal moisture should use lubricants ■ Avoid sex immediately after awakening as secretions accumulate during sleep and may cause coughing ■ Prolonged kissing and oral sex worsen breathing

FIGURE 3.3

Evaluation of the Infertile Couple

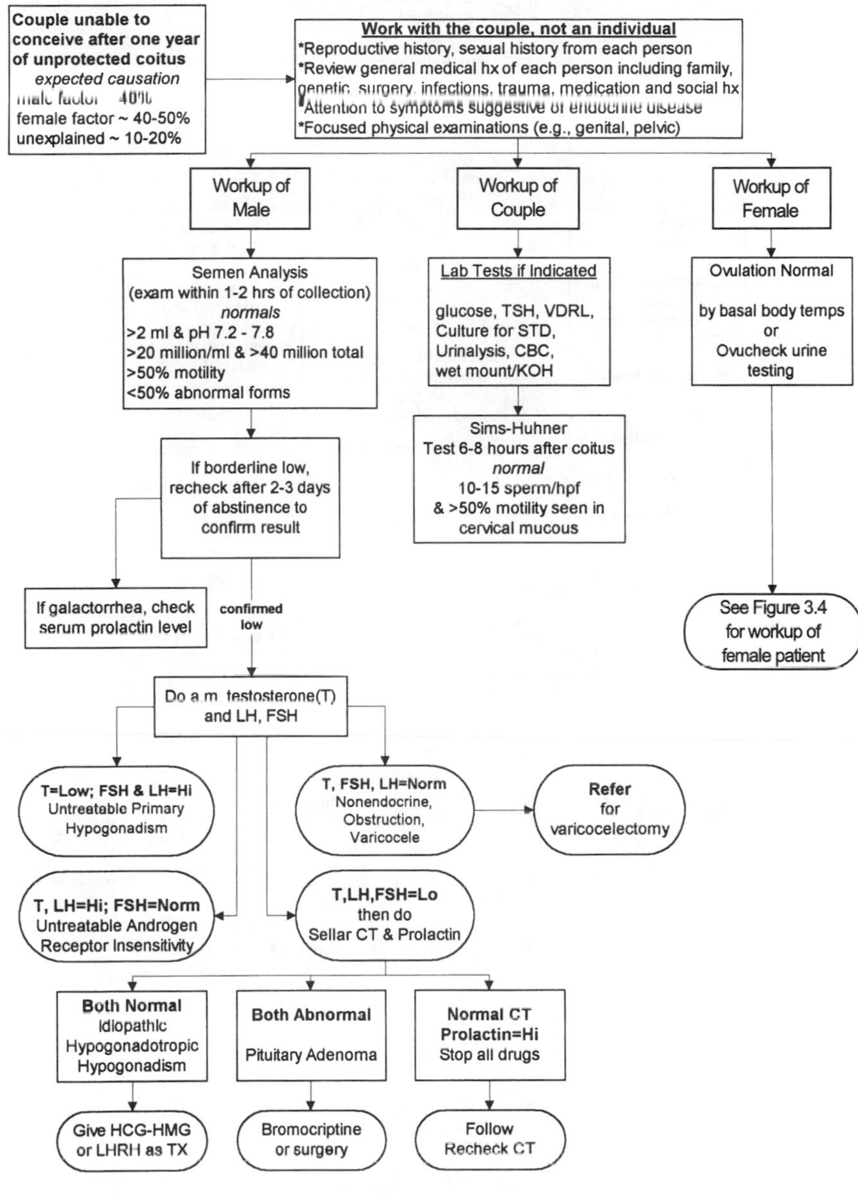

FIGURE 3.4

Evaluation of the Infertile Couple: Female

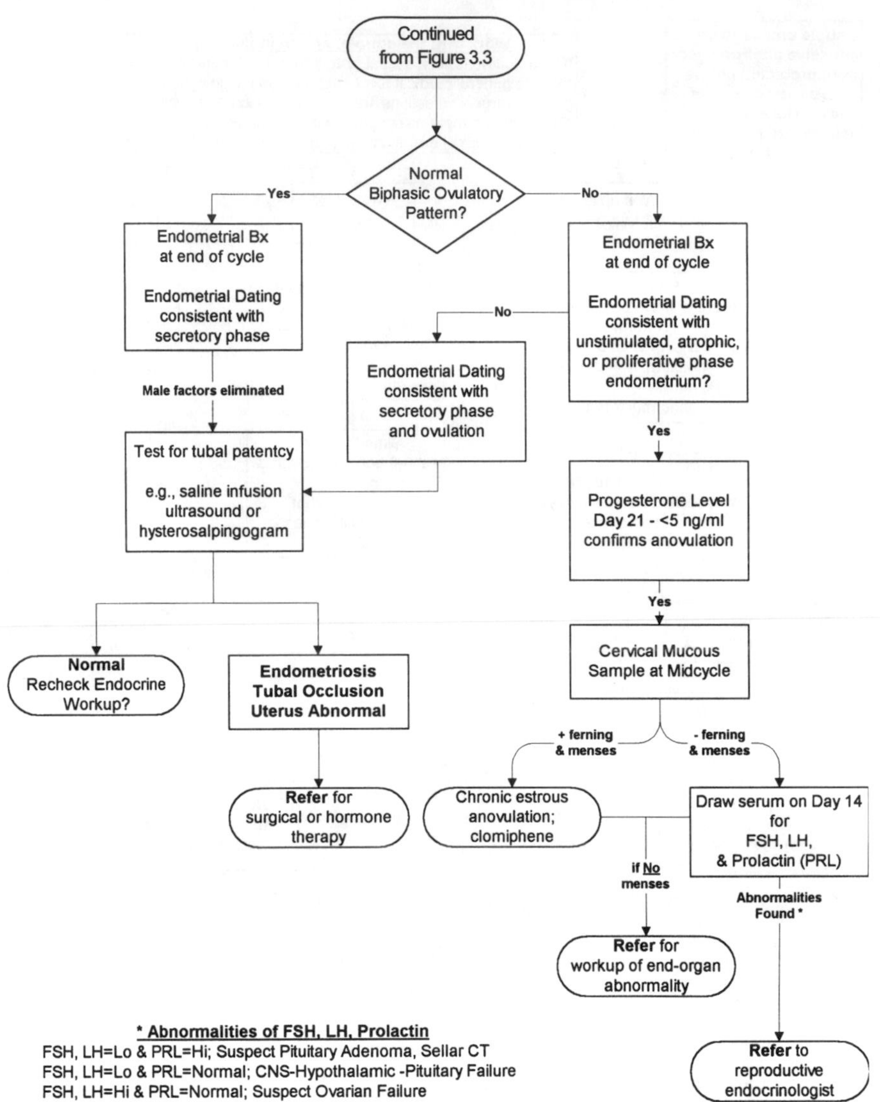

*** Abnormalities of FSH, LH, Prolactin**

FSH, LH=Lo & PRL=Hi; Suspect Pituitary Adenoma, Sellar CT
FSH, LH=Lo & PRL=Normal; CNS-Hypothalamic -Pituitary Failure
FSH, LH=Hi & PRL=Normal; Suspect Ovarian Failure

chapter 4

Hereditary Diseases

Michael L. Madden, MD, and H. Dale Meade, MD

IN THIS CHAPTER

- The science of hereditary disorders
- The diagnosis of genetic disease
- Obtaining a family history for genetic disease
- Colon cancer: a mendelian model
- Examples of syndromic cancer
- Dyslipoproteinemias
- Commercial laboratories offering diagnostic tests
- Disorders that have genetic tests available
- Genetic counseling
- Perinatal genetic screening
- Primary care problems with complex genetic traits
- Polygenic threshold inheritance
- Known causes of abortion and newborn syndromes
- Pedigree case studies
- Web site resources

BOOKSHELF RECOMMENDATIONS

- Mahowald MB, Scheuerle AS, McKusick VA. *Genetics in the Clinic: Clinical, Ethical, and Social Implications for Primary Care*. St Louis: Mosby, Inc; 2001.
- Nora JJ. *Medical Genetics: Principles and Practice*. 4th ed. Philadelphia: Lea and Febiger; 1993.
- Thurmon TF. *A Comprehensive Primer on Medical Genetics*. London: Parthenon Publishing; 1999.

THE SCIENCE OF HEREDITARY DISORDERS

DNA is the basis of inheritance. Nuclear DNA is of paternal and maternal origin. Mitochondrial DNA is of maternal origin. The DNA molecule is a long double helical ladder. The sides of the ladder are composed of deoxyribose and phosphate moieties. Each rung is a base pair: adenine-thymine or guanine-cytosine. Each sequence of three bases is a *codon*. Each codon encodes a specific amino acid or is a *stop codon*. A stop codon signals the termination of the polypeptide. Genes are long segments of DNA separated by noncoding segments, which regulate gene expression. A gene is composed of alternating *introns* and *exons*. Only the exons are destined to code for a protein. One strand of the DNA chain called the *sense strand* transcribes a complementary strand of RNA. In RNA, ribose is substituted for deoxyribose and uracil for thymine. After the introns are cleaved and the exons spliced, mature messenger RNA travels to the ribosome. In the ribosome, the code is translated into a protein.

When cells divide, DNA is compacted into paired homologous chromosomes. The average chromosome has 1000 genes. Humans have 46 chromosomes: 22 pairs of autosomes plus either XX or XY. During mitosis, DNA has already doubled itself so that each daughter cell receives 46 chromosomes, a full complement of DNA. During meiosis, the sperm and ovum receive only 23 chromosomes. Fertilization of the ovum restores the full complement of DNA.

A child inherits two copies of each gene, one from each parent. Each copy is called an *allele*. In the case of a mutation, the mutant allele can be dominant or recessive. For autosomal dominant inheritance, if one parent carries the *disease-causing gene*, 50% of the progeny will inherit the disease. If the disorder is recessive and each parent carries one copy of the mutant allele, 25% of the progeny will be normal, 50% will be carriers, and 25% will inherit the disease. If a parent carries a mutant gene on an X chromosome it is called X-linked. If recessive, the mother will transmit the disease to half her sons. Half her daughters will be carriers. If X-linked dominant, a male will transmit the disease to all his daughters but to none of his sons.

Mutations can result from a substitution of one base pair. There is no change if the new codon codes the same amino acid. If the mutation changes one amino acid, it is a missense mutation. If the protein still performs its function, no harm has been done. Sometimes, a change of one amino acid can markedly change the conformation of the protein. A good example is sickle cell disease. If the new codon is a stop codon, the protein will be shortened and likely nonfunctional. This is a nonsense mutation.

Deletion or *addition* of a base pair causes a frame shift. The wrong amino acids will be encoded until a stop codon causes a truncated protein. Marfan syndrome is autosomal dominant. In some cases, a frame-shift causes truncation of fibrillin. Connective tissues then contain only 50% of the normal amount of fibrillin.

Meiotic instability can cause expansion of short tandem repeats of triplet bases. Huntington's disease and fragile X syndrome are examples.

DIAGNOSIS OF GENETIC DISEASE

The diagnosis of genetic disease is based on complete history, physical examination, and laboratory tests. The most important element is a thorough family history. (See Table 4.1.) The inquiry into the health of family members must often extend beyond parents, siblings, and children to grandparents, uncles, aunts, and even cousins. Careful questioning about pregnancy outcomes on both sides of the family is important. Family photographs can be helpful. The family history is recorded by mapping a pedigree depicting the family tree. Once the symbols are learned and with some practice, the pedigree saves time. (See Figure 4.1.) It also provides an image of the family that can by serendipity diagnose a genetic disease (eg, discovering a cancer family or familial dyslipoproteinemia from drawing the pedigree of a child with Down syndrome).

During the physical exam, a cluster of unusual features might clue in the astute clinician to a particular syndrome. The finding of an unusual appearance should at least trigger referral to a medical geneticist.

TABLE 4.1

Questions to Ask When Obtaining a Family History

General

1. Current or past history relevant to the problem
2. Information about relatives: names, birth dates, any health or developmental problems, causes of death, surgeries, and so on
3. Information about miscarriages, stillbirths, and children who died in infancy
4. Racial and ethnic background
5. Family origin: as in England, Taiwan, Guatemala, and so on

Specific

1. "Who do you look like in the family?" Remember that others in the family might be affected too.
2. "Is there anyone in the family with birth defects, mental retardation, or learning problems?"
3. "Are you aware of any miscarriages or stillbirths in your mother/sisters/daughters?"
4. "Are there any early infant deaths or children who died before 1 year of age?"
5. "Are you and your spouse related?" and "Do you share distant cousins or grandparents?" The physician should ask politely and preface this with, "I ask everyone this question." There are cultures, including some in the United States, in which it is not taboo for one's spouse to be a cousin. Person's in these cultures will not be offended by the question and will probably know their family history well. People who are not related will not be offended. If the patient refuses to answer, the physician should consider incest.
6. "Are you interested in having more children?" This can be awkward to ask immediately after the birth of an affected child; the physician can defer if necessary. However, it is good to know the answer to this question because it can help the physician determine how important recurrence risk information is for this family.

Adapted from Mahowald MB, Scheuerle AS, McKusick VA. *Genetics in the Clinic: Clinical, Ethical, and Social Implications for Primary Care.* St Louis: Mosby, Inc; 2001.

TABLE 4.2

Mendelian Colon Cancer

Disorder (gene): McKusick Number	Tumors	Etiology
Cancer family-Lynch I (APC|KRAS|p53|DCC): 114500	Colorectal cancer arising from a cascade of mutations in which the p53 is transitional	Autosomal dom chromosome 17p
Familial colorectal cancer (DCC): 120470	Colorectal cancer	Autosomal dom chromosome 18q
Nonpolyposis colon cancer (FMSL1): 600258	Colon cancer; genomic instability	Autosomal dom chromosome 2q
Nonpolyposis colon cancer (FMSL2): 600259	Colon cancer; genomic instability	Autosomal dom chromosome 7p
Nonpolyposis colon cancer 1, cancer family-Lynch II, Muir-Torre syndrome (MSH2): 120435	Breast cancer, colon cancer, endometrial cancer, ovarian cancer, soft tissue sarcomas, sebaceous skin tumors, keratoacanthoma, genomic instability	Autosomal dom chromosome 2p
Nonpolyposis colon cancer 2 (MLH1): 120436	Colon cancer; genomic instability	Autosomal dom chromosome 3p
Familial adenomatous polyposis, Turcot syndrome, Gardner syndrome (APC): 175100	Epidermoid cysts, cutaneous fibromas, osteomas, supernumerary teeth, duodenal polyps, duodenal cancer, colon polyps, colon carcinoma, glioma, astrocytoma	Autosomal dom chromosome 5q
Familial juvenile polyposis: 174900	Intestinal polyposis onset in childhood; colon cancer in fourth decade	Autosomal dom

Adapted from Thurmon TF. *A Comprehensive Primer on Medical Genetics*. London: Parthenon Publishing; 1999.

TABLE 4.3

Examples of Syndromic Cancer

Syndrome, Synonyms (Gene): McKusick Number	Findings	Etiology
Basal cell nevus syndrome (NBCCS): 109400	Calcified falx cerebri, telecanthus, odontogenic cysts of jaw, rib anomalies, vertebral anomalies, palmar pits, multiple basal cell nevi	Autosomal dom; chromosome 9q22.3
Beckwith-Wiedeman (BWS): 130650	Macrosomia, macroglossia, organomegaly, omphalocele, Wilms tumor	Autosomal dom; chromosome 11p15
Cowden syndrome: 158350	Multiple hamartomas of skin and mucous membranes, fibroadenomatous enlargement of breasts, breast cancer	Autosomal dom
Denys-Drash syndrome (WTI): 194070	Pseudohermaphroditism, progressive nephropathy, Wilms tumor	Autosomal dom; chromosome 11p
Familial atypical mole melanoma, dysplastic nevus syndrome (CMM1): 155600	Fair complexion, freckles, multiple reddish brown irregular 5- to 15-mm nevi on upper trunk and limbs, melanoma around age 45	Autosomal dom; chromosome 1p
Li-Fraumeni syndrome (53): 191170	Breast cancer, medulloblastoma, leukemia, adenocarcinoma of lung, rhabdomyosarcoma, adrenocortical carcinoma	Autosomal dom; chromosome 17p

Syndrome, Synonyms (Gene): McKusick Number	Findings	Etiology
Multiple endocrine neoplasia III (MENIIB): 162300	Mucosal neuromas, patulous lips, marfanoid habitus, prognathism, megacolon, pheochromocytoma, medullary carcinoma of thyroid	Autosomal dom; chromosome 10q11.2
Peutz-Jeghers syndrome (PJS): 175200	Melanin spots of lips, buccal mucosa, digits; intestinal polyposis; polyps of respiratory tree and urinary tract; breast cancer; pancreatic cancer	Autosomal dom
Von Hippel-Lindau syndrome (VHL): 193300	Cerebellar hemangioblastoma, retinal angioma, renal cell carcinoma, pancreatic carcinoma, pheochromocytoma	Autosomal dom; chromosome 3p26
WAGR syndrome (WTI): 194070	Aniridia, hypogenitalism, mental retardation, Wilms tumor	Autosomal dom; chromosome 11p

Adapted from Thurmon TF. *A Comprehensive Primer on Medical Genetics*. London: Parthenon Publishing; 1999.

WAGR indicates Wilms tumor, aniridia, genitourinary malformations, and mental retardation.

TABLE 4.4

Dyslipoproteinemias

Disorder, Synonyms: Features (all cause premature coronary disease)	McKusick Number*	Profile	Cholesterol	Triglycerides
Apolipoprotein E defect, broad-beta disease, dysbetalipoproteinemia: xanthomas (planar, tendon, tuberous, tuberoeruptive), peripheral vascular disease	107741	3	Elevated	Elevated
Analphalipoproteinemia, Tangier disease: large orange tonsils, neuropathy, weakness, lymphadenopathy, hypersplenism	205400	Low HDL-C, abnormal LDL and chylomicrons	Low	Normal
Combined hyperlipidemia	144250	2a**, 2b**, 4, 5 (rare)	Elevated	Elevated
Familial hypercholesterolemia, LDL receptor defect: corneal arcus, xanthelasma, xanthomas (tendon in heterozygotes)	143890	2a**, 2b (rare)**	Elevated	Normal
Familial hypercholesterolemia B: xanthomas (tendon in heterozygotes and planar in homozygotes) corneal arcus, xanthelasma	144010	Abnormal LDL	Elevated	Normal
Familial hypertriglyceridemia: abnormal glucose tolerance, atheroeruptive xanthoma	145750	4, 5 (rare)	Normal	Elevated
Hyperlipoproteinemia II, hyperbetalipoproteinemia: corneal arcus, xanthomas (tendon and tuberous)	144400	2a** 2b**	Elevated Elevated	Normal Elevated
Hyperlipoproteinemia IV: abnormal glucose tolerance, atheroeruptive xanthoma	144600	4	Normal	Elevated
Hyperlipoproteinemia V	144650	5 low LDL and HDL	Normal	Elevated

Adapted from Thurmon TF. *A Comprehensive Primer on Medical Genetics*. London: Parthenon Publishing; 1999.

HDL-C indicates high-density lipoprotein cholesterol; LDL, low-density lipoprotein.

*Adapted from McKusick VA. *Mendelian Inheritance in Man: Catalogues of Autosomal Dominant, Autosomal Recessive, and X-Linked Phenotypes*. 11th ed. Baltimore: Johns Hopkins University Press; 1995.

**Profile 2a, and rarely, 2b, also characterizes the common polygenic type of hypercholesterolemia, which is many times more prevalent than the dyslipoproteinemias.

GENETIC TESTING

Genetic testing is labor intensive. Like any testing, the sensitivity and specificity depend on the population being tested. Genetic testing should be done if warranted by the family history or clinical picture. The patient should have pretest counseling and give informed consent. Contact the laboratory for specific instructions before obtaining the specimen. The laboratory should conform to quality standards such as those set by the College of American Pathologists. A list of labs is included as Table 4.6.

Cytogenetic testing uses dividing cells to identify chromosome abnormalities. Prenatal samples are from chorionic villi or amniotic fluid. After birth, blood lymphocytes are used. The cells must be kept alive. Blood should be collected in tubes with sodium heparin. The cells are arrested in metaphase. They are lysed and Giemsa stain is applied. The chromosomes are identified by size and banding patterns. They are photographed and cut out. A karyotype is constructed. The paired autosomes are arranged 1 to 22 in declining order of size followed by XX or XY. Aneuploidies are abnormal numbers of chromosomes. Examples include Down's syndrome (trisomy 21) and Turner's syndrome (45, XO).

Molecular genetic testing does not require living cells. Blood is collected in purple-top tubes with EDTA. Tissue can be preserved in formalin. Direct techniques are used to detect mutations after both the gene and mutations within the gene are known. Techniques used to detect mutations include allele-specific oligonucleotide hybridization analysis, direct sequencing, heteroduplex analysis, multiplex polymerase chain reaction analysis, and Southern blot analysis. Direct testing does not require testing of other family members. A limitation of direct analysis is that some diseases are caused by many mutations, some of which are not detected by any single genetic test. A large number of different mutations at a single locus is called allelic heterogeneity. Mutations at two or more genetic loci that result in identical phenotypes is called locus heterogeneity.

Indirect analysis, also called linkage analysis, does not require that the gene be identified or its function known. It is also used when the gene is known, but the mutations are too numerous and heterogeneous to make direct analysis practical. Limitations of this type of analysis include the requirement of testing more than one affected individual in a particular generation and more than one generation.

Some connective tissue diseases are more easily diagnosed by measuring the protein in tissue from a skin biopsy. Inborn errors of metabolism cause metabolic enzyme defects. These diseases are identified by screening for metabolites in urine or blood.

TABLE 4.5

Disorders That Have Genetic Tests to Help in Diagnosis

Disorder	Transmission	Gene Location	Comments
Adult Polycystic Kidney	Autosomal Dominant	PKD1(16p13.3) PKD2(4q13–23) PKD3	Occurs in 1/400 to 1/1000 live births. Other associated abnormalities include liver cysts, berry aneurysms, and mitral valve prolapse.
Familial Adenomatous Polyposis	Autosomal Dominant	APC tumor-suppressor gene chonchromosome 5q21	While a minimum of 100 mucosal polyps are required for diagnosis, some affected have as many as 2500.
Hereditary Nonpolyposis Colon Cancer	Autosomal Dominant	2p22, 3p, 21, 2q31–33, 7p22	These individuals develop multiple colonic malignancies. Adenoma formation is earlier than in general population.
Cystic Fibrosis	Autosomal Dominant	7q31–32	There are known and unknown mutations. The common denominator is defective transport of chloride across the cell membrane.
Duchenne Muscular Dystrophy	X-Linked Disorder	xp21	This mutation decreases the production of a protein called dystrophin causing muscle abnormalities.
Hemophilia A (Factor VIII Deficiency)	X-Linked Disorder	xq28	Clinical severity is determined by varying levels of factor VIII.

Disorder	Transmission	Gene Location	Comments
Familial Hypercholesterolemia	Autosomal Dominant	Chromosome 19 with more than 150 mutations, which are divided into 5 classes	LDL receptors are defective in some way in classes I–V
Fragile X Syndrome	X-Linked Disorder	Familial mental retardation, 1 gene on the long arm of the X chromosome	One of most common known causes of inherited mental retardation. As many as half of the carrier females are mentally retarded.
Sickle Cell Disease	Autosomal Recessive	Point mutation on the β-globulin chain of hemoglobin	Mutation results in hemoglobin that aggregates and polymerizes when the hemoglobin deoxygenates. In hemozygotes almost all of hemoglobin is HbS. In heterozygotes 40% of hemoglobin is HbS.
Tay-Sachs Disease	Autosomal recessive Affected frequency 1:2500 Carrier frequency 1:25	Chromosome 15	Decrease in hexaminidase A α-subunit results in accumulation of GM2 ganglioside in cells. Most devastating is accumulation in the CNS.
Breast Cancer	Autosomal Dominant	BRCA1 and BRCA2 mutations	5–10% of all breast cancer is inherited. The two mutations account for 50% of the inherited cases.
Huntington Disease	Autosomal Dominant	1T15 on chromosome 4p	A degenerative brain disorder with frequency of 10/100 000. Hallmarks are chorea and behavioral disturbance.

CNS indicates central nervous system; LDL, low-density lipoprotein.

TABLE 4.6

Commercial Laboratories Offering Diagnostic Tests

Code	Name	Location	Telephone
A	Athena Diagnostics	Worchester, MA	800 394-4493
Bd	Baylor DNA Diagnostic Laboratory	Houston, TX	800 226-3624
Bk	Baylor Kleberg Cytogenetics Laboratory	Houston, TX	800 441-4363
Bo	Boston University Human Genetics	Boston, MA	617 638-7083
C	Corning Nichols Institute	San Juan Capistrano, CA	800 642-4657
J	Jefferson Institute of Molecular Medicine	Philadelphia, PA	215 955-4830
L	Laboratory Corporation of America	Research Triangle Park, NC	800 334-5161
M	Mayo Medical Laboratories	Rochester, MN	800 533-0567

Disorder	A	Bd	Bk	Bo	C	J	L	M
Achondrogenesis II						+		
Achondroplasia		+						
Adrenal hypoplasia			+					
Adrenal hypoplasia								
Amyloidosis								+
Amyotrophic lateral sclerosis	+							
Angelman syndrome		+	+	+	+			
Canavan disease		+						
Charcot-Marie-Tooth 1A			+		+			
Chondrodysplasia						+		
Chronic granulomatous disease				+				
Citrullinemia				+				
Colorectal cancer							+	
Cystic fibrosis		+		+	+		+	+
Dentatorubral pallidoluysian atrophy		+						
DiGeorge syndrome			+	+	+		+	
Duchenne/Becker muscular dystrophy	+	+		+	+			+
Fragile X syndrome		+		+	+		+	
Friedreich ataxia				+				
Gaucher disease		+		+			+	
Hemophilia A		+		+				+
Hereditary neuropathy	+		+					
Huntington disease	+	+		+				

Disorder	A	Bd	Bk	Bo	C	J	L	M
Kallman syndrome			+					
Kearns-Sayre syndrome	+							
Kennedy spinal bulbar atrophy	+	+						
Kniest syndrome						+		
Leber optic atrophy	+							
Leigh syndrome	+							
Machado-Joseph syndrome	+	+		+				
MELAS syndrome	+							
MERRF	+							
Miller-Dieker syndrome			+	+	+		+	
Multiple endocrine neoplasia 2				+				+
Myelogenous leukemia				+				+
Myotonic dystrophy		+		+				+
Neurofibromatosis 1				+			+	
Neurofibromatosis 2	+							
Norrie disease	+							
Ornithine transcarbamalase deficiency				+				
Phenylketonuria				+				
Polycystic kidney disease				+				
Polyposis coli				+			+	+
Prader-Willi syndrome		+	+	+			+	+
Sickle cell/SC anemia		+		+			+	
Smith-Magenis syndrome			+				+	
Spinal muscular atrophy				+				
Spinocerebellar ataxia 1	+	+		+				+
Spondyloepiphyseal dysplasia						+		
Stickler syndrome	+					+		
Tay-Sachs disease		+		+			+	
Thalassemia α							+	+
Uniparental disomy							+	
Vas deferens absence				+				
Velocardiofacial syndrome			+	+			+	
Von Hippel-Lindau disease				+				
Waardenburg syndrome 1				+				
Williams syndrome			+	+			+	
Wilson disease				+				
Y chromosome DNA				+		+		+

Adapted from Thurmon TF. *A Comprehensive Primer on Medical Genetics*. London: Parthenon Publishing; 1999.

MELAs indicates myopathy, encephalopathy, lactic acidosis, and stroke-like episodes; MERRF, myoclonic epilepsy and ragged red fibers.

TABLE 4.7

Genetic Counseling

Medical geneticists and genetic counselors do most genetic counseling. There are over 1000 medical geneticists and 1800 genetic counselors in the United States. In the future, family physicians with added training will do genetic counseling. Genetic counseling helps a counselee understand the medical facts of a genetic problem. He or she is given the probability of occurrence of the disease in the unborn child or future progeny. Management alternatives are explored with the counselee in a nondirective way. The counselee chooses a course based on the facts and his/her beliefs.

Case 1: Trisomy

Trisomy 18 occurs in 1/8000 live births. The babies have multiple anomalies, failure to thrive, and severe mental retardation. Most die in infancy.

A 19-year-old gravid 2 has 15-week gestation triple screen indicating increased risk of trisomy 18. She is referred to a genetic counselor. After counseling, she agrees to level II ultrasound and amniocentesis.The perinatologist reports a normal ultrasound study. Cytogenetic study of the amniotic fluid determines the fetus is 46, XX. The result was a healthy female infant.

Case 2: Hypertrophic Cardiomyopathy

Hypertrophic cardiomyopathy is the most common cause of sudden death in adolescent athletes. The disease is autosomal dominant with variable penetrance. Nine genes and 100 mutations explain 50% of the cases. The variability in expression depends on the mutation and other unknown genetic factors.

A 15-year-old high school football player sees his family physician for a preparticipation sports physical exam. History reveals a paternal uncle who died suddenly at age 35. The youth has no history of exercise-induced chest pain or syncope. A systolic murmur is heard along the left sternal border accentuated by standing and Valsalva maneuver. His physician suspects hypertrophic cardiomyopathy. A cardiologist confirms the diagnosis and recommends avoidance of competitive sports. The family physician counsels the concerned parents and their son. The potential for sudden death due to ventricular tachyarrhythmias and the variable progression of the disease are discussed. An autopsy report on the paternal uncle confirmed hypertrophic cardiomyopathy. This means the boy's father carries the gene unless there is mistaken paternity. He may or may not have clinically detectable disease. All first-degree relatives should be clinically evaluated for hypertrophic cardiomyopathy. (See Case 3 pedigree, Figure 4.1.) The family is offered referral to a geneticist for possible identification of the mutation. More knowledge of the genetics of this disease may lead to new treatment in the future.

Case 3: Clubfoot

Clubfoot is a polygenic disorder. The risk to a sibling or a child of the proband is 3%. Case 3 is born with clubfeet requiring multiple surgeries. Her older sister had normal feet. There was no family history of clubfoot. She had four more sisters and a daughter without clubfoot. (See Case 2 pedigree, Figure 4.1.)

Case 4: Early Onset Alzheimer

Early-onset familial Alzheimer disease accounts for 5% of all cases of Alzheimer disease. Mutations of three genes have been identified. Transmission is autosomal dominant. The most prevalent type, AD 3 accounts for 20–70% of kindreds. The gene, presenilin 1, on chromosome 14q24 encodes a transmembrane protein. Genetic testing for presenilin 1 mutations is available in clinical laboratories. AD 1 accounts for 10–15% of families. It is caused by mutations in the gene that enclodes amyloid precursor protein. Testing is available on a research basis only. AD 4 is rare. The gene, presenilin 2, on chromosome 1 encodes a protein similar to presenilin1. One laboratory offers testing. A young married woman seeks counseling. Her mother, age 45, has early Alzheimer disease. Her maternal grandfather had Alzheimer disease. He died at age 55 in a nursing home. The counselee asks: "Could I be carrying the gene?" It is recommended that her mother be tested for the presenilin 1 mutation. If the test is positive, the daughter has a 50% chance of carrying the mutant gene. If negative, the risk is much lower. (See Case 4 pedigree, Figure 4.1.)

TABLE 4.8

Perinatal Genetic Screening

Disease	Target Population	Timing of Test
Cystic Fibrosis	Offered to all women	Preconception
Down Syndrome, Trisomines, Neural Tube Defect	AFP offered to all <35 years; amniotic fluid cells for >35 years	16–18 Gestational weeks
Hemoglobinopathies	Asian, Black, and Mediterranean Women	Preconception
Tay-Sachs Disease/Jewish Genetic Disease Panel	Ashkenazi couples	Preconception

AFP indicates α-fetoprotein.

TABLE 4.9

Known Fetal Genetic Causes of Abortion and Newborn Syndromes

Newborns		Abortuses		
Aberrations	**Percent**	**Frequency**	**Percent**	**Frequency**
Trisomy 13			0.005	1/20 000
Trisomy 14	2.2	1/45		
Trisomy 15	2.5	1/40		
Trisomy 16	9.8	1/10		
Trisomy 18	1.8	1/56	0.0125	1/8000
Trisomy 21	5.0	1/20	0.143	1/700
Trisomy 22	3.4	1/29		
XXY			0.1 males	1/1000
XYY			0.1 males	1/1000
45,X	5.4 females	1/19	0.01 females	1/10 000
XXX			0.1 females	1/1000
Balanced translocations			0.2	1/500
Unbalanced translocations	1.8	1/56	0.05	1/2000
Triploidy	10.2	1/10		
Tetraploidy	3.6	1/28		
Other	10.4	1/10	0.11	1/900

Adapted from Thurmon TF. *A Comprehensive Primer on Medical Genetics*. London: Parthenon Publishing; 1999.

TABLE 4.10

Primary Care Problems with Complex Genetic Traits

- Affective disorders
- Allergy
- Asthma
- Autoimmune disorders
- Cancers
- Connective tissue disease
- Coronary artery disease
- Diabetes
- Epilepsy
- Gout
- Inflammatory bowel disease
- Obesity
- Peptic ulcer disease
- Rheumatoid arthritis

TABLE 4.11

Common Diseases and Malformations Whose Distributions Conform to Expectations of Polygenic Threshold Inheritance

Disorder	Rate (%)	h^2	Sex Ratio M:F	Normal Parents: Rate of 2nd affected child (%)	Affected Parents: Rate of having affected child (%)	Affected Parents: Rate of 2nd affected child (%)
Ankylosing spondylitis	0.2	0.70				
Asthma	0.4	0.80				
Cleft lip/palate	0.1	0.76		2		
Bilateral				6		
Clubfoot	0.1	0.68	2:1	3	3	10
Congenital heart defect	0.5	0.35		2 (same type)	14 (if mother)	
Additional risk				4 (other type)		
Coronary heart disease	3	0.65				
Hip dislocation	0.07	0.60	1:6	6	12	36
Hirschsprung disease	0.02		4:1			
Short segment				3	2	
Long segment				12		
Hypertension	5	0.62				

Disorder	Rate (%)	h^2	Sex Ratio M:F	Normal Parents: Rate of 2nd affected child (%)	Affected Parents: Rate of having affected child (%)	Affected Parents: Rate of 2nd affected child (%)
Hypospadias (males)	0.2			10	10	
Neural tube defect	0.5	0.60		4	4	8
Peptic ulcer	4	0.37				
Pyloric stenosis	0.3	0.75	5:1			
Male proband				2	4	13
Female proband				10	17	38
Renal agenesis bilateral	0.01		3:1			
Male proband				3		
Female proband				7		
Schizophrenia	1					
Scoliosis adolescent	0.22	1:6	1:6	7	5	
Tracheoesophageal fistula	0.03	1:1	1:1	1	1	

Adapted from Thurmon TF. *A Comprehensive Primer on Medical Genetics*. London: Parthenon Publishing; 1999.

TABLE 4.12

Useful Web Site Resources

Resource	Web site
American College of Medical Genetics	www.faseb.org/genetics/acmg/
Center for Medical Genetics	http://research.marshfieldclinic.org/genetics/
Cedars-Sinai Medical Center Division of Medical Genetics	www.csmc.edu/genetics
GeneTests/GeneClinics	www.genetests.org www.geneclinics.org
National Center for Biotechnology Information	www.ncbi.nlm.nih.gov/Omim

FIGURE 4.1

Pedigree Case Studies

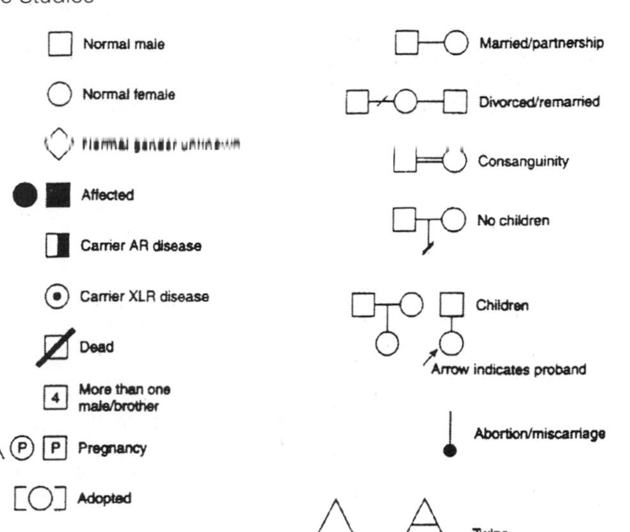

Case 2

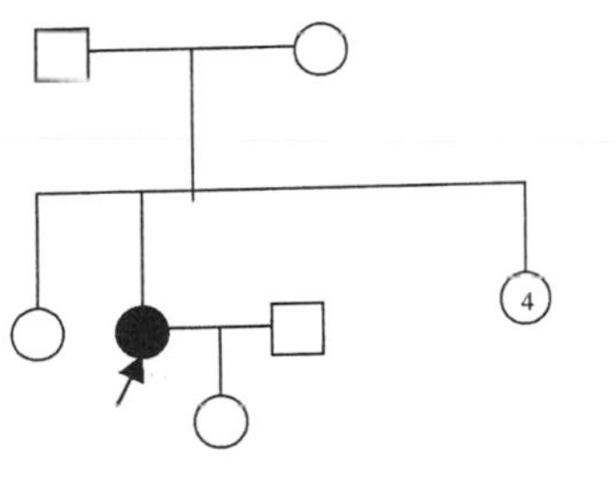

Case 3

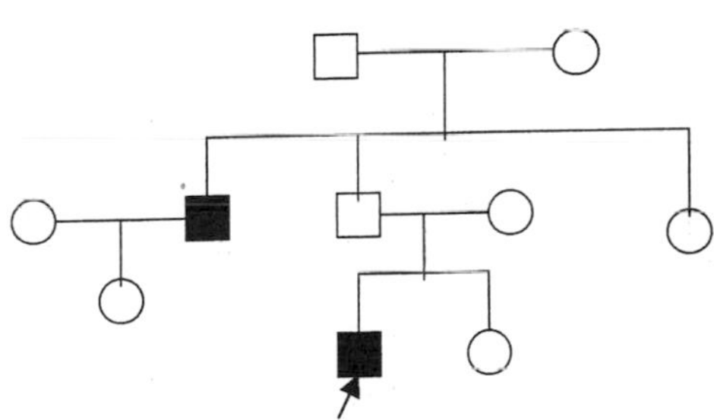

Case 4

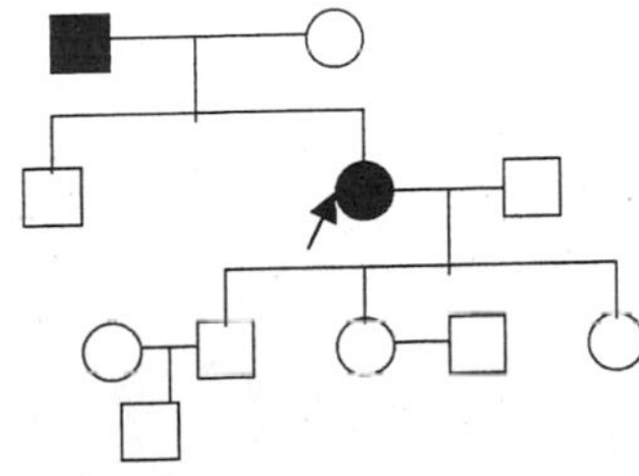

Reproduced with permission from Elsevier Science. (Mahowald MB, Scheuerle AS, McKusick VA. *Genetics in the Clinic: Clinical, Ethical, and Social Implications for Primary Care*. St Louis: Mosby, Inc; 2001.)

AR indicates autosomal recessive.

chapter 5

Maternity Care

Brenda L. Stokes, MD

IN THIS CHAPTER

- Preconception care and evaluation
- Routine prenatal care
- Genetic counseling and medications in pregnancy
- Medical complications of pregnancy
- Obstetrical complications of pregnancy
- Hypertension in pregnancy
- Antepartum fetal surveillance
- Fetal heart rate monitoring, scalp sampling, and assessment of fetal maturity
- Bishop score and induction of labor
- Vaginal birth after cesarean section (VBAC)
- Stages of labor, dysfunctional labor, and labor curves
- Shoulder dystocia, use of forceps, and vacuum extractor
- Indications for cesarean delivery, postpartum hemorrhage, and RhoGAM
- Common breastfeeding problems

BOOKSHELF RECOMMENDATIONS

- American College of Obstetricians and Gynecologists. *Compendium of Selected Publications*. Washington, DC: The American College of Obstetricians and Gynecologists; 2002 (updated yearly).
- Cunningham F, Gant N, Gilstrap L, Hauth J, Leveno K, Wenstrom K. *Williams Obstetrics*. 21st ed. New York: McGraw Hill; 2001.
- Gabbe SG, Niebyl JR, Simpson JL, eds. *Obstetrics: Normal & Problem Pregnancies*. 4th ed. New York: Churchill Livingstone; 2002.

- Briggs CC, Freeman RK, Yaffe SJ. *Drugs in Pregnancy and Lactation: A Reference Guide to Fetal and Neonatal Risk*. 6th ed. Philadelphia: Lippincott Williams & Wilkins; 2002.
- Hauth JC, Merenstein GB. *Guidelines for Perinatal Care*. 4th ed. Washington, DC and Elk Grove Village, IL: American College of Obstetricians and Gynecologists and American Academy of Pediatrics; 1997.

TABLE 5.1

Preconception Care and Evaluation

Preconception care identifies health risks to the mother and/or the fetus and modifies these before conception in the hope of preventing or reducing birth defects and complications related to pregnancy. Ideally all women receive preconception evaluation and counseling; however, about half of all pregnancies are unplanned. Therefore, this should be done at other routine office visits for all sexually active women.

Evaluation	Screening	Comments
Medical history	Chronic conditions, such as diabetes, hypertension, asthma, genetic history, surgical history	Control chronic medical conditions
Family history	Chronic conditions, genetic history (maternal and paternal)	Screening tests if high risk for genetic disease such as hemoglobinopathies, cystic fibrosis, Tay-Sachs
Reproductive history	Any STDs, previous OB history, gynecologic history	Identify risk of preterm labor, incompetent cervix
Nutrition history	Vegetarian diet, appropriate vitamin supplements, pica, eating disorders, PKU	Adequate calories and vitamin supplements, prevent neural tube defects (0.4 mg of folic acid recommended), dietary control of PKU
Medications	Prescribed, OTC, illicit drug use	Identify known teratogens and change if possible
Environmental	Work and/or home exposures	High-risk jobs (daycare worker or medical), toxic chemical or radiation exposures
Social history	Alcohol, tobacco, and illicit drug use, high-risk sexual practices, history of past or present abuse, financial	Referrals as needed
Physical examination	Attention to breast, pelvic, cardiovascular, pulmonary exams	Identify malformations, high blood pressure, heart murmurs, wheezing
Laboratory as indicated	CBC, rubella titer, RPR, HIV, hepatitis B, Pap smear, genital and urine cultures, genetic screen, PPD	

Continued

TABLE 5.1

Preconception Care and Evaluation, cont'd

Evaluation	Screening	Comments
Education	Exercise, nutrition, safety, substance use, menstrual calendar	
Immunizations as indicated	Rubella, hepatitis B, varicella, influenza	

CBC indicates complete blood cell count; HIV, human immunodeficiency virus; OB, obstetric; OTC, over-the-counter; PKU, phenylketonuria; PPD, purified protein derivative; RPR, rapid plasma reagin; and STDs, sexually transmitted diseases.

ROUTINE PRENATAL CARE

TABLE 5.2

Diagnosis of Pregnancy

β-HCG is detected in urine or blood.

β-HCG can be detected in blood by day 11 of pregnancy.

Quantitative β-HCG in blood:	<5 IU/mL negative
	5–25 indeterminate
	>25 positive

In normal pregnancy the quantitative β-HCG will approximately double in 72 hours.

HCG indicates human chorionic gonadotropin.

TABLE 5.3

Pregnancy Dating

An accurate estimated date of delivery (EDD) is very important in assessing the gestational age of the fetus. A final EDD should be based on the following:

- Dating by last menstrual period (LMP) using a wheel, table, or Naegele's rule (first day of LMP minus 3 months plus 1 week)
- Estimated size of uterus at first prenatal exam
- Appearance of fetal heart tones (FHTs) on Doppler (10–12 weeks)
- Quickening (16–20 weeks)
- Appearance of FHTs with unamplified fetoscope (19–20 weeks)
- Uterus at the navel at 20 weeks

When there are discrepancies in the dates or if LMP is unknown or considered inaccurate, then ultrasound should be used to determine EDD. Later ultrasound measurements are inaccurate and can be confirmed with a repeat ultrasound 4 weeks after the first.

Measurement	Gestational Age	Accuracy
Crown-rump length	5–12 weeks	Within 4–5 days
Biparietal diameter and femur length	12–28 weeks	Within 14 days
Biparietal diameter and femur length	>28 weeks	Within 21 days

FIGURE 5.1

Assessing Gestational Age by Uterine Growth

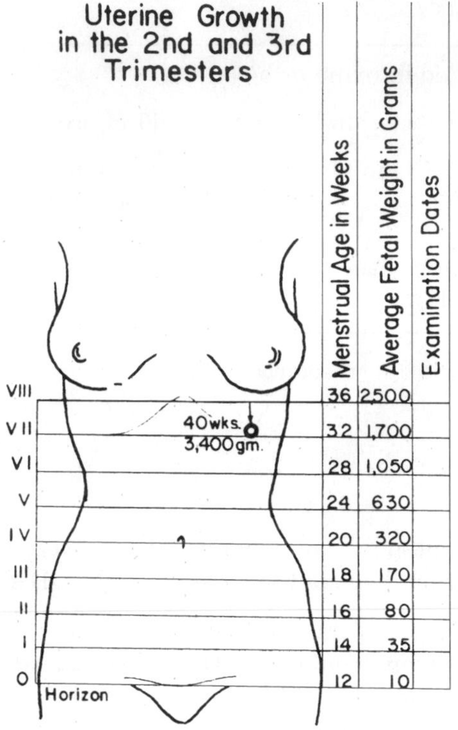

Reproduced with permission from Iffy L. *1982–1983 Modern Medicine Ob-Gyn Pocket Guide.* New York: Harcourt Brace Javanevich; 1982.

TABLE 5.4

Pregnancy Table for Expected Date of Delivery

Find the date of the last menstrual period in the top line (light type) of the pair of lines. The dark number (bold type) in the line below will be the expected day of delivery.

Jan	1	2	3	4	5	6	7	8	9	10	11	12	13	14	15	16	17	18	19	20	21	22	23	24	25	26	27	28	29	30	31	
Oct	**8**	**9**	**10**	**11**	**12**	**13**	**14**	**15**	**16**	**17**	**18**	**19**	**20**	**21**	**22**	**23**	**24**	**25**	**26**	**27**	**28**	**29**	**30**	**31**	**1**	**2**	**3**	**4**	**5**	**6**	**7**	**Nov**
Feb	1	2	3	4	5	6	7	8	9	10	11	12	13	14	15	16	17	18	19	20	21	22	23	24	25	26	27	28				
Nov	**8**	**9**	**10**	**11**	**12**	**13**	**14**	**15**	**16**	**17**	**18**	**19**	**20**	**21**	**22**	**23**	**24**	**25**	**26**	**27**	**28**	**29**	**30**	**1**	**2**	**3**	**4**	**5**				**Dec**
Mar	1	2	3	4	5	6	7	8	9	10	11	12	13	14	15	16	17	18	19	20	21	22	23	24	25	26	27	28	29	30	31	
Dec	**6**	**7**	**8**	**9**	**10**	**11**	**12**	**13**	**14**	**15**	**16**	**17**	**18**	**19**	**20**	**21**	**22**	**23**	**24**	**25**	**26**	**27**	**28**	**29**	**30**	**31**	**1**	**2**	**3**	**4**	**5**	**Jan**
April	1	2	3	4	5	6	7	8	9	10	11	12	13	14	15	16	17	18	19	20	21	22	23	24	25	26	27	28	29	30		
Jan	**6**	**7**	**8**	**9**	**10**	**11**	**12**	**13**	**14**	**15**	**16**	**17**	**18**	**19**	**20**	**21**	**22**	**23**	**24**	**25**	**26**	**27**	**28**	**29**	**30**	**31**	**1**	**2**	**3**	**4**		**Feb**
May	1	2	3	4	5	6	7	8	9	10	11	12	13	14	15	16	17	18	19	20	21	22	23	24	25	26	27	28	29	30	31	
Feb	**5**	**6**	**7**	**8**	**9**	**10**	**11**	**12**	**13**	**14**	**15**	**16**	**17**	**18**	**19**	**20**	**21**	**22**	**23**	**24**	**25**	**26**	**27**	**28**	**1**	**2**	**3**	**4**	**5**	**6**	**7**	**Mar**
June	1	2	3	4	5	6	7	8	9	10	11	12	13	14	15	16	17	18	19	20	21	22	23	24	25	26	27	28	29	30		
Mar	**8**	**9**	**10**	**11**	**12**	**13**	**14**	**15**	**16**	**17**	**18**	**19**	**20**	**21**	**22**	**23**	**24**	**25**	**26**	**27**	**28**	**29**	**30**	**31**	**1**	**2**	**3**	**4**	**5**	**6**		**April**
July	1	2	3	4	5	6	7	8	9	10	11	12	13	14	15	16	17	18	19	20	21	22	23	24	25	26	27	28	29	30	31	
April	**7**	8	**9**	**10**	**11**	**12**	**13**	**14**	**15**	**16**	**17**	**18**	**19**	**20**	**21**	**22**	**23**	**24**	**25**	**26**	**27**	**28**	**29**	**30**	**1**	**2**	**3**	**4**	**5**	**6**	**7**	**May**
Aug	1	2	3	4	5	6	7	8	9	10	11	12	13	14	15	16	17	18	19	20	21	22	23	24	25	26	27	28	29	30	31	
May	**8**	**9**	**10**	**11**	**12**	**13**	**14**	**15**	**16**	**17**	**18**	**19**	**20**	**21**	**22**	**23**	**24**	**25**	**26**	**27**	**28**	**29**	**30**	**31**	**1**	**2**	**3**	**4**	**5**	**6**	**7**	**June**
Sept	1	2	3	4	5	6	7	8	9	10	11	12	13	14	15	16	17	18	19	20	21	22	23	24	25	26	27	28	29	30		
June	**8**	**9**	**10**	**11**	**12**	**13**	**14**	**15**	**16**	**17**	**18**	**19**	**20**	**21**	**22**	**23**	**24**	**25**	**26**	**27**	**28**	**29**	**30**	**1**	**2**	**3**	**4**	**5**	**6**	**7**		**July**
Oct	1	2	3	4	5	6	7	8	9	10	11	12	13	14	15	16	17	18	19	20	21	22	23	24	25	26	27	28	29	30	31	
July	**8**	**9**	**10**	**11**	**12**	**13**	**14**	**15**	**16**	**17**	**18**	**19**	**20**	**21**	**22**	**23**	**24**	**25**	**26**	**27**	**28**	**29**	**30**	**31**	**1**	**2**	**3**	**4**	**5**	**6**	**7**	**Aug.**
Nov	1	2	3	4	5	6	7	8	9	10	11	12	13	14	15	16	17	18	19	20	21	22	23	24	25	26	27	28	29	30		
Aug.	**8**	**9**	**10**	**11**	**12**	**13**	**14**	**15**	**16**	**17**	**18**	**19**	**20**	**21**	**22**	**23**	**24**	**25**	**26**	**27**	**28**	**29**	**30**	**31**	**1**	**2**	**3**	**4**	**5**	**6**		**Sept.**
Dec.	1	2	3	4	5	6	7	8	9	10	11	12	13	14	15	16	17	18	19	20	21	22	23	24	25	26	27	28	29	30	31	
Sept.	**7**	**8**	**9**	**10**	**11**	**12**	**13**	**14**	**15**	**16**	**17**	**18**	**19**	**20**	**21**	**22**	**23**	**24**	**25**	**26**	**27**	**28**	**29**	**30**	**1**	**2**	**3**	**4**	**5**	**6**	**7**	**Oct.**

Adapted from Venes D, Thomas CL, eds. *Taber's Cyclopedic Medical Dictionary*. Philadelphia: FA Davis; 2001.

TABLE 5.5

Routine Prenatal Care

History
Current medical history, chronic conditions, past surgeries, previous obstetrical history, gynecologic history (including sexually transmitted diseases and surgeries), significant family history, social history, maternal and paternal genetic history (hemoglobinopathies, cystic fibrosis, Tay-Sachs, Down syndrome, mental retardation, neural tube defects), medications, allergies, tobacco, alcohol and drug use, nutrition, activity, occupation with any significant exposures

Physical Exam
General exam to include height, weight, blood pressure, thyroid, cardiac, pulmonary, breasts, abdomen, pelvic with clinical pelvimetry, and rectum

Laboratory
First visit: complete blood cell count, rapid plasma reagin (RPR), or Venereal Disease Research Laboratories (VDRL) test, rubella titer, blood type with Rh, antibody screen, hepatitis B surface antigen, human immunodeficiency virus screen, Pap smear, urinalysis with culture, genital cultures to include gonorrhea and chlamydia, and hemoglobin electrophoresis or other tests when indicated; consider ultrasound for dating

15–20 weeks' gestation (ideally 16–18 weeks): serum α-fetoprotein or multiple marker screen, chorionic villous sampling or amniocentesis if indicated; consider ultrasound for dating and/or anatomic survey

24–28 weeks' gestation: 1-hour 50-g Glucola screen, if >140 mg/dL then need a 3-hour glucose tolerance test, repeat hemoglobin or hematocrit

28 weeks' gestation: repeat RPR or VDRL, reassess hemoglobin or hematocrit if indicated, repeat genital cultures for gonorrhea or chlamydia if indicated, ultrasound if indicated

36 weeks' gestation: rectovaginal group B streptococcal culture

Patient Education
Medications, diet, exercise, smoking, alcohol, illicit drug use, weight gain, travel, intercourse, expected plan for care, costs, expected fetal development, signs and symptoms to call immediately, seatbelts, environmental or workplace hazards, toxoplasmosis precautions, breast care, infant feeding, childbirth and other offered classes, indications for cesarean delivery, antepartum fetal surveillance, analgesia/anesthesia options, infant care, infant car seat, newborn circumcision, sibling jealousy, postpartum contraception, postpartum depression, postpartum care

TABLE 5.6

Estimates for Dietary Needs for Pregnancy and Lactation (US RDA)

Nutrient	RDA or ESADDI for Pregnant Adult Women[a]	US RDA[b] Adults and Children Over 3 years Old[c]	Pregnant or Lactating Women[d]
	RDA:		
Protein	60 g	65 g	65 g
Vitamin A	800 mg RE[e]	5000 IU	8000 IU
Vitamin D	10 μg[f]	400 IU	400 IU
Vitamin E	10 mg of α-TE[g]	30 IU	30 IU
Vitamin K	65 μg	—*	—
Vitamin C	70 mg	60 mg	60 mg
Thiamin	1.5 mg	1.5 mg	1.7 mg
Riboflavin	1.6 mg	1.7 mg	2.0 mg
Niacin	17 mg NE[h]	20 mg	20 mg
Vitamin B_6	2.2 mg	2.0 mg	2.5 mg
Folacin	400 μg	400 μg	800 μg
Vitamin B_{12}	2.2 μg	6 μg	8 μg
Calcium	1200 mg	1000 mg	1300 mg
Phosphorus	1200 mg	1000 mg	1300 mg
Magnesium	300 mg	400 mg	450 mg
Iron	30 mg	18 mg	18 mg
Zinc	15 mg	15 mg	15 mg
Iodine	175 μg	150 μg	150 μg
Selenium	65 μg	—	—
	ESADDI:		
Biotin	30–100 μg	300 μg	300 μg
Pantothenic acid	4–7 mg	10 mg	10 mg
Copper	1.5–3.0 mg	2 mg	2 mg
Manganese	2.0–5.0 mg	—	—
Fluoride	1.5–4.0 mg	—	—
Chromium	50–200 μg	—	—
Molybdenum	75–250 μg	—	—

Continued

Adapted from The National Academy of Sciences. *Nutrition in Pregnancy.* Washington, DC: National Academy Press; 1990.

RDA indicates recommended daily allowance; ESADDI, estimated safe and adequate daily dietary intake.

[a]From National Research Council, 1989

[b]From National Nutrition Consortium, 1975

[c]Used in the labeling of most foods (eg, ready-to-eat cereals and vitamin and mineral supplements for adults)

[d]Used in the labeling of vitamin-mineral supplements designed for pregnant and lactating women

[e]1 RE (retinol equivalent) = 1 μg of retinol, 6 μg of β-carotene, or 12 μg of other provitamin A carotenoids, whereas 1 IU is usually equated to 0.3 μg of retinol and to 0.6 μg of β-carotene. By calculation, 8000 IU of vitamin A from vitamin supplements or cereal fortified with retinol equals 2400 RE

[f]1 μg of vitamin D (cholecalciferol) = 40 IU

[g]1 α-TE (tocopherol equivalent) = 1 mg of RRR-α-tocopherol = 1.49 IU RRR-α-tocopherol = 0.74 IU of all-*rac*-α-tocopherol (the synthetic form)

[h]1 NE (niacin equivalent) is equal to 1 mg of niacin or 60 mg of dietary tryptophan

*Not established

FIGURE 5.2

Pregnancy Weight Gain and Perinatal Mortality

Overweight mothers had the fewest fetal and neonatal deaths with a 15- to 16-lb weight gain in term pregnancies. The optimal gain for normally proportioned mothers was 20 lbs and for underweight mothers was 30 lbs. With weight gains of more than 20 lbs, underweight mothers had significantly lower perinatal mortalities than did mothers who were not underweight ($P < .005$). The underweight mothers in question had fewer losses to amniotic fluid infections, premature rupture of fetal membranes, and major congenital anomalies.

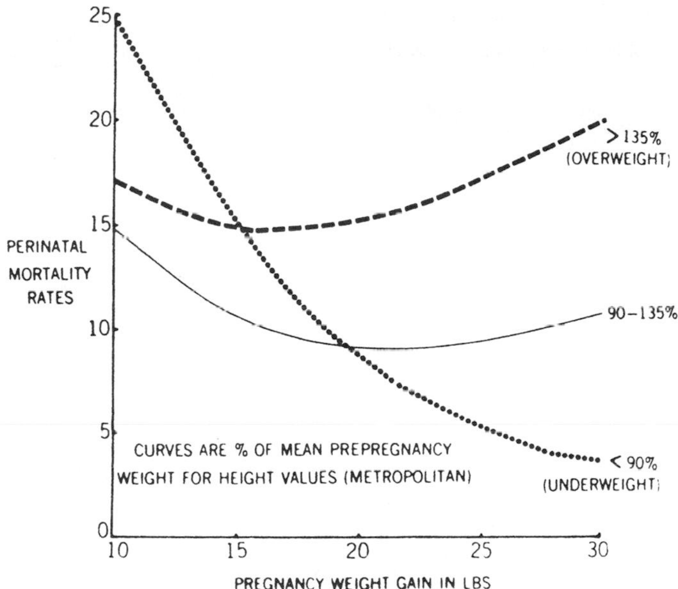

Reproduced with permission from Elsevier Science. (Naeye RL. Weight gain and the outcome of pregnancy. *Am J Obstet Gynecol.* 1979;135:3–9.)

TABLE 5.7

Target Weight Gain During Pregnancy Based on BMI for Singleton Gestation*

Prepregnancy BMI	Category	Recommended Weight Gain (lb)	Recommended Weight Gain (kg)
<19.8	Low	28–40	12.5–18.0
19.8–26.0	Normal	25–35	11.5–16.0
26.1–29.0	High	15–25	7.0–11.5
>29.0	Obese	<15	<7.0

Adapted from The National Academy of Sciences. *Nutrition in Pregnancy*. Washington, DC: National Academy Press; 1990.

BMI indicates body mass index (weight/height^2).

*Young adolescents should gain at the upper ends of the range.

TABLE 5.8

Physiological Norms of Pregnancy (32–36 Weeks)

Parameter	Nonpregnant	Pregnant
Thyroid		
T_4 (μg/dL)	3.4–6.4	5.5–10.0
T_3 (%)	25–38	12–25
FTI (μg/dL)	1.2–1.6	0.9–1.4
Blood Count		
Hb (g/dL)	12–16	10–14
HCT (%)	37–47	32–42
WBC (total/mm^3)	4500–10 000	5000–15 000
ESR (mm/hr)	20	30–90
Iron Studies		
Serum Fe (μg)	75–150	65–120
TIBC	240–450	300–500
Blood Pressure	120/80	114/65
Pulse	70	80
Cardiac Output (L/min)	4.5	6.0
ECG	Normal	15° left axis deviation
V_1 and V_2	Normal	Inverted T wave
V_4	Normal	Low T
III	Normal	Q and inverted T
aV_R	Normal	Small Q
Respiratory		
Respirations (rate/min)	15	16
Tidal volume (mL)	475	675
Vital capacity (mL)	3150	3300–3400
Residual volume (mL)	950	750
Pao_2 (mm Hg)	95–100	95–100
$Paco_2$ (mm Hg)	35–40	25–35
Renal		
GFR (creatinine clearance, mL/min)	80–120	110–180
BUN (mg/dL)	10–18	4–12
Creatinine (mg/dL)	0.6–1.2	0.4–0.9
Uric acid (mg/dL)	2.0–6.4	2.0–5.5

Adapted from Henry JB. *Postgrad Med.* 1972;52:110.

BUN indicates blood urea nitrogen; ECG, electrocardiogram; ESR, erythrocyte sedimentation rate; Fe, iron; FTI, free thyroxine index; GFR, glomerular filtration rate; Hb, hemoglobin; HCT, hematocrit; T_3, triiodothyronine; T_4, thyroxine; TIBC, total iron binding capacity; WBC, white blood cells.

GENETIC COUNSELING AND MEDICATIONS IN PREGNANCY

TABLE 5.9

Maternal Age-Specific Risk Estimates for Significant Chromosomal Disorders*

Maternal Age (years)	Down Syndrome per 1000 Liveborn	Other Chromosomal Disorders per 1000 Liveborn	Total Significant Chromosomal Disorders per 1000 Liveborn	As Fraction†
15	1.0	1.3	2.3	1/450
16	0.9	1.3	2.2	1/450
17	0.8	1.3	2.1	1/500
18	0.7	1.3	2.0	1/500
19	0.6	1.3	1.9	1/500
20	0.6	1.3	1.9	1/500
21	0.6	1.3	1.9	1/500
22	0.6	1.3	1.9	1/500
23	0.7	1.3	2.0	1/500
24	0.8	1.3	2.1	1/500
25	0.8	1.3	2.1	1/500
26	0.9	1.3	2.2	1/450
27	1.0	1.3	2.3	1/450
28	1.0	1.3	2.3	1/450
29	1.1	1.4	2.5	1/400
30	1.1	1.4	2.5	1/400
31	1.2	1.5	2.7	1/350
32	1.4	1.6	3.0	1/333
33	1.7	1.7	3.4	1/300
34	2.2	1.8	4.0	1/250
35	2.7	2.2	4.9	1/200
36	3.5	2.4	5.9	1/170
37	4.5	2.8	7.3	1/140
38	5.7	3.2	8.9	1/110

Maternal Age (years)	Down Syndrome per 1000 Liveborn	Other Chromosomal Disorders per 1000 Liveborn	Total Significant Chromosomal Disorders per 1000 Liveborn	As Fraction†
39	7.2	3.7	10.9	1/90
40	9.2	4.5	13.7	1/70
41	11.7	5.4	17.1	1/60
42	14.9	6.6	21.5	1/50
43	19.0	8.1	27.1	1/37
44	24.2	10.1	34.3	1/30
45	30.8	12.6	43.4	1/25
46	39.3	16.0	55.3	1/20
47	50.0	20.3	70.3	1/14
48	63.8	26.1	89.9	1/10
49	81.2	33.7	114.9	1/9

Adapted from Iffy L, Kaminetzky H. *Principles and Practice of Obstetrics and Perinatology*. Vol 1. New York: John Wiley & Sons; 1981: 398.

*Numbers are based on various estimates, especially those of Hook and Cross. Clinically significant conditions include Down syndrome, trisomies 18 and 13, XXY, and XYY, but not XXX.

†This column provides useful approximations for genetic counseling.

TABLE 5.10

Maternal Serum α-Fetoprotein Screening (MSAFP)

Elevated Levels Caused By: (occurs in 5% of those tested)

Fetus

Anencephaly, spina bifida (80–85%), encephalocele, omphalocele, gastroschisis, cystic hygroma, edema

Maternal

Hepatitis, persistent AFP production, hepatocellular carcinoma, herpes infection, African American race

Pregnancy

Incorrect estimate of gestational age, preeclampsia, multiple gestation, fetal to maternal bleed, abruption, Rh is isoimmunization, ataxia-telangiectasia, congenital nephrosis, epidermolysis bullosa simplex, severe oligohydramnios, spontaneous abortion, fetal demise, prematurity, acardiac twin, cyst or chorioangiomata of the placenta

Depressed Levels Caused By:

Fetus

Trisomies 21 and 18 (percent detected improved by using the multiple-marker screen [MSAFP, β-HCG, estriol, and PAPP-A]), sex-chromosomal aneuploidy

Maternal

Insulin-dependent diabetes mellitus, obesity If screening test is abnormal, order an ultrasound for an anomaly scan at 18–20 weeks. Consider amniocentesis for chromosome analysis, α-fetoprotein, and acetylcholinesterase assay.

TABLE 5.11

Indications for Amniocentesis for Genetic Diagnosis

- Abnormal maternal serum α-fetoprotein screening or multiple marker screen
- Abnormal ultrasound
- Advanced maternal age (>35 at time of delivery); risk is 1 in 270 for trisomy 21
- Previous child with a chromosomal abnormality
- Known parental chromosomal rearrangement
- Other suspected genetic disorder or inborn error of metabolism based on parental or family history
- Parent or previous child with a neural tube defect

TABLE 5.12

Potential Effects of Maternal Drug Ingestion on the Fetus or Neonate

Drug	Effect
ACE inhibitors and ARBs	IUGR; oligohydramnios; hypotension; anuria; renal failure; fetal demise
Alcohol	Fetal alcohol syndrome; IUGR
Aminoglycosides	Cranial nerve VIII toxicity
Amiodarone	IUGR, transient bradycardia, prolonged QT interval
Amphetamines	Cardiac defects; irritability; poor feeding
Androgens	Masculinization of female
Antineoplastics	Congenital anomalies; IUGR
Barbiturates and benzodiazepines	Withdrawal
β-blockers	Bradycardia; hypoglycemia; IUGR; respiratory depression
Carbamazepine	Fetal anomalies, fetal hydantoin syndrome, spina bifida, cardiac defects
Cephalothin	Positive direct Coombs test
Chloramphenicol	"Gray baby" syndrome
Diethylstilbestrol	Vaginal adenosis or adenocarcinoma
Heroin, other narcotics, and propoxyphene	Withdrawal; convulsions; neonatal death; IUGR
HMG-CoA reductase inhibitors	Recommended to stop in pregnancy as is, no fetal effects observed
Iodide	Goiter; mental retardation
Isotretinoin	Fetal anomalies; fetal demise
Lithium	Congenital heart disease; cleft palate or lip
Misoprostol	Abortifacient
Novobiocin	Hyperbilirubinemia
NSAIDs	Oligohydramnios; premature closure of the ductus arteriosus; prolonged labor; postmaturity
Phenylpropanolamine HCl	Eye and ear problems; hypospadias
Phenytoin	Cleft lip and palate; congenital small stature; hydantoin syndrome; IUGR; skeletal anomalies
Progestins	Clitoromegaly and labial fusion; septal defects; limb reduction anomalies; hypospadias; VACTERL syndrome
Propylthiouracil	Goiter; cretinism
Quinine	Thrombocytopenia
Radioactive iodine	Thyroid ablation

Continued

TABLE 5.12

Potential Effects of Maternal Drug Ingestion on the Fetus or Neonate, cont'd

Drug	Effect
Reserpine	Nasal congestion; drowsiness
Salicylates	Neonatal and maternal bleeding; postmaturity; abruption
Warfarin sodium	Fetal demise; hemorrhage; blindness; mental retardation; nasal hypoplasia; stippled epiphyses
Spironolactone	Cleft palate, masculinization (in theory; not observed)
Sulfonamides	Hyperbilirubinemia; kernicterus
Tetracyclines	Discoloration of teeth; inhibition of bone growth
Thiazides	Thrombocytopenia; hyperbilirubinemia; hypokalemia; SGA
Thiocarbamides	Goiter; hyperthyroidism
Tobacco	SGA; spotaneous abortion; preterm delivery; placental abruption; SIDS
Tricyclic antidepressants	Cardiac defects
Trimethadione	Cleft lip and palate; congenital heart disease; hydantoin syndrome; skeletal anomalies; IUGR
Trimethoprim	Hyperbilirubinemia at term
Valproic acid	Neural tube defects

ACE indicates angiotensin-converting enzyme; ARBs, angiotensin II receptor blockers; HMG-CoA, hydroxymethyl glutaryl coenzyme A; IUGR, intrauterine growth retardation; NSAIDs, nonsteroidal anti-inflammatory drugs; SGA, small for gestational age; SIDS, sudden infant death syndrome; and VACTERL, vertebral, anal, cardiac, tracheal, esophageal, renal, and limb anomalies.

TABLE 5.13

FDA Drug Categories for Pregnancy

A	Safety established using controlled human studies
B	Safety established using controlled animal studies and no risk observed in humans
C	Uncertain safety; animal studies show an adverse effect, but it is not seen or not studied in humans
D	Unsafe; benefit may outweigh risk
X	Highly unsafe; risk outweighs benefit in all situations

MEDICAL COMPLICATIONS OF PREGNANCY

TABLE 5.14

Prevention of Transmission of HIV From Mother to Infant

Patient Selection

- All known HIV-positive pregnant patients
- Any CD4 count and viral load
- If not on previous antiretroviral therapy, consider delaying treatment until after the first trimester based on the risks and benefits
- If already on antiretroviral therapy, consider continuing therapy in the first trimester based on the risks and benefits

Drug Selection

- Depends on the gestational age at presentation and if the mother has had prior therapy
- Avoid efavirenz and hydroxyurea due to potential teratogenic effects
- Avoid the combination of didanosine and stavudine due to possible maternal hepatotoxicity or lactic acidosis
- See the following table for appropriate drugs

ZDV Regimen

- **Antepartum:** ZDV 200 mg tid or 300 mg bid starting at week 14 until delivery
- **Intrapartum:** ZDV 2 mg/kg IV over 1 hour, then continuous infusion of 1 mg/kg/hr until delivery
- **Postpartum:** Infant gets ZDV syrup 2 mg/kg PO every 6 hours until 6 weeks old, first dose at 6–12 hours old. Culture infant's blood at birth and at 12, 24, and 78 weeks and test for antibodies at 15 and 18 months.

---

bid indicates twice daily; HIV, human immunodeficiency virus; IV, intravenous; PO, orally; tid, three times daily; and ZDV, zidovudine.

TABLE 5.15

Selected Regimens for Prevention of Transmission of HIV From Mother to Infant

Gestational Age at Presentation	Prior Anti-HIV Therapy	Viral Load (Colonies/ mL)	Treatment Regimen	Delivery Mode
<36 weeks	No	>1000	Standard combination therapy and ZDV regimen starting at 10–12 weeks	Consider elective cesarean section at 38 weeks if viral load still >1000
<36 weeks	No	<1000	ZDV regimen starting at 10–12 weeks	No evidence to support elective cesarean delivery if viral load <1000
<36 weeks	Yes	Any	At 12 weeks continue therapy and add ZDV if not part of current therapy. Less At 12 weeks consider risks and benefits of continuing therapy, restart same regimen and add ZDV after 12 weeks.	Same considerations as above based on viral load
>36 weeks	Yes	Any	Continue all current medications. ZDV regimen during labor	Same as above
In labor	No	Any	Several options: single dose of nevirapine (200 mg PO) at onset of labor and for newborn (2 mg/kg PO) when 48 hours old, ZDV and 3TC during labor and continue for 1 week in newborn, ZDV regimen, or 2 doses of	No evidence to support cesarean delivery for HIV-infected women who present in labor

Gestational Age at Presentation	Prior Anti-HIV Therapy	Viral Load (Colonies/ mL)	Treatment Regimen	Delivery Mode
			nevirapine combined with the ZDV regimen	
Postpartum	Yes or no	Any	ZDV regimen for the newborn	N/A

Information based on the May 4, 2001 Department of Health and Human Services guidelines available online at www.hivatis.org.

HIV indicates human immunodeficiency virus; N/A, not applicable; PO, orally; 3TC, lamivudine; and ZDV, zidovudine.

DIABETES IN PREGNANCY

Diabetes is a significant cause of perinatal morbidity and mortality. Tight control of blood sugars reduces this. It is recommended to screen all pregnant women between 24 to 28 weeks of gestation for gestational diabetes with a 50-gram Glucola test. If the one-hour Glucola result is more than 140 mg/dL, then a three-hour glucose tolerance test using a 100-g glucose load should be done. Gestational diabetes is diagnosed if two values on the three-hour glucose tolerance test are above the normal limits. Risk factors for gestational diabetes include a history of elevated blood sugar, glycosuria, family history of diabetes, prior delivery of large-for-gestational-age infant, anomalous or stillborn infant, polyhydramnios, habitual abortion, or maternal obesity.

TABLE 5.16

Diagnosis of Gestational Diabetes Using a Three-Hour Glucose Tolerance Test with a 100-gram Glucose Load

Fasting blood sugar	95 mg/dL
1 hour	180 mg/dL
2 hour	155 mg/dL
3 hour	140 mg/dL

TABLE 5.17

White Classification of Diabetes in Pregnancy

Class	Age at Onset (year)	Duration (year)	Complications	Insulin
A1	Any	Pregnancy	None	No
A2	Any	Pregnancy	None	Yes
B	>20	<10	None	Yes
C	10–19	10–19	None	Yes
D	<10	20	Benign retinopathy	Yes
F	Any	Any	Nephropathy	Yes
R	Any	Any	Proliferative retinopathy	Yes
H	Any	Any	Heart disease	Yes

Adapted from White P. *Am J Med.* 1949;7:609.

TABLE 5.18

Cardiovascular Disease During Pregnancy

Cardiac disease occurs in approximately 1% of all pregnancies. It remains a significant cause of maternal and fetal morbidity and mortality. Rheumatic heart disease is still the most common problem. Management needs to be coordinated with a cardiologist and is aimed at the prevention of congestive heart failure.

Prevention Factors

Infection	Nutritional deficiencies
Anemia	Physical stress
Venous congestion	Fluid retention

Peak cardiac output occurs at 25–32 weeks (30–50% above nonpregnant levels).

Steps in Management

- Diagnose early and classify heart condition according to the New York Heart Association criteria
- Auscultate heart frequently; check for anemia often
- Class 1 and 2: Frequent rest, housekeeping aid, avoid stairs
- Class 3: Greatly reduced activity, bed rest for mild failure
- Class 4: Consider therapeutic abortion
- Diet low in salt, lower water intake to 800–1000 mL/day for failure
- Diuretics for moderate or advanced disease plus edema or venous congestion
- Digitalis for failure apparent by signs and symptoms
- Hospitalize patient before EDC to evaluate cardiac status
- Careful monitoring during labor; avoid hypotension
- Shorten second stage with forceps; regional block (caudal) recommended
- SBE prophylaxis

TABLE 5.19

Differential Diagnosis of the Dermatoses Associated with Pregnancy

Disease	Gestational Age at Onset	Type of Lesions	Distribution of Rash	Symptoms	Associated Laboratory Abnormalities	Therapy	Maternal and Fetal Morbidity and Mortality
Herpes gestationis	First month to postpartum	Erythematous papules, vesicles, and bullae	Extremities, abdomen, buttocks, or generalized (10% mucous membranes)	Severe pruritus	Eosinophilia, biopsy with immunofluorescence of the basement membrane between the dermis and epidermis	Systemic corticosteroids	No maternal, reports of prematurity; growth restriction, and stillbirth in fetus
Impetigo herpetiformis	Any	Small pustules that may coalesce	Genitalia, inner thigh, axilla, breasts, umbilicus, extremities	Pruritus, pain, severe systemic symptoms (fever, chills, vomiting, diarrhea, lymphadenopathy, septicemia)	Hypocalcemia, hyperphosphatemia	Systemic corticosteroids, antibiotics for secondary infections, fetal surveillance and deliver when fetal lungs mature	Increased mortality in mother and fetus, maternal cardiac and renal failure in severe cases

Disease	Gestational Age at Onset	Type of Lesions	Distribution of Rash	Symptoms	Associated Laboratory Abnormalities	Therapy	Maternal and Fetal Morbidity and Mortality
PUPPP (pruritic urticarial papules and plaques of pregnancy)	Third trimester	Erythematous urticarial papules and plaques	Abdomen to thighs, buttocks, and occasionally arms and legs	Severe pruritus	None, biopsy to distinguish from herpes gestationis	Topical steroids, antipruritics, occasionally systemic corticosteroids	None
Prurigo gestationis (papular dermatitis)	Late second and third trimesters	Small papules, some with excoriations	Earlier onset on extensor surfaces of extremities, later onset on abdomen	Pruritus	None reliably	Antipruritics	None
Cholestasis of pregnancy	Third trimester	None or excoriations	Generalized	Pruritus	Elevated bilirubin	Antipruritics	No maternal; reports of stillbirths

FIGURE 5.3

How to Diagnose Rubella in Pregnancy

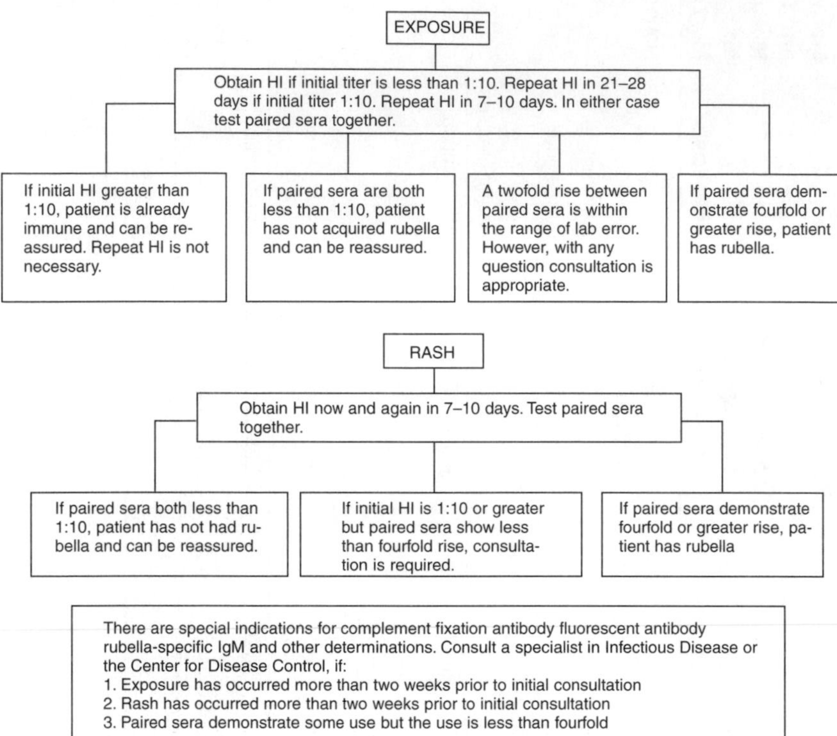

Adapted from The American Academy of Family Physicians. McCubbin JH, Smith JS. How to diagnose rubella during pregnancy. *Am Fam Phys.* 1981;23:205.

TABLE 5.20

Back Pain During Pregnancy

There are three common back pain syndromes in pregnancy:

1. High-back pain (above the lumbar area) associated with muscle strain and fatigue.
2. Low-back pain (lumbar area) associated with muscle strain and related to lifting and bending.
3. Sacroiliac pain (buttock/thigh) associated with subluxation at the SI joint.

The first two usually will decrease in frequency as the patient nears term. The third will usually increase in frequency near term and can be associated with radicular pain. Sacroiliac pain is treatable.

Criteria for Diagnosis of Sacroiliac Subluxation

Sacral pain—usually unilateral, radiates like sciatica

Positive Piedallu's sign—forward flexion results in asymmetrical movement of posterosuperior iliac spines; one becomes higher than the other

Positive pelvic compression—pain provoked by direct, downward pressure on anterosuperior iliac spines

Asymmetry of anterosuperior iliac spines—examine in the supine position; one appears higher than the other

Confirmatory Signs of Sacroiliac Subluxation

Straight leg raise—causes pain at highest elevation

Flexion block—with patient supine, flex knee at 90°, then passively flex knee toward chest; flexion of thigh is blocked to one-half the expected range on painful side

Positive Patrick's test—pain is provoked by placing one heel on the opposite knee in the supine position and simultaneously rotating the leg outward

Pain at Baer's point—tenderness just to the side and 2–3 inches below the umbilicus on the painful side, one third of the distance between the umbilicus and the anterosuperior iliac spine

Management of Sacroiliac Subluxation

One to two rotational manipulations of the SI joint and lumbar spine is usually sufficient to resolve the SI pain. Patient is placed supine, and the ipsilateral shoulder is held to the table. The patient's painful side is manipulated by flexing the thigh toward the abdomen with the knee in full flexion, then internally rotating the knee toward the contralateral side.

Adapted from Ostgaard HC, Anderson GBJ, Karlsson K. Prevalence of back pain in pregnancy. *Spine.* 1991;16:549; and Daly JM, Frame PS, Rapoza PA. Sacroiliac subluxation: a common, treatable cause of low-back pain in pregnancy. *Fam Pract Res J.* 1991;11:149.

OBSTETRICAL COMPLICATIONS OF PREGNANCY

TABLE 5.21

Possible Causes for Spontaneous Abortion*

Chromosomal abnormalities	Incompetent cervix
Abnormal zygote	Smoking
Age of gametes	Moderate/heavy alcohol use
Advanced maternal age	Excessive caffeine
Antiphospholipid syndromes	Environmental chemical exposure
Rh isoimmunization	Radiation
Anti-P antibodies	Uncontrolled diabetes
Uterine anomalies/defects (synechiae, leiomyomas)	Infections (*Mycoplasma hominis, Ureaplasma urealyticum*, herpes simplex, HIV, syphilis, group B streptococcus, toxoplasmosis)
Lupus erythematosus	Thyroid disease
Severe maternal disease	Progesterone deficiency
IUD in place	

HIV indicates human immunodeficiency virus; IUD, intrauterine device.

*Defined as loss of products of conception before 20 weeks of gestation or weighing less than 500 grams. Occurs in approximately 15% of all pregnancies.

TABLE 5.22

Management of Spontaneous Abortion

Type	Definition	Evaluation and Treatment
Complete	Passage of all products of conception	Administer RhoGAM if Rh negative; follow β-HCG levels to zero
Threatened	Vaginal bleeding prior to 20 weeks of gestation without the passage of tissue	Pelvic rest; RhoGAM if indicated
Inevitable	Vaginal bleeding prior to 20 weeks gestation and cervical os is open	Evacuation of the uterus; RhoGAM if indicated
Incomplete	Vaginal bleeding and cramping with the passage of tissue but some tissue remains in the uterine cavity or the endocervical canal	Surgical evacuation of the uterus; RhoGAM if indicated
Missed	Nonviable fetus with retained products of conception	Evacuation of the uterus; evaluation for coagulopathy; RhoGAM if indicated
Septic	Infection associated with abortion, usually induced	Appropriate antibiotics and supportive care
Habitual	Three or more consecutive spontaneous abortions	Need to evaluate for cause; labs include CBC, glucose, liver and renal function tests, thyroid test, TORCH titers, Coombs' test, antiphospholipid antibodies, cervical cultures for *Ureaplasma* and *T. mycoplasma*

β-HCG indicates β-human chorionic gonadotropin; CBC, complete blood cell count; TORCH, toxoplasmosis, other viruses, rubella, cytomegalovirus, and herpes simplex.

TABLE 5.23

Sites and Incidence of Ectopic Pregnancy

Site	Percent of Cases	Incidence
Ampular	47.0	The incidence of ectopic pregnancy is increasing and is between 1 in 100 and 1 in 200 pregnancies. The typical high-risk patient is older, has a higher parity, has had prior infertility, and has had a prior ectopic pregnancy or PID. Also current IUD use and prior tubal surgery.
Isthmic	21.6	
Fimbrial	5.8	
Interstitial	3.7	
Infundibular	2.5	
Other	19.4	

PID indicates pelvic inflammatory disease; IUD, intrauterine device.

TABLE 5.24

Signs and Symptoms Associated with an Ectopic Pregnancy

Signs or Symptoms	Incidence
Pain	80%
Irregular vaginal bleeding	60–80%
Adnexal mass	50%
Nonspecific gastrointestinal complaints	80%
Dizziness or syncope	55%
Uterine enlargement	30%

TABLE 5.25

Use of β-Human Chorionic Gonadotropin (β-HCG), Ultrasound, and Progesterone Levels in the Diagnosis of an Ectopic Pregnancy

- In a normal gestation the β-HCG will double in approximately 2 days.
- The lower limit of normal rise in β-HCG in 2 days is 66%.
- A gestational sac can be visualized by transvaginal ultrasound at a β-HCG level of 1500–2000 mIU/mL.
- Transabdominal ultrasound will show a gestational sac at a β-HCG level of 6000–6500 mIU/mL.
- The absence of a gestational sac above these levels suggests an ectopic pregnancy until proven otherwise.
- Serum progesterone levels can be helpful in that a level <5 ng/mL is associated with a nonviable pregnancy and >25 ng/mL is associated with a viable intrauterine pregnancy.
- Most ectopic pregnancies have a serum progesterone level of 10–20 ng/mL.
- Suction curettage may be helpful to differentiate from a spontaneous abortion.

FIGURE 5.4

Diagnosis of Suspected Ectopic Pregnancy

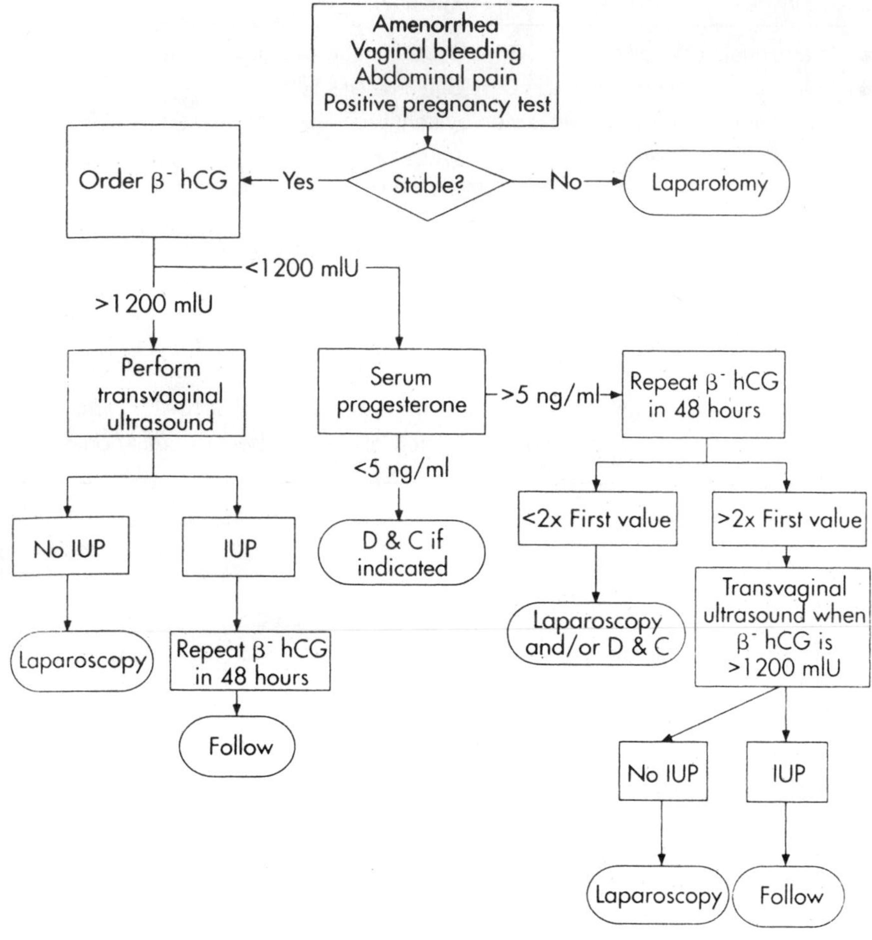

TABLE 5.26

Culdocentesis Technique

Obtain informed consent; risks are hemorrhage and organ puncture.
Swab vagina and cervix with povidine-iodine.
Grasp posterior lip of cervix with tenaculum, and apply gentle traction.
Subcutaneous lidocaine anesthetic may be used in posterior fornix.
Insert spinal needle on a 10-mL Luer-lock syringe in posterior fornix into transitional fold.
Keep parallel to uterus and apply continuous, gentle negative pressure while inserting into cul-de-sac.
More than 5 mL of nonclotting blood is 99% diagnostic of ectopic pregnancy.
If bowel is inadvertently punctured, no harm should result; withdraw needle and observe.

TABLE 5.27

Therapy for Ectopic Pregnancy

Surgical Treatment

- Laparoscopic salpingostomy or salpingectomy
- Laparotomy for unstable patient

Medical Treatment (Methotrexate)
Patient selection

- Diagnosis made without surgery
- Stable with no signs of active bleeding
- Ectopic mass measures 3.5 cm or less on ultrasound
- Desire for future fertility
- Reliable for follow-up
- β-HCG less than 15 000 mIU/mL
- No contraindications for methotrexate

Contraindications to methotrexate

- Hepatic dysfunction: AST > 2x normal
- Renal disease: serum creatinine >1.5 mg/dL
- Active peptic ulcer disease
- Blood dyscrasia: leukocytes <3.0 or platelets <100
- Immunodeficiency
- Breastfeeding
- History of hepatic, renal, or hematologic disease
- Active pulmonary disease
- Known sensitivity to drug
- Fetal cardiac activity (relative contraindication)

Dosing schedule and lab testing

- Initial labs include quantitative β-HCG, CBC, chemistry screen to check liver and kidney function, blood type and antibody screen
- Rh-negative patients receive Rh immune globulin
- Two dosing schedules
    1. Single dose of IM methotrexate 50 mg/m^2 divided in two doses on day 1
    2. Four serial doses of IM methotrexate 1 mg/kg on days 1, 3, 5, and 7 and leucovorin rescue 0.1 mg/kg on days 2, 4, 6, and 8
- Day 4 after first injection, repeat quantitative β-HCG (may increase with single dose)
- Day 7 after first injection, repeat quantitative β-HCG, CBC, chemistry screen
- If β-HCG levels do not decrease by at least 15% from day 4 to day 7, need to repeat methotrexate dose or recommend surgery

- Need to abandon medical therapy for surgical intervention if significantly worsening abdominal pain, hemodynamically unstable, increasing or plateau of β-HCG by day 7
- Follow β-HCG titers weekly until undetectable

Patient instructions and cautions

- Potential side effects: impaired liver function, stomatitis, gastritis, or enteritis, bone marrow suppression, dizziness, pneumonitis, reversible alopecia
- Avoid alcohol, NSAIDs, vitamins containing folic acid, and sexual intercourse
- Abdominal pain may get worse before improvement, but severe pain needs to be evaluated
- May experience vaginal bleeding
- Contact physician if any signs of rupture develop, such as sudden onset of severe abdominal pain, significant worsening of abdominal pain, heavy vaginal bleeding, dizziness, syncope, or tachycardia

---

AST indicates aspartate aminotransferase; CBC, complete blood cell count; β-HCG, β-human chorionic gonadotropin; IM, intramuscular; NSAIDs, nonsteroidal anti-inflammatory drugs.

TABLE 5.28

Differential Diagnosis of Hyperemesis Gravidarum

Multiple gestation	Hepatitis
Molar pregnancy	Peptic ulcer disease
Cholecystitis	Pancreatitis
Pyelonephritis	Gastroenteritis
Fatty liver of pregnancy	

TABLE 5.29

Treatment Options for Hyperemesis Gravidarum

Hydration and correction of electrolyte abnormalities

- Try PO but may require IV or TPN if severe

Dietary counseling

Vitamin supplementation

- Folic acid 0.4 mg
- Consider adding vitamin B_6

Antiemetics

- Antiemetics: metaclopramide, ondansetron, droperidol
- Phenothiazines: promethazine, prochlorperazine, chlorpromazine
- Antihistamines: doxylamine, trimethobenzamide, diphenhydramine, chlorpheniramine, meclizine
- Alternative medicine: ginger, acupressure, acupuncture

Emotional support

IV indicaes intravenous; PO, oral; TPN, total parenteral nutrition.

TABLE 5.30

Management of the Incompetent Cervix

Facts

Most common cause of second-trimester spontaneous abortions

Etiological factors include congenital, cervical trauma due to surgery or laceration at prior delivery, overzealous D&C or therapeutic abortion, and exposure to DES in utero

Diagnosis

History of recurrent second-trimester spontaneous abortions

Painless dilation and effacement of the cervix

Bulging membranes

Feeling of vaginal pressure with associated discharge

Premature rupture of membranes

Transvaginal ultrasound shows cervical length <2 cm, funneling of internal os, or bulging of membranes into the endocervical canal

Treatment

Cultures for gonorrhea, *Chlamydia*, group B *Streptococcus*

Antibiotic prophylaxis for positive group B *Streptococcus* or as indicated

Bedrest as indicated

Possible short-term use of indomethacin (usually only with emergency cerclage)

Surgical cerclage (McDonald—purse-string with Mersilene band, modified Shirodkar—submucosal suture, or abdominal cerclage)

D&C indicates dilation and curettage; DES, diethylstilbestrol.

TABLE 5.31

Third-Trimester Bleeding

Any third-trimester bleeding is presumed to be caused by the placenta, and the fetus should be considered endangered until proven otherwise. As a general rule, any third-trimester bleeding should be evaluated in the hospital where surgical care is immediately available. The bleeding may be painful or painless.

Common causes of third-trimester bleeding	
Placenta previa	Implantation of the placenta over the cervical os; complete, partial, or marginal; painless bleeding; 1 in 200 pregnancies
Abruptio placentae	Premature separation of the placenta; 1 in 120 pregnancies; mild to severe; significant fetal mortality (25–30%)
Velamentous insertion of the cord/vasa previa	Bleeding from rupture of a fetal vessel; rare; sudden deterioration of fetal heart rate with painless bleeding; significant fetal mortality (>50%)
Ruptured uterus or dehiscence of previous uterine scar	Rare, but more common if previous uterine scar; painful vaginal bleeding
Lesion or infection	Cervical, vaginal, or vulvar
Bloody show	Cervical dilation

General Rules

- First assess maternal and fetal stability
- Do not do a vaginal exam in an unprepared setting; avoid inserting a finger into the cervix
- Establish intravenous access and have blood available for transfusion
- Alert surgical team and have them stand by if performing a double set-up exam
- Can establish whether bleeding is maternal or fetal in origin by using the Apt test

Apt test

- Mix 1 part of blood from the vagina with 5 parts tap water and centrifuge; mix 5 parts of the pink supernatant with 1 part of 1% sodium hydroxide and centrifuge
- Fetal blood results in no color change (pink)
- Maternal blood results in color change to light brown or yellow-brown

FIGURE 5.5

Painful Third-Trimester Bleeding

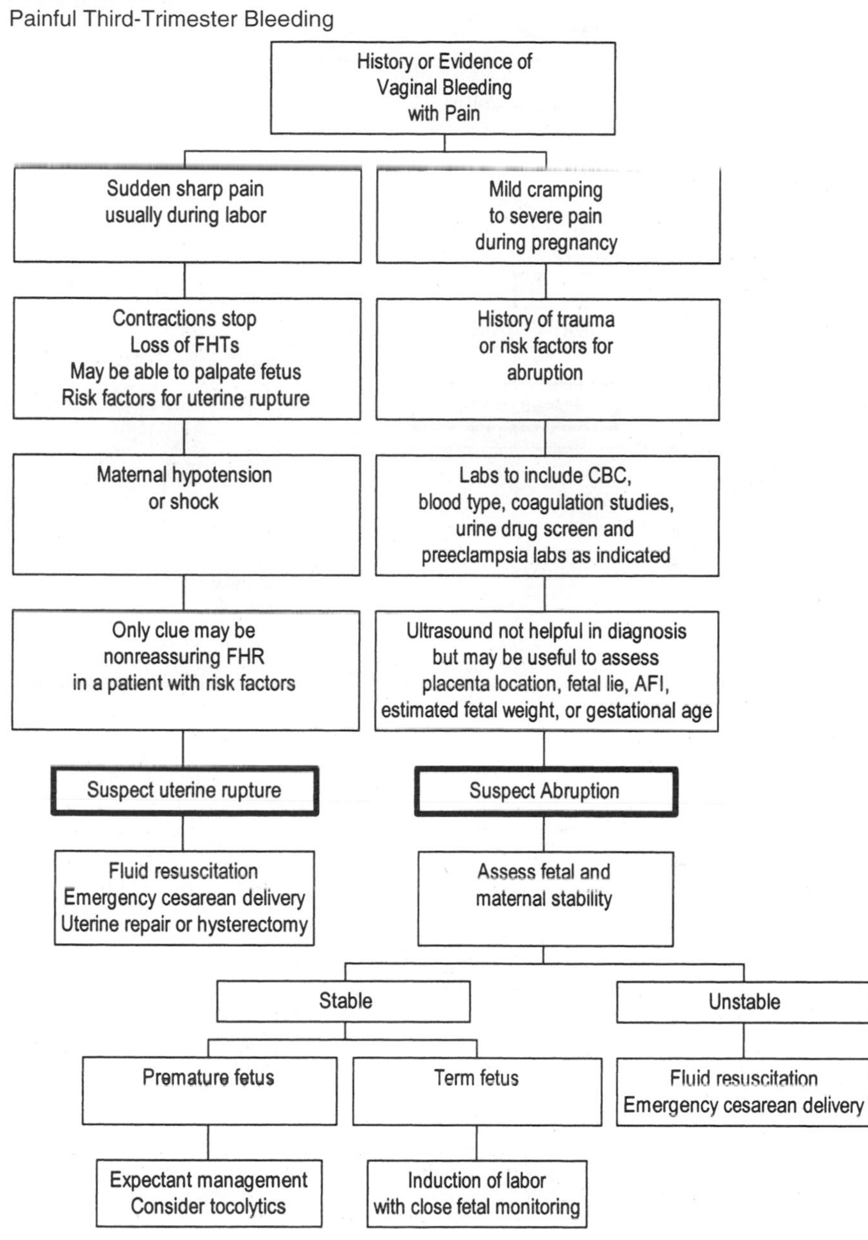

FIGURE 5.6

Painless Third-Trimester Bleeding

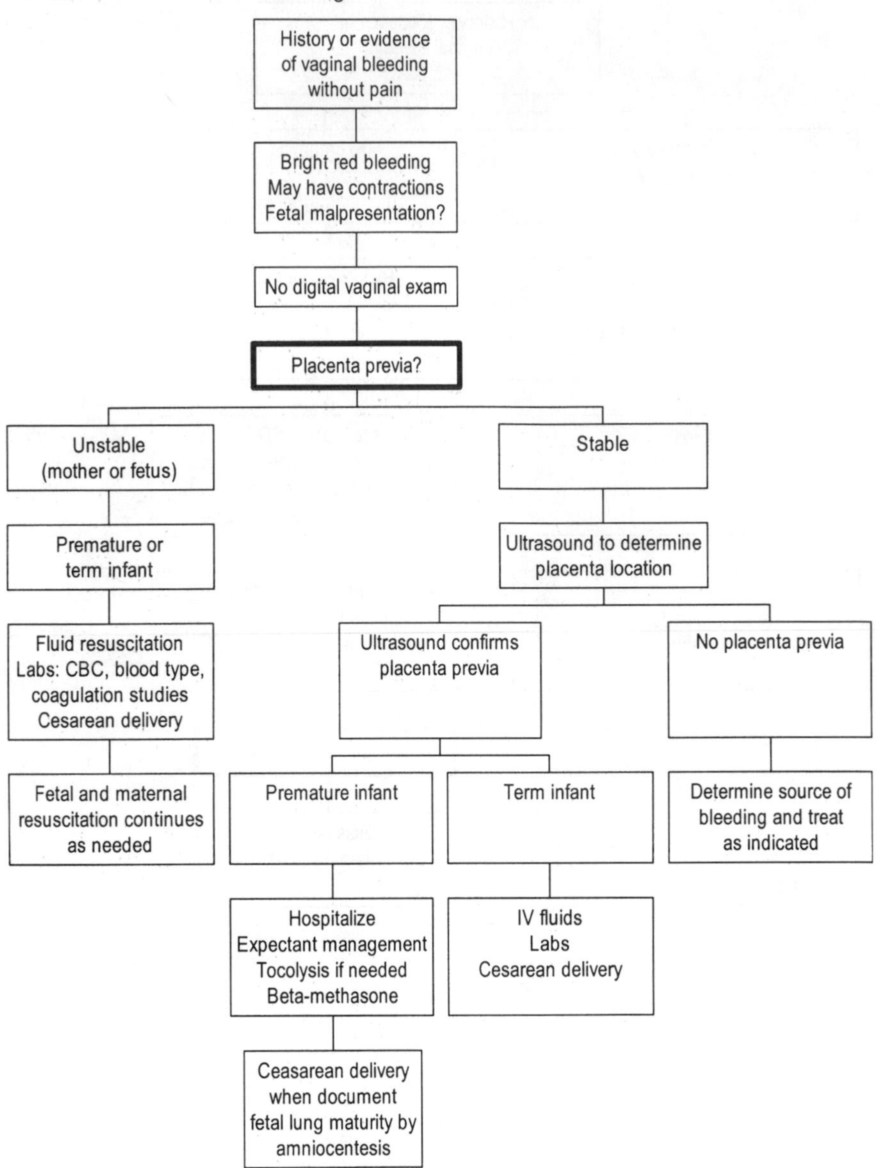

FIGURE 5.7

Abnormalities of Amniotic Fluid Volume: Causes and Complications

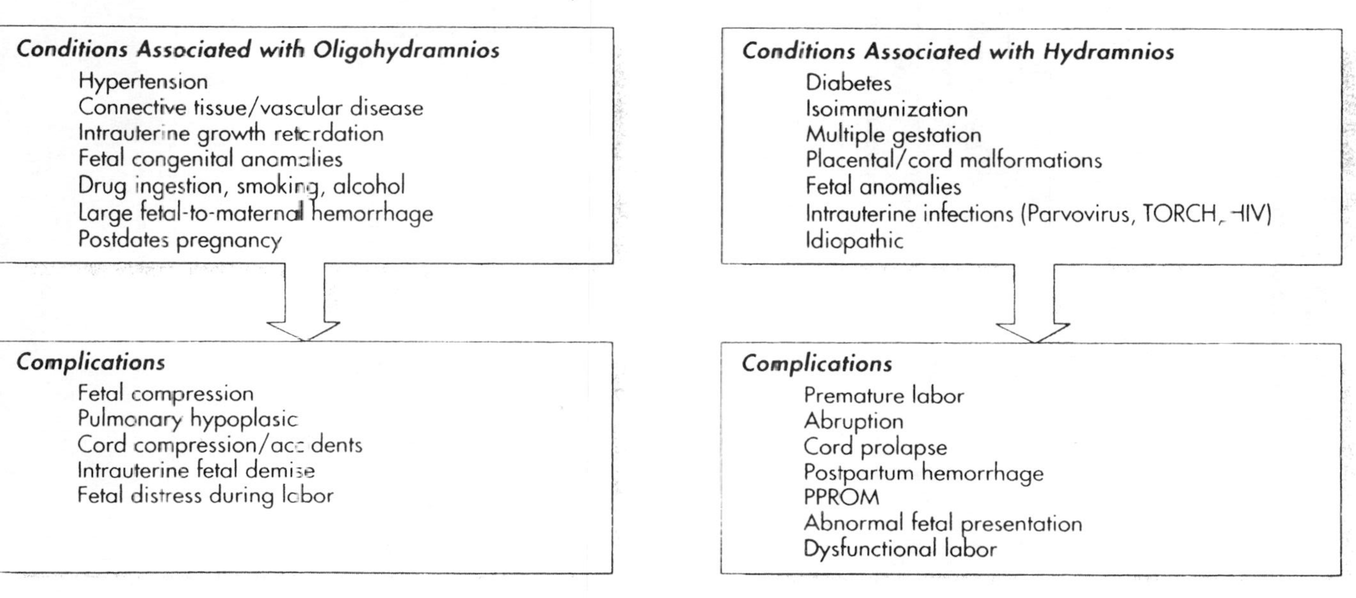

Adapted from Smith CS, Weiner S, Bolognese RJ. Amniotic fluid volume: importance and assessment. *The Female Patient.* 1990;15:87.

FIGURE 5.8

Management of Abnormalities of Amniotic Fluid Volume

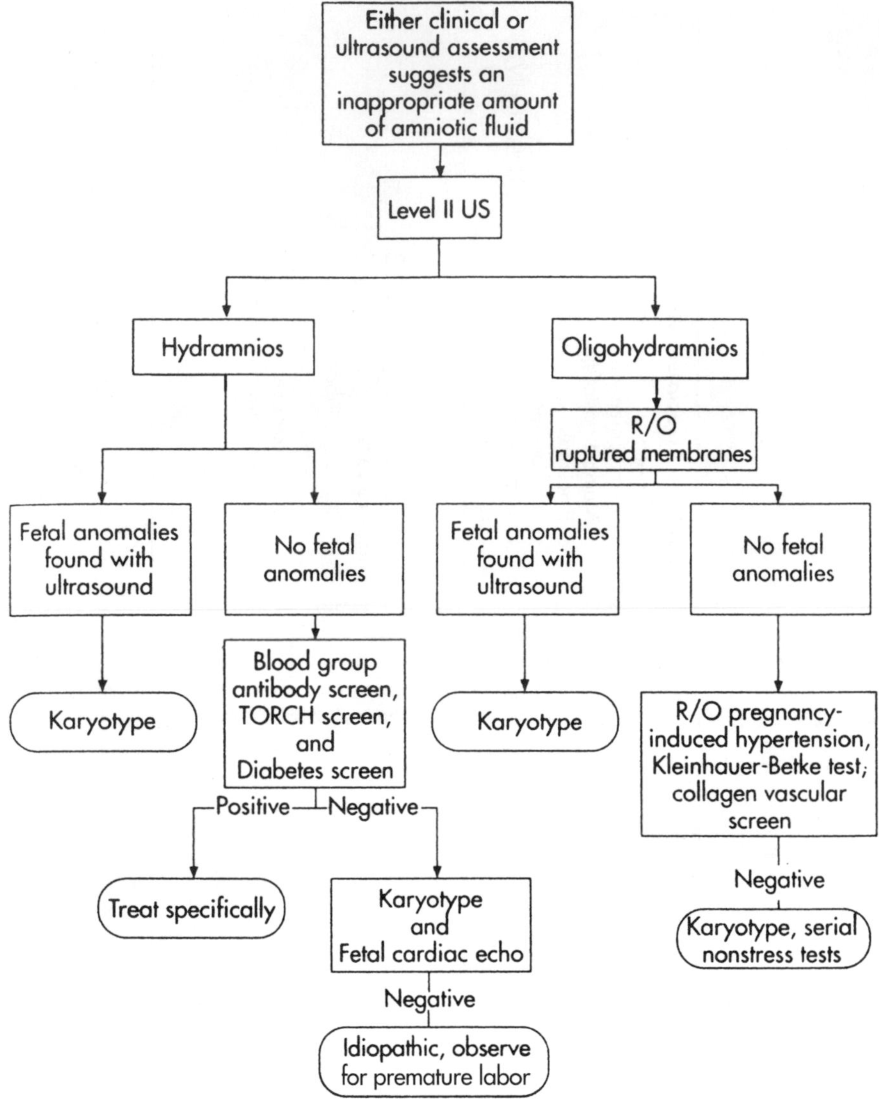

Adapted from Smith CS, Weiner S, Bolognese RJ. Amniotic fluid volume: importance and assessment. *The Female Patient*. 1990;15:87.

TABLE 5.32

Diagnosis of Preterm Premature Rupture of Membranes (PPROM)

Spontaneous premature rupture of membranes usually occurs at or near term. Ninety-five percent of term pregnancies and 50% of preterm pregnancies will enter labor in the first 24 hours. Seventy-five percent of preterm pregnancies will deliver within 1 week. Increased incidence of malformations with PPROM. Intra-amniotic infection is common. There is an increased risk of fetal malpresentation, abruption, cesarean delivery, and complications related to prematurity. PPROM at less than 26 weeks is associated with an increased risk of pulmonary hypoplasia. Evidence of fetal compromise or chorioamnionitis is an indication for immediate delivery regardless of gestational age.

Diagnosis

History of sudden gush of fluid or continuous leaking of fluid
Palpate uterus for estimation of fetal size
External fetal monitoring for contractions and fetal heart rate tracing
Sterile speculum examination to visualize the cervix, look for pooling of amniotic fluid or meconium staining, and collect samples:

- Cultures for gonorrhea, chlamydia (cervical), and group B *Streptococcus* (rectovaginal)
- Vaginal fluid allowed to air dry onto glass slide for fern test (amniotic fluid crystallizes and looks like a fern); false positive with cervical mucus
- Nitrazine paper to check for alkaline pH (paper turns blue if positive [false positives in presence of semen, blood, alkaline antiseptics, or bacterial vaginosis])
- Wet prep of vaginal fluid
- Sample of fluid from external os on a glass slide then heated; amniotic fluid turns white and cervical mucus turns brown
- Sample for evaluation for fetal lung maturity (phosphatidylglycerol and lecithin/sphingomyelin [L/S] ratio)

If rupture is uncertain, ultrasound to evaluate for oligohydramnios is useful.

If still uncertain, indigo carmine dye can be infused transabdominally with ultrasound guidance into amniotic fluid, with observation for passage of blue fluid vaginally.

TABLE 5.33

Management of Preterm Premature Rupture of Membranes without Evidence of Amnionitis

Gestational Age	Management
<24 weeks (nonviable fetus)	Counsel parents regarding the risks of induction of labor verses expectant management; hospitalization not shown to be beneficial
24–30 weeks	Expectant management to include bed rest, pelvic rest, hospitalize and monitor for signs and symptoms of infection and/or labor; consider corticosteroids and antibiotics; tocolytics have unclear benefit
30–32 weeks	Expectant management; consider corticosteroids and antibiotics; maternal and fetal monitoring
32–36 weeks	Induction after establishing positive fetal lung maturity; expectant management prior to this; antibiotics beneficial
>36 weeks	Induction of labor if not spontaneous after 12–28 hours

TABLE 5.34

Diagnosis of Amnionitis

Clinical	Laboratory
Maternal fever	Amniocentesis with positive gram stain, culture, or glucose >20 mg/dL is diagnostic
Maternal tachycardia	Leukocytes in amniotic fluid are nondiagnostic
Fetal tachycardia	Leukocytosis is nonspecific
Uterine tenderness	

FIGURE 5.9

Strategies for Prevention of Perinatal Group B Streptococcal (GBS) Infections*

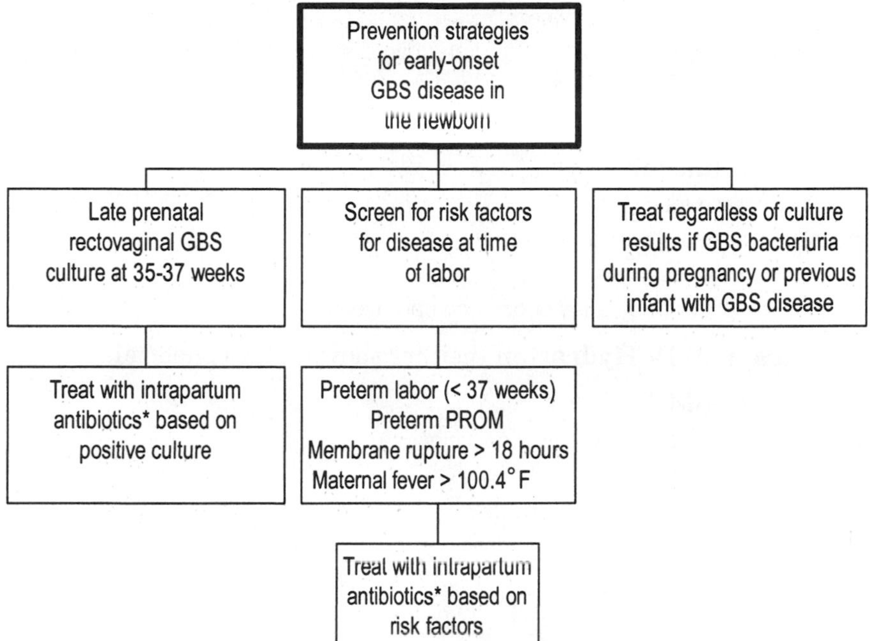

* Based on the current CDC recommendations from MMWR, 1996. See www.cdc.gov for updated recommendations.

** CDC recommends intravenous Penicillin G 5 million units initially then 2.5 million units every 4 hours until delivery (IV ampicillin is also acceptable). Use clindamycin or erythromycin if allergic to penicillin.

TABLE 5.35

Management of Premature Labor

- Onset of labor prior to 37 weeks
- Occurs in approximately 10% of all pregnancies
- Associated with a high rate of neonatal morbidity and mortality
- Presence of cervical change with dilation of at least 2 cm or effacement of 80%

Initial Evaluation

- Maternal and fetal stability
- Determine gestational age
- Imminence of delivery
- Potential underlying cause or other complications

Bed Rest and IV Hydration (neither shown to be beneficial)

Corticosteroids

- Appropriate at 24–34 weeks of gestation
- No contraindications
- Shown to reduce the incidence of RDS, IVH, and infant mortality
- Betamethasone, 12 mg IM in 2 doses, 24 hours apart
- Dexamethasone, 6 mg IM in 4 doses, 12 hours apart

Tocolytics

- Effective for delaying delivery for 24–48 hours (allow time for corticosteroids or patient transfer if needed)
- No proven benefit to long-term therapy
- Given if definite preterm labor, maternal and fetal stability established, no contraindications (maternal or fetal), and cervix is <4 cm dilated

IM indicates intramuscular; IV, intravenous; IVH, intraventricular hemorrhage; RDS, respiratory distress syndrome.

TABLE 5.36

Management of Preterm Labor with Tocolytics

Drug	Dose	Side Effects	Contraindications
Terbutaline	0.25 mg SQ q1–4 hours or 2.5–5 mg PO q 6 hours	Maternal or fetal tachycardia, palpitations, chest pain, anxiety, tremor, nausea, dyspnea, headache, pulmonary edema	Hypertension, cardiovascular disease, uncontrolled diabetes, hyperthyroidism, hemorrhage
Ritodrine	IV infusion started at 0.1 mg/min then titrated by 0.05 mg/min q 10 min until labor suppressed, max dose is 0.35 mg/min	Same as terbutaline and hypokalemia, hyperglycemia, cardiac ischemia	Same as terbutaline and multiple gestation and hypovolemia
Magnesium sulfate	IV infusion started as a 4–6 g bolus then run at 1–4 g/hr, therapeutic level is 5.5–7.5 mg/dL	Depends on serum levels; loss of DTRs, somnolence, slurred speech, respiratory depression, decreased urine output, pulmonary edema	Impaired renal function, myasthenia gravis, recent MI
Nifedipine	10–20 mg PO q 4–8 hours	Edema, hypotension, tachycardia, nausea, flushing, dizziness, bowel changes	Concurrent use with $MgSO_4$, CHF, aortic stenosis
Indomethacin	25–100 mg PR initially then 25 mg PO q 4–6 hours	Oligohydramnios, premature closure of the ductus arteriosus, edema, bleeding, GI upset, nausea, vomiting	Renal disease, peptic ulcer disease, coagulopathy, hypersensitivity to drug, gestational age over 30 weeks

CHF indicates congestive heart failure; DTRs, deep tendon reflexes; GI, gastrointestinal; IV, intravenous; $MgSO_4$, magnesium sulfate; MI, myocardial infarction; PO, orally; PR, rectally; SQ, subcutaneously.

HYPERTENSION IN PREGNANCY

- Most common medical disorder of pregnancy.
- Occurs in 5–10% of all pregnancies.
- Major cause of maternal and fetal morbidity and mortality.
- Preeclampsia has classic triad of elevated blood pressure, edema, and proteinuria.
- Chronic hypertension has documented hypertension prior to pregnancy or prior to 20 weeks of gestation; can have superimposed preeclampsia.
- Transient hypertension is defined as blood pressure elevation in pregnancy without evidence of preeclampsia.
- Eclampsia is defined as seizures or coma in the presence of preeclampsia without other neurological cause.

TABLE 5.37

Classification of Preeclampsia

Parameter	Mild to Moderate	Severe
CNS	Hyperreflexia, headache	Seizures, blurred vision, scotomas, headache, clonus, irritability
Renal	Proteinuria of 300 mg to 4 g/24 hours	Proteinuria >5 g/24 hours
Hepatic	LFTs normal	LFTs elevated, epigastric pain, ruptured liver
Hematological	Hemoglobin normal	Hemoglobin elevated
Blood pressure	<160/110 mm Hg	>160/110 mm Hg
Fetal	No evidence of IUGR, oligohydramnios, or fetal distress	IUGR, oligohydramnios, fetal distress

CNS indicates central nervous system; IUGR, intrauterine growth retardation; LFTs, liver function tests.

FIGURE 5.10

Management Strategies for Mild to Moderate Preeclampsia

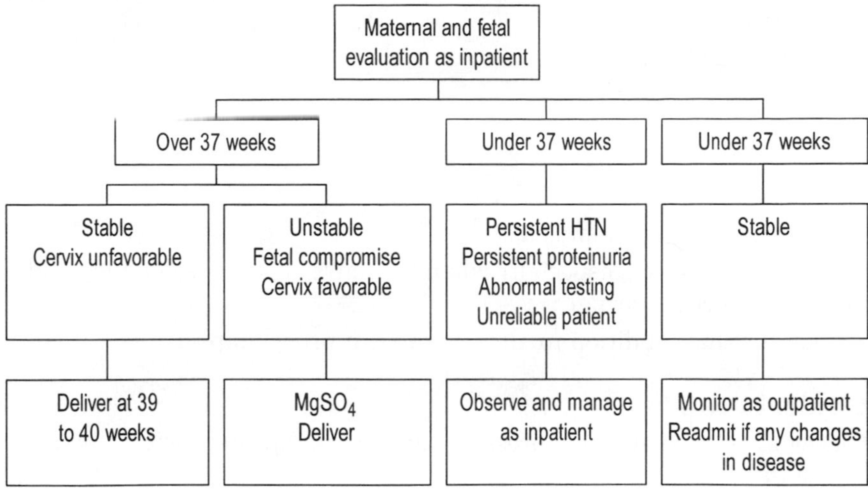

FIGURE 5.11

Management Strategies for Severe Preeclampsia

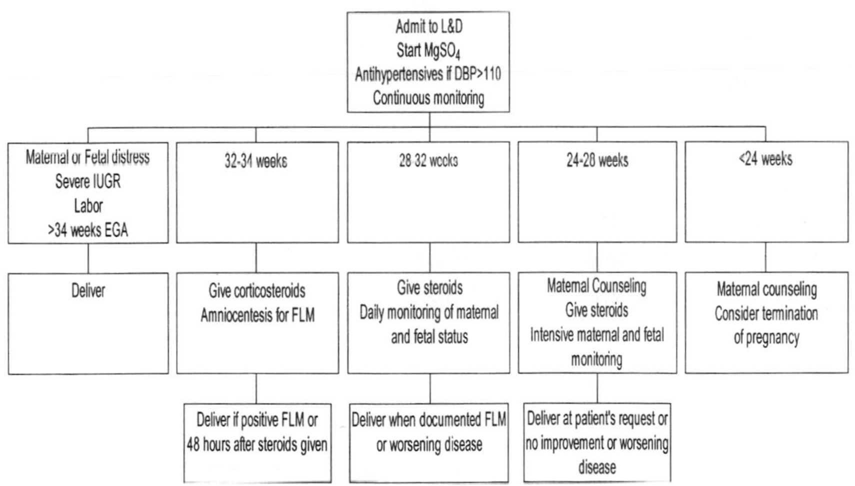

TABLE 5.38

HELLP Syndrome

Definition
Intravascular **H**emolysis
Elevated **L**iver enzymes
Low **P**latelet count
Syndrome
Form of severe preeclampsia
Often misdiagnosed, especially when it occurs early in pregnancy and blood pressure is normal
Screen for this condition in all women with preeclampsia
Clinical Features
Classic triad of high blood pressure, edema, and proteinuria
Platelets $<100\ 000/\mu L$
Elevated AST (SGOT)
Documented hemolysis (elevated LDH and bilirubin, abnormal peripheral blood smear)
Complications
Disseminated intravascular coagulation (DIC), most common
Placental abruption
Acute renal failure
Eclampsia
Management
Assess cardiovascular status and support as needed
Monitor liver enzymes and platelet count
Start $MgSO_4$ for seizure prophylaxis
Treat DIC
Continuous fetal monitoring
Deliver as soon as possible

AST indicates aspartate aminotransferase; DIC, disseminated intravascular coagulation; LDH, lactic denydrogenase; $MgSO_4$, magnesium sulfate; SGOT, serum glutamic oxaloacetic transaminase.

TABLE 5.39

Drugs Used in Preeclampsia

Magnesium Sulfate

- Used for seizure prophylaxis
- Continued post partum
- Start as 4–6 g bolus, then continue as an infusion usually at 2 g/hour
- Therapeutic levels are 4–8 mg/dL
- Watch for signs and symptoms of toxicity
- Calcium gluconate given as 1 gram over 2 minutes to reverse toxicity

Hydralazine

- Used for diastolic BP >110 mm Hg or systolic BP >180 mm Hg
- Give as 5–10 mg IV bolus every 20 minutes
- Keep diastolic BP between 90 and 110 mm Hg
- Watch for tachycardia and hypotension

Labetalol

- Used as a second-line agent to hydralazine
- Give as 20 mg IV every 10 minutes to a maximum of 300 mg

BP indicates blood pressure; IV, intravenous.

FIGURE 5.12

Management of Trauma in Pregnancy

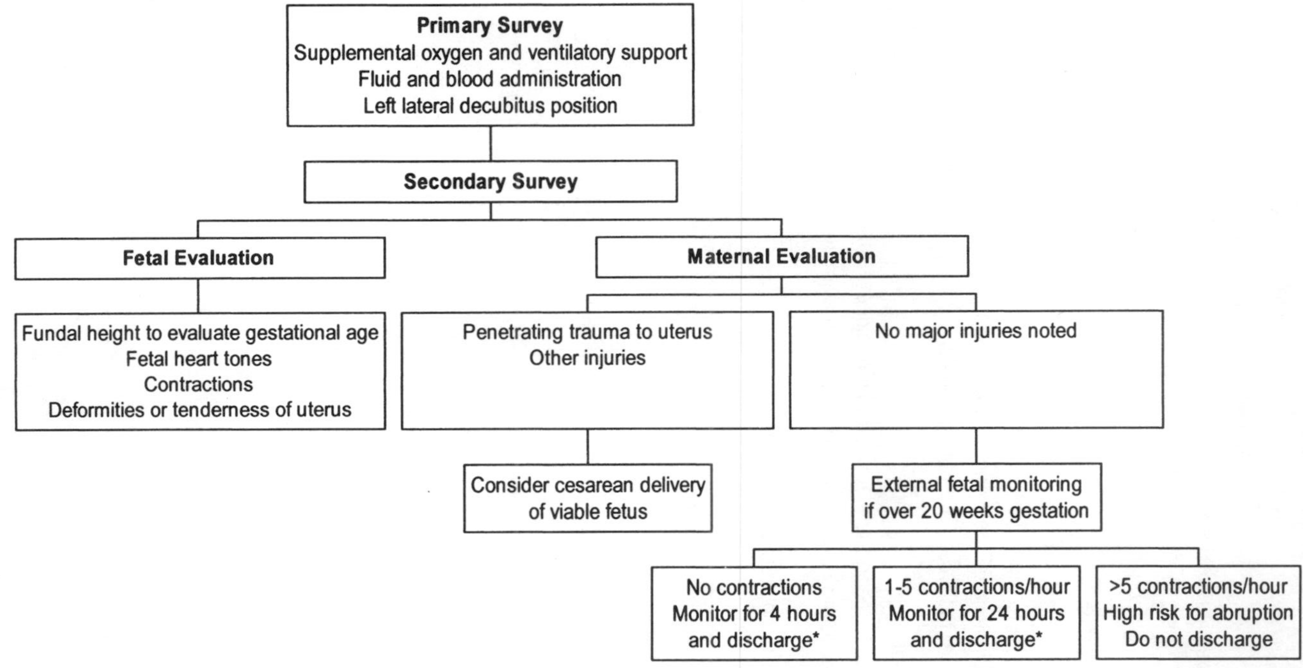

*Discharge criteria: Reassuring fetal heart rate tracing, intact membranes, no uterine tenderness, no vaginal bleeding, and no uterine irritability. Rh-negative mothers receive 300 μg of Rh immune globulin, unless Kleihauer-Betke testing indicates more is needed. (Give 300 μg for every 30 cc of transfused fetal blood.)

TABLE 5.40

Antepartum Fetal Surveillance

COMMENTS

- Usually initiated at 32–34 weeks in selected patients, may need earlier testing for certain high-risk patients
- Frequency of testing depends on the reason for the testing, weekly or biweekly if condition that prompted the testing persists
- Purpose is to decrease the risk of fetal death, although there is only observational data to support this
- Oligohydramnios or abnormal test results may indicate the need for delivery; clinical judgment should be used in these cases

INDICATIONS FOR TESTING

- High-risk pregnancy (maternal or fetal)
- Decreased fetal movements
- Oligo- or polyhydramnios
- Intrauterine growth restriction
- Postterm pregnancy
- Previous fetal demise

METHODS OF TESTING

Fetal Kick Counts

- Assessment of fetal movement
- Different methods: 10 movements in 2 hours, counts three times a week

Nonstress Test (NST)

- Fetal heart rate accelerates with fetal movements in the nonacidotic and not neurologically depressed fetus
- Fetal heart rate tracing reactive when accelerations peak at least 15 beats per minute above the baseline and last for at least 15 seconds from baseline to baseline
- Reactive tracing has at least two accelerations in a 20-minute period
- Nonreactive tracing has less than two accelerations during a 40-minute period
- Acoustic stimulation may be needed to elicit an acceleration
- Nonreactive NST may occur in a normal fetus, especially at earlier gestational ages

Contraction Stress Test (CST)

- Need to have at least 3 contractions lasting at least 40 seconds in a 10-minute period
- May need to induce contractions with nipple stimulation or intravenous oxytocin
- Interpretation based on the presence or absence of late decelerations
- Negative: no late or significant variable decelerations
- Positive: late decelerations following at least 50% of contractions

Continued

TABLE 5.40

Antepartum Fetal Surveillance, cont'd

- Equivocal: intermittent late or significant variable decelerations or decelerations in the presence of uterine hyperstimulation
- Unsatisfactory: less than three contractions in a 10-minute period or tracing is uninterpretable
- Relative contraindications: risk of preterm labor, preterm rupture of membranes, previous uterine surgery, placenta previa

Biophysical Profile (BPP)

- Five components with either 2 points if present or 0 points if absent
- Components 2–5 are done by ultrasound of the fetus
    1. Nonstress test
    2. Fetal movement: three or more discrete body or limb movements in a 30-minute period
    3. Fetal tone: one or more episodes of extension and then flexion of an extremity or opening and closing a hand
    4. Amniotic fluid volume: one vertical pocket measuring at least 2 cm
    5. Fetal breathing movements: one episode lasting 30 seconds in a 30-minute period
- Score of 8 or 10 is normal, 6 is equivocal, and 4 or less is abnormal (if amniotic fluid volume is absent, need further evaluation regardless of other components)

Umbilical Artery Doppler Velocimetry

- Useful in growth-restricted fetuses
- High rate of perinatal mortality if flow is absent or reversed
- Need to assess multiple waveforms by an experienced ultrasound technologist

Adapted from The American College of Obstetricians and Gynecologist, Practice Bulletin No. 9, *Antepartum Fetal Surveillances*, September 1999.

TABLE 5.41

Fetal Heart Rate Monitoring

Baseline

Normal is 120–160 bpm

<120 over a 10-minute period is bradycardia (normal [usually not <90 bpm], congenital heart block, drugs, hypothermia, hypoxia)

>160 over a 10-minute period is tachycardia (infection, fever, drugs, asphyxia, prematurity, thyrotoxicosis, arrythmia)

Variability

Short-term or beat-to-beat requires a fetal scalp electrode

Long-term

- normal is 6- to 25-beat variation around the baseline
- decreased is 3 to 6 beat variation
- absent is <3-beat variation
- marked is >25-beat variation

Accelerations

Fetal heart rate increases 15 beats above the baseline with a return to baseline in ≥15 seconds

Decelerations

Early

- Mirrors the contraction
- Usually from head compression

Variable

- Occurs at any time and is variable in appearance
- Usually a sign of cord compression

Late

- Onset is after the start of the contraction and ends after the contraction
- Uniform in shape
- Indication of uteroplacental insufficiency

Special Considerations

Reassuring FHR pattern when all parameters are normal

Nonreassuring pattern when persistent late or variable decelerations, decreased or absent variability, or other persistent abnormal FHR tracings

Sinusoidal pattern of smooth, regular sine wave pattern, ominous FHR pattern

Pseudosinusoidal pattern of regular sine wave pattern of low amplitude, seen with maternal narcotic administration

Saltatory pattern of marked variability with a bizarre pattern

bpm indicates beats per minute; FHR, fetal heart rate.

FIGURE 5.13

Changes in Fetal Heart Rate Patterns due to Various Causes

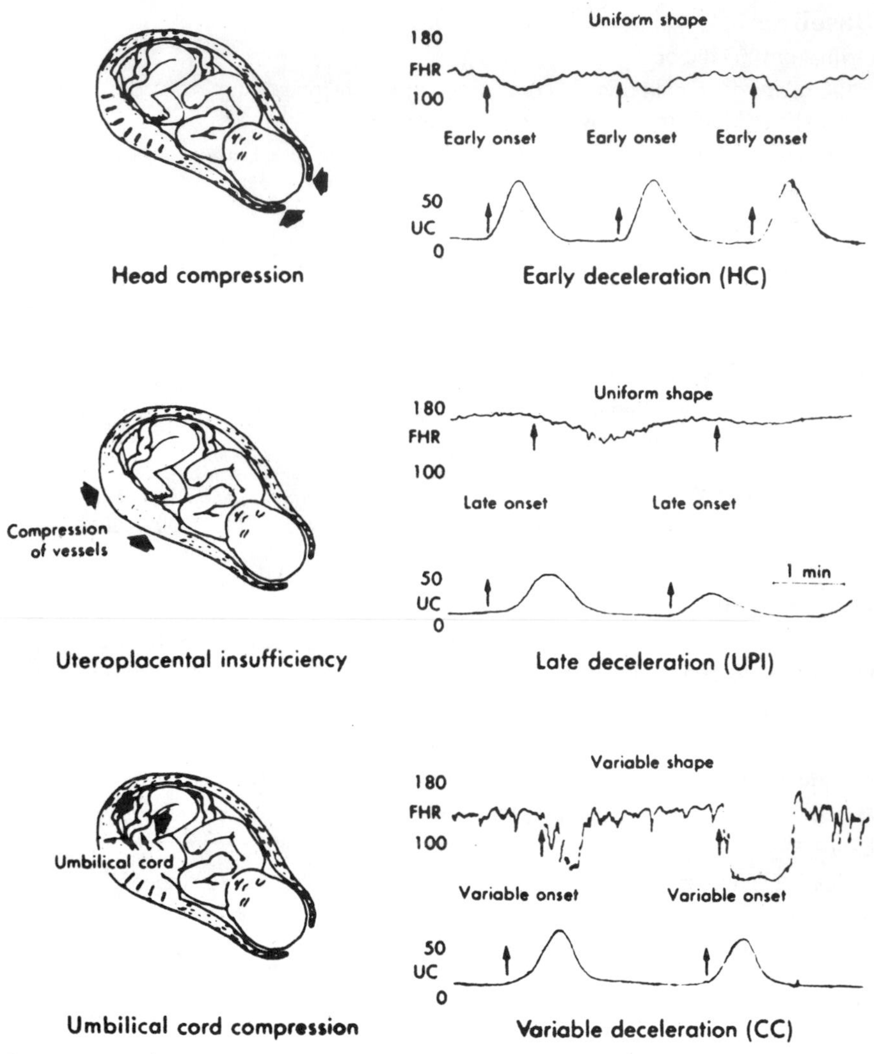

Reproduced with permission from Hon EH. *An Atlas of Fetal Heart Rate Patterns.* New Haven, Ct: Harty Press;1968.

TABLE 5.42

Fetal Blood Scalp Sampling

Indications

Abnormal fetal heart rate tracing
Suspected fetal acidosis

Contraindications

Bleeding disorder
Amnionitis

Procedure

Cervix must be dilated at least 2 cm with patient in the dorsal lithotomy position
Endoscope is passed through the cervix and the fetal scalp is visualized
Scalp is swabbed with ethyl chloride and then silicon
A 2–3 mm puncture is made with a small scalp blade
Blood is drawn into a collection tube for analysis

Interpretation

Scalp pH of 7.25 to 7.40 is normal, pH <7.2 is ominous
Po_2 is usually 18–25 mm Hg and Pco_2 is usually 40–50 mm Hg

TABLE 5.43

Intrauterine Resuscitation of Nonreassuring Fetal Heart Rate Pattern

Place mother in right or left lateral decubitus position
Start mask O_2 at 8 L/min
Start IV fluids with D_5NS or D_5LR, bolus then run at 125–200 mL/hr
Stop oxytocin if infusing and consider terbutaline to arrest labor
Do vaginal exam to assess for prolapsed cord and cervical dilation, effacement, and fetal station
Place intrauterine pressure catheter and fetal scalp electrode if indicated
Consider amnioinfusion

IV indicates intravenous; D_5NS, 5% dextrose in 0.9% sodium chloride; D_5LR, 5% dextrose in lactated ringer solution.

TABLE 5.44

Assessment of Fetal Maturity

Assessment	Criteria
Clinical assessment of fetal maturity (based on ACOG guidelines)	■ Documented fetal heart tones for 30 weeks by Doppler or 20 weeks by nonelectronic fetoscope ■ 36 weeks have lapsed since a positive serum or urine β-HCG pregnancy test ■ Ultrasound at 6–11 weeks shows a crown-rump length measurement consistent with a gestational age of ≥39 weeks ■ Ultrasound measurement at 12–20 weeks supports a gestational age ≥39 weeks based on clinical criteria
Amniocentesis	■ L/S ratio of 2.0 or higher (higher in diabetics) ■ Phosphatidylglycerol is present

ACOG indicates American College of Obstetricians and Gynecologists; β-HCG, β-human chorionic gonadotropin; L/S, indicates lecithin to sphingomyelin ratio.

TABLE 5.45

Bishop Score for Labor Inducibility

Score ≥9 indicates induction of labor should be successful. Score of 0–4 indicates a success rate of 50–55%, 5–9 indicates 90% success rate, ≥10 is almost 100% success rate.

Factor	0	1	2	3
Cervical dilation (cm)	Closed	1–2	3–4	≥5
Effacement (%)	0–30	40–50	60–70	≥80
Fetal station	−3	−2	−1	+1 or +2
Consistency of cervix	Firm	Medium	Soft	—
Position of cervix	Posterior	Mid	Anterior	—

TABLE 5.46

Induction of Labor*

Document reason, gestational age, fetal position, fetal lung maturity, if indicated, and fetal heart tones prior to induction.

Agent	Dosage	Special Considerations
PGE_2 gel	0.5 mg applied every 6 hours for 2–3 doses	Increases the Bishop score but no decrease in rate of cesarean delivery 1% rate of hyperstimulation Wait at least 6–12 hours prior to starting oxytocin Fetal monitoring for 30 min to 2 hours after application
PGE_2 insert (cervidil)	10 mg released as 0.3 mg/hr	Single application placed in posterior vaginal fornix 5% rate of hyperstimulation Wait 30–60 min after removal to start oxytocin Continuous fetal monitoring
PGE_1 (misoprostol)	25 μg every 4–6 hours for 1–3 doses	Increase rate of uterine rupture in VBAC candidates Wait 4 hours after application prior to starting pitocin More studies needed to determine recommended dose, frequency of administration, and recommended fetal monitoring
Mechanical dilators	Laminaria Foley catheter	Forcibly dilates cervix by pressure Increased risk of infection
Rupture of membranes		High rate of success if high Bishop score Risk of prolonged rupture of membranes, prolapsed cord or compression of cord, infection, and rupture of vasa previa
Oxytocin	Start infusion at 0.5–2 mU/min and increase by 1– 2 mU/min every 15–30 min until adequate labor	Different protocols for preparation and infusion Half-life 4 min, can stop infusion if hyperstimulation occurs Continuous fetal monitoring is recommended Water intoxication if prolonged administration or high doses (40 mU/min)

FDA indicates Food and Drug Administration; PG, prostaglandin; VBAC, vaginal birth after cesarean.

*Data based on American College of Obstetricians and Gynecologists Practice Bulletin No. 10, Induction of Labor, November 1999.

TABLE 5.47

Cervical Dilation: Translating Fingers into Centimeters

Fingers	Centimeters
1 (tight)	1
1 (loose)	2
2 (tight)	3
2 (loose to slightly spread)	4
2 (spread)	5–7
1 fingerbreadth of lateral cervix	8
1/2 fingerbreadth of lateral cervix remaining on each side	9
Only anterior cervix palpable	9+ (anterior lip)
No palpable cervix	10 (complete dilation)

Adapted from Iffy L, Kaminetzky H. *Principles and Practice of Obstetrics and Perinatology*. Vol 2. New York: John Wiley & Sons; 1981: 818.

TABLE 5.48

Vaginal Birth After Cesarean Section (VBAC)*

Advantages

- Lower maternal morbidity and mortality if successful (no randomized trials)
- Success rate about 60–80%
- Shorter hospital stay
- Better immediate bonding with the infant
- Less blood loss
- Lower cost

Disadvantages

- Increased risk of complications with unsuccessful trial of labor
- Potential for uterine rupture (4–9% risk with classic incision/0.2–1.5% risk with low transverse incision)
- Risk of rupture increases with increased number of uterine scars
- Poor outcome for mother and fetus if uterine rupture

Guidelines for lowering the risk

- Accurate number and type of prior cesarean sections (1 or 2)
- Prior incision was low transverse and no other uterine scars or previous rupture
- No recurrent indications (cephalopelvic disproportion, maternal herpes, maternal systemic disease)
- No new indication (placenta previa, fetal distress, malpresentation)
- Patient counseled carefully for informed consent with documentation
- Admit when in active labor
- Have IV in place
- Type and cross for 2 units of packed RBCs
- Continuous fetal monitoring
- Emergency cesarean section can be performed within 30 minutes of decision with availability of anesthesia and personnel
- Primary physician in constant attendance during labor

Contraindications

- Prior classic or "T"-shaped uterine incision
- Prior transfundal uterine surgery
- Contracted pelvis
- Medical or obstetrical complication that requires a cesarean delivery
- Inability to perform an emergency cesarean section

IV indicates intravenous; RBCs, red blood cells.

*Data from American College of Obstetricians and Gynecologists Practice Bulletin No. 5, *Vaginal Birth After Previous Cesarean Delivery*, July 1999.

TABLE 5.49

Stages of Labor

Stage of labor	Definition	Duration/Rate Nulliparas	Multiparas
First stage: Latent	Dilation up to 4–5 cm, slow dilation	21 hours, ≤0.5 cm/hour	14 hours, ≤0.5 cm/hour
First stage: Active	Phase of maximal dilation followed by a deceleration phase that ends with complete dilation	1.0 cm/hour	1.0–2.0 cm/hour
Descent	Occurs in the first and second stages but mostly in the second	1.0 cm/hour	1.5 cm/hour
Second stage	From full dilation to delivery	2 hours	1 hour
Third stage	From delivery of fetus to delivery of placenta	<15–30 min	<15–30 min
Total labor	Onset of labor to delivery of placenta	25.8 hours (mean 10.0)	19.5 hours (mean 6.2)

Adapted from Iffy L, Kaminetzky H. *Principles and Practice of Obstetrics and Perinatology*. New York: John Wiley & Sons; 1981.

TABLE 5.50

Dysfunctional Labors: Diagnosis and Management

Latent Phase Disorders (Before 4 cm of Cervical Dilation)

Dx: Prolonged latent phase is >20 hours in nulliparas; >14 hours in multiparas

Causes

Unripe cervix 18%	Sedation 19%	Unknown 17%
False labor 10%	Anesthesia 7%	
Uterine inertia 9%	CPD rare	

Rx

False labor observed (10%): Discharge

Observed to progress: Expect NSVD or cesarean

Fail to progress (5%): Oxytocin stimulation

Active Phase Disorders (From ≥4–5 cm of Cervical Dilation)

Dx: Primary dysfunctional labor is <1.2 cm/hr nullipara; <1.5 cm/hr multipara

Causes

CPD 28%	Sedation 42%
Malposition 74%	Anesthesia 14%

Rx

CPD: Cesarean section

Other causes: Observed and two out of three progress to vaginal delivery

If cervical dilation not progressing and you suspect uterine inertia, try oxytocin stimulation

Dx: Secondary arrest of labor is in active phase but without full dilation

Causes

CPD 45%	Malposition 73%	Exhaustion
Sedation 63%	Anesthesia 19%	

Rx

CPD: Cesarean section

Other causes: Try oxytocin; many will require cesarean delivery.

NOTE: All dysfunctional labors should be monitored with internal fetal scalp electrode and uterine pressure catheter as soon as insertion is possible.

Adapted from Friedman EA, et al. *Obstet Gynecol.* 1965; 25:845.

CPD indicates cephalopelvic disproportion; Dx, diagnosis; NSVD, normal spontaneous vaginal delivery; Rx, treatment.

FIGURE 5.14

Friedman Labor Curves Typifying Various Normal and Abnormal Patterns of Cervical Dilation.

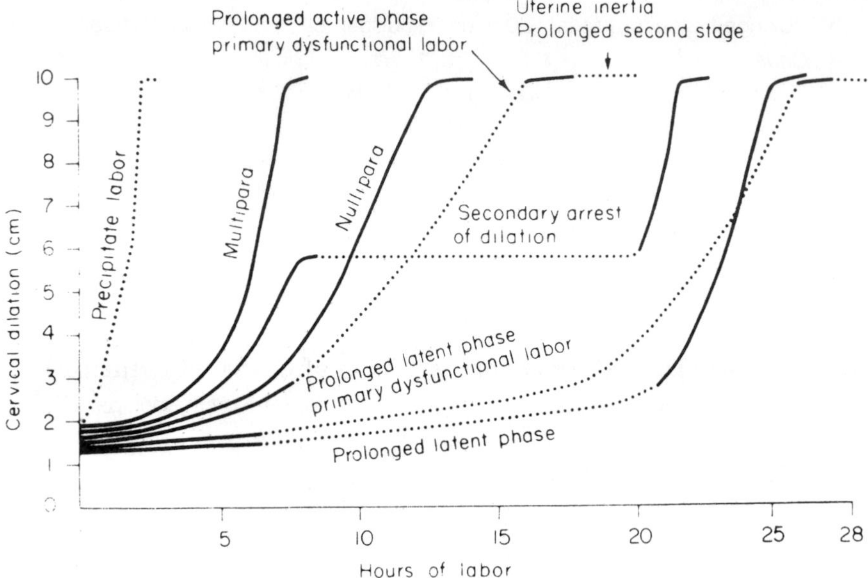

Reproduced with permission from Vorherr H. Disorders of uterine function during pregnancy. In: Assali NS, ed. *Pathophysiology of Gestation*. New York: Academic Press; 1972:191.

FIGURE 5.15

Management of Shoulder Dystocia

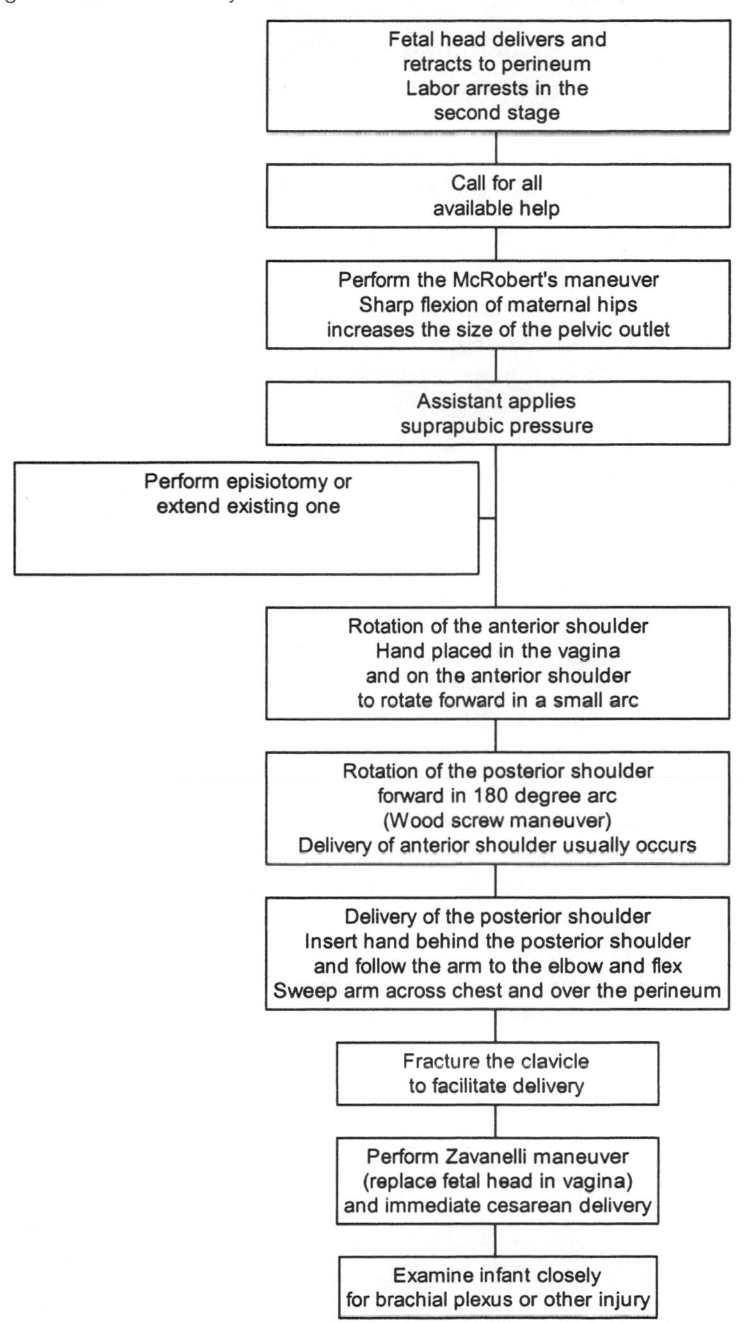

TABLE 5.51

Guidelines for the Use of Forceps

Use in the Event of the Following:

- Cervix dilated to 10 cm, membranes ruptured
- Fetal head on or just above pelvic floor (below interspinous plane), eg, low or outlet forceps
- Vertex or face presentation, or aftercoming head of a breech

Indications

- Obliterated perineal reflex, as with conduction anesthesia
- Maternal heart disease, hypertension, neurological disorder, vascular anomaly
- Abruptio placentae or vasa previa
- Second stage fails to progress (>2 hours) and head is well into pelvis, maternal exhaustion
- Rotatory arrest
- Some cases of fetal distress
- Breech and delivery of aftercoming head

Technique

- Use Simpson's, DeWeese, or Tarnier's forceps for primipara with fetus with long, molded head; Elliot (fenestrated) or Tucker-McLean (nonfenestrated) forceps for multipara with rounded fetal head; Kielland's forceps (no pelvic curve) for rotation; Piper forceps (long blades with deep curve) for breech
- Wash genitalia, empty bladder by straight catheterization
- Assess position of head, sutures, and fontanelles
- Give adequate anesthetic (pudendal, conduction, general)
- Insert left blade (lies to your right) first, then right, keeping hand between maternal tissue and blade
- Close forceps and check position by palpation of fetal head, maternal vaginal and cervical tissues
- Cut generous episiotomy
- Gently test pull, then pull for effect in a downward and outward axis, moving to almost vertical upward as head emerges, then remove forceps

TABLE 5.52

Use of the Vacuum Extractor for Prolonged Second Stage of Labor

Use of Mityvac Device or Silastic Cup

Indications

- Fetal distress (if delivery imminent)
- Prolonged second stage of labor
- Maternal exhaustion, weak uterine expulsive force

Contraindications

- Malpresentation (breech, face, brow); must be vertex
- Premature infant
- Intact membranes
- Incomplete cervical dilation; head not engaged
- Presenting part requires rotation
- Cephalopelvic disproportion
- Prior fetal scalp sampling

Technique

- Connect cup to pump
- Ascertain fetal head in normal vertex position and well engaged; remove scalp electrode if present
- Spread labia, fold cup, and insert into position over posterior fontanelle
- Sweep finger around edge to check for entrapped maternal tissue
- Reduce pressure to − 100 mm Hg (10–20 cm H_2O)
- With next contraction rapidly reduce pressure to −380–580 mm Hg (maximum 65 cm H_2O), and begin traction in line with the pelvic axis
- When contraction subsides, take pressure up to −100 mm Hg
- Recheck with finger sweep
- Episiotomy may be needed
- Once head delivered, remove cup; cephalohematoma occurs in about 15% of cases

Discontinue Under the Following Circumstances

- Delivery not accomplished after 10 minutes at maximum pressure or 30 minutes from start of procedure
- Cup disengages three times
- No progress after three consecutive pulls
- Fetal scalp traumatized by extractor

Complications

- Injury to maternal tissue (cervix, vaginal wall)
- Fourth-degree extension of episiotomy

Continued

TABLE 5.52

Use of the Vacuum Extractor for Prolonged Second Stage of Labor, cont'd

- Cephalohematoma (red or blue circular scalp discoloration)
- Skin swelling, petechiae, or injury to fetal scalp
- Failure to extract promptly

Adapted from The American Academy of Family Physicians. Epperly TD, Breitinger ER. Vacuum extraction. *Am Fam Phys*. 1988;38:205–210.

TABLE 5.53

Indications for Cesarean Delivery

- Previous cesarean section or uterine surgery
- Nonreassuring FHR pattern
- Cephalopelvic disproportion
- Failure to progress/descend
- Malpresentation (breech, transverse, face-mentum posterior)
- Multiple gestation, especially if malpresentation
- Obstruction of birth canal (eg, extensive condylomata acuminata)
- Placenta previa
- Prolapsed cord
- Active herpes infection
- Invasive cervical carcinoma
- Severe abruption with nonreassuring FHR pattern

FHR indicates fetal heart rate.

FIGURE 5.16

Management of Postpartum Hemorrhage

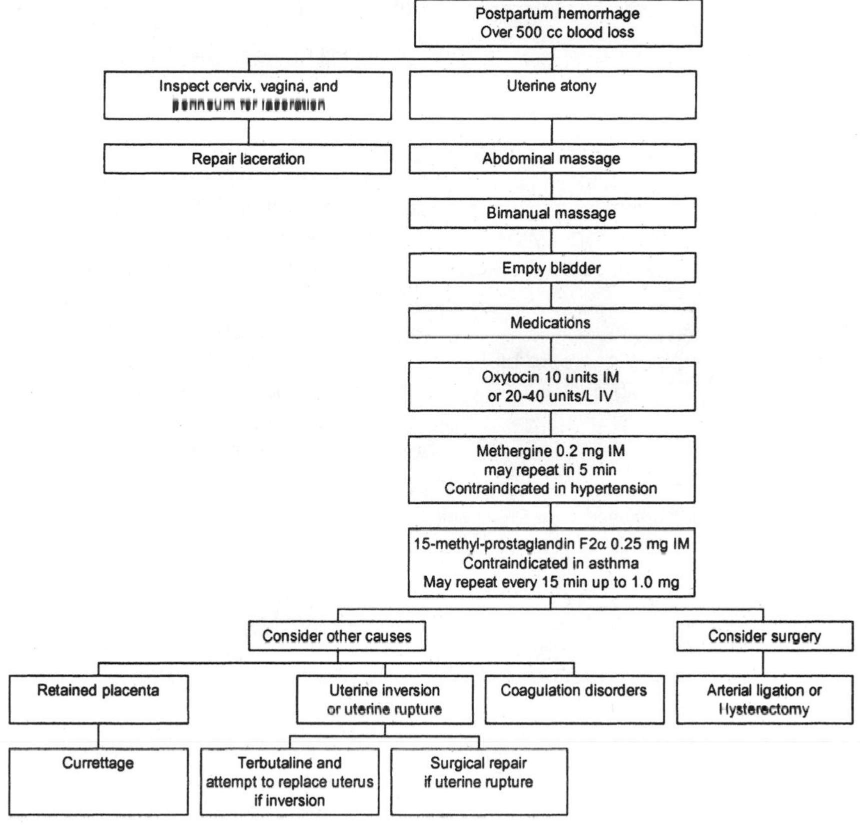

TABLE 5.54

Protocol for the Administration of RhoGAM

Office	Blood Bank
Initial Visit Draw clotted blood for ABO group, Rh type, and antibody screening test	If patient is Rh negative, and antibody screen is negative for anti-Rh_0(D), report as candidate for RhoGAM at 28 weeks and at delivery
28 Weeks *If patient is Rh negative*: Draw clotted blood for antibody screen; inject RhoGAM, 300-μg dose	If antibody screen is negative or antibody other than anti-Rh_0(D) is detected, report as candidate for RhoGAM at delivery if infant is not Rh negative
Following Delivery Collect mother's blood and cord blood; inject RhoGAM, 300-μg dose	Perform fetal cell screen on maternal sample using micro-D^u procedure. Type cord blood. If not Rh negative (D and D^u negative), issue appropriate amount of RhoGAM

Courtesy Johnson and Johnson, New Brunswick, NJ.

TABLE 5.55

Managing Common Breastfeeding Problems

Condition	Symptoms	Treatment
Sore nipples	Cracking, bleeding, pain, bruising	Proper latch-on, rinse nipple with water after feeding, express milk onto nipple and let air-dry, lanolin ointment to nipple
Engorgement	Breast large and hard	Warm water on breasts in shower, hand express or pump milk before feeding
Blocked ducts	Smooth, tender lump in breast that does not decrease after nursing	Warm compresses, massage lump toward nipple, frequent nursing
Mastitis	Fever, myalgias, warm, red, tender, wedge-shaped area on breast, usually caused by *S. aureus*, streptococcus, or *E. coli*	Frequent nursing, fluids, rest, antibiotics, warm soaks, and pain control
Breast abscess	Fever, warm, red, hard, tender mass	Usually requires incision and drainage
Candida infection	Red, tender, nipples with papules, check infant for thrush or diaper rash	Topical nystatin for mother and nystatin suspension for infant
Breast milk jaundice	Jaundice in infant at third day of life; bilirubin ≤15 mg/dL	Increase frequency of feeds, change to formula for about 24–48 hours while mother pumps in severe cases
Inhibited letdown or lactation failure	No letdown felt by mother, no uterine cramping	Frequent nursing, quiet, relaxed environment, proper infant latch-on, oxytocin nasal spray to enhance letdown
Return to work	Missed feedings	On-site feeding or breast pump,* can refrigerate breast milk for up to 48 hours and can freeze for 3–4 months
Poor infant weight gain	Infant not appropriately gaining weight	May supplement with formula, weigh infant before and after feedings to monitor intake, evaluate infant for other causes of failure to thrive

Continued

TABLE 5.55

Managing Common Breastfeeding Problems, cont'd

Condition	Symptoms	Treatment
Medications		Check for compatibility for breastfeeding, not all medications that are safe to use in pregnancy are safe to use in breastfeeding

*Check with a lactation consultant or reliable source for appropriate breast pumps.

chapter 6

Women's Health

Patricia A. Pletke, MD

IN THIS CHAPTER

- Health screening
- Breast disease
- Pap smears
- Colposcopy
- Menstrual disorders
- Endometrial aspiration
- Endometriosis
- Endometrial and ovarian cancer
- Vaginitis
- Pelvic inflammatory disease
- Contraception
- Premenstrual syndrome and PMDD
- Menstrual migraines
- Menopause

BOOKSHELF RECOMMENDATIONS

- Hatcher RA, Trussell J, Stewart F, et al, eds. *Contraceptive Technology*. 17th ed. New York: Ardent Media, Inc; 1998.
- Johnson CA, Johnson BE, Murray JL, Apgar BS, eds. *Women's Health Care Handbook*. Philadelphia: Hanley and Belfus, Inc; 1996.
- Pfenninger JL, Fowler GC, eds. *Procedures for Primary Care Physicians*. St Louis: Mosby Yearbook, Inc; 1994.
- Smith MA, Shimp LA, eds. *20 Common Problems in Women's Health Care*. New York: McGraw-Hill; 2000.
- Stosur H, Hatcher RA, Nelson A, Zieman M, Darney P, Crenin MD, eds. *A Pocket Guide to Managing Contraception*. Tiger, GA: Bridging the Gap Foundation; 2001.

TABLE 6.1

Routine Health Screening Recommendations for Women

Monitor Annually

- Height and weight
- Blood pressure
- Breast examination

Testing

- Pap Test
  - —Start with onset of sexual activity or age 18
  - —Yearly in high-risk women (multiple sexual partners, early onset of first sexual intercourse, tobacco use, low socioeconomic status)
  - —At least every 3 years in other women
  - —May discontinue after hysterectomy for benign disease or in women over 65 who have had regular normal Pap smears
- Chlamydia
  - —Screening for high risk women (age less than 25, new or multiple partners, history of prior sexually transmitted disease, unmarried, low socioeconomic status)
- Rubella Screening
  - —Done once to determine immunity; vaccinate if nonimmune and not pregnant
- Cholesterol
  - —Over age 45, monitor every 5 years if normal
- Fecal Occult Blood
  - —Annually starting at age greater than 50
- Sigmoidoscopy
  - —Every 5 years, or colonoscopy every 10 years
- Mammography
  - —Annually starting at age 40 through to age 69–75; no evidence for or against doing later in life
  - —Reasonable to consider in women with at least 5-year life expectancy
- Thyrotropin
  - —Once over age 50
- Bone Density
  - —See Chapter 17

Adapted from the USPSTF Guidelines, American College of Physicians Recommendations.

TABLE 6.2

Special Nutritional Recommendations for Women

Folic Acid

- All women of reproductive age should get 400 mcg of folic acid daily

Calcium

- Young adults: 1200–1500 mg daily
- Pregnant/nursing: 1300 mg daily
- 25–50 years old: 1000 mg daily
- Over 50 years on hormone replacement therapy: 1000–1200 mg daily
- Over 50 years not on HRT: 1500 mg
- Over 65 years: 1500 mg daily

Iron

- 10–15 mg daily

Vitamin D

- Adolescent–age 50: 200 IU daily
- Age 50–65: 400 IU daily
- Age >65: 600 IU daily

TABLE 6.3

Breast Pain

Breast Pain

- Most common breast symptom for which women seek treatment
- Breast cancers rarely present as breast pain (less than 5%)
- Can be classified as cyclic or noncyclic

Cyclic Breast Pain

- Usually bilateral and poorly localized
- Peaks premenstrually and significantly decreases with onset of menses
- Characterized as dull, heavy, soreness
- In women in their 20s to 30s and postmenopausally with estrogen therapy
- Spontaneously resolves with menopause or sometimes with pregnancy
- High response to hormonal manipulation

Noncyclic Breast Pain

- Tends to be unilateral and well localized
- Unrelated to menstrual cycle
- Sharp, stabbing quality
- Tends to occur in women in their 40s
- May resolve spontaneously
- Less response to hormonal manipulation
- Usually idiopathic but may be associated with begin lesions such as macrocysts or fibroadenomas; rarely associated with cancer

Evaluation

- Breast exam (physical findings correlate poorly); if mass present evaluate
- Mammogram in women aged 35 or older

Treatment

- Before treatment patient records symptoms and intensity (preferably using a pain scale) through one menstrual cycle
- Sports bras improve symptoms with minimal side effects (some initial discomfort)
- Nonsteroidal anti-inflammatory drugs used in usual analgesic to anti-inflammatory doses
- Danazol
  - —Only drug with Food and Drug Administration approval for breast pain
  - —Side effects (menstrual irregularity, hirsutism, acne, weight gain) limit use to those with severe, activity-limiting symptoms
  - —100 mg twice daily to start, for 2 months; with complete resolution of symptoms decrease to 100 mg/d for 2 months; then 100 mg every other day for 2 months; then discontinue

—For persistent symptoms continue 100 mg twice daily for 2 more months before any change in dose. If needed, at 4 months can increase to 200 mg twice daily

- **Evening Primrose Oil**

—Over-the-counter herbal preparation

—Low incidence of side effects; most common is nausea

—Dose 3 g/d

—May take 3–4 months to see benefit

TABLE 6.4

Breast Masses

Definition: A dominant breast mass is a palpable abnormality that differs from surrounding breast tissue and the corresponding area in the other breast. It persists throughout the menstrual cycle.

Differential Diagnosis

- Cyst
- Fibroadenoma
- Prominent area of fibrocystic change
- Fat necrosis
- Cancer

Evaluation

- Physical examination: location, size, consistency, mobility, presence of similar finding in opposite breast, skin changes
- Aspiration or ultrasound if cyst suspected; must be further evaluated if fluid is bloody, cyst recurs, or palpable mass present after aspiration
- Mammography: all women age greater than 40; younger women if clinically suspicious
- Any dominant mass, other than nonrecurring cyst, requires biopsy regardless of mammography findings

---

TABLE 6.5

Nipple Discharge

Characteristics That Help Distinguish Physiologic From Pathologic (Either type may be clear, white, or dark green)

Physiologic	Pathologic
Occurs only with compression	Spontaneous
Frequently bilateral	Usually unilateral
May involve multiple ducts	Confined to single duct
No palpable abnormality	May be associated with a mass
Nonbloody	May be bloody

Evaluation

- Breast exam, checking for masses, nipple discharge characteristics
- Mammography for women > 35 or any age with palpable abnormality
- Hemoccult any nipple fluid
- Surgical referral for any woman with spontaneous, unilateral, serous, or bloody nipple discharge
- Stop all nipple/breast stimulation for woman with physiologic discharge. Should resolve with lack of stimulation

TABLE 6.6

Pap Smears

Absence of Endocervical Cells: In a patient with no known risk factors, who has had three normal, consecutive, annual Pap tests and whose current test has no other abnormalities, the Pap test may be repeated in 12 months. If the patient is at increased risk, repeat test at patient convenience. (American College of Obstetricians and Gynecologists Committee opinion #153 March 1995)

Bethesda System 2001: Standardized system for reporting results of Pap test. Includes up to five components:

1. Specimen adequacy
2. General categorization
3. Interpretation/results
4. Automated review and ancillary testing (include as appropriate)
5. Educational notes and suggestions

1. Specimen Adequacy

Satisfactory for evaluation-slide meets four criteria:

- Patient and specimen identified
- Pertinent clinical history is available
- Sample is technically interpretable (no more than 75% of cells obscured by blood, inflammation, or debris) and is of proper cellular composition
- There is evidence that the cervical transformation zone has been sampled

2. General Categorization (optional)

- Negative for intraepithelial lesion or malignancy
- Epithelial cell abnormality (see interpretation/results)
- Other (see interpretation/results)
- Category of benign cellular changes has been eliminated

3. Interpretation/Results

- Negative for intraepithelial lesion or malignancy
  - —Organisms
    - *Trichomonas vaginalis*
    - Fungal organisms morphologically consistent with *Candida* species
    - Shift in flora suggestive of bacterial vaginosis
    - Bacteria morphologically consistent with *Actinomyces* species
    - Cellular changes associated with herpes simplex virus
  - —Other nonneoplastic findings (optional)
    - Reactive cellular changes
      - Inflammation (includes typical repair)
      - Radiation
      - Intrauterine contraceptive device

Continued

TABLE 6.6

Pap Smears, cont'd

Glandular cells status post hysterectomy

Atrophy

- Epithelial cell abnormalities
  - —Squamous cell
    - Atypical squamous cells (ASC)
      Of undetermined significance (ASC-US)
      Cannot exclude HSIL (ASC-H)
      Category of favor reactive change has been eliminated
    - Low grade squamous intraepithelial lesion encompassing human papilloma virus/mild dysplasia/cervical intraepithelial neoplasia (CIN) I
    - High-grade squamous intraepithelial lesion (HSIL) encompassing moderate and severe dysplasia, carcinoma in situ; CIN 2 and CIN 3
  - —Glandular cell
    - Atypical glandular cells (AGC) (specify endocervical, endometrial, or not otherwise specified)
    - Atypical glandular cells (ACG) favor neoplastic (specify endometrial or not otherwise specified)
    - Endocervical adenocarcinoma in situ (AIS)
    - Other

4. Automated Review and Ancillary Testing (include as appropriate)

- If automated review or other testing (such as HPV) is done, the type of testing and results are noted

5. Educational Notes and Suggestions (optional)

- Opportunity for pathologist to communicate comments about the cytology results and make suggestions about further evaluation

Pap Smears and Cervical Cancer

- 13,000 women develop cervical cancer annually in the United States.
- 50% of these women have never had a Pap smear.
- 10% have not had a Pap smear within 5 years of diagnosis.
- 10% of these women had some errors in follow-up.
- 30% of these women had errors in the interpretation or obtaining of their pap smears.

Techniques to Optimize Collection of a Good Pap Smear

- If possible advise patients not to douche for at least 24 hours prior to exam.
- Use speculum lubricated only with water.

- Visualize entire cervix.
- If needed gently wipe away vaginal discharge.
- Take Pap smear before cultures or wet preps.
- Obtain separate ecto- and endocervical specimens (can use the same slide for both).
- Obtain ectocervical specimen first with wooden or plastic spatula.
- Sample endocervix with brush or broom rotated one fourth to full turn; avoid vigorous manipulation as it may cause bleeding that will obscure cells.
- Apply uniformly to slide and fix immediately.

New Pap Technologies

- Liquid based: thin layer preparations: sample placed in a small bottle of fixative solution. Centrifuged in cytology laboratory and cells transferred as a monolayer onto slide
- Computer-assisting screening: two methods available using conventionally obtained and stained Pap smears
  —Autopap-video microscope linked to computers that use an algorithum to score as to likelihood of abnormality. Abnormal slides manually rescreened
  —Auto Cyte Screen-video microscope computer system presents all images to human reviewer who determines whether manual review required based on images seen. System then compares its determination with the reviewer. If both agree no further review is needed, slide read as within normal limits. If either computer or cytotechnologist determine need slide is manually reviewed

- **HPV testing: Hybid Capture II**
  —Detects 13 high-risk types of HPV
  —Sample obtained with cervical swab of transformation zone and placed in liquid transport medium
  —Test can also be done on residual material from liquid used to transport specimens for monolayer preparation
  —HPV testing of ASCUS Pap smears approximately 90% sensitive in women with high-grade lesions. May have a role in determining which women with ASCUS need colposcopy

- **Clinical issues**
  —Encourage regular Pap screening of all women; as family physicians we have many opportunities to address this with our patients
  —Clinical implications of new testing currently being studied (ALTS trial)
  —Costs of newer technologies significantly higher than conventional Pap testing and may represent burden to patients
  —One option is to discuss available techniques, address patient's risk factors and concerns, and jointly decide on type of screening.

TABLE 6.7

Colposcopy

Definition: The examination of the cervix under magnification. Used to direct biopsies when there is reason to suspect an abnormality of the cervix

Indications

- Abnormal Pap smear
- Abnormal appearance of the cervix
- Follow-up of previously treated cervical abnormalities
- History of in utero diethylstilbestrol exposure

Contraindications

- Actively menstruating
- Acute gonorrhea or chlamydia cervicitis
- Noncooperative patient

Precautions

- Avoid endocervical curettage during pregnancy due to risk of inducing rupture of membranes
- Biopsy with caution during pregnancy due to increased risk of bleeding

Procedure (Follow These Steps)

1. Repeat Pap smear if needed.
2. Gently remove cervical mucus with cotton-tipped applicator (moistened with saline).
3. Inspect entire cervix as a whole under low power.
4. Repeat with green filter.
5. Apply acetic acid and inspect cervix again under low, then high power.
6. Manipulate cervix with cotton-tipped applicator or Kevorkian curette to visualize entire transformation zone.
7. Choose the most abnormal areas to biopsy.
8. Start with most dependent biopsy site (eg, inferior and work superiorly).
9. Place each specimen in separate container labeled as to location.
10. Stop bleeding at biopsy sites with Monsel solution if needed.
11. Do endocervical curettage and place specimen in separate container.
12. Document findings. With map of cervix label findings and location of biopsies.
13. Patient education: may spot or bleed for several days; nothing in vagina for 1 week after biopsy; may have brown/black discharge from the Monsel solution.
14. Discuss findings with patient and arrange follow-up to discuss biopsy results and initiate therapy if indicated.

TABLE 6.8

Colposcopy Findings

Normal Colposcopic Findings

- **Original Squamous Epithelium:** Smooth pink, featureless; covers most of ectocervix
- **Columnar Epithelium:** Irregular, beefy appearing, usually at least partially visible during reproductive age; mildly acetowhite; lies between squamous epithelium and endometrium
- **Transformation Zone:** Area between original and new squamo-columnar junction; may contain gland openings, nabothian cysts, islands of columnar epithelium
- **Squamous Metaplasia:** Normal physiologic process whereby columnar epithelium changes to squamous epithelium; occupies transformation zone

Abnormal Colposcopic Findings

- **Acetowhite Epithelium:** Area which transiently appears white, following the application of acetic acid; correlates with high nuclear density
- **Mosaicism:** Pattern of blood vessels resembling chicken wire or mosaic tiles
- **Punctation:** Area of fine red dots, often within an acetowhite area; caused by seeing blood vessels on end
- **Abnormal Blood Vessels:** Blood vessels not following a normal tree branch pattern of larger to smaller vessels; appear as cork screws, commas; may indicate severe lesion
- **Leukoplakia (or Hyperkeratosis):** Elevated white area clearly seen before application of acetic acid
- **Suspect Invasive Cancer:** Roughened irregular cervical epithelium, abundant abnormal vessels, dense acetowhite change, may see ulcerated/necrotic tissue

Unsatisfactory Colposcopy

- Squamocolumnar junction not visible
- Entire lesion not seen (goes into endocervical canal)
- Unable to visualize whole cervix

TABLE 6.9

Menstruation

Normal: Definition

Normal menstrual cycles occur regularly every 21–35 days, with bleeding lasting 3–8 days. Blood loss averages 30–80 mL.

Abnormal: Definitions

- **Dysfunctional Uterine Bleeding:** Excessive uterine bleeding without demonstrable organic cause. Most frequently due to endocrine abnormalities, particularly anovulation.
- **Intermenstrual Bleeding:** Bleeding of variable amounts occurring between regular menstrual periods.
- **Menometrorrhagia:** Prolonged uterine bleeding occurring at irregular intervals.
- **Menorrhagia:** Prolonged (more than 7 days) or excessive (greater than 80 mL) uterine bleeding occurring at regular intervals. (Synonym: hypermenorrhea.)
- **Metrorrhagia:** Uterine bleeding of variable amount occurring at irregular but frequent intervals.
- **Oligomenorrhea:** Uterine bleeding at intervals from 35 days to 6 months.
- **Polymenorrhea:** Uterine bleeding occurring at regular intervals of less than 21 days.
- **Primary Amenorrhea:** Absence of any spontaneous menses in an individual older than $16\frac{1}{2}$ years of age.
- **Secondary Amenorrhea:** Absence of menses for a length of time equivalent to at least three normal cycles or 6 months.

Definitions adapted from Sterchever MA, Droegumeller W, Mishell D, eds. *Comprehensive Gynecology*. St Louis: Mosby, Inc; 1997.

TABLE 6.10

Treatment of Primary Dysmenorrhea

Nonsteroidal Anti-inflammatory Drugs (NSAIDs)

- First-line therapy
- Effective pain relief in 64–100% of subjects
- For examples of recommended drugs and dosages see Table 6.11
- Try an agent from another class of NSAIDs if first agent ineffective

Oral Contraceptives

- First-line therapy if contraception is desired, otherwise second-line therapy
- Up to 90% effective
- May take up to three cycles for noticeable decrease in pain

Failure to respond to one or both of these regimens may indicate a secondary cause for the dysmenorrhea.

TABLE 6.11

Prescription NSAIDs for Dysmenorrhea

Drug (Trade Name)	Available Dosage	Initial Dosage	Subsequent Dosage	24-h Maximum	First-Day Maximum
Diclofenac (Cataflam)	50 mg	100 mg	50 mg tid	150 mg	200 mg
Ibuprofen (Motrin)	400 mg 600 mg 800 mg	NA	400 mg q 4 h	3.2 g	NA
Ketoprofen (Orudis)	25 mg 50 mg 75 mg	NA	25–50 mg q 6–8 h	300 mg	N/A
Meclofenamate sodium	50 mg 100 mg	NA	100 mg tid	300 mg	NA
Mefenamic acid (Ponstel)	250 mg	500 mg	250 mg q 6 h	1 g	1.25 g
Naproxen (Naprosyn)	250 mg 375 mg 500 mg	500 mg	500 mg q 12 h (or) 250 mg q 6–8 h	1.25 g	NA
Naproxen sodium (Anaprox, Anaprox DS)	275 mg 550 mg	550 mg	550 mg q 12 h (or) 275 mg q 6–8 h	1.1 g	1.375 g
Rofecoxib (Vioxx)	25 mg 50 mg	NA	50 mg q d	50 mg	NA

NSAIDs indicates nonsteroidal anti-inflammatory drugs; NA, not applicable; tid, three times daily; q 4 h, every 4 hours; q d, daily.

TABLE 6.12

Differential Diagnosis of Abnormal Vaginal Bleeding

Pregnancy Related

- Spontaneous abortion (threatened, incomplete, complete)
- Ectopic pregnancy
- Trophoblastic disease
- Postpartum conditions (retained products of conception, subinvolution of uterus)

Uterine Abnormalities/Conditions

- Leiomyoma
- Adenomyosis
- Intrauterine device

Endometrial Abnormalities

- Endometrial hyperplasia
- Endometrial carcinoma
- Endometrial polyp
- Endometritis

Cervical Abnormalities

- Cervicitis
- Cervical carcinoma
- Cervical polyp

Vaginal

- Trauma/foreign body
- Neoplasm

Ovarian

- Ovarian neoplasm
- Polycystic ovary syndrome

Systemic

- Coagulopathy (including leukemias, thrombocytopenia, von Willebrand)
- Thyroid disorder
- Adrenal disorders
- Hepatic disease
- Renal disease
- Diabetes mellitus

Dysfunctional Uterine Bleeding

- Most common etiology for abnormal vaginal bleeding
- Abnormal bleeding in the absence of structural pathology, pregnancy, or systemic disease; hormonally related
- Most common type is anovulatory (see Table 6.13)

TABLE 6.13

Anovulatory Bleeding

Definition: Noncyclic menstrual bleeding associated with failure of ovulation. May vary from scant spotting to excessive prolonged bleeding. Accounts for about 85% of DUB.

Diagnosis

- Made by the exclusion of anatomic pathology in the presence of irregular bleeding

Causes

- Adolescence (cycles become ovulatory on average about 20 months after menarche)
- Perimenopause
- Premature ovarian failure
- Hypothyroidism
- Hypothalamic dysfunction (eg, anorexia nervosa)
- Primary pituitary disease
- Hyperandrogenic states (eg, polycystic ovary syndrome, congenital adrenal hyperplasia, androgen-secreting tumor)
- Hyperprolactinemia

Evaluation

- **Lab:** CBC, TSH, HCG
- **Physical Exam:** Looking for evidence of infection, uterine size, trauma, polyps, cervicitis
- **Endometrial Biopsy:** Women over age 35 and those with history of risk factors for endometrial cancer. If secretory endometrium on biopsy, further evaluate for intracavitary uterine lesions
- **Ultrasound:** Useful when physical exam unsatisfactory for determining uterine size and shape; if ovaries not well identified or abnormality suspected; to assess endometrial thickness
- Saline infusion sonography or hysteroscopy may be needed to assess intrauterine pathology

Treatment

- **Chronic:** To establish a regular bleeding pattern
  - —Cyclic progestogen: example, 10 mg medroxyprogesterone q d for 10 days each month; does not protect against pregnancy
  - —Combined oral contraceptive pills: one pill each day; provides pregnancy protection

- **Acute (moderately heavy bleeding):** To stop bleeding
  - —Medroxyprogesterone 10 mg po q d for 10 days
  - —Progesterone in oil 100 mg im injection for one dose
  - —Combined oral contraceptive pills, one pill three to four times daily for 3–5 days then complete package at one pill/day
  - —With either method bleeding should stop; patient will bleed again at end of therapy but should be a more limited bleed
  - —After treatment of acute episode consider chronic treatment basing choice on patient's desire for avoiding or becoming pregnant
- Acute (uncontrolled, very heavy bleeding): To stop bleeding
  - —May require hospitalization
  - —Intravenous estrogen 25 mg every 4 hours until bleeding slows; maximum three doses
  - —Oral conjugated estrogens 2.5 mg qid

CBC indicates complete blood cell count; DUB, dysfunctional uterine bleeding; HCG, human chorionic gonadotropin; po, orally; d, daily; qid, four times daily; TSH, thyrotropin.

TABLE 6.14

Evaluation of Perimenopausal Abnormal Vaginal Bleeding

History

- Possibility of pregnancy (contraceptive use, etc)
- Pattern of bleeding
- Other medical illness (DM, HTN)

Physical

- Weight (obesity increases risk for endometrial hyperplasia and cancer)
- Blood pressure
- Uterine size/shape (enlarged? fibroids?)
- Obvious site of bleeding (cervical polyp, friable cervix)

Lab

- CBC (assess for anemia)
- HCG (R/O pregnancy)

Further Evaluation (Required)

- Endometrial aspiration (Pipelle): High sensitivity and specificity for endometrial cancer; less sensitive for other diseases; uncomfortable
- Transvaginal ultrasonography: High negative predictive value; endometrial stripe greater than 5 mm needs further evaluation (endometrial biopsy, hysteroscopy); may be better tolerated than biopsy

CBC indicates complete blood cell count; DM, diabetes mellitus; HCG, human chorionic gonadotropin; HTN, hypertension; R/O, rule out.

TABLE 6.15

Endometrial Sampling (Pipelle)

Indications

- Abnormal vaginal bleeding
- AGUS Pap Smear
- High risk for endometrial cancer (patients on unopposed estrogen or tamoxifen therapy)

Contradictions

- Pregnancy
- Infection of the genital tract

Four Preliminary "P's"

- Premedicate with 800 mg ibuprofen, 1 hour prior to procedure if not contraindicated
- Rule out pregnancy
- Obtain permission (informed consent)
- Prophylaxis with antibiotics for patients with artificial heart valves

Procedure

- See Table 6.16.

Results

- Benign
  —Proliferative endometrium: Indicates estrogen effect without progesterone. If biopsy done late in cycle, indicates anovulatory cycle
  —Secretory endometrium: Indicates ovulation has occurred; reflects estrogen and progesterone influence on endometrium
  —Atrophic endometrium: Indicates lack of estrogen stimulation of endometrium
- Hyperplasia: Indicates excess estrogen stimulation; requires treatment
  —With atypia (25% of these progress to cancer if untreated)
  —Without atypia
- Endometrial cancer

TABLE 6.16

Endometrial Aspiration: Procedure*

1. Perform bimanual exam to determine uterine size, shape.
2. Visualize cervix using speculum.
3. Cleanse cervix with Betadine.
4. Apply tenaculum to anterior aspect of cervix (optional).
5. Insert the sampling device into the uterus. Resistance may be felt at the angle between the cervix and body of the uterus. If so, apply gentle traction to tenaculum to straighten out angle.
6. Once device has been inserted to the fundus, record depth of uterus.
7. Stabilize the sampling device with one hand and withdraw the plunger in one swift motion to create suction.
8. Rotate sheath between the fingers while also moving it back and forth from fundus to internal os several times until tissue is seen filling the lumen.
9. Withdraw the device; using the plunger, expel contents into container of preservative to be sent to pathology.
10. Control any bleeding.
11. Remove excess Betadine or blood from vaginal vault with large cotton-tipped applicators or sponge forceps with gauze.
12. Remove speculum.
13. Discuss findings with patient and arrange follow-up.

*Aspiration may be done as a clean rather than sterile procedure as long as the part of the endometrial aspiration device entering the uterus remains sterile.

TABLE 6.17

Endometriosis

Endometriosis

- Presence of endometrial tissue outside of the uterine cavity.
- Presents as pelvic pain, dysmenorrhea, and/or infertility.

Diagnosis

- Suspected in women with secondary dysmenorrhea (most common cause), pelvic pain, infertility, and dyspareunia.
- Physical exam may reveal uterosacral nodularity, retroversion of uterus, adnexal masses, diffuse or local tenderness, or decreased pelvic mobility. Findings nonspecific and may be absent.
- Diagnosis requires visualization by laparoscopy or laparotomy.

Treatment

- Mildly symptomatic women who do not desire pregnancy in whom endometriosis is suspected may be treated with NSAIDs or OCPs without confirming diagnosis by laparoscopy.
- No medical treatment clearly superior to another or placebo for infertility associated with endometriosis.
- Surgical treatment associated with increased fertility but effect may be small.
- Some women desiring pregnancy benefit from assisted reproduction.
- Hormonal therapy, surgery, or both can be used to treat pain. Combination treatment may offer an advantage but extent of benefit unclear.
- Hormonal therapy attempts to shrink endometrial implants through androgen-induced atrophy or estrogen deprivation.
- Side effects of hormonal therapy include mood changes, increased hair growth, irregular bleeding, weight gain, and decreased libido.
- See Table 6.18 for commonly used drugs in management of endometriosis.
- Estrogen-progestin add-back therapy (at usual postmenopausal replacement doses) has been used to counteract side effects of GnRH-agonist therapy.

GnRH indicates gonadotropin-releasing hormone; NSAIDs, nonsteroidal anti-inflammatory drugs; OCPs, oral contraceptive pills.

TABLE 6.18

Drugs Used in the Treatment of Endometriosis

Drug (Brand Name)	Drug Class	Dosage	Comments
Combination OCPs (various)	Estrogen/ progestin	One tablet daily po	Contraceptive; may help dysmenorrhea
Medroxy-progesterone acetate depot (Depo-Provera)	Progestin	150 mg IM q 3 mo	Contraceptive; spotting, menstrual irregularity, possible amenorrhea
Medroxypro-gesterone acetate (Provera)	Progestin	10–50 mg po q d	Irregular bleeding and weight gain common
Danazol (Danocrine)	Synthetic steroid	400–800 mg q d po	Menstrual irregularities, weight gain, androgenic effects
Goserelin (Zoladex)	GnRH agonist	3.6 mg SC implant q mo	Side effects are those of hypoestrogenism: vaginal dryness, hot flashes, decreased libido, insomnia, depression, fatigue, headache
Leuprolide (Lupron)	GnRH agonist	3.75 mg IM/mo	Side effects are those of hypoestrogenism: vaginal dryness, hot flashes, decreased libido, insomnia, depression, fatigue, headache
Nafarelin (Synarel)	GnRH agonist	200 μg intranasal bid	Side effects are those of hypoestrogenism: vaginal dryness, hot flashes, decreased libido, insomnia, depression, fatigue, headache

Adapted from Parent-Stevens L, Burns EA. Menstrual disorders. In: Smith MA, Shimp LA, eds. *20 Common Problems in Women's Health Care.* New York, NY: McGraw-Hill; 2000.

GnRH indicates gonadotropin-releasing hormone; IM, intramuscularly; OCPs, oral contraceptive pills; po, orally; q 3 mo, every 3 months; q d, daily; SC, subcutaneous.

TABLE 6.19

Endometrial Cancer

Epidemiology

- Most common gynecologic malignancy
- Fourth most common cancer in women
- 72 cases per 100 000 women
- Approximately 32 000 women diagnosed per year
- About 80% detected in localized stages
- 5-year survival rate of 80% for stage 1

Presentation

- 90% present with abnormal bleeding
- Any bleeding in postmenopausal woman needs to be evaluated
- Perimenopausal women may have intermenstrual spotting, increased menstrual flow, decreased menstrual interval. Abnormal bleeding should be evaluated
- Pap smears: No pathognomonic finding but certain findings need evaluation, including any endometrial cells in postmenopausal women or atypical glandular cells of undetermined significance

Risk Factors (Most Related to Increased Uterine Exposure to Estrogens)

- Nulliparity
- Early menarche
- Late menopause
- Tamoxifen therapy
- Anovulatory cycles
- Unopposed estrogen stimulation
- Estrogen-secreting tumors
- Diabetes mellitus
- Hypertension
- Age greater than 40

Protective Factors

- Progesterone added to estrogen replacement therapy
- Oral contraceptive use
- Hysterectomy

TABLE 6.20

Ovarian Cancer

Epidemiology (United States)

- Fifth most common malignancy in women
- 25 000 new cases each year
- 1/70 women
- 14 000 deaths per year
- Peak age 55–65

Risk Factors

- Most cases, no identifiable risk factors
- Higher rates with nulliparity and late (age greater than 35) first pregnancy
- Breast cancer (2–4 times increased risk)
- Family history: 10% chance of developing ovarian cancer with one first-degree relative and 50% chance with two first-degree relatives
- Familial cancer syndromes account for 3%–5% of ovarian cancer
  —Familial breast-ovary cancer syndrome—autosomal dominant
  —Lynch syndrome II—cancers of colon, lung, prostate, uterus, and ovary

Protective Factors (Reduces Risk)

- High parity
- Breastfeeding
- Oral contraceptives
- Hysterectomy or BTL
- Oophorectomy
- Some indications that diet high in plant foods may reduce risk

Screening

- No effective screening available
- CA 125—may be normal in half of women with stage 1 disease; may be elevated in endometriosis or PID
- Transvaginal US—expensive
- CA 125 with sonography achieves high specificity and sensitivity but is too expensive for screening

Presentation

- 70% present with advanced disease
- Clues to early diagnosis: palpable ovary in postmenopausal women; cystic ovary more than 1 year after menopause
- Common symptoms: abdominal fullness and early satiety
- Ascites in postmenopausal women; must rule out ovarian cancer
- Bowel obstruction may result from tumor implants on omentum or small bowel
- Most early-stage cancers found incidentally during workup for another problem or routine pelvic exam

BTL indicates bilateral tubal ligation; CA 125, cancer antigen 125; PID, pelvic inflammatory disease; US, ultrasound.

TABLE 6.21

Diagnosis and Treatment of Vaginitis

Bacterial Vaginosis: A clinical syndrome characterized by malodorous vaginal discharge resulting from the replacement of the normal flora, lactobacillus, with high concentrations of anaerobic bacteria.

Diagnosis (Requires Meeting 3 of 4 Criteria)

- Homogeneous, white, noninflammatory discharge that smoothly coats the vaginal walls
- Presence of clue cells on microscopic exam of discharge
- pH of vaginal fluid greater than or equal to 4.5
- Fishy odor of vaginal discharge before or after addition of 10% potassium hydroxide.

Treatment

1. Recommended regimens for nonpregnant women:
   —Metronidazole 500 mg po bid for 7 days
   —Clindamycin cream 2% one full applicator intravaginally for 7 days
   —Metronidazole gel 0.75% one applicator intravaginally bid for 7 days
2. Alternate regimens:
   —Metronidazole 2 g orally in a single dose
   —Clindamycin 300 mg po bid for 7 days
3. Treatment in pregnancy:
   —Metronidazole 250 mg po bid for 7 days

Trichomoniasis: A vaginal infection caused by the protozoan *Trichomonas vaginalis*. May be asymptomatic but often characterized by a diffuse malodorous yellow-green discharge. May also be accompanied by vulvar irritation and inflammation of the cervix.

Diagnosis

Wet prep showing flagellated mobile organisms

Treatment

1. For nonpregnant women:
   —Metronidazole 2 g orally in a single dose
2. Alternative treatment:
   —Metronidazole 500 mg bid for 7 days
3. Treatment in pregnancy:
   —Patients can be treated with metronidazole 2 g orally in a single dose

Vulvovaginal Candidiasis: A vaginal infection characterized by itching and a thick white vaginal discharge caused usually by *Candida albicans* and occasionally by other *Candida* species or *Torulopsis*.

Continued

TABLE 6.21

Diagnosis and Treatment of Vaginitis, cont'd

Diagnosis (suggested by pruritus and erythema of the vulvovaginal area)

- Wet prep or potassium hydroxide preparation showing yeast or pseudohyphae or culture can be used to make the diagnosis. Vaginal pH usually less than or equal to 4.5.

Treatment

- Butoconazole 2% (Femstat, Mycelex) cream: 5 g intravaginally for 3 days*
- Clotrimazole (Lotrimin) 1% cream: 5 g intravaginally for 7–14 days*
- Clotrimazole: 100-mg vaginal tablet for 7 days*
- Clotrimazole: 100-mg vaginal tablet, two tablets for 3 days*
- Clotrimazole: 500-mg vaginal tablet, one tablet, once
- Miconazole (Monistat) 2% cream: 5 g intravaginally for 7 days*
- Miconazole: 200-mg vaginal suppository, one qd for 3 days*
- Miconazole: 100-mg vaginal suppository, one qd for 7 days*
- Nystatin: 100 000-unit vaginal tablet, one qd for 14 days
- Terconazole: 6.5% (Vagistat-1) ointment, 5 g intravaginally in a single application*
- Terconazole (Terazol) 0.4% cream: 5 g intravaginally for 7 days
- Terconazole 0.8% cream: 5 g intravaginally for 3 days
- Terconazole: 80 mg vaginal suppository, one q d for 3 days
- Diflucan: 150 mg oral tablet, one tablet as a single dose

bid indicates twice daily; po, orally; q d, daily.

*Available over the counter

TABLE 6.22

Recurrent Vulvovaginal Candidiasis

Definition: Four or more episodes of vulvovaginal candidiasis (confirmed microscopically or by culture) within 1 year.

Risk Factors

- Uncontrolled DM
- Immunosuppression
- Corticosteroid therapy

Most women with RVVC have no risk factors.

Treatment

- 14-day course of a standard oral or topical treatment, followed by a 6-month prophylactic regimen

Prophylaxis Regimens

- Clotrimazole: Two 100-mg suppositories intravaginally twice a week or one 500-mg suppository once a week
- Terconazole 0.8% vaginal cream: one applicator full once a week
- Fluconazole (Diflucan): 100–200 mg po once a week or 150 mg po once a month
- Itraconazole (Sporanox): 50–100 mg po daily or two 200 mg tablets po once a month
- Ketoconazole (Nizoral): 100 mg po daily or two 200-mg tablets po q d × 5 days at the end of the menstrual period
- Boric acid: 600-mg vaginal suppository daily during menstruation

DM indicates diabetes mellitus; po, orally; RVVC, recurrent vulvovaginal candidiasis.

TABLE 6.23

Pelvic Inflammatory Disease

Definition: Inflammatory disease of the female upper genital tract including any combination of endometritis, salpingitis, tubo-ovarian abscess, and pelvic peritonitis. Often caused by *N gonorrhoeae* or *C trachomatis,* but may also be caused by microorganisms that can be part of vaginal flora (such as anaerobes, *G vaginalis, H influenza,* enteric gram-negative rods, and *Streptococcus agalactiae*). *M hominis* and *U urealyticum* may also be causal agents.

Diagnosis

Diagnosis is imprecise and difficult; symptoms may be mild or nonspecific. Empiric treatment of PID should be initialized in sexually active young women and others at risk of STD if all of the following minimum criteria are present and no other cause of the illness can be identified.

- Lower abdominal tenderness
- Adnexal tenderness
- Cervical motion tenderness

Additional criteria supporting a diagnosis of PID:

- Oral temperature greater than 100°F
- Abnormal cervical or vaginal discharge
- Elevated erythrocyte sedimentation rate
- Elevated C-reactive protein
- Laboratory documentation of cervical infection with *N gonorrhoeae* or *C trachomatis*

Definitive criteria for diagnosing PID include the following:

- Histopathologic evidence of endometritis on endometrial biopsy
- Transvaginal sonography or other imaging techniques showing thickened, fluid-filled tubes, free pelvic fluid, or tubo-ovarian complex
- Laparoscopic abnormalities consistent with PID

Treatment

Hospitalization: criteria

- Surgical emergencies such as appendicitis cannot be excluded
- The patient is pregnant
- The patient does not respond clinically to oral antimicrobial therapy
- The patient is unable to follow or tolerate an outpatient oral regimen
- The patient has severe illness, nausea and vomiting, or high fever
- The patient has a tubo-ovarian abscess
- The patient is immunodeficient (ie, has HIV infection with low CD4 counts, is taking immunosuppressive therapy, or has another disease)

Parenteral Regimens for Pelvic Inflammatory Disease*

Regimen A

Cefotetan 2 g IV every 12 hours plus Doxycycline 100 mg IV or orally every 12 hours

(or)

Cefoxtin 2 g IV every 6 hours plus Doxycycline 100 mg IV or orally every 12 hours

Regimen B

Clindamycin 900 mg IV every 8 hours

(plus)

Gentamicin loading dose IV or IM (2 mg/kg body weight) followed by a maintenance dose (1.5 mg/kg) every 8 hours

Alternative Parenteral Regimens

- Ofloxacin 400 mg IV every 12 hours

  (plus)

  Metronidazole 500 mg IV every 8 hours

(or)

- Ampicillin/Sublactum 3 g IV every 6 hours

  (plus)

  Doxycycline 100 mg IV or orally every 12 hours

(or)

- Ciprofloxicin 200 mg IV every 12 hours

  (plus)

  Doxycycline 100 mg IV or orally every 12 hours

  (plus)

  Metronidazole 500 mg IV every 8 hours

Oral Regimens

Regimen A

Ofloxacin 400 mg orally twice a day for 14 days

(plus)

Metronidazole 500 mg orally twice a day for 14 days

Regimen B

Ceftriaxone 250 mg IM plus Doxycycline 100 mg orally twice a day for 14 days

(or)

Cefoxitin 2 g IM plus probenecid 1 g orally plus Doxycycline 100 mg orally twice a day for 14 days

(or)

Other parenteral third-generation cephalosporin plus Doxycycline 100 mg orally twice a day for 14 days

HIV indicates human immunodeficiency virus; IM, intramuscularly; IV, intravenously; PID, pelvic inflammatory disease; STD, sexually transmitted disease.

*For more information refer to www.cdc.gov/nchstp/dstd.

TABLE 6.24

Comparative Contraceptive Efficacy

Percent of Women Experiencing an Unintended Pregnancy During First Year of Use

Method	Typical Use	Perfect Use
Chance (no method)	85	84
Spermicides	26	6
Periodic Abstinence	25	–
■ Calendar	—	9
■ Ovulation Method	—	3
■ Sympto-thermal	—	2
■ Postovulation	—	1
Cap		
■ Parous women	40	26
■ Nulliparous women	20	9
Diaphragm	20	6
Withdrawal	19	4
Condom		
■ Female	21	5
■ Male	14	3
Pill	5	
■ Progestin only	—	0.5
■ Combined	—	0.1
IUD		
■ Progesterone T	2.0	1.5
■ Cooper T 380A (Paragard)	8	0.6
Depo-Provera	0.3	0.3
Female Sterilization	0.5	0.5
Male Sterilization	0.15	0.10

Adapted from Hatcher RA. *Contraceptive Technology*. 17th ed. New York: Ardent Media, Inc; 1998.

IUD indicates intrauterine device.

TABLE 6.25

World Health Organization Categories for Oral Contraceptives

WHO Category #4 (should not use—condition represents unacceptable health risks)

- DVT or PE or history of these (estrogens promote blood clotting)
- CVA, CAD, ischemic heart disease
- Structural heart disease complicated by pulmonary hypertension, artrial fibrillation, or history of SBE
- DM with retinopathy, neuropathy, vascular disease or duration of diabetes for more than 20 years
- Breast cancer
- Pregnancy
- Liver problems: benign hepatic adenoma or liver cancer; active viral hepatitis; severe cirrhosis
- Headaches, including migraines, with focal neurological symptoms (may be indication of increased risk of strokes)
- Lactation, less than 6 weeks post partum (some concern regarding neonatal exposure to hormones during first 6 weeks; oral contraceptives can decrease volume of milk production)
- Major surgery with prolonged immobilization or any surgery on the legs (increased risk of DVTs and PE)
- Over 35 years old and currently smoking 20 or more cigarettes a day (increased risk for cardiovascular disease)
- Hypertension with blood pressures greater than 160/100 or with vascular disease

WHO Category #3 (should not use—theoretical or proven risk outweighs advantages; may be chosen as last resort)

- Post partum less than 21 days (theoretical concern regarding possible increased risk of clotting)
- Lactation 6 weeks to 6 months (may decrease the quantity of milk)
- Undiagnosed abnormal vaginal/uterine bleeding
- Past history of breast cancer with no evidence of recurrence for 5 years
- Use of drugs that affect liver enzymes: rifampin, rifabutin, and griseofulvin; anticonvulsants such as phenytoin, carbamazepine, barbiturates, topiramate, and primidone (may decrease the efficacy of OCPs)
- Gallbladder disease: current biliary tract disease or history of oral contraceptive-related cholestasis

WHO Category #2 (can use—advantages outweigh known or theoretical risk; may need closer-than-usual follow up)

- Severe headaches that definitely start after initiation of oral contraceptives; migraine headaches without focal neurologic symptoms
- Diabetes mellitus: gestational diabetes or diabetes without vascular disease
- Major surgery without prolonged immobilization
- Sickle cell disease

Continued

TABLE 6.25

World Health Organization Categories for Oral Contraceptives, cont'd

- Moderate blood pressure elevation (140–159/100–109 mm Hg); monitor blood pressure periodically
- Unexplained vaginal bleeding
- Undiagnosed breast mass
- Cervical cancer and CIN
- Over age 50
- Conditions likely to make it difficult to take oral contraceptives consistently and correctly (mental retardation, major psychiatric illness, alcoholism)
- Family history of hyperlipidemia (may be at increased risk of heart disease)
- Family history of death of a parent or sibling due to myocardial infarction before age 50 (suggests a need for lipid evaluation)

WHO Category #1 (can use—no increased risk; no restrictions)

- Postpartum greater that 21 days
- Postabortion after first or second trimester or immediately after post-septic abortion
- History of gestational diabetes
- Varicose veins
- Mild headaches
- Irregular vaginal bleeding
- Past history of pelvic inflammatory disease
- Current or recent history of PID or STD
- Vaginitis
- Increased risk of STD
- HIV positive, AIDS or high risk of HIV
- Benign breast disease
- Family history of breast cancer
- Cervical ectropion
- Endometrial or ovarian cancer
- Viral hepatitis carrier
- Uterine fibroids
- Past ectopic pregnancy
- Obesity
- Thyroid conditions: simple goiter, hyper- or hypothyroidism
- Benign or malignant gestational trophoblastic disease
- Iron-deficiency anemia
- Epilepsy
- Current use of antibiotics
- Severe dysmenorrhea
- Endometriosis

- Benign ovarian tumors
- Prior pelvic surgery
- Tuberculosis
- Malaria

AIDS indicates acquired immunodeficiency syndrome; CAD, coronary artery disease; CIN, cervical intraepithelial neoplasia; CVA, cerebrovascular accident; DM, diabetes mellitus; DVT, deep venous thrombosis; HIV, human immunodeficiency virus; OCPs, oral contraceptive pills; PE, pulmonary embolism; PID, pelvic inflammatory disease; SBE, subacute bacterial endocarditis; STD, sexually transmitted disease.

TABLE 6.26

Noncontraceptive Benefits of Oral Contraceptives

- Decreased dysmenorrhea
- Decreased menstrual flow
- Prevention of dysfunctional uterine bleeding and endometrial hyperplasia in women with chronic anovulation
- Improvement in acne
- Decreased incidence of pelvic inflammatory disease
- Decreased incidence of ectopic pregnancy
- Decreased incidence of benign breast disease (fibroadenoma and cystic changes)
- Decreased risk of ovarian and endometrial carcinomas
- Other possible benefits include decreasing the severity of rheumatoid arthritis; prevention and suppression of functional ovarian cysts; increased bone mineral density in perimenopausal women

Adapted from American College of Obstetricians and Gynecologists. Hormonal contraception. *ACOG Tech Bull.* 1994;198 and American College of Obstetricians and Gynecologists. Oral contraceptives for adolescents: benefits and safety. *ACOG Tech Bull.* 1999;256.

TABLE 6.27

Emergency Postcoital Contraception

Instructions for Use: Take first dose within 72 hours of unprotected intercourse and a second dose 12 hours later. Consider pretreatment 1 hour before each equal dose with an orally administered antiemetic such as prochlorperazine (Compazine) (5–10 mg), promethazine (Phenergan) (12.5–25 mg), or trimethobenzamide (Tigan) (250 mg).

Combined Oral Contraceptive Pills

Trade Name	Pill/Dose
Ovral	2 white pills
Alesse	5 pink pills
Levlite	5 pink pills
Nordette	4 light orange pills
Levlen	4 light orange pills
Levora	4 white pills
Lo/Ovral	4 white pills
Triphasil	4 yellow pills
Trivora	4 pink pills
Preven*	2 blue pills

Progesterone-Only Methods

Trade Name	Pill/Dose
Ovrette	20 yellow pills
Plan B*	1 white pill

*Marketed specifically for this purpose.

Contraindications

- The only contraindication is pregnancy

Efficacy

- 74.1% reduction in risk of pregnancy

Side Effects

- Nausea (50%)
- Vomiting (20%)

Less Common Side Effects

- Heavy menses and mastalgia (38%)
- Bleeding before next menstrual period due.

Some women (8%) are 4 or more days late for period.

Adapted from Wertheinmer RE. Emergency postcoital contraception. *Am Fam Physician*. 2000; 62:2287–2292.

TABLE 6.28

Premenstrual Syndrome

Definition: Premenstrual syndrome (PMS) is a cluster of affective and somatic symptoms recurring during the luteal phase of the menstrual cycle. Diagnosis is made clinically, by concurrent charting of symptoms and menses on a daily calendar through two or more cycles

Key Features

- Symptoms occur within most menstrual cycles
- Symptoms relieved within 4 days of onset of menses
- Symptoms absent in first half of menstrual cycle
- Symptoms vary from woman to woman but tend to stay the same for an individual
- Symptoms not explained by another disorder

Examples of PMS Symptoms

Affective/Cognitive	Somatic
Anxiety	Breast tenderness
Irritability	Bloating
Tension	Dependent edema
Anger	Fatigue
Tearfulness	Insomnia
Depression	Headache
Loneliness	Low backache
Difficulty concentrating	
Food cravings	
Appetite change	

Treatments for PMS

Lifestyle

- Aerobic exercise at least three times weekly
- Complex carbohydrate diet

Dietary Supplements

- Calcium: 1000–1200 mg daily
- Magnesium: 200–400 mg daily
- Vitamin E: 400 IU mg daily*

Drugs

- SSRIs: Initial drug of choice for severe PMS; PMDD

  Fluoxetine (Paxil, Sarafem) 20–60 mg

  Sertraline (Zoloft) 50–150 mg

  Paroxetine (Paxil) 20–50 mg

Continued

TABLE 6.28

Premenstrual Syndrome, cont'd

- Spironolactone: 100 mg a day (25 mg q.i.d) during luteal phase
- Oral Contraceptives: Effectiveness not well established, may improve physical symptoms

PMDD indicates premenstrual dysphoric disorder; SSRIs, selective serotonin reuptake inhibitors.

*Evidence for effectiveness not as strong as calcium and magnesium but no adverse effect at recommended dose.

TABLE 6.29

Premenstrual Dysphoric Disorder (PMDD)

Premenstrual dysphoric disorder represents the severe emotional and behavioral extreme of premenstrual syndrome (PMS). Diagnostic criteria are outlined in the DSM HIV section on Criteria Sets and Axes Provided for Further Study.

- Symptoms occur during the week before the onset of menses and resolve within a few days after the menstrual period has started
- Symptoms must be of sufficient severity to interfere with usual activities such as work, domestic functioning, or social relationships
- Five of the following symptoms must be present, including one of the first four:
  —Feelings of sadness, low self worth, or hopelessness
  —Feelings of anxiousness or tension
  —Mood lability
  —Feelings of anger and irritability
  —Loss of interest in usual activities; social withdrawal
  —Problems with concentration
  —Decreased energy; feeling fatigued
  —Change in appetite, food cravings, or overeating
  —Hypersomnia or insomnia
  —Feelings of being out of control or overwhelmed
  —Physical symptoms associated with PMS such as breast tenderness, bloating, or headache
- Symptoms are not secondary to a medical condition and do not represent premenstrual exacerbation of existing mental disorder
- Selective serotonin reuptake inhibitors are usually well tolerated and effective in treating PMDD

Adapted from American Psychiatric Association. *Diagnostic and Statistical Manual of Mental Disorders.* 4th ed. Washington, DC: American Psychiatric Association; 1994.

TABLE 6.30

Menstrual Migraines

Menstrual Migraines

- Appear to be triggered by falling estrogen levels
- Reported frequency 26–70%
- True menstrual migraines occur only during time of menses (typically 2 days before to 3 days after start of period)
- Menstrually triggered migraines are headaches that occur with increased frequency, severity, and duration in someone who also has migraines throughout the cycle

Treatments: Prophylactic

- Traditional migraine prophylactic therapy given on a daily basis for menstrually triggered migraines or perimenstrually for true menstrual migraine
- Other therapies that can be taken perimenstrually for true menstrual migraine headaches

  —NSAIDs (eg, ketoprofen long acting 100–200 mg daily for 1–2 days before expected onset of menses and continued during menses)
  —Ergotamines (eg, DHE nasal spray every 8 hours for 3 days before and after starting menses; total 6 days therapy)
  —Triptans (eg, sumatriptan 25 mg tid 2–3 days before expected onset of headache and continued for a total of 5 days)
  —Magnesium 360 mg orally
- Hormone therapy may be indicated if other treatments fail

  —Active pills of combination OCPs administered daily for 6–12 weeks (skip placebo pills during this time) helpful for some women
  —Transdermal estradiol patches, danazol, and tamoxifen have also been used.

Treatments: Acute

- Effective or commonly used drugs include

  —NSAIDs
  —Dihydroergotamine
  —Triptans
  —Combination of aspirin, caffeine and acetaminophen
- For severe headaches not controlled by above

  —Analgesics combined with narcotics
  —Narcotics alone
  —Major tranquilizers (haldol, chlorpromazine, thiothixene, droperidol)
  —Intravenous dihydroergotamine

DHE indicates dihydroergotamine mesylate; NSAIDs, nonsteroidal anti-inflammatory drugs; OCPs, oral contraceptive pills; and tid, three times daily.

TABLE 6.31

Premature Ovarian Failure/Premature Menopause

Premature Ovarian Failure

- Loss of ovarian functioning before age 40
- Hypergonadotropic amenorrhea
- Usually associated with premature menopause but idiopathic and autoimmune-related types may have one or more spontaneous remissions

Premature Menopause

- Last menstrual period before age 40

Causes

- Surgical oophorectomy
- Chromosomal abnormalities, such as Turner mosaic
- Radiation to the ovaries
- Autoimmune diseases (thyroid, parathyroid, or adrenal disorders; SLE, diabetes mellitus)
- Idiopathic

Evaluation

- Weekly FSH, LH, estradiol for 4 consecutive weeks
- Karyotype
- ESR, RF, ANA, total protein and serum albumin/globulin ratio, ovarian antibodies
- TSH
- AM cortisol

Complications

- Increased mortality rate
- Possible increased cardiovascular morbidity and mortality
- More severe vertebral bone loss and greater incidence of hip fracture

ANA indicates antinuclear antibody; ESR, erythrocyte sedimentation rate; FSH, follicle-stimulating hormone; LH, luteinizing hormone; RF, rheumatoid factor; SLE, systemic lupus erythematosus; TSH, thyrotropin.

TABLE 6.32

Menopause

Menopause

- Defined as the last menstrual period
- Diagnosed retrospectively after 1 year of amenorrhea
- 95% of women reach menopause between ages 45 and 55 (mean age, 51.4)
- Considered premature menopause if occurs before age 40 (see Table 6.31)
- Endometrial biopsy recommended for women with periods beyond 55
- FSH levels higher than 30 to 40 IU/L usually indicate menopause; however, single elevated FSH level does not reliably diagnose menopause

Climacteric

- The perimenopausal time period during which the ovary progressively reduces estrogen production and ceases ovulatory function

Menopausal and Perimenopausal Symptoms

- Menstrual irregularities
  —Common during perimenopause
  —Shorter or longer cycles common and do not necessarily require evaluation
  —Evaluate intermenstrual bleeding, bleeding without a discernible pattern, or excessively heavy bleeding
  —Women without contraindications may use low-dose oral contraceptive pills to control cycles
- Vasomotor symptoms
  —Hot flash (sudden onset of warmth)
  —Hot flush begins about a minute after hot flash; characterized by redness of upper body and profuse sweating
  —Often occur at night, disturbing sleep
  —Incidence: about 85% of women experience; number and severity vary
  —Related to low estrogen levels and respond well to estrogen therapy
- Psychological symptoms
  —Depression, irritability, anxiety, insomnia, forgetfulness, and difficulty in concentration have been associated with menopause
  —Timing of menopause often coincides with other significant changes in a woman's life (children leaving home, divorce, need to care for parents)
  —Estrogen has been helpful in some women with mild symptoms
  —Significant anxiety or depression needs to be treated regardless of menopausal status

Treatment: Basic Principles

- Symptoms, risk factors, and concerns: menopause is not a disease and medical treatment is not necessarily the best option for an individual
- Treatments are directed at relieving symptoms (such as hot flashes) or preventing complications of prolonged hypoestrogenic state (osteoporosis, urogenital atrophy)

- Hormonal therapy with estrogen or estrogen plus progestin has been the standard treatment but significant controversies exist regarding many aspects of therapy
  —Clear benefits include decreased hot flashes and flushes (by 80%); decreased bone loss; decreased risk of vertebral (by 50%) and hip (by 25%–30%) fractures
  —Definite risks include increased risk of DVT (by a factor of 2.7) and increased risk of endometrial cancer (only in women not taking a progestin as part of therapy)
  —Breast cancer risk does not seem to be increased with use of hormone therapy less than 5 years; longer use seems to increase risk by a factor of 1.35
  —For example of hormone regimens see Table 6.33

- Alternatives to traditional hormone therapy of menopause can be found in Table 6.35

DVT indicates deep venous thrombosis; FSH, follicle-stimulating hormone.

TABLE 6.33
Postmenopausal Hormone Therapy Regimens

Type	Regimen	Comments
Cyclic-sequential	■ Estrogen for 25 days ■ Progestin for last 12–14 days of estrogen ■ Last 5–6 days of each month hormone-free	■ Longest used method of postmenopausal hormone therapy ■ 97% of women will have withdrawal bleeding through age 60; drops to 60% after age 65 ■ No cases of endometrial cancer with sufficient dosing (10 mg MPA or 5 mg norethindrone) or duration (12–14 days) of progestin ■ Endometrial biopsy if bleeding during days taking hormones
Continuous-sequential	■ Estrogen each day ■ Progestin 12–14 days each month (usually first 12–14 days)	■ No estrogen withdrawal symptoms ■ 80%–90% have withdrawal bleeding ■ Endometrial biopsy if bleeding occurs before 10th day of progestin
Continuous Combined	■ Daily estrogen ■ Daily progestin	■ Some concern about ability of this method to protect against endometrial cancer ■ Goal is to achieve amenorrhea ■ May need to increase progestin dose to obtain amenorrhea ■ Endometrial biopsy if bleeding after 6 months of therapy
Cyclic Combined	■ Estrogen for 25 days each month ■ Progestin for same 25 days each month	■ Allows for shedding of any endometrial buildup ■ Amenorrhea often develops (75% by 4 months) ■ Amenorrhea less common before age 55

Type	Regimen	Comments
Widely Spaced Progestin Therapy	■ Daily estrogen ■ Progestin for 14 days every third to fourth month using higher progestin doses (MPA 10–20 mg)	■ Longer, heavier (but less frequent) withdrawal bleed ■ Some women have in-between bleeding ■ Decreasing interval between progestin administration or reserving method for women greater than 3 years after menopause, decreases unscheduled bleeding ■ Associated with 6%–20% incidence of endometrial hyperplasia in one study

TABLE 6.34

Contraindications for Hormone Replacement Therapy

Absolute Contraindications	Relative Contraindications
Estrogen-responsive breast cancer	Chronic liver disease
Endometrial cancer	Severe hypertriglyceridemia
Undiagnosed abnormal vaginal bleeding	Endometriosis
Active thromboembolic disease	Previous thromboembolic disease
Prior complications from estrogen	Gallbladder disease
	Acute intermittent porphyria
	Uterine fibroid tumors
	Risk for thromboembolic disease

TABLE 6.35

Alternatives to Traditional Hormone Therapy for Perimenopausal and Menopausal Symptoms

Vasomotor Symptoms

- SSRIs: Venlafaxine (Effexor) 60% reduction in hot flashes; Paroxetine (Paxil) similar reduction
- Clonidine: most studies show no benefit
- Progesterone cream: 20 mg ($\frac{1}{4}$ tsp) massaged into skin of arms, thighs, or breasts improved vasomotor symptoms
- Soy protein: natural phytoestrogens, effective in decreasing vasomotor symptoms, total cholesterol and LDL, and bone loss
- Black cohosh: an herbal remedy that may reduce symptoms. German Commission E recommends using no more than 6 months secondary to lack of clinical data on long-term use.

Bone Loss Prevention/Treatment

- SERMs (selective estrogen-receptor modulators): reduces risks of new vertebral fractures by 30%; no significant effect on nonvertebral fractures. Raloxifene approved for treatment and prevention of postmenopausal osteoporosis. Associated with hot flashes and increased thromboembolic events. Studies under way to assess role in prevention of breast cancer.
- Bisphosphonates: decrease risks of new vertebral, hip, and other nonvertebral fracture by 50%. May cause esophageal and GI side effects. Examples: alendronate (Fosamax) 10 mg daily or 70 mg weekly; risendronate (Actonel) 5 mg daily.

Urogenital Atrophy

- Vaginal estrogen cream: used daily to treat symptomatic vaginal dryness, atrophy. After 4–8 weeks can taper to several times weekly. An estrogen vaginal ring inserted and left in place for 90 days is an alternative.
- Vaginal lubricants may also be helpful.

GI indicates gastrointestinal; LDL, low-density lipoprotein; SSRIs, selective serotonin reuptake inhibitors.

chapter 7

Men's Health

John W. Hedrick, MD

IN THIS CHAPTER

- Lifespan facts
- Exercise prescription
- Recommended cancer screening
- Testosterone replacement therapies
- Monitoring testosterone replacement therapy
- Clinical signs and symptoms of andropause
- Andropause evaluation and treatment
- Tanner stages
- Depression in men
- Treatment of androgenic alopecia in men
- Renal disease in men
- Diagnosing nephrotic syndrome
- Renal stone disease
- Benign disease of the male anogenital tract
- Evaluation of scrotal or testicular mass
- Cystitis
- Microhematuria evaluation and treatment
- Bladder dysfunction
- Urinary incontinence treatment
- Genital trauma
- Inguinal hernia evaluation and treatment
- Neoplasia of the male anogenital tract and breast
- Prostate carcinoma staging system
- Urinary bladder cancer staging
- History, physical examination, and labs for male fertility workup
- Male contraception options

- Sexual problems: ejaculatory dysfunction
- Male genital and breast exam
- Circumcision
- Urethral culture for sexually transmitted disease
- Bladder catheterization
- Vasectomy

BOOKSHELF RECOMMENDATIONS

- Behrman RE, Kliegman R, Jenson HB, eds. *Nelson Textbook of Pediatrics*. 16th ed. Philadelphia, PA: WB Saunders Company; 2000.
- Bickley LS, ed. *Bates' Pocket Guide to Physical Examination and History Taking*. 3rd ed. Philadelphia, PA: Lippincott, Williams & Wilkins; 2000.
- Cotran RS, Kumar V, Collins T, et al. *Robbins Pathologic Basis of Disease*. 6th ed. Philadelphia, PA: WB Saunders Company; 1999.
- Nieh P. *Case Studies in Urology for the House Officer*. Philadelphia, PA: Lippincott, Williams & Williams; 1989.
- Pfenninger JL. *Procedures for Primary Care Physicians*. St Louis, MD: Mosby, Inc; 1994.
- Venes D, Thomas CL, eds. *Taber's Cyclopedic Medical Dictionary*. 19th ed. Philadelphia, PA: FA Davis Company; 2001.

WELLNESS

TABLE 7.1

Male Life Expectancy

All races	73.8 years
White	74.5 years
Black	67.6 years

TABLE 7.2

Exercise Prescription: Five Elements

1. **Aerobic activity:** specify type (ie, walking, cycling, running, swimming, rowing, etc).
2. **Frequency:** minimum every other day. Ideal is every day with sensible exceptions to rest and prevent overuse injury
3. **Duration:** at least 30 minutes of sustained activity. Longer regimens have additional health benefits (45–60 minutes)
4. **Intensity:** based on target heart rate. Target heart rate is determined by calculating maximal heart rate (HR) (220 bpm − age = max HR in bpm) then obtaining relative exercise intensity by percentage of maximal heart rate (low intensity: 55%–64% max HR; high intensity: 75%–90% max HR)
5. **Warm up and cool down:** gentle stretching or walking lasting up to 5 minutes for each portion

TABLE 7.3

Recommended Cancer Screening

Lung Cancer Screening

There are no recommendations for lung cancer screening in low risk or high-risk patients. Rather, the US Preventive Services Task Force recommends counseling patients against smoking. Sputum cytologies and screening chest x-rays have not been accurate in screening for lung cancer.

Oral Cancer Screening

Low-risk patient: Insufficient evidence for or against screening in these patients. However, visual inspection and cytology are the methods most commonly used to screen. Reducing alcohol and tobacco use is cited as the emphasis in low-risk populations.
High-risk patient: (history of heavy smoking or drinking) a regular oral exam by a physician or dentist is recommended.

Colorectal Cancer Screening

Average-risk persons over 50 years old:

Annual fecal occult blood testing or flexible sigmoidoscopy every 5 years;

Annual fecal occult blood testing and flexible sigmoidoscopy every 5 years; or

Double-contrast barium enema every 5–10 years; or

Colonoscopy every 10 years

High-risk person: first-degree relative with colorectal cancer or adenomatous polyps. Screening applies at age 40 or 10 years before the age at time of diagnosis in affected relative, whichever is earlier. Strongly consider colonoscopy for high-risk patient whose first-degree relative was less than 50 at time of diagnosis.

Skin Cancer

No consensus: American Cancer Society recommends skin exam every 3 years between ages 20 and 40 and annually thereafter. US Preventive Services Task Force found insufficient evidence to recommend for or against screening for skin cancer.

Testicular Cancer

American Cancer Society recommends testicular exam but does not give frequency of exam: US Preventive Services Task Force finds insufficient evidence for or against routine screening of low-risk patients. American Cancer Society recommends monthly self-exams in high-risk patients (testicular atrophy, ambiguous genitalia, cryptorchidism).

Prostate Cancer Screening

Low-risk patients: Insufficient evidence to support annual digital rectal exam (DRE) and prostate specific antigen (PSA) in asymptomatic patients. However, some recommend DRE and PSA for patients who are over age 50, have life expectancy of at least 10 years, who request screening and are fully informed of the limitations of screening.

High-risk patients (African Americans and patients with prostate cancer in two or more first-degree relatives): American Cancer Society (ACS) and American Urological Association (AUA) recommend DRE and PSA at age 45. However, others recommend discussing the limitations with patients and individualizing the approach.

TABLE 7.4

Testosterone Replacement Therapies

Generic	Trade	Dose	Comments
Oral			
Testosterone undecanoate	Andriol	120–200 mg divided tid	Monitor liver function and H/H if uses large doses
Fluoxymesterone	Halotestin	5–20 mg qd	May decrease the anticoagulant requirements in patients requiring oral anticoagulants
Methyl-testosterone	Metandren Testred Android	10–30 mg qd 10–50 mg/d 10–50 mg/d	May decrease glucose and insulin requirements
Parenteral (IM)			
Testosterone propionate		qod injection (rarely used)	Can cause hepatocellular neoplasms, hepatitis, polycythemia, increased cholesterol, and suppression of clotting factors II, V, VII, and X
Testosterone cypionate	Depo Testosterone Cypionate	200–400 mg q 3–4 wk	
Testosterone enanthate	Delatestryl	200–400 mg q 4 wk	
Transdermal			
Transdermal patch	Androderm	5 mg daily application to skin	Absorption is erratic
	Testoderm	4, 6 mg daily application to scrotum	Higher risk of hepatotoxicity
	Testoderm TTS Androgel 1%	5 mg daily to skin 5 mg daily applied to skin	Monitor liver function

TABLE 7.5

Monitoring Testosterone Replacement Therapy

- Annual liver function tests
- Fasting lipid panel (particular emphasis with inpatients with significant coronary risk factors)
- Annual digital rectal exam and prostate specific antigen
- Monitor for exacerbations for worsening of sleep apnea

Adapted from Morales A, Heaton JP, Carson CC III. Andropause: a misnomer for a true clinical entity. *J Urol.* 2000;163:705–712.

TABLE 7.6

Clinical Signs and Symptoms of Andropause

Subsequent to middle age androgen levels in men decline. This male climacteric is manifested variably among men with fatigue, depression, decreased libido, erectile dysfunction, mood, and cognitive disturbances.

- Gradual onset and progression
- Decreasing libido
- Erectile dysfunction
- Mood fluctuations (fatigue, depression, anger)
- Decreased intellectual activity
- Decreased muscle volume and strength
- Decreased body hair
- Skin changes
- Osteoporosis
- Increased visceral fat

Adapted from Morales A, Heaton JP, Carson CC III. Andropause: a misnomer for a true clinical entity. *J Urol.* 2000;163:705–712.

FIGURE 7.1

Andropause Evaluation and Treatment

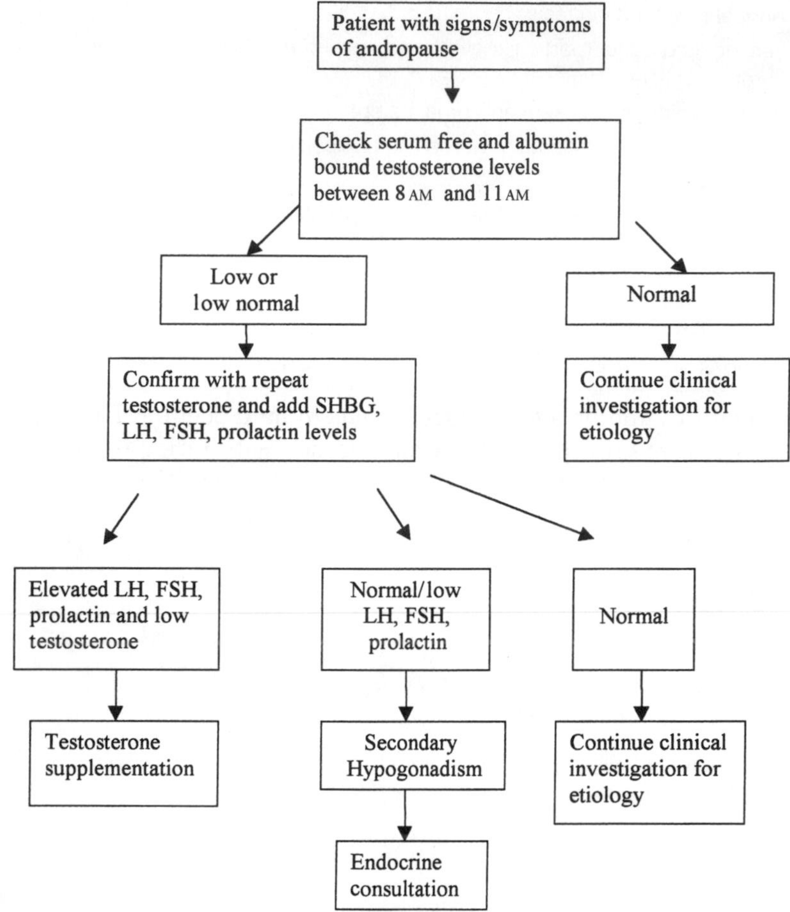

Adapted from Morales A, Heaton JP, Carson CC 3rd. Andropause: a misnomer for a true clinical entity. *J Urol.* 2000;163:705–712.

FSH indicates follicle stimulating hormone; LH, luteinizing hormone; SHBG, serum hormone binding globulin.

TABLE 7.7

Tanner Stages: Classification of Sex Maturity Stages in Boys

SMR Stage	Pubic Hair	Penis	Testes
1	None	Preadolescent	Preadolescent
2	Scanty, long, slightly pigmented, texture altered	Slight enlargement	Enlarged scrotum, pink
3	Darker, starts to curl, small amount	Longer	Larger
4	Resembles adult type but less in quantity; coarse, curly	Larger, glans and increase in breadth	Larger, scrotum dark
5	Adult distribution, spread to medial surface of thighs	Adult size	Adult size

Adapted from Behrman RE, Kliegman R, Jenson HB, eds. *Nelson Textbook of Pediatrics*. 16th ed. Philadelphia, PA: WB Saunders Company; 2000.

MENTAL HEALTH

TABLE 7.8

Depression in Men

Risk Factors for Depression in Men

- Alcohol abuse
- Comorbid disease
- Family history of depression
- History of depression
- Physical disabilities
- Psychosocial stressors
- Side effects of medications (beta blockers, antihistamines, methyldopa, benzodiazepines, reserpine, barbiturates)
- Social isolation
- Single marital status

Most Frequent Symptoms of Depression in Men*

- Change in bowel habits
- Fatigue
- Multiple somatic complaints
- Sleep disturbances
- Weight fluctuation

Selective Serotonin Reuptake Inhibitor (Preferred Drug Therapy)

- Citalopram (Celexa)
- Fluoxetine (Prozac)†
- Paroxeline (Paxil)†
- Setraline (Zoloft)†

*Depressed mood is less common in elderly patients.

†Preferred in elderly men due to shorter half life.

TABLE 7.9

Treatment of Androgenic Alopecia in Men

Topical Therapy

- Minoxidil: Best in younger patients with limited hair loss occurring less than 5 years; must be used indefinitely; 30%–40% success rate

Oral Therapy

- Finasteride: 1 mg/d; 70%–80% response rate; must be used indefinitely

Surgical

- Transplant
- Flap procedure

Artificial Techniques

- Hair weave
- Toupee

TABLE 7.10

Renal Diseases More Common in Men

Renal Cell Carcinoma Male preponderance of 3:1. 85%–90% of all renal cancer in adults usually diagnosed in 60s and 70s. Higher frequency in cigarette, pipe, and cigar smokers. *Clinical presentation*: Classic triad—CVA pain, palpable abdominal mass, hematuria. Hematuria in 90% cases. More advanced cases present with fever, malaise, weakness, and weight loss. Unfortunately, tumors have grown up to 10 cm in diameter and have metastasized before symptoms are noted. May be associated with the following paraneoplastic syndromes: polycythemia, hypercalcemia, hypertension, feminization, Cushing syndrome, eosinophilia, leukemoid reactions, amyloidosis. 25% of patients present with metastasis on diagnosis. 50% of these are metastasis to lung, 33% to bone, and 10%–15% to the contralateral kidney. *Prognosis*: The average 5-year survival is about 45%, while the average 5-year survival without distant metastasis is about 70%. With renal vein or perinephric fat invasion, the 5-year survival is 15%–20%. *Treatment*: Nephrectomy is the treatment of choice.
Membranous Glomerulonephritis *Incidence*: Peak age 35–50 years old; male to female ratio is 2:1. *Clinical presentation*: Usually asymptomatic with proteinuria discovered on routine UA. *Diagnosis*: Nephrotic range proteinuria. Kidney biopsy required for diagnosis. *Lab*: C3, C4, CH50, ANA, RF, ESR, anti-GBM titer, Hep panel ANCA, ASO titer or strep screen, HIV serology, antithyroid ABs, RPR, anti-DNA. Evaluate for common malignancies (lung, colon, prostate, etc). *Etiology*: Usually idiopathic. However, 25% of cases have underlying disease such as SLE, hepatitis B and C, tumors, drug toxicity, and parasitic infection. *Treatment*: Steroids, cytotoxic agents, or combination. *Prognosis*: One third of patients progress to dialysis 10 years from diagnosis and one third regress or completely resolve.
Postinfectious Proliferative Glomerulonephritis *Incidence*: 2:1 male predominance, rare prior to 2 years. Most common cause of nephritic urine in school-aged children with glomerulonephritis. No age predilection in adults. *Clinical presentation*: Most commonly follows group A, β-hemolytic streptococcal upper respiratory or skin infection. However, may also occur in patients with subacute bacterial endocarditis, visceral abscesses, osteomyelitis, or bacterial sepsis, hematuria, hypertension,

edema, proteinuria, and acute renal failure. Not all patients will have severe presentation and many patients may be asymptomatic, particularly in household contacts of index cases. Nephrotic range proteinuria is uncommon. 8–14 day latency after infection and may be long as 21–28 days following skin infections.

Diagnosis: Culture, ASO titer, complement profile, ANA, RF, ESR, anti-GBM ABs, Hep panel, ANCA, HIV serology. Renal biopsy in all adults and in children who present atypically or in whom disease persists.

Treatment: Blood pressure treatment is addressed with fluid and sodium restriction and antihypertensive agents as indicated. Azotemia is addressed with protein restriction. Close contacts to index cases should receive throat cultures and treatment as indicated.

Prognosis: Complete recovery is common in children, but adults with decreased creatinine clearance, persistent proteinuria >2 mg per day, or who are elderly have decreased chance of return to normal renal function.

Goodpasture Syndrome (Antiglomerular Basement Membrane Disease)

Incidence: Peak age in 30s, second peak over 60 years; 2:1 male predominance.

Clinical presentation: Pulmonary hemorrhage and nephritis are classic. Hemorrhage varies in severity from hemoptysis to CXR infiltrates and may occur remote from nephritis. Smoking, infections, and fluid overload are common exacerbating agents.

Diagnosis: Presence of serum anti-GBM ABs on renal biopsy.

Etiology: Autoantibodies to GBM antigen, which cross-reacts with pulmonary tissue antigens.

Treatment: 14-day course of albumin plasma exchange, systemic steroids, and cytotoxic therapy. Patients typically recover fully unless near end-stage failure when treatment is begun. Recurrence rarely occurs but usually responds to repeat therapy. It is important to note, however, that a significant number of patients progress to complete renal failure.

IgA Nephropathy (Berger Disease)

Incidence: Occurs most frequently in 20s and 30s with a 3:1 male predilection. The most common form of glomerulonephritis (20%–40% of biopsy-proven cases).

Clinical presentation: Macroscopic hematuria following a URI is the typical presentation. It may also present with microscopic hematuria on routine UA. Nephrotic range proteinuria is seen in some cases, but proteinuria typically is mild.

Diagnosis: Renal biopsy.

Etiology: Due to deposition of IgA in the glomerular mesangium.

Continued

TABLE 7.10

Renal Diseases More Common in Men, cont'd

Treatment: Aggressive steroid and cytotoxic agents are used only in acute renal failure or if glomerular crescents are seen on electron microscopy.

Prognosis: Usually slowly progress to chronic renal failure. Some patients, however, escape renal failure. 20-year kidney survival is 75%.

ANA indicates antinuclear antibody; ESR, erythrocyte sedimentation rate; HIV, human immunodeficiency virus; IgA, immunoglobulin; RPR, rapid plasma reagin; SLE, systemic lupus erythematosus; UA, urinalysis.

TABLE 7.11

Diagnosing Nephrotic Syndrome

Criteria for Diagnosis

- Proteinuria ≥3.5 g /24 hr/1.73 m
- Serum albumin <3.5 g/dL
- Serum total cholesterol >200 mg/dL
- Edema

Primary Causes

- Membranous glomerulonephritis
- Postinfectious proliferative glomerulonephritis
- Goodpasture syndromes
- IgA nephropathy (Berger disease)

Secondary Causes

- Autoimmune: Goodpasture syndromes; polyarteritis nodosa
- Infectious: postinfectious glomerulonephritis
- Neoplastic: Hodgkin disease, non-Hodgkin lymphoma, chronic lymphogenous leukemia, hairy cell leukemia

TABLE 7.12

Renal Stone Disease More Common in Men

Idiopathic Hypercalciuria: Unknown etiology. Appears heritable, more prominent in men and more common during the third decade of life.

Diagnosis: 24-hour urine calcium excretion exceeds 300 mg/24 h. Serum calcium is normal.

Treatment: Long-acting thiazide diuretics, increase fluids to produce >2 L urine per day. Monitor for hypokalemia and supplement as indicated or add potassium-sparing diuretic. Avoid triamterene due to its stone-forming propensity. Low sodium and protein diet. Normal calcium diet. Follow-up by repeat 24 urine calcium.

TABLE 7.13

Benign Disease of the Male Anogenital Tract

Selected Penile Anomalies
■ *Epispadias*: Congenital opening of the urethra on the dorsal penile surface
■ *Hypospadias*: Congenital opening of the urethra on the ventral penile surface
■ *Peyronie Disease*: Fibrous thickening and contracture of the cavernous sheaths of the penile corpora resulting in penile deviation with erections
Scrotal Pathology
■ *Cryptorchidism*: Condition of prenatally undescended testicle/testicles. The cryptorchid testis is at higher risk for future cancer development.

FIGURE 7.2
Evaluation of Scrotal or Testicular Mass

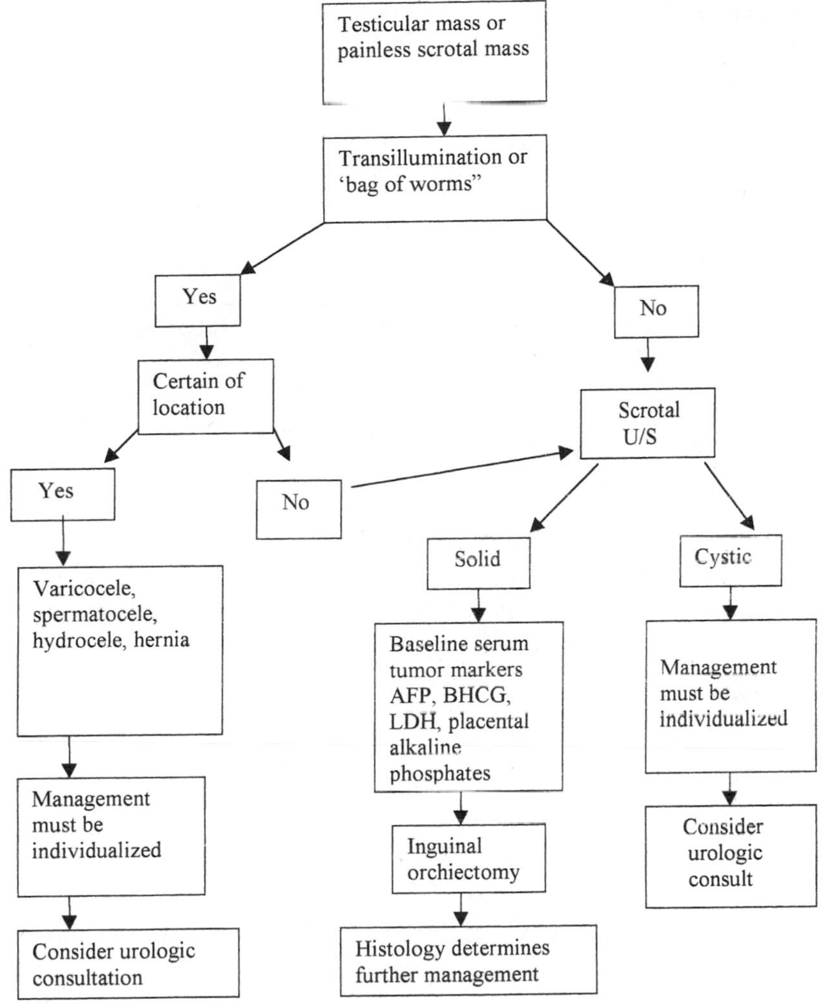

TABLE 7.14

Cystitis in Men*

Irritative Symptoms

- Frequency
- Urgency
- Nocturia
- Dysuria

Low Back Pain

Suprapubic Pain

*Men are at higher risk of concomitant urinary tract pathology (ie, prostatitis, urethritis, strictures, benign prostatic hypertrophy, etc).

TABLE 7.15

Uncomplicated UTI in Healthy Men Aged 15–50

Risk Factors for Urovirulent Strains

- Insertive anal intercourse
- Intercourse with a vaginally infected or colonized female partner
- Noncircumcised patient

Diagnosis

- Clinical symptoms are the same as in women
- Rule out urethritis with gram stain and culture
- $\geq 10^4$ CFU/mL on urine culture
- *Escherichia coli*, Enterobacteriaceae are most common pathogens

Treatment

- Fluoroquinolones are recommended initial empiric treatment
- Add amoxicillin to empiric treatment if enterococcus suspected on initial gram stain
- 7-day treatment course for uncomplicated UTI
- 10–14 days treatment for pyelonephritis
- Obtain pretreatment and posttreatment culture
- 4–6 week course of therapy if recurrent species due to potential prostatic or upper urinary source

Further Urologic Studies

- Adolescents and men with pyelonephritis, recurrent infections, or if complicated infection (catheter related, etc)

UTI indicates urinary tract infection; CFU, colony-forming units.

FIGURE 7.3

Microhematuria Evaluation and Treatment

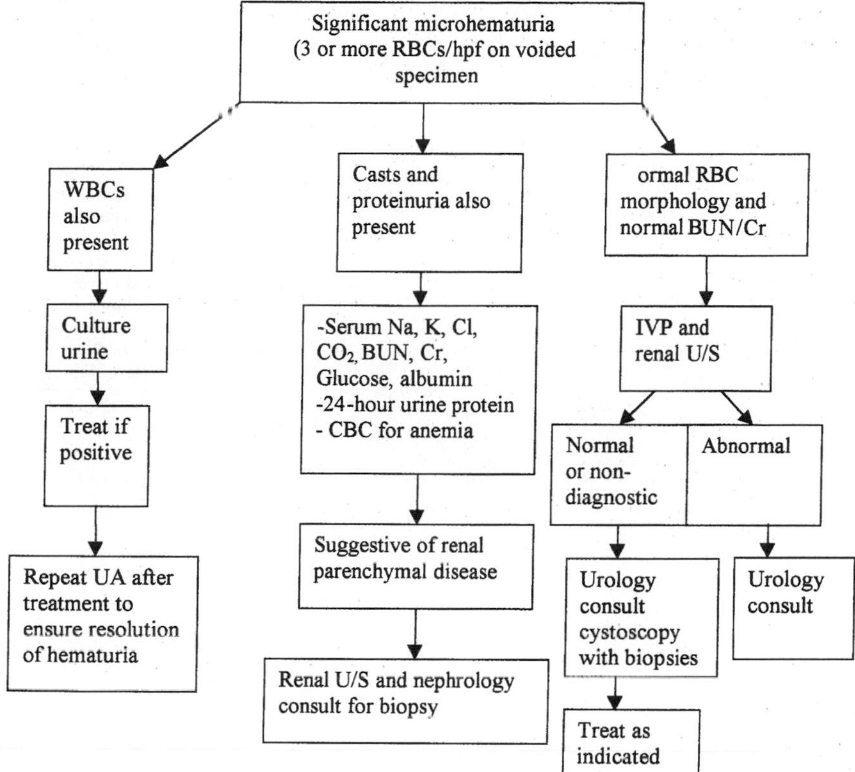

FIGURE 7.4

Bladder Dysfunction

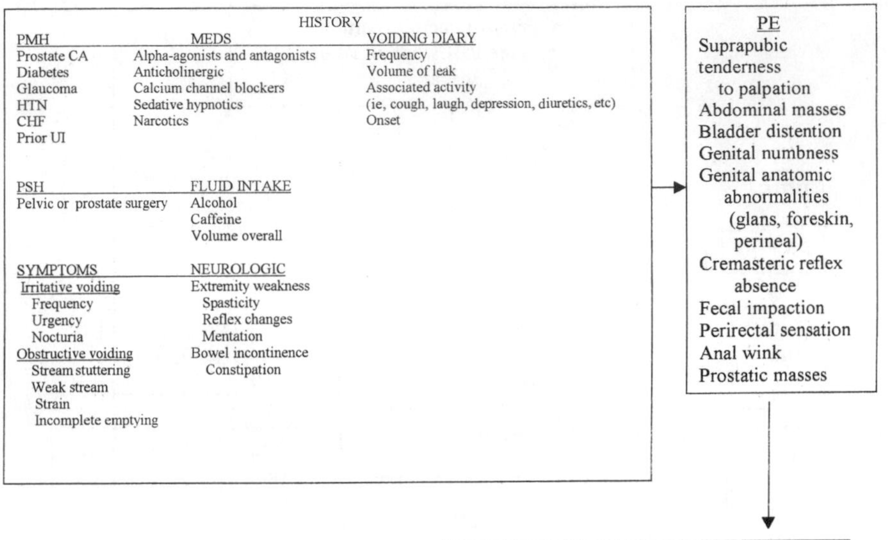

LABS

UA: infection, diabetes, tumor

Post void Residual: obstruction or weak detrussor muscle

Uroflowmetry: obstruction or weak detrussor muscle

UROLOGIC CONSULTATION IF:

Prior pelvic surgery or irradiation

Frequent UTI

Severe hesitancy

Post void residual >200 mL

Inability to catheterize

Persistent hematuria

Initial treatment failure

TABLE 7.16

Urinary Incontinence Treatment

Overflow Incontinence

- Remove the etiology of obstruction (TURP; alpha-blockers; terazosin [titrate to 10 mg qhs], Finasteride 5 mg qhs)
- Discontinue implicated medications

Functional Incontinence

- Prompted voiding
- Timed voiding
- Diapers

Urge Incontinence

- Anticholinergic medication (Oxybutynin 2.5–5 mg tid; tolterodine [Detrol] 1–2 mg bid)
- Bladder training
- Biofeedback

Stress Incontinence

- Biofeedback (except total incontinence)
- Collagen injections
- Artificial sphincter placement

TABLE 7.17

Male Genital Trauma

Superficial Penile/Scrotal Lacerations: Reapproximate with 4.0 chromic or Vicryl suture.

Penile Degloving or Scrotal Skin Loss: Immediate urologic and plastic surgery consultation for intraoperative cleansing debridement, grafting, and skin flaps.

Traumatic Penile Amputation: If recovered, the amputated distal penis should be placed in a clean plastic bag and immersed in cold saline. For proximal stump hemorrhage, direct pressure and temporary circumferential Penrose drain placement at the penile base may be used until urologic and plastic surgery consultants arrive. Reanastomosis of a severed penis is possible up to 6 hours after amputation. Otherwise, local reshaping is advised.

Penile Fracture (Corpus Cavernosum Rupture): Usually associated with vigorous intercourse. The tearing of the tunica albuginea results in immediate pain, detumescence, and subsequent development of an enlarging penile hematoma. Nonoperative management with ice packs and bed rest for 24–48 hours followed by heat and pressure dressings is rarely used and is not generally advised. 10% of patients with fractured penis, particularly managed nonoperatively, will have permanent deformity, decreased sexual pleasure, and erectile dysfunction. Operative management consists of repairing the torn tunica with subsequent application of a pressure dressing.

Traumatic Lymphangitis: Clinically presents as translucent, nodular, mobile, nontender subcutaneous mass at the level of the coronal sulcus that may be semicircular or may encircle the entire penis. Associated with prolonged intercourse or masturbation, it is treated with sexual abstinence and nonsteroidal anti-inflammatory drugs (NSAIDs). Resolution typically occurs within 2–3 weeks.

Human Penile Bite: Obtained during sexual activity. Treatment in immunocompetent patients is with outpatient cephalexin, NSAIDs, and reexam in 2–3 days. Immunocompromised patients should be treated as inpatients with broad-spectrum systemic antibiotic coverage for anaerobic and aerobic bacteria particularly if cellulitis is apparent at exam.

Testicular Trauma: Ultrasound with Doppler is the study of choice to completely evaluate testicular integrity.

- *Testicular contusion*: Treat with bed rest, ice packs, NSAIDs, and urologic consultation.
- *Testicular dislocation, laceration, disruption*: Intraoperative hematoma evacuation, testicular parenchymal debridement and repair of the tunica albuginea is ideal treatment. Note that with

testicular dislocation, associated injuries such as pelvic fracture, hip dislocation, and contusions are common.

Urethral Injury: Any blood at the urethral meatus is indication for retrograde urethrography to rule out urethral laceration. Failure to identify urethral trauma may contribute to subsequent development of urethral strictures and incontinence.

FIGURE 7.5

Inguinal Hernia Evaluation and Treatment

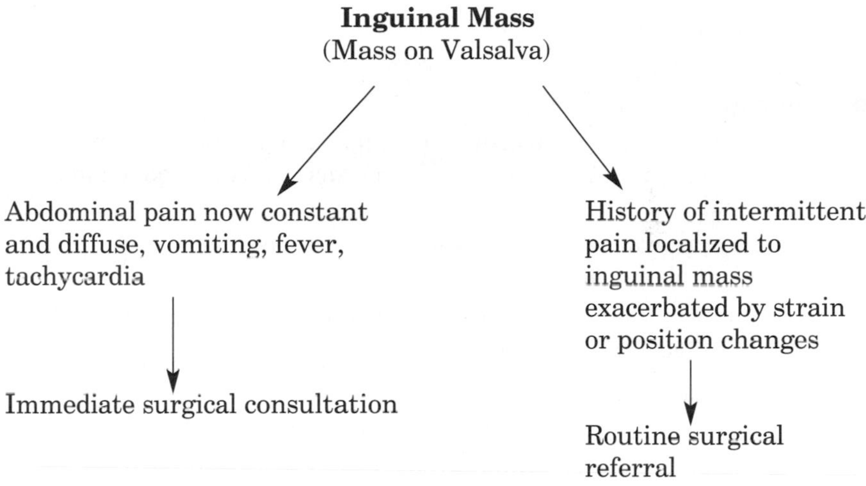

TABLE 7.18

Neoplasia of the Male Anogenital Tract and Breast

Breast Cancer in Men

- Fewer than 1% of cancers in men
- Highest incidence 40s–70s
- Clinically presents as unilateral, nontender, firm, immobile, eccentric breast mass; some cases have associated spontaneous nipple discharge, lymphadenopathy, or skin dimpling overlying the mass
- Evaluation is via ultrasound, mammography, needle biopsy, and surgical consultation

Penile Carcinoma

- <1% of cancer in men
- Unknown etiology
- Circumcision is effective preventive measure if done in infancy; the same is apparently not true if circumcision is postponed into adulthood
- Clinical appearance is red, velvety, moist-appearing, well-delineated plaque or papule
- Located most often on the glans or prepuce; may have foul-smelling purulent discharge from foreskin

Testicular Cancer

- Relatively rare cancer with 2–3/100,000 cases annually
- Over 95% are germ cell tumors; remainder are either stromal or metastatic
- More common in whites than African Americans
- Most common in right testicle; likely related to the fact that cryptorchidism is mostly on the right
- Older individuals have higher incidence of seminoma and testicular lymphoma
- Orchiopexy does not decrease cancer risk for cryptorchid testes, but rather keeps testicle accessible for surveillance and screening
- Increased risk of developing cancer in contralateral testicle if present in one testicle
- Testicular cancer is 20–50 times more common in immunosuppressed patients
- Additional testicular cancer risks: sedentary lifestyle, diagnosis of neonatal jaundice and microsomia, and excess in utero estrogen exposure
- 2 times greater risk in son of father with testicular cancer and higher risk to brothers of cancer patient

- Present with painless testicular mass or may be found on screening exam
- Ultrasound is diagnostic
- Serum markers are used to moniter treatment response
- α-Fetoprotein, B-HCG, LDH, and placental alkaline phosphatase are obtained
- Treatment is via orchiectomy; subsequent radiation and or chemotherapy are decided based on histologic findings

Prostate Cancer (see Table 7.19 for treatment)

Demographics

- Most common US male cancer
- 1 in 10 will develop prostate CA
- Highest incidence in men over 50
- Japanese-Americans have lowest incidence
- African-Americans have highest incidence

Risk Factors

- Three times higher risk of cancer if first-degree relative with disease
- 10 times risk if first- and second-degree relative with disease
- Patients with hereditary prostate cancer 1 locus (HPC-1) demonstrate earlier age, more aggressive cancers, and higher-grade tumors at time of diagnosis
- STDs are not risk
- Slightly increased risk in men with BPH
- No causal relationship between vasectomy and prostate CA
- PSA and DRE are available screening resources
- Histologic grade correlates with prognosis

Urinary Bladder Cancer (see Table 7.20 for staging)

- 2.5 times more common in men than women
- Over 90% of bladder cancer is transitional cell type
- 70% higher incidence in whites than African Americans
- Presents with gross hematuria or microhematuria in over 75% of cases; may also have irritative symptoms (dysuria, urgency, frequency), flank pain, and be totally asymptomatic
- Diagnosis with IVP and cystoscopy
- Treatment (see Table 7.19)
- Reconstructive procedures after radical cystoprostatectomy include ilioconduit procedure with cutaneous urinary ostomy

Continued

TABLE 7.18

Neoplasia of the Male Anogenital Tract and Breast, cont'd

and neobladder construction; these reconstructions require frequent self-catheterization and involve recurrent infection

Scrotal Cancer

- Rare male cancer
- Usually squamous cell carcinoma treated with local excision
- Malignant melanoma and basal-cell carcinoma may be rarely seen and are treated as in other dermatologic locations

Urethral Cancer

- Usually squamous cell carcinoma in bulbar or pendulous urethra
- Associated with benign urethral stricture
- Presents with obstructive voiding symptoms or as tender urethral mass
- Treatment is based on tumor location and stage and involves local excision with radiation and chemotherapy as indicated

BPH indicates benign prostatic hyperplasia; DRE, digital rectal examination; IVP, intravenous pyelogram; LDH, lactate dehydrogenase; PSA, prostate-specific antigen; STD, sexually transmitted disease.

TABLE 7.19

Prostate Carcinoma Staging System

American (Whitmore-Jewett)	TNM	Criteria	Treatment
A	T1	Incidental tumor found on TURP specimen	Observation
A1	T1a	Three or fewer microscopic foci seen in TURP specimen	Radical retropubic prostatectomy and radiotherapy
A2	T1b	More than three microscopic foci seen in TURP specimen	Radical retropubic prostatectomy and radiotherapy
B	T2	Tumor confined to the prostate	Radical retropubic prostatectomy and radiotherapy
B1	T2a	Tumor is 1.5 cm or less and surrounded by normal tissue on three sides	Radical retropubic prostatectomy and radiotherapy
B2	T2b	Tumor is >1.5 cm or present in both lobes	Radical retropubic prostatectomy and radiotherapy
C	T3	Tumor invading the capsule, apex, bladder neck, or seminal vesicle but is not fixed	Radical retropubic prostatectomy and radiotherapy
C1	T3	No invasion of seminal vesicles	Radical retropubic prostatectomy and radiotherapy
C2	T3	Seminal vesicle invasion	Radical retropubic prostatectomy and radiotherapy
C2	T4	Pelvic wall fixed to seminal vesicle	Radical retropubic prostatectomy and radiotherapy
C2	T4	Tumor invading adjacent structures other than those listed for T3	Radical retropubic prostatectomy and radiotherapy
D	N	Lymph node metastasis	Hormonal therapy with Lupron or orchiectomy (chemotherapy rarely effective)
D1	N	May or may not be grossly confined to gland with regional pelvic lymph node metastasis	Hormonal therapy with Lupron or orchiectomy (chemotherapy rarely effective)

Continued

TABLE 7.19

Prostate Carcinoma Staging System, cont'd

American (Whitmore-Jewett)	TNM	Criteria	Treatment
D2	M	Distant metastasis	Hormonal therapy with Lupron or orchiectomy (chemotherapy rarely effective)
D3	M	Advanced metastatic diseases with progression after hormonal therapy	Hormonal therapy with Lupron or orchiectomy (chemotherapy rarely effective)

Adapted from Epperson W, Frank W. Male genital cancers. *Prim Care*. 1998;25:459–472.

TURP indicates transurethral prostatectomy, TNM, tumor, nodal, metastasis involvement from the International Tumor Classification.

TABLE 7.20

Urinary Bladder Cancer Staging

American (Marshall)	TNM	Criteria	Treatment
Stage 0	ta	Tumor limited to mucosa; papillary noninvasive	Transurethral resection and follow up with intravesicle chemotherapy or immunotherapy for multifocal or recurrent tumor
	Tis	Carcinoma in situ	Transurethral resection and follow up with intravesicle chemotherapy or immunotherapy for multifocal or recurrent tumor
Stage A	T1	Tumor through lamina propria, but not the muscularis propria	Transurethral resection and follow up with intravesicle chemotherapy or immunotherapy for multifocal or recurrent tumor
Stage B1	T2	Tumor one half or less of the bladder wall	Radical cystoprostatectomy
Stage B2	T3a	Tumor into more than one half of the bladder wall, but still contained within the muscularis propria	Radical cystoprostatectomy
Stage C	T3b	Tumor into the perivesical fat	Radical cystoprostatectomy
Stage D1	T4a	Invasion of the prostate	Radical cystoprostatectomy
	T4b	Invasion of the pelvic or abdominal wall	Radical cystoprostatectomy
Stage D2		Widespread metastasis	Radical cystoprostatectomy

Adapted from Epperson W, Frank W. Male genital cancers. *Prim Care*. 1998;25:459–472.

TNM indicates tumor, nodal, metastasis involvement from the International Tumor Classification.

TABLE 7.21

History for Male Fertility Workup

Infertility	Sexual	Childhood
Length of infertility Prior fathered children Prior infertility evaluation Female partner evaluation and treatment	Erectile dysfunction Lubricant use Intercourse timing and frequency Masturbation frequency	Congenital anomalies Cryptorchidism/orchiopexy Testicular torsion or trauma Puberty onset
Surgical	**Medical**	**Family**
Orchiectomy Retroperitoneal trauma Pelvic trauma Pelvic, inguinal, or scrotal surgery Herniorrhaphy Y-V plasty TURP	Systemic illness Prior/current therapy Viral/febrile infections Mumps orchitis STDs TB Smallpox	Cystic fibrosis Androgen receptor deficiency First-degree relatives w/infertility
Medications/Gonadotoxins		**ROS**
Drugs ■ Chemotherapy ■ Cimetidine ■ Sulfasalazine ■ Nitrofurantoin Alcohol, marijuana, tobacco Androgenic steroids *Chemicals (pesticides)* *Thermal exposure* ■ Radiation		Anosmia Galactorrhea Visual field defects Respiratory infections

TABLE 7.22

PE for Male Fertility Workup

Habitus	Abdominal/Inguinal
Hair presence	Surgical scars
Gynecomastia	Orchiopexy
Eunuchoid appearance	Herniorrhaphy Y-V plasty
Rectum	**Phallus**
Prostate size, masses	Hypospadias/epispadias
Seminal vesicle presence, dilation, induration	Chordee
Scrotum	
Testicular size, consistency (firm, 20 cm^3)	
Epididymis presence, dilation, induration	
Vas deferens presence, induration, granuloma	
Varicocele	

TABLE 7.23

Labs for Male Fertility Workup

Semen Analysis	Endocrine Testing (Morning Collection)
Adequate	LH
Volume-1.5 to 5.0 mL	FSH
Density > 20 million/mL	Serum testosterone
Motility > 60%	Prolactin (if galactorrhea)
Forward progression > 2 (scale 0 to 4)	
Morphology > 60% normal	
No significant sperm agglutination	
No significant pyospermia	
No hyperviscosity	

TABLE 7.24

Interpretation of Male Infertility Testing

Condition	Findings	Treatment
Primary testicular failure	Elevated FSH, LH, severe oligospermia or azospermia, low testosterone	None
Varicocele	Elevated FSH, borderline oligoasthenospermia in the presence of varicocele, LH, and testosterone normal	Varicocelectomy
Hypogonadotropic hypogonadism	Low FSH, LH, testosterone, and anosmia	HGC-HMG
Prolactinoma	Elevated prolactin level	Bromocriptine or surgery
Androgen receptor resistance	Elevated testosterone, borderline LH elevation, FSH NL, oligospermia or azospermia; 5 alpha-reductase deficiency is suspected with additional history of ambiguous genitalia	Untreatable

TABLE 7.25

Male Contraceptive Options

Condom

- Readily accessible. Available in polyurethane for patients with latex allergy. Protects also against STDs.

Vasectomy

- Offers permanent sterility with option of potential reversibility. MINS (minimally invasive, no scalpel) technique offers less postoperative edema and discomfort. 29% of all vasectomies in the US are with MINS technique.

Experimental Options

- *Hormonal*: Decrease spermatogenesis via combination of hormonal agents to suppress FSH and intratesticular testosterone effects. Examples include DMPA and testosterone enanthate.
- *Gonadal toxins*: Examples include gossypol, nitrofuran derivatives, and sulfasalazine. Currently side effects such as hypokalemia and pulmonary fibrosis preclude marketed use.
- *Immunotherapy*: Vaccines to develop antibodies to FSH and LHRH.

TABLE 7.26

Sexual Problems: Ejaculatory Dysfunction

Premature Ejaculation

- *Definition*: Orgasm within 1 minute after vaginal penetration or ejaculation prior to effecting anticipated partner pleasure
- *Treatment (medical)*:
  —SSRIs (in order of greatest ejaculatory delay)
  Paroxetine (Paxil) 20 mg/d
  Fluoxetine (Prozac) 20 mg/d
  Sertraline (Zoloft) 50 mg*
  —Tricyclic
  Clomipramine (Anafranil) 25 mg/d
  —Local
  - Topical 2% lidocaine jelly (no literature recommended guidelines for use)
  - 2.5 lidocaine/2.5 procaine cream (Emla): apply to penis and occlude with condom 30 minutes prior to intercourse. Recommend washing off with soap and water prior to penetration to prevent excess vaginal and penile anesthesia. This method may be titrated to obtain optimal desensitization for the patient.
  - SS cream (herbal topical preparation, which reportedly increases ejaculatory latency 10-fold)

  —Behavioral modification therapy
  - Usually with sex therapist
  - Usually concomitantly with medical and or local therapies

Retrograde Ejaculation

- *History*: Presence of aspermia (no ejaculate from penile meatus with orgasm)
- *Diagnosis*: Postmasturbatory urinalysis with spermatozoa in the specimen
- *Etiologies*:
  —Diabetes mellitus: May cause retrograde and anejaculation secondary to autonomic neuropathies
  —Spinal cord injuries: Due to damage of nerves that coordinate ejaculation
  —Transurethral resection of the prostate (TURP): secondary to incomplete bladder neck closure
  —Abdominopelvic surgery (colorectal resection, ileoanal anastomosis, retroperitoneal lymphadenectomy): secondary to nerve damage

—Pediatric congenital pelvic anomalies: Due to anatomic abnormality or from the surgical correction of the anomaly

—Drug induced: SSRIs, MAOIs, TCAs, antihypertensives, NSAIDs, alcohol, methadone, bethanidine, chlordiazepoxide, epsilon-aminocaproic acid, guanethidine sulfate, hexamethonium, pargyline, phentolamine

Treatment

—Discontinue offending medication

—Medical:

- Pseudoephedrine: Sudafed Plus (120 mg 90 minutes prior to ejaculation or 60 mg qid × 3 days prior to ejaculation)
- Phenylpropanolamine: Ornade or nasal-D (75 mg bid 3 days prior to ejaculation)
- Imipramine: Tofranil (25 mg qhs or bid × 1 month)
- Phenylephrine: Neo-Synephrine (dose 1–2 hours prior to ejaculation)
- Ephedrine: Ventolin, Alupent, Proventil (30–60 mg 1–2 hours prior to ejaculation)

Ejaculatory Duct Obstruction

- *History*: Low-volume ejaculation, painful ejaculation, hematospermia, perineal or testicular pain
- *Physical Exam*: Normal vasa deferentia bilaterally, semen volume <2 mL, pH <7.2, and no sperm or fructose in semen
- *Diagnostic Testing*: Transrectal ultrasound showing seminal vesicle dilated >1.5 cm or dilated ejaculatory ducts >2.3 mm; may show associated intraductal cyst, calcifications, or stones (other methods include transrectal seminal vesicle sperm aspiration, transrectal seminal vesiculography, and vasography)
- *Treatment*: Guided by the etiology of the obstruction (ie, stones are removed after transurethral resection of the ejaculatory ducts)

MAOI indicates monoamine oxidase inhibitor; NSAIDs, nonsteroidal anti-inflammatory drugs; SSRI, selective serotonin reuptake inhibitor; TCA, tricyclic antidepressant.

*A study suggests Zoloft may be as effective on an as-needed basis.

PROCEDURES/SKILLS

TABLE 7.27

Male Genital and Breast Exam

Penis (standing)

- Inspection: For appearance of age-appropriate virilization, normal prepuce, normal glans, and urethral meatus
- Palpation: Particularly the shaft for stricture or masses

Scrotum (standing)

- Inspection: Any appearance of masses or skin abnormalities
- Palpation: Note any testicular, epididymal, or vas deferens masses or tenderness

Hernia (standing)

- Inspection: Look for any femoral/inguinal masses with Valsalva maneuver
- Palpation: Note any advancing mass or tissue contacting examining finger through external inguinal ring

Digital Rectal Exam (lateral decubitus or supine with knees flexed to chest)

- Inspection: Note any sacrococcygeal or perianal abnormalities
- Palpation: Sweep the rectal walls for masses or tenderness; examine the prostate for mass or tenderness

Breasts

- Inspection: Note normal nipple and areola
- Palpation: Examine areola and breast tissue for masses; palpate axilla for adenopathy

TABLE 7.28

Neonatal Circumcision Anesthesia

Dorsal Penile Nerve Block

- Cleanse the 2 o'clock and 10 o'clock positions at the base of the penile shaft with alcohol.
- Using a tuberculin syringe, insert the needle about 0.3 mm beneath the skin surface, oriented parallel to the penile shaft.
- Inject 0.3 mL of lidocaine without epinephrine.
- Repeat to opposite site.

TABLE 7.29

Neonatal Gomco Circumcision

Consent

Most institutions have printed literature on risks and benefits of elective circumcision—be sure to cover decreased incidence of HIV, STDs penile cancer, UTIs, and balanitis. Also female partners of uncircumcised males have a higher incidence of cervical cancer. Inquire regarding a family history of hemophilia.

Contraindications

- Hypospadias
- Penile anatomic pathology
- Ambiguous genitalia
- Age <12 hours old
- Severe illness
- Prematurity (until ready for discharge)

HIV indicates human immunodeficiency virus; STD, sexually transmitted disease; UTI, urinary tract infection.

TABLE 7.30

Procedure for Circumcision

After local anesthesia (if desired), prepare and sterilize, drape the penis and scrotum.

- Using hemostats, stabilize the foreskin by clamping it at the 10 o'clock and 2 o'clock positions.
- Using a straight hemostat, carefully enter the foreskin and bluntly dissect adhesions of the glans to the foreskin by opening the hemostats. Adhesions should be lysed down to the corona.
- Next, insert the lower tip of the hemostat into the foreskin opening (be sure to angle the tip upward) and advance one half to one third to the corona.
- Close the hemostat and crush the dorsal foreskin parallel to the penile shaft.
- Remove the hemostat and cut the foreskin down the middle of the dorsal crush using iris scissors.
- Retract the foreskin proximally, exposing the glans.
- Using a single layer of gauze, bluntly lyse any coronal adhesions and inspect the glans for anatomic pathology (ie, hypospadias, etc).
- Place the appropriate bell (1.0, 1.3, 1.45) over the glans and reapproximate the foreskin over the glans and bell.
- Using a sterile safety pin, pierce the foreskin just proximally to the hemostat attachments still remaining at 10 and 2 o'clock and close the safety pin.
- Now insert the safety pin and bell shaft through the hole in the distal base of the Gomco clamp.
- Assemble the top portion of the clamp with the base and seat the bell shaft into its position.
- Using gauze, or a hemostat, pull foreskin through the hole in the base of the clamp until apex of the dorsal foreskin incision is above the base plate of the clamp.
- Tighten the clamp firmly.
- Remove the foreskin using a scalpel and discard.
- Disassemble the clamp and use gauze to separate the foreskin from the bell.
- Wrap the glans in petroleum gauze.
- Instruct parents to purchase a small container of petroleum jelly to be used only on the glans until healed and epithelialized.
- Advise the parents to allow the petroleum dressing to fall off on its own.
- Reevaluate at the 2-week well-baby exam.
- Gently retract foreskin during baths.

TABLE 7.31

Urethral Culture for Sexually Transmitted Disease

- Obtain before first AM void if possible.
- With patient standing, grasp the penis around the shaft and insert the urethral culture swab 1–2 cm into the urethral meatus. Let it absorb secretions for 5–10 seconds before removing and sending to lab.

TABLE 7.32

Bladder Catheterization

Contraindications

- Known stricture
- Recent bladder neck or urethral reconstruction
- Uncooperative patient
- Suspected or known urethral disruption with pelvic trauma
- Acute prostatic or urethral infection

Technique

- With the patient in supine position sterilely prepare the urethral meatus, holding the penis with one hand and keeping the other hand sterile.
- Inject 10 mL of 2% lidocaine jelly into the urethra using a syringe without a needle.
- After 5–10 minutes, insert the 16 or 18 Foley catheter until the junction of the catheter and inflation port are at the urethral meatus.
- (Note: be sure to check the Foley balloon integrity prior to insertion.) Inflate the balloon with 5 mL of normal saline and gently retract the catheter to seat the balloon against the bladder neck. If there is resistance to inflation or the patient complains of pain during inflation, deflate and advance the catheter to ensure the balloon is beyond the urethra fully in the bladder.

TABLE 7.33
Vasectomy

Indication

- To provide sterility in a man capable of giving informed consent.
- Be sure the patient understands that reversal is not guaranteed.

Contraindications

- Skin infections
- Nonpalpable vas deferens bilaterally
- Bleeding disorders
- Psychosocial stress relating to a decision to choose vasectomy (eg, divorce)
- Inadequate informed consent

Complications

- Failure rate 1 in 300 (failure to document azoospermia 4 months out from procedure)
- Sperm granuloma
- Congestive epididymitis
- Hematoma
- Infection

Review

- Past history: Bleeding disorders, allergy to lidocaine, history of orchitis, history of accessory vas deferens, abnormal genital anatomy, any aspirin or NSAIDs daily, any HTN, any bleeding disorders
- PE: Normal vital signs; palpable vas deferens bilaterally

Procedure

- Detailed explanation of vasectomy techniques is beyond the scope of this chapter. (Refer to Pfenninger JL. *Procedures for Primary Care Physicians*. St Louis, MO: Mosby, Inc; 1994, for details on scalpel and no-scalpel vasectomy techniques.)

Postoperative Care

- Motrin 800 mg q 8 h with food
- Narcotic for 2–3 days if needed for breakthrough pain
- Ice × 24 (on for 20 minutes/off for 20 minutes), athletic supporter for 1 week then as needed
- Intercourse with barrier protection after 1 week
- Follow up semenalysis in 6 weeks
- If sperm remain, repeat in 1 month
- If initial semenalysis shows azoospermia, then confirm with repeat in 4 months

chapter 8

Care of the Older Adult

Patricia A. Pletke, MD

IN THIS CHAPTER

- Screening
- Prevention
- Functional assessment
- Preoperative assessment
- Weight loss/malnutrition
- Medication use and the older adult
- Pain
- Insomnia
- Dementia
- Depression
- Medicare

BOOKSHELF RECOMMENDATIONS

- Adelman AM, Daly MP, eds. *20 Common Problems in Geriatrics*. New York: McGraw-Hill; 2001.
- Cobbs EL, Duthie EH, Murphy TB, eds. *Geriatric Review Syllabus: A Core Curriculum in Geriatric Medicine*. 4th ed. Dubuque, Iowa: Kendall/Hunt Publishing Company for the American Geriatrics Society; 1999.
- Guttman R, Seleski M. *Diagnosis, Management and Treatment of Dementia*. Chicago: AMA Press; 1999.
- Reuben DB, Herr K, Pacala JT, Potter JF. *Geriatrics at Your Fingertips, 2001 Edition*. Belle Mead, NJ: Excerpta Medica, Inc, for the American Geriatrics Society; 2001.

TABLE 8.1

Screening Recommendations for Older Adults

Cardiovascular Diseases

- Lipid disorders
  - —Test and treat those with known coronary disease
  - —Probably beneficial to screen those 65–74 years at high risk (hypertensive, diabetics, smokers) every 5 years and treat if indicated.
- Hypertension
  - —Check blood pressure at each visit; at least once yearly in those who are candidates for treatment of hypertension

Cancer

- Breast cancer
  - —Mammograms annually through age 70–85
  - —Increasing consensus to continue annual mammograms as long as life expectancy greater than 3 years
  - —Medicare covers annual screening mammograms
- Colorectal cancer
  - —Yearly fecal occult blood testing (3 consecutive stools)

    plus
  - —Flexible sigmoidoscopy every 5 years

    (or)
  - —Colonoscopy every 10 years
  - —No upper age limit; consider patient's medical condition and probable life expectancy
  - —Medicare covers yearly FOBT, biennial flexible sigmoidoscopy, or colonoscopy every 10 years
- Cervical cancer
  - —Pap smears every 1–3 years through age 70 depending on risk factors
  - —Older women who have never had a Pap smear or who have not had regular screening should be screened until 2 negative Pap tests a year apart
  - —Women with a hysterectomy without removal of cervix should follow usual screening approach
  - —Women with a total hysterectomy for benign disease do not need Pap smear testing
  - —A woman's physical condition, life expectancy, ability to cooperate with Pap testing, or ability to undergo treatment need to be considered in deciding to perform Pap smear
  - —Medicare covers screening Pap smears every 2 years

- Prostate cancer
  —Recommendations vary about routine PSA
  —Healthy men up to age 65–70 should receive counseling about the potential benefits and harms associated with screening
  —Screening in the very old or frail person is not indicated
  —ACS recommendation is to do annual screening as long as there is a 10-year life expectancy

- Lung cancer
  —The USPSTF, the ACS, the AAFP, and the ACP all recommend against screening for lung cancer with chest x-rays or sputum cytologies
  —Encourage smokers to quit

- Skin cancer
  —USPSTF states insufficient evidence for or against screening for skin cancer
  —Clinicians urged to remain alert for skin lesions with malignant features

- Ovarian cancer
  —USPSTF recommends against screening for ovarian cancer

Other

- Diabetes
  —USPSTF: insufficient evidence to recommend for or against screening the general population
  —ADA recommends fasting plasma glucose every 3 years for those at high risk for type II diabetes mellitus (family history of disease, obesity, nonwhite race, HTN, history of impaired glucose tolerance, age greater than 45)

- Thyroid
  —Routine screening not recommended by USPSTF
  —TSH every year for women aged greater than 65
  —Maintain low threshold clinically for ordering TSH; disease fairly common, symptoms may be atypical in elderly

- Sensory disorders
  —Visual screening with standard chart
  —Question elderly people and/or family members about hearing; otoscopy, and hearing tests on those with suspected problems

- Bone density (see Chapter 17)

AAFP indicates American Academy of Family Physicians; ACS, American Cancer Society; ACP, American College of Physicians; ADA, American Diabetes Association; TSH, thyrotropin.

TABLE 8.2

Prevention for the Older Adult

Immunizations

- Influenza: vaccine yearly mid October to November; avoid in persons with allergy to egg protein
- Pneumococcal vaccine: vaccinate most elderly once; revaccinate those who received initial vaccine prior to age 65 if more than 5 years since vaccinated
- Tetanus: booster every 10 years in persons who have received primary series; provide initial three-dose series in those who have never received it
- Medicare covers the cost of above immunizations

Behaviors

- Encourage and provide assistance for cessation of smoking
- Assess alcohol use (see Table 8.10)
- Encourage maintenance of weight within 10% of ideal body weight
- Counsel on healthy nutrition
- Encourage brushing and flossing of teeth

Injury Prevention

- Encourage seat belt use and avoidance of alcohol when driving, ask if having any difficulties with driving
- Discuss risks for falls and arrange for assistive devices if needed (tub rail, etc)
- Discuss risk factors for burns or fire: water temperatures, smoking in bed; encourage use of smoke detectors

Chemoprophylaxis

- Women into their 70s should be counseled about the risks and benefits of estrogen therapy
- Patients with multiple risk factors for myocardial infarction should be counseled about the potential risks and benefits of aspirin prophylaxis

TABLE 8.3

Functional Assessment of the Older Adult*

Purpose

- Identify signs, symptoms, risk factors for common problems; to help maintain or improve functioning and allow maximal independence and quality of life

Definition

- Questions, observations, and simple tests used to identify patients at risk

Implementation

- Include screen as part of a routine physical exam, or components can be done separately over the course of multiple office visits

Target Population

- All community-dwelling adults. In particular, frail or older elderly benefit from comprehensive assessment. Perform cognitive function evaluation in high-risk persons

*Note: Examples of screening assessments and follow-up of abnormalities found in Tables 8.4 and 8.5.

TABLE 8.4
Functional Assessment Screening

Domain	Assessment	Follow-up
ADLs	■ Ask about ability to perform ADLs and IADLs (Table 8.6)	■ Evaluate for cognitive disorders ■ PT/OT for neurological or musculoskeletal disorder ■ Assess need for more structured/supportive living situation
Mobility	**Gait/balance**	
	■ Ask about falls ■ "Get up and go" test (Table 8.7) ■ Modified Romberg (Table 8.8) ■ Functional Reach Test (Table 8.9)	■ Gait training, exercise or balance training ■ Gait aids (cane, walker) ■ Treat underlying musculoskeletal, neurologic disorders
	Shoulder function	
	■ Have patient put hands together behind head and then behind waist	■ Consider x-ray studies ■ PT for ROM, decrease pain
	Hand function	
	■ Squeeze 2 fingers of examiner's hands with each hand (grasp strength) ■ Squeeze a sheet of paper between thumb and index finger; examiner tries to pull out (pinch strength) ■ Have patient pick up small object (tests dexterity)	■ Consider adaptive equipment ■ Treat pain if present ■ PT for pain relief/strengthening
Cognitive function	■ Folstein MMSE (Table 8.30) ■ Clock drawing (Table 8.33)	■ Evaluate for reversible causes ■ See Tables 8.24–8.33 dementia
Depression	■ Question "do you feel sad or depressed often?"	■ Depression scale (see Tables 8.39–8.41)

Domain	Assessment	Follow-up
Nutrition	■ Questions: "Have you lost 10 or more pounds in the last 6 months without trying?" and "Are your clothes getting loose?"	■ See Table 8.12
Vision	■ Question: "Do you have trouble watching TV or driving because of your eyesight?" ■ Have patient read a headline and a sentence from the newspaper	■ Ophthalmologist exam
Hearing	■ "Whisper test" (10 words whispered 6 inches behind the patient) ■ Ability to hear watch ticking or sound of rubbing fingers together	■ Cerumen impaction? ■ Refer for audiometry
Continence	■ Ask patient if he/she ever has urine or stool leakage	■ Evaluate for causes of incontinence, refer if necessary
Alcohol use	■ Question: "Tell me about your drinking" ■ CAGE Questionnaire (Table 8.10)	■ Treat appropriately ■ Arrange counseling if appropriate
Needs assessment	■ Assess ADLs ■ Interview caregivers and assess burden	■ Arrange for home assistance, adaptive equipment, adult day care, meal service ■ Discuss advance directives

ADLs indicates activities of daily living; IADLs, instrumental activities of daily living; MMSE, mini-mental state examination; PT/OT, physical therapy/occupational therapy; ROM, range of motion.

TABLE 8.5

Ten-Minute Screen for Geriatric Conditions

Problem	Screening Measure	Positive Screen
Vision	■ Question: "Because of your eyesight, do you have trouble driving a car, watching television, reading, or doing any of your daily activities?" ■ If the patient answers "yes," test each eye with the Snellen eye chart while the patient wears corrective lenses (if applicable)	■ "Yes" to question and inability to read at greater than 20/40 on the Snellen eye chart
Hearing	■ Use an audioscope set at 40 dB. Test the patient's hearing using 1000 and 2000 Hz	■ Inability to hear 1000 or 2000 Hz in both ears or inability to hear frequencies in either ear
Leg mobility	■ Time the patient after giving these directions: "Rise from the chair. Then walk 20 feet briskly, turn, walk back to the chair and sit down."	■ Unable to complete task in 15 seconds
Urinary incontinence	■ Question: "In the past year, have you ever lost your urine and gotten wet?" ■ If the patient answers "yes," ask this question: "Have you lost urine on at least 6 separate days?"	■ "Yes" to both questions
Nutrition and weight loss	■ Question: "Have you lost 10 pounds over the past 6 months without trying to do so?" ■ If the patient answers "yes," weigh the patient	■ "Yes" to the question or a weight of less than 45.5 kg (100 lb)
Memory	■ Three-item recall	■ Unable to remember all three items after 1 minute
Depression	■ Question: "Do you feel sad or depressed?"	■ "Yes" to the question

Problem	Screening Measure	Positive Screen
Physical disability	■ Ask the patient these six questions: 1. "Are you able to do strenuous activities, like fast walking or bicycling?" 2. "Are you able to do heavy work around the house, like washing windows, walls or floors?" 3. "Are you able to go shopping for groceries or clothes?" 4. "Are you able to get to places that are out of walking distance?" 5. "Are you able to bathe: sponge bath, tub bath, or shower?" 6. "Are you able to dress: put on a shirt, button and zip your clothes, put on your shoes?"	■ "No" to any of the questions

Adapted from Moore A, Siu AL. Screening for common problems in ambulatory elderly: clinical confirmation of a screen instrument. *Am J Med.* 1996;100:438–443.

TABLE 8.6

Activities of Daily Living

Physical Activities of Daily Living (ADL)

- Dressing
- Bathing
- Grooming
- Toileting
- Transferring (bed to chair)
- Ambulation
- Eating

Instrumental Activities of Daily Living (IADL)

- Telephone use
- Shopping
- Meal preparation
- Housekeeping
- Managing money
- Traveling (transportation)
- Taking medication
- Laundry

TABLE 8.7

The "Get Up and Go" Test for Gait Assessment in Elderly Patients

Procedure

- Have the patient sit in a straight-backed high-seat chair and say:
  —*Get up (without using armrests)*
  —*Stand still momentarily*
  —*Walk forward 10 feet*
  —*Turn around and walk back to chair*
  —*Turn and be seated*
- **Assess**
  —Sitting balance
  —Transfers from sitting to standing
  —Pace and stability of walking
  —Ability to turn without staggering

Interpretation

- No formal scoring
- Useful for serial comparisons in same patient

Problem Observed	Suspect
Unable to rise up out of chair	Overall strength decline or decreased proximal muscle strength (eg, PMR, MD)
Unstable to stand still	Postural hypotension, weakness, balance (central) disorder
Gait abnormal	Trouble initiating movement (eg, Parkinson)
Unable to turn around	Cerebellar ataxia, normal-pressure hydrocephalus; balance difficulty

- If patient appears at risk for falling at any point, indicates that severe abnormalities are present
- Also assesses ability to hear, understand, and follow simple directions

TABLE 8.8

Modified Romberg

- Patient standing does each maneuver first with eyes open, then closed:
    1. Feet comfortably apart
    2. Feet together
    3. One foot slightly in front of the other (heel to instep)
    4. One foot directly in front of the other
- Observe stability with each position
- Assesses standing balance; may help identify causative factors

TABLE 8.9

Functional Reach Test

- Patient stands with one shoulder alongside wall, extends arm straight out with fist extended. Patient then leans forward as far as possible alongside wall (with fist remaining extended) without taking a step or losing stability
- Should be able to reach forward at least 6 inches; measure distance from original hand position to new position
- Shorter distances indicate risk for falling

TABLE 8.10

"CAGE" Questionnaire for Screening for Alcoholism in Elderly Patients

Questions

- **C**ut down
  Have you ever tried to cut down on your drinking?
- **A**nnoyed or angered
  Have others annoyed or angered you by criticizing your drinking?
- **G**uilty
  Have you ever felt guilty about your drinking?
- **E**ye-opener
  Have you ever used alcohol to steady your nerves or reduce the effects of a hangover?

Interpretation

- Two or more positive answers, 75% positive predictive value for alcoholism
- One positive answer, further evaluate patient's alcohol use. Michigan Alcoholism Screen test may be used

TABLE 8.11

Preoperative Assessment of the Older Adult

Cardiovascular Assessment

- Determine presence of underlying cardiac disease that could adversely affect outcome
- All patients need medical history, functional status, and ECG results
- Additional cardiac workup unnecessary if:
  1. Patient has in the last 5 years undergone coronary artery bypass grafting or angioplasty and stent placement and is asymptomatic, or
  2. Noninvasive cardiac testing was done within the last year with normal results
- Other patients can be stratified according to risk
  —High risk (unstable angina, uncompensated CHF, symptomatic ventricular arrhythmias): need cardiac condition stabilized before elective surgery
  —Intermediate risk (mild angina, compensated or prior CHF): can proceed to surgery if functional status is good. Need additional cardiac workup if poorly functional
  —Low risk: may proceed to surgery without additional cardiac evaluation unless:
    1. Scheduled for high-risk procedure (aortic or major vascular operation, peripheral vascular procedures, prolonged surgical procedures associated with large fluid shifts and/or blood clots), or
    2. Have poor functional capacity (inability to walk 2–3 blocks, unable to climb stairs or perform light housework)

Pulmonary Evaluation

- Patients with good exercise tolerance are good candidates for surgery
- Control COPD or asthma prior to surgery
- Pulmonary function testing recommended prior to surgery for patients with asthma or COPD and those scheduled for pneumonectomy
- Obtain intraoperative monitoring of arterial blood gases in COPD patients

Hematologic Evaluation

- Obtain coagulation studies in patients unable to give a history of bleeding disorders, those with personal or family history of bleeding disorders, and patients under going high risk-neurologic procedures.

Continued

TABLE 8.11

Preoperative Assessment of the Older Adult, cont'd

- Platelets should be greater than 100,000 mm^3 for major surgery and greater than 50,000 mm^3 for minor surgery
- Aspirin should be withheld 5–7 days prior to surgery and ibuprofen 2 days prior to surgery
- Warfarin can be withheld 2 days prior to surgery and restarted post operatively. Use heparin if patient requires continuous anticoagulation

Endocrine Evaluation

- Check for diabetes with fasting blood sugar
- Fasting blood sugar target is less than 200 mg/dL (lower risk of postoperative infection and faster rate of healing)
- Maintain low threshold for obtaining TSH (atypical presentation of thyroid disease common in the elderly). Stabilize thyroid conditions prior to elective surgery
- Obtain history of steroid use especially in patients with arthritis, COPD. Adrenal suppression occurs with chronic use (even in small doses) and patients will require additional perioperative supplementation with steroids

Rheumatologic Evaluation

- Obtain cervical spine radiographs in patients with rheumatoid arthritis to rule out atlantoaxial subluxation
- Obtain history of steroid use

Gastrointestinal Evaluation

- Obtain PT/INR testing in patients with history of liver disease
- Make anesthesiologist aware of abnormal LFTs and/or hepatitis so that selection and dosage of anesthetic agents can be adjusted
- Patients with constipation need to be placed on a bowel regimen preoperatively

Urologic Evaluation

- Evaluate and treat UTI in symptomatic patients
- Perform routine urinalysis in patients scheduled for genitourinary surgery; orthopedic procedures involving implantation; recent UTIs

Neurologic Evaluation

- Inform anesthesiologist if patient has a history of seizures
- Dementia patients are at increased risk of delirium postoperatively. Correct any factors that may also contribute to risk of delirium (hypoxia, urinary retention, pain, infection, electrolyte abnormalities, hypotension)

Psychiatric Issues

- Screen for alcohol and drug use. Detoxification prior to elective surgery

Functional Status

- Assessment of activities of daily living and instrumental activities of daily living provide a baseline for evaluating rehabilitation goals
- Consider patients' support system and possible need for long-term care postoperatively

Advance Directives

- Discuss and document patients' directives regarding resuscitation and other end-of-life issues

---

Adapted from Clark E. Preoperative assessment: primary care work-up to identify surgical risks. *Geriatrics.* 2001; 56:36–40.

CHF indicates congestive heart failure; COPD, chronic obstructive pulmonary disease; ECG, electrocardiogram; TSH, thyrotropin; UTI, urinary tract infection.

TABLE 8.12

Weight Loss/Malnutrition

Involuntary Weight Loss: Percentages triggering need for evaluation

- >5% in 1 month
- >7% in 3 months
- >10% in 6 months

History

- Assess appetite, interest in eating
- Assess factors affecting access to food: transportation to grocery store, economic issues, ability to prepare meals, ability to feed self
- Ask patient or caregiver if clothing seems looser, especially if trying to assess person without previous weights available
- Ask about symptoms that can lead to weight loss: nausea and vomiting, decreased sense of taste, difficulty swallowing
- Ask about symptoms of diseases associated with weight loss (diabetes mellitus, thyroid disease)

Physical Examination

- Measure weight at each visit and height once a year
- Signs that may indicate malnutrition: alopecia, confusion, dry skin, dependent edema, dry hair, glossitis, generalized muscle weakness, and wasting
- Look for oral lesions, poorly fitting dentures
- Look for signs of illness that can cause weight loss: hyperthyroidism, cancers, chronic infections, other chronic diseases such as CHF, renal failure

Lab

- Albumin: level <3.5 g/dL suggestive of malnutrition; levels 3.5–4 g/dL (institutionalized, frail elderly) and <5 g/dL (community-dwelling elderly) associated with increased mortality
- Transferrin <200 mg/dL; shorter half-life than albumin so may be more sensitive indicator of recent-onset of undernutrition; influenced by iron status
- Prealbumin levels <11 mg/dL suggest significant undernutrition; half life ~2 days
- TSH testing to rule out thyroid disease as etiology of weight loss
- CBC to look for signs of anemia or infection; anemia can indicate poor nutritional intake or be a result of GI blood loss

- Assess renal and liver function, total protein, calcium
- Hemoccult testing
- Chest x-ray

Treatments

- Address any and all underlying issues (may be multifactorial)
- Consult dietitian if needed for nutritional counseling, patient education
- Ensure patient has adequate access to food
- Appetite stimulants
  —Megestrol acetate (Megace): 800 mg once daily
  —Dronabinol (Marinol): 2.5 mg bid before lunch and dinner; may increase if necessary up to 20 mg/d
  —Mirtazapine (Remeron): antidepressant with appetite stimulant side effects. Usual dose 15–30 mg q hs

---

bid indicates twice daily; CBC, complete blood cell count; CHF, congestive heart failure; GI, gastrointestinal; TSH, thyrotropin.

TABLE 8.13

Changes in the Older Adult Affecting Medication Use

Absorption

- Generally complete but slower among elderly persons; affects symptom-relieving drugs such as analgesics or anxiolytics
- Drug and drug-food interactions may influence absorption; decreased absorption of fluoroquinolones with antacids, iron, or sucralfate
- Disease states may alter absorption; for example, decreased hepatic blood flow from CHF decreases first-pass effect leading to increases in concentrations of drugs such as levodopa, nifedipine, omeprazole, labetalol, and lidocaine

Body Composition

- Aging associated with decrease in total body water and body mass
- Reduce loading dose of drugs that are mainly water soluble (eg, lithium, aminoglycosides) or those that bind to skeletal muscle (eg, digoxin)

Metabolism

- Marked variability in hepatic drug metabolism with advancing years secondary to decline in hepatic blood flow
- Biotransformation through cytochrome P-450 system occurs more slowly in older persons (affects metabolism of warfarin, phenytoin, and diazepam)

Distribution

- Albumin is the binding protein for acidic drugs (eg, phenytoin, warfarin, naproxen); L-acid glycoprotein binds mainly basic drugs (eg, tricyclic antidepressants, quinidine, lidocaine)
- Chronic disease can decrease albumin levels; acute illness may affect L-acid glycoprotein levels
- Important for drugs with narrow therapeutic index; serum concentrations reflect both bound and unbound drug
- Example: phenytoin; if albumin low and serum concentration of phenytoin is normal, the unbound portion is increased and patient may develop toxicity with normal serum concentration

Elimination

- Primary factor is reduced glomerular filtration and renal blood flow rate that occurs with age or as a consequence of disease
- BUN and creatine may not reflect GFR due to age-related decreased muscle mass or protein-calorie malnutrition
- Monitor drug levels for medications with narrow therapeutic window

Pharmacodynamic Changes Associated With Aging

- Alteration in sensitivity to a medication that may occur at the receptor or organ level
- Examples: enhanced sedation with benzodiazepines, greater pain relief with narcotics, greater cardiac and CNS toxicity with theophylline

---

BUN indicates serum urea nitrogen; CHF, congestive heart failure; CNS, central nervous system; GFR, glomerular filtration rate.

TABLE 8.14

Guidelines for Prescribing for Elderly Patients

- Review current medications (preferably by visual inspection of patients' medication containers) and indications and directions for use at each visit
- Ask about over-the-counter medications and supplements including vitamin and herbal preparations
- Look for potential drug interactions
- Review drug allergies and history of adverse reactions
- Keep dosing regimens as simple as possible
- Provide instructions verbally and in writing
- Include spouse/caregiver (if appropriate) when giving instructions
- Start with lowest dose and titrate up slowly
- Discontinue medications that seem to be no longer needed
- Try to make only one change at a time
- Monitor for adverse effects
- Explore issues regarding difficulty in obtaining medication
- Use newer drugs with caution (elderly not well represented in clinical trials)

TABLE 8.15

Selected Drug Interactions

- Tricyclic antidepressants and type I antiarrhythmics have potentially fatal interactions
- Coumadin interacts with multiple medications; consult drug prescribing information
- Erythromycin may increase levels of theophylline and digoxin
- Intravenous contrast contraindicated in patients taking metformin; discontinue metformin for several days prior to contrast studies and withhold for 48 hours afterward
- Quinidine increases digoxin levels
- Selegiline taken with some antidepressants can cause severe delirium
- Rhabdomyolysis may occur when statins are used with other lipid-lowering medications
- Sucralfate interferes with absorption of quinolones

TABLE 8.16

Medications to Use With Caution or Avoid in the Elderly

- Barbiturates: Highly addictive, more side effects than other sedative hypnotics
- Meperidine: Increased accumulation of metabolite, not very effective as oral analgesic
- Ticlopidine: Potential toxic side effects including TTP; not significantly better than aspirin in preventing clotting
- Indomethacin: Central nervous system side effects
- Propoxyphene: Little analgesic advantage over acetaminophen; narcotic-type side effects
- Phenylbutazone: May produce serious hematologic side effects
- Meprobamate: Highly addictive and sedating
- Benzodiazepines: Long-acting ones cause increased sedation and risk of falls; use short- and intermediate-acting benzodiazepines in small doses if used at all
- Disopyramide: Negative ionotrope, strongly anticholinergic
- Dipyridamole: Orthostatic hypotension
- Chlorpropamide: Prolonged half-life, can cause serious hypoglycemia; may cause SIADH
- Muscle relaxants: Anticholinergic side effects, sedation, and weakness; questionable effectiveness
- Pentazocine: CNS side effects including confusion and hallucinations
- Amitriptyline: Anticholinergic and sedating
- Doxepin: Strongly anticholinergic and sedating
- Reserpine: Orthostatic hypotension, depression, impotence, sedation
- Methyldopa: May cause bradycardia and exacerbate depression
- Digoxin: Decreased renal clearance in elderly may lead to toxicity; avoid doses greater than 0.125 mg daily except when treating atrial arrhythmias
- Trimethobenzamide: May cause extrapyramidal side effects; less effective than other antiemetics
- Gastrointestinal antispasmodics: Highly anticholinergic
- Antihistamines: Potent anticholinergic effects in many
- Hydergine: Has not been shown to be effective
- Diphenhydramine: Strong anticholinergic; avoid as hypnotic; use in smallest possible dose for acute allergic reactions
- Iron supplements: Exceeding dose of 325 mg increases constipation without substantial increase in total absorption

Adapted from Beers MH. Explicit criteria for determining potentially inappropriate medication use by the elderly: an update. *Arch Intern Med.* 1997;157(14):131–136.

CNS indicates central nervous system; SIADH, syndrome of inappropriate secretion of antidiuretic hormone; TTP, thrombotic thrombocytopenic purpura.

TABLE 8.17

Medications to Avoid or Use With Caution in Older Patients With Certain Disease States

Disease	Medication	Comments
Heart failure	■ Disopyramide ■ Drugs with high sodium content (sodium bicarbonate, etc)	■ Negative ionotrope ■ Leads to fluid retention
Diabetes	■ β-blockers ■ Corticosteroids	■ May block hypoglycemia symptoms ■ Worsen diabetic control
HTN	■ Diet pills; amphetamines	■ Elevate blood pressure
COPD	■ β-blockers ■ Sedative-hypnotics	■ May worsen respiratory function ■ May slow respiratory rate and lead to CO_2 retention
Asthma	■ β-blockers	■ May worsen respiratory function
Ulcers	■ NSAIDs ■ Aspirin ■ Potassium	■ Exacerbates ulcer disease, gastritis, or GERD
Seizures/epilepsy	■ Clozapine, thorazine, thioridazine	■ Lower seizure threshold
Peripheral vascular disease	■ β-blockers	■ May worsen peripheral artery blood flow and precipitate claudication
Blood clotting disorders (on anticoagulant therapy)	■ Aspirin, NSAIDs ■ Dipyridamole and ticlopidine	■ May cause bleeding ■ Same
BPH	■ Anticholinergic antihistamines ■ Gastrointestinal antispasmodics ■ Muscle relaxants ■ Narcotic drugs ■ Flavoxate, oxybutynin ■ Bethanechol ■ Anticholinergic antidepressants	■ Impair micturition and cause obstruction
Incontinence	■ β-blockers	■ Relaxes external bladder sphincter ■ May increase incontinence

Disease	Medication	Comments
Constipation	■ Anticholinergic drugs	■ May worsen constipation
Syncope or falls	■ β-blockers	■ Negative chronotrope and ionotrope, which may precipitate syncope or falls
	■ Long-acting benzodiazepines	■ Contributes to increased falling
Arrhythmias	■ Tricyclic antidepressants	■ May induce arrhythmias
Insomnia	■ Decongestants, SSRIs, theophylline, desipramine, methylphenidate, and MAOs, β-agonists	■ May cause or worsen insomnia

Adapted from Beers MH. Explicit criteria for determining potentially inappropriate medication use by the elderly: an update. *Arch Intern Med.* 1997;157(14):131–136.

BPH indicates benign prostatic hyperplasia; COPD, chronic obstructive pulmonary disease; GERD, gastroesophageal reflux disease; MAO, monoamine oxidase; NSAIDs, nonsteroidal anti-inflammatory drugs; SSRIs, selective serotonin reuptake inhibitor.

TABLE 8.18

Summary of AGS Recommendations for Assessment of Chronic Pain in Older Persons

- Assess older persons for pain with each presentation for health care services
- Recognize persistent or recurrent pain that has a significant impact on function or quality of life
- Use a variety of terms (burning, discomfort, aching, soreness) in screening older persons for pain
- Use behavior changes, facial expressions, changes in functioning, and caregivers' observations as clues that patients with cognitive or language impairments are experiencing pain
- Identify and treat conditions requiring specific interventions: manage underlying disease, treat or refer for psychiatric conditions if present, refer to pain clinic for intractable/life-altering pain, identify drug or alcohol abuse and refer for treatment
- Comprehensive pain assessment for all patients with chronic pain (see Table 8.19)
- Have patient or caregiver use a pain log or diary to record pain intensity, duration, medication use, and response to treatment
- Reassess patients with chronic pain for improvements, deterioration, or complications related to treatment

TABLE 8.19

Comprehensive Geriatric Pain Assessment

- Goal of assessment is to use history, physical exam, and patient labs to ascertain sequence of events leading to present pain complaint and to establish a diagnosis, plan for care, and estimate of prognosis
- Identify characteristics of current pain: intensity, type of pain, location, duration, precipitating, and relieving factors
- Review analgesic history including use of over-the-counter and "natural" preparations, record of side effects, and usefulness of previous and current treatments
- Complete physical exam with focus on neuromuscular system (weakness, paresthesias, neurologic impairments, numbness) and musculoskeletal system (palpate for tenderness, inflammation, deformity, trigger points)
- Evaluate physical functioning: assess impact of pain on activities of daily living. Use range of motion testing and/or more formalized testing such as the "Get Up and Go" test (see Table 8.7)
- Evaluate psychosocial functioning including evaluation for depression, assessment of patient's support system and identification of any dysfunctional relationships
- Quantify pain with a standard pain scale

TABLE 8.20

Pain Management in the Older Patient

- Older patients with chronic pain impairing quality of life are candidates for pharmacologic therapy
- Utilize least invasive route of administration
- Utilize fast-onset, short-acting analgesics for episodic (chronic recurrent or noncontinuous) pain
- Acetaminophen in doses up to 4000 mg per day is the drug of choice for mild to moderate musculoskeletal pain
- Use NSAIDs with caution:
  —Avoid high-dose, long-term use
  —Use prn rather than around the clock
  —Avoid dose accumulation by using short-acting NSAIDs
  —Avoid in patients with abnormal renal function, peptic ulcer disease history, bleeding disorder
  —Do not use more than one NSAID at a time
  —Cox 2 inhibitor agents, decreased adverse GI effects; renal adverse effects similar to the other NSAIDs
- Opioids for moderate to severe pain
  —Use prn dosing for episodic pain
  —Long-acting, sustained-release preparations used for continuous pain only
  —Use short-acting, fast onset analgesics for breakthrough pain
  —Titrate long-acting medication based on (1) need for use of medication for breakthrough pain and (2) adverse effects related to medication
  —Prevent constipation with encouragement of adequate fluids, physical activity, and prophylactic bowel regimen
  —Caution patients and caregivers about probability of mild sedation, impaired cognition. Warn about potential for falls and have patient avoid driving until tolerance to this side effect develops
  —Nausea usually resolves within a few days but may be treated until then with an antiemetic
  —Avoid meperidine because of accumulation of toxic metabolite
- Fixed-dose combinations: dose limited by acetaminophen or NSAID component
- Other medications
  —Carbamazepine: medication of choice for trigeminal neuralgia; may be useful with other neuropathic pain
  —Gabapentin: also useful for neuropathic pain
  —Tricyclic antidepressants: may be helpful with neuropathic pain
    Avoid with glaucoma, benign prostatic hypertrophy
    Significant anticholinergic effects (constipation, dry mouth, urinary retention, blurred vision)
    Nortriptyline and desipramine least anticholinergic and are preferred agents for the elderly in this category

- Nonpharmacologic treatments
  - —Local heat or cold application may be helpful; avoid in patients with impaired sensation
  - —Massage
  - —Topical lidocaine or capsaicin can be used for postherpetic neuralgia
  - —Topical salicylates may provide some relief in musculoskeletal pain

GI indicates gastrointestinal; NSAIDs, nonsteroidal anti-inflammatory drugs; prn, when necessary.

TABLE 8.21

Sleep Disorders in Older Adults

Normal Sleep: Sufficient to maintain alertness through the day. Averages 8 hours per night. Occurs in cycles of REM (rapid eye movement) sleep and non-REM

Aging Changes: Slightly delayed onset, less deep sleep, less REM sleep, more frequent awakenings

Evaluation of Sleep Complaints

- History: sleep pattern; medications that may disrupt sleep; pain, nocturia, or other sleep-disturbing symptoms; snoring; symptoms of dementia
- Physical exam: obesity, signs of CHF, COPD; arthritis or other potential causes of pain; screening for depression/dementia
- Lab: TSH, metabolic profile, drug levels if indicated
- Sleep laboratory: if sleep apnea or nocturnal myoclonus a strong consideration or if significant insomnia persists

Nonpharmacologic Approaches to Treatment

- Wait until sleepy before going to bed
- Maintain a bedtime ritual and perform consistently at same time
- Avoid watching TV in bed or reading for long periods
- Perform relaxation techniques if needed; massage may be helpful
- Avoid heavy meals, alcohol prior to bedtime
- Limit caffeine to early in the day and limit total amount
- Create an environment conducive to sleep: eliminate noise, maintain a comfortable temperature
- Get up at same time each day

Pharmacologic Treatment

- Use smallest effective doses for short periods of time
- Examples of some agents used in Table 8.23

CHF indicates congestive heart failure; COPD, chronic obstructive pulmonary disease; TSH, thyrotropin.

TABLE 8.22

Common Sleep Disorder Syndromes in the Older Adult

Medication Side Effects

- Aminophylline, phenytoin, serotonin reuptake inhibitors, levodopa, decongestants, caffeine, and nicotine can disrupt sleep
- Quinidine, glucocorticoids, and some β-blockers can cause nightmares.
- Treatment: counsel patients about side effects of caffeine and OTC medications on sleep; attempt to reduce or discontinue medications that may be disrupting sleep

Psychophysiologic Insomnia

- Tension/anxiety impairs ability to fall asleep
- Often starts with an external cause (financial concerns, family problems) but may become self-perpetuating
- May be exacerbated by caffeine or alcohol
- Relaxation techniques may be useful

Advanced Sleep Phase Syndrome

- Person goes to bed early (fatigue, boredom) and wakens early (but usually has slept a fairly normal length of time)
- Treatment geared toward keeping patient awake in the evening with activity, exercise, or bright light therapy.

Nighttime Awakening

- Need to urinate, SOB, or pain interfere with normal sleep cycle
- Treatment: identify and treat cause if possible

Institutional Insomnia

- Environment not conducive to sleep: too noisy, too bright, or too many interruptions
- Treatment: attempt to reduce sleep-disrupting practices. Nonpharmacologic interventions such as relaxing music, warm milk, or massage may be helpful

Psychiatric

- Dementia: disturbances in sleep-wake rhythms common. Patients may respond to evening dose of anxiolytic or risperidone
- Depression: associated with frequent arousals and early morning awakening. Treat depression; may benefit from dose of a sedating antidepressant at bedtime

Nocturnal Myoclonus

- Periodic repetitive jerking movements of limbs may cause arousal
- Restless leg syndrome is related and characterized by intense discomfort in legs
- Uremia, sleep apnea, and chronic arthritis associated with nocturnal myoclonus
- Antihistamines, caffeine, anemia, diuretics, and antidepressants can aggravate both nocturnal myoclonus and restless leg syndrome

Sleep Apnea

- Five apneic (cessation of nasobuccal airflow for 10 seconds or more) or 10 hypopneic (50% reduction in airflow for same for same amount of time) episodes per hour of sleep
- Prominent symptoms: excessive daytime somnolence and snoring
- Diagnosis by sleep study at a sleep laboratory
- Treatment: CPAP; weight loss and/or surgical widening of airway may help

Sundowning

- Somnolence during day with alertness and agitation in the evening and early night
- More common in hospitalized patients or nursing home residents
- Treatment: treat reversible causes of delirium if present. Increase daytime activity and prevent napping if possible

REM Behavior Disorder

- Intense muscular activity during REM sleep (normally inhibited)
- Treatment: long-acting benzodiazepine such as clonazepam

CPAP indicates continuous positive airway pressure; OTC, over-the-counter; REM, rapid eye movement.

TABLE 8.23

Sleep Medications for the Elderly

Drug/Dosage	Advantages	Disadvantages/ Problems
Chloral hydrate 250 mg starting dose, up to 1000 mg	■ Available in capsules, syrup, or suppository ■ Well tolerated	■ Hypnotic effect lost after 2 weeks of continuous use ■ Contraindicated with significant renal, cardiac, or hepatic impairment ■ Rebound insomnia
Lorazepam (Ativan) 0.25 mg starting dose, up to 2 mg/d	■ Effective in initiating and maintaining sleep ■ Generic inexpensive ■ Good anxiolytic	■ Associated with falls in elderly ■ Some rebound insomnia ■ May see some memory loss and performance problems
Nefazodone (Serzone) 50 mg starting dose, up to 200 mg/d	■ No morning hangover ■ Tolerance doesn't develop ■ Anxiolytic	■ Mild oversedation ■ Mild orthostasis ■ May cause nausea ■ Black box warning
Trazodone (Desyrel) 25 mg starting dose, up to 150 mg/d	■ No tolerance ■ No morning hangover ■ Useful if depression present ■ Can be combined with SSRIs	■ Moderate orthostasis ■ Administration of this medication with food may decrease the orthostasis
Zolpidem (Ambien) 5 mg starting dose, may increase to 10 mg	■ No hangover ■ Rapid onset of action	■ Rare confusional state or psychosis
Melatonin Optimal dose controversial, 2–3 mg suggested	■ Decreases sleep latency and improved quality of sleep in some patients ■ No morning hangover	■ Nonprescription: quality/content of active ingredient not guaranteed ■ Not well studied; inconsistent results

SSRIs indicates selective serotonin reuptake inhibitor.

Medication that should probably be avoided in the elderly:

- Barbiturates: Use leads to dependency
- Sedating antihistamines: Anticholinergic effect; may also interfere with new learning and/or access to memory
- Long-acting benzodiazepines: Cause daytime sedation, lethargy, ataxia, falls, cognitive and psychomotor impairment
- Triazolam (short-acting benzodiazepine): Causes transient amnesia and confusion. Not effective in maintaining sleep
- Some would consider chloral hydrate in this category secondary to gastrointestinal side effects, morning hangover, and potential interaction with protein-bound medications

TABLE 8.24

Dementia

Dementia: A condition with impairment in cognitive function (memory, reasoning abilities, language skills, praxis) that may be accompanied by behavioral changes, personality changes, hallucinations, delusions, and deterioration in functioning.

Alzheimer Disease

- Most common form of dementia
- Progressive impairment in memory
- Changes in behavior, personality, and ability to function as disease progresses

Multi-infarct Dementia

- Second most common form of dementia
- Often difficult to distinguish from Alzheimer and may coexist
- May progress in stepwise rather than gradual fashion
- May be associated with signs of stroke
- Patient usually has underlying hypertension

Frontal Lobe Dementia

- Characterized by prominent behavioral disturbances (inappropriate social behavior, disturbed judgment)

Diffuse Lewy Body Dementia

- Characterized by extrapyramidal motor symptoms similar to Parkinson disease
- Delusions and hallucinations

Dementia Associated With Parkinson Disease

- Occurs in up to 40% of Parkinson patients over time
- General slowing of cognition in patients with typical Parkinson (bradykinesia, rigidity, gait, and balance problems)

Normal-Pressure Hydrocephalus

- Triad of apraxia, dementia, and urinary incontinence
- Gait disorder characterized by "magnetic gait"; each step taken deliberately as though foot stuck to the ground

Alcohol-Related Dementia

- May occur along with other causes of dementia
- Patients often apathetic and irritable

Dementia Associated With Depression

- Up to 15% of patients presenting with memory impairment or inability to perform higher cognitive functions have some degree of underlying depression

Thyroid Disease

- Older patients with hyperthyroidism or hypothyroidism may have dementia
- Hyperthyroidism-related dementia associated with apathy

Others

- Vitamin B_{12} and folate deficiency can lead to changes in higher cognitive functioning
- Tertiary syphilis can cause a dementia-like illness
- Human immunodeficiency virus–associated dementia—consider in persons who received blood transfusion between 1978 and 1985 or who have other risk factors
- Medication-related dementia: sedating agents such as benzodiazepines, major tranquilizers, sedating antihistamines, and beta-blockers.

TABLE 8.25

Diagnostic Workup for Memory Loss/Possible Dementia

History

- Patient and caregivers report of symptoms including rate of progression, effect on ability to function (see Table 8.26): signs and symptoms that indicate the need for evaluation for dementia
- Review of medications, including over-the-counter, prescriptions, nutritional supplements, and herbal remedies
- Assessment of risk factors: medical history, family history, history of alcohol or drug abuse, history of head trauma or falls, dietary history

Examination

- General physical exam: usually normal with Alzheimer disease; may see weight loss in some patients as early sign
- Neurologic exam: focal changes suggest an underlying neurologic cause
- Mental status testing: screen with clock drawing test or the Mini-Mental State Examination (MMSE) (see Tables 8.28 and 8.29)
- MMSE may be normal early in highly educated persons
- Neuropsychological testing: more comprehensive testing indicated in patients with signs or symptoms of dementia with normal scores on screening testing. May be helpful in differentiating AD from other types of dementias or depression; provides a baseline to monitor progression of disease and evaluate effectiveness of interventions; costly
- Functional assessment: assess patient's ability to perform activities of daily living and instrumental activities of daily living

Laboratory Studies

- CBC
- Metabolic profile
- Vitamin B_{12} and folic acid
- Syphilis serology
- TSH
- Other lab as indicated by patient's history, symptoms

Neuroimaging

- Indications: recent onset of symptoms, dementia with focal or atypical symptoms
- CT cheaper and better tolerated than MRI but less sensitive to detecting cerebrovascular disease and ischemic white matter changes
- "Functional" neuroimaging studies (SPECT and PET) may be useful in distinguishing types of dementia; expensive and not yet widely available

AD indicates Alzheimer's dementia; CBC, complete blood cell count; CT, computed tomography; MRI, magnetic resonance imaging; PET, positron emission tomography.

TABLE 8.26

Signs and Symptoms That May Indicate the Need for Evaluation for Dementia

Cognitive Changes

- New forgetfulness
- More trouble understanding spoken and written communication
- Difficulty finding words
- Not knowing current facts such as current president
- Disorientation

Personality Changes

- Inappropriate friendliness
- Blunting and disinterest
- Societal withdrawal
- Excessive flirtatiousness and hypersexuality
- Easy frustration
- Explosive spells

Psychiatric Symptoms

- Withdrawal or apathy
- Depression
- Suspiciousness
- Anxiety
- Insomnia
- Fearfulness
- Paranoia
- Abnormal beliefs
- Hallucinations

Changes in Day-to-Day Functioning

- Difficulty driving
- Getting lost
- Forgetting recipes
- Neglecting household chores
- Difficulty handling money
- Making mistakes at work
- Trouble with shopping

Problem Behaviors

- Wandering
- Agitation
- Noisiness
- Restlessness
- Being out of bed at night

Adapted from Rabbins PV, Ketsos CG, Steel CD. *Practical Dementia Care*. New York: Oxford University Press; 1999:23.

TABLE 8.27

Dementia Treatments

Cognitive Impairment: Cholinesterase Inhibitors

- Improve cognitive and behavioral functions and slow progress of disease; do not reverse memory loss
- Indicated for Alzheimer-type dementia but may be effective in vascular dementia as well. Decreases hallucinations and delusions in patients with Lewy body disease
- Donepezil (Aricept)
  —Start 5 mg at hs; increase to 10 mg after 4–6 weeks
  —May give with or without food
  —Increased cholinergic side effects if dose increased too rapidly
  —Metabolized by the cytochrome P-450 system; consider potential for drug-drug interactions
- Galantamine (Reminyl)
  —Start with 4 mg bid with meals; increase to 8 mg bid after 4 weeks. May increase to 12 bid after additional 4 weeks
  —Do not exceed 16 mg daily with moderate renal or hepatic impairment. Do not use with severe hepatic impairment
  —Low incidence of GI side effects
- Rivastigmine (Exelon)
  —Start with 1.5 mg bid; increase to 3 mg bid after 4 weeks
  At 4 or more–week intervals may increase to 4.5 mg, then 6 mg bid
  —20% of patients unable to tolerate 6–12 mg daily
  —Nausea, vomiting, diarrhea, abdominal pain, and anorexia most common side effects
  —Available in liquid form
- Tacrine (Cognex)
  —Not a first-line agent secondary to GI side effects and risk of hepatotoxicity: rarely used now that newer agents available
  —Start with 10 mg qid between meals
  —Maintain dose for 4 weeks then may increase slowly to maximum dose 160 mg daily
  —Monitor transaminase levels every other week starting at 4 weeks. May decrease to monthly monitoring for 2 months at week 16 and then every 3 months
  —Take with meals if stomach upset

Cognitive Impairment: Nontraditional Therapies

- None approved yet by FDA for treatment of dementia
- NSAIDs may decrease risk of Alzheimer disease secondary to anti-inflammatory effect. Increased risks with using these medications in the elderly (GI ulceration and bleeding, renal impairment, interference with medications). Not recommended at this time

- Vitamin E, 1000 mg bid delayed progression of disease and nursing home placement; did not improve cognition
- Ginkgo biloba may be effective in delaying symptom progression in patients with Alzheimer disease

Vascular Dementia: Treatment

- Goal of treatment is to prevent further cerebrovascular insult by treating stroke risk factors (hypertension, diabetes mellitus, elevated lipids, smoking, and obesity)
- Aspirin prophylaxis for patients at risk
- Anticoagulation for patients with atrial fibrillation unless contraindicated

Behavioral Symptoms

- Nonpharmacological interventions: provide routines, reduce choices, modify environment to reduce excess stimulation
- Pharmacologic treatments:
  —Delusions, hallucinations, and disordered thinking, risperidone and olanzapine
  —Agitation and aggression antipsychotic medications. Atypical antipsychotics associated with decreased risk of extrapyramidal symptoms
  —Depression: SSRIs effective for depression associated with dementia
  —Evaluate and treat for pain in dementia patient with new-onset behavior changes

---

bid indicates twice daily; FDA, Food and Drug Administration; GI, gastrointestinal; NSAIDs, nonsteroidal anti-inflammatory drugs; qid, four times daily; SSRIs, selective serotonin reuptake inhibitors.

TABLE 8.28

Characteristics Distinguishing Changes of Typical Aging From Dementia

Typical Aging	Dementia
Independence in daily activities preserved	Person becomes critically dependent on others for key independent living activities
Complains of memory loss but able to provide considerable detail regarding incidents of forgetfulness	May complain of memory problems only if specifically asked; unable to recall instance where memory loss was noticed
Patient is more concerned about alleged forgetfulness than are close family members	Close family members much more concerned about incidents of memory loss than patient
Recent memory for important events, affairs, conversations not impaired	Notable decline in memory for recent events and ability to converse
Occasional word finding difficulties	Frequent word finding pauses and substitutions
Does not get lost in familiar territory; may have to pause momentarily to remember way	Gets lost in familiar territory while walking or driving; may take hours to eventually return home
Able to operate common appliances even if unwilling to learn how to operate new appliances	Becomes unable to operate common appliances; unable to learn to operate even simple new appliances
Maintains prior level of interpersonal social skills	Exhibits loss of interest in social activities; exhibits socially inappropriate behaviors
Normal performance on mental status examinations, taking education and culture into account	Abnormal performance on mental status examination not accounted for by educational or cultural factors

Table developed by David Knopman, MD. Reproduced with permission from the American Medical Association. (Guttman R, Seleski M, eds. *Diagnosis, Management, and Treatment of Dementia*. Chicago: AMA Press; 1999.)

TABLE 8.29

Dementia Evaluation Tools

Mini-Mental State Examination (MMSE)

- Evaluates orientation, registration, attention, memory, and language
- Standard questions and scoring (see Table 8.30)
- Score less than 25 considered abnormal; score less than 23 traditional indication of dementia
- Consider patient's educational level and baseline intellectual function
- See Table 8.31 for age and education level median scores

Hachinski Ischemic Score for Multi-infarct Dementia

- 13-item scale that may help distinguish multi-infarct or mixed-type dementia from Alzheimer
- See Table 8.32

Clock Drawing Test

- See Table 8.33

TABLE 8.30

Mini-Mental State Examination

ORIENTATION **Where Are You?** (Ask the general first, then the specific questions below) 1. Name this place (building or hospital). 2. What floor are you on now? 3. What state are you in? 4. What county are you in? (If not in a county, score if city is correct.) 5. What city are you in (or near) now? **What is the date today?** (Ask the general question first, then the specific questions below) ■ What year is it? ■ What season is it? ■ What month is it? ■ What is the day of the week?	Score 1 for each correct (Max = 10)
REGISTRATION ■ Name three objects (such as ball, flag, and tree) and have patient repeat them. (Say objects at about 1 word per second. If patient misses object, ask him/her to repeat back to you until he/she learns. Stop at 6 repeats.)	Score 1 for each object correctly repeated (Max = 3)
ATTENTION AND CALCULATION ■ Subtract 7s from 100 in a serial fashion to 65	Score 1 for each correct to 65 (Max = 5)
Alternatively, ■ Ask the subject to spell the word WORLD. Then have the subject spell it backward.	Score 1 for each correctly placed letter
RECALL ■ Do you recall the names of the three objects?	Score 1 for each (Max = 3)
LANGUAGE ■ Ask patient to provide names of a watch and pen as you show them to him or her	Score 1 for each object correct (Max = 2)

■ Repeat "no ifs, ands, or buts" (only one trial)	Score 1 if correct
■ Give patient a piece of plain blank paper and say "take the paper in your right hand, fold it in half, and put it on the floor."	Score 1 for each part done correctly (Max =3)
■ Ask patient to read and perform task written on paper, "close your eyes."	Score 1 if patient closes eyes
■ Ask patient to write a sentence on a piece of paper	Score total of 1 if sentence has a subject, object, and verb (Max = 1)

CONSTRUCTION

■ Ask patient to copy the following design of the interlocking five-sided figures.	Score 1 if all 10 angles are present and two angles intersect; ignore tremor and rotation (Max = 1)

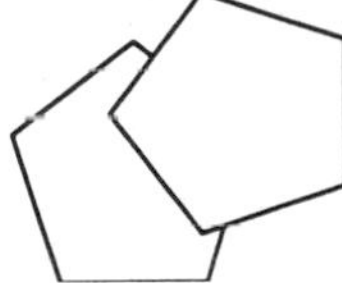

Total Score	Maximum score = 30

Source: "Mini-Mental State," a practical method for grading the cognitive state of patients for the clinician. *J Psychiatr Res.* 1975;12:189–198.

TABLE 8.31

Median Score on Mini-Mental State Examination by Age and Educational Level

Educational Level

Age (years)	4th Grade	8th Grade	High School	College
18 to 24	22	27	29	29
25 to 29	25	27	29	29
30 to 34	25	26	29	29
35 to 39	23	26	28	29
40 to 44	23	27	28	29
45 to 49	23	26	28	29
50 to 54	23	27	28	29
55 to 59	23	26	28	29
60 to 64	23	26	28	29
65 to 69	22	26	28	29
70 to 74	22	25	27	28
75 to 79	21	25	27	28
80 to 84	20	25	25	27
>84	19	23	26	27

Reproduced with permission from the American Medical Association. (Crum RM, Anthony JC, Bassett SS, Folstein MF. Population-based norms for the Mini-Mental State Examination by age and educational level. *JAMA.* 1993;269(18):2386–2391.)

TABLE 8.32

Hachinski Ischemic Score for Multi-infarct Dementia*

Points	Score	Item
2†		1. Abrupt onset of symptoms
1		2. Stepwise deterioration
2†		3. Fluctuating course
1		4. Nocturnal confusion
1		5. Relative preservation of personality
1		6. Depression
1		7. Somatic complaints
1		8. Emotional incontinence
1		9. History or presence of hypertension
2†		10. History of strokes
1		11. Evidence of associated atherosclerosis
2†		12. Focal neurologic symptoms
2†		13. Focal neurologic signs
Total		

*Total score (items 1–13) of 7 points or higher suggests multi-infarct dementia or mixed dementia. Total score of 4 or less indicates dementia is not likely to be due to vascular causes.
†Weighted with 2 points. Do not assign 1 point to any of these. Score either 0 or 2 points.

TABLE 8.33

Clock Drawing Task

- Brief screening test for cognitive impairment
- Patient instructed to draw the face of a clock, put the numbers in the correct positions, then draw the hands at a particular time such as 10 minutes after 11
- Various methods for scoring have been used/described
- Important considerations
  —Grossly distorted circle or extraneous markings are rarely produced by cognitively intact persons
  —A perfectly drawn clock unlikely to be drawn by cognitively impaired person
- Any difficulty with this task indicates need for complete diagnostic evaluation for dementia

TABLE 8.34

Diagnosis of Depression in the Elderly

Important Indicators

- Decreased interest in activities
- Feelings of helplessness, hopelessness, guilt
- Feeling that life is empty
- Avoidance of social interactions
- Psychomotor agitation or retardation
- Difficulty making decisions or initiating projects
- Recurrent thoughts of death or suicide
- Sad, downcast mood

Less Reliable Indicators
(may be associated with aging or concomitant medical illness)

- Fatigue
- Weight loss/appetite change
- Poor sleep pattern
- Difficulty with memory

Medical Evaluation

- H & P with neurologic exam
- TSH, chemistry screen, CBC, consider Vitamin B_{12} and folate levels
- Assess for alcohol use/abuse
- Medications: look for those that may be contributing to or causing depression (see Table 8.36)

Psychosocial Issues

- Cognitive functioning: screen for dementia
- Grief/loss
- Changes in role/responsibilities (eg, change from work to retirement; need to assume new responsibilities after death of spouse)
- Living environment, support system
- Assess suicide risk

Depression Rating Scales

- Hamilton Rating Scale for Depression (all ages)
- Cornell Scale for Depression in Dementia (see Table 8.40)
- Geriatric Depression Scale (see Table 8.39)

CBC indicates complete blood cell count; TSH, thyrotropin.

TABLE 8.35

Risk Factors for Suicide in the Older Adult

- White male over age 80, highest risk
- Psychotic depression
- Recent loss/bereavement
- Firearms in the home
- Development of a disability
- Feeling of hopelessness
- Increased severity of depression

TABLE 8.36

Some Medications Contributing to or Causing Depression

Methyldopa	Digitalis
Clonidine	Progesterone
Propranolol	Tamoxifen
Reserpine	Estrogens
Hydralazine	Corticosteroids
Benzodiazepines	Propoxyphene
Cimetidine	

TABLE 8.37

Treatment of Depression in the Older Adult

Goals

- Improve symptoms (sleep, appetite, energy level, mood)
- Improve functioning and quality of life
- Reduce suicide rates
- Decrease family/caregiver distress
- Lower need for health care services
- Improve medical conditions and mortality

Pharmacotherapy

- Medications as effective in older persons as in younger adults
- Recommendation to start low, go slow, and monitor side effects
- No one medication clearly more effective than another
- Consider side effect profile, prior response to a specific medication, medical illness, and patients' most prominent symptoms (sleep disturbance, apathy, agitation, etc) in choosing antidepressant
- Approximately 30% do not respond to first medication; recommendation is to switch to a different antidepressant after an adequate trial at a therapeutic dose of the initial medication
- Continue medication at dose effective in inducing remission of symptoms at least 6 months beyond remission for first episode and at least 12 months in those with a recurrent episode
- If insomnia persists in patient with an otherwise good response, consider addition of a sedating antidepressant such as trazodone
- Treat comorbid conditions that may be contributing to depression (eg, acute infections, thyroid disease). Some recommend doing this prior to using antidepressant medication if depression is mild and reserving antidepressant medication for persistent depression. Reasonable to consider severity of systems and expected length of time needed to control medical illness in decision to treat concurrently or sequentially
- Serotonin syndrome: cognitive symptoms (confusion, anxiety, irritability, drowsiness, autonomic nervous system overactivity, hyperthermia, diaphoresis, tachycardia, hypertension, gastrointestinal symptoms) and neuromuscular symptoms (myoclonus, hyperreflexia, rigidity tremor, ataxia, clonus, and nystagmus); can occur with SSRIs, MAOIs, or selegiline. May be precipitated by meperidine or dextromethorphan in patients on SSRIs, MAOIs

Psychotherapy

- Counseling an important component in treatment of older adults with depression
- Some patients cannot tolerate or will not take medication
- Older adults with depression and significant psychosocial stressors (loss of loved ones, decreased social support, isolation)
- No single type of therapy clearly superior to others
- Primary care physician can provide empathy by listening to patient, encouraging patient to become involved in social activities, and educating patient about depression
- Primary physician can use specific types of therapy such as cognitive behavioral, problem solving, or interpersonal or refer to therapist

Electroconvulsive Therapy

- Safe and effective
- Consider in severe or psychotic depression; patients with contraindications to medications or poor response to medications, patients needing rapid response
- Contraindications: patient not candidate for anesthesia; increased intracranial pressure, intracranial tumor
- Relative contraindications: stroke within 1 month or MI within 3 months
- Side effects: memory loss, confusion; usually temporary

MAOIs indicates monoamine oxidase inhibitors; MI, myocardial infarction; SSRIs, selective serotonin reuptake inhibitors.

TABLE 8.38
Antidepressants in the Elderly

Medication	Indication/ Advantages	Side Effects/ Precautions
SSRIs	■ Mild to moderate depression ■ Minimal cardiac effects ■ Not anticholinergic (OK with BPH, glaucoma) ■ Low sedation	■ Potential drug-drug interactions
Citalopram (Celexa)	■ May have less effect on P450 system than other SSRIs	■ Sedation, dry mouth
Fluoxetine (Prozac)	■ Generally not indicated in the elderly because of long half-life	■ Anxiety, agitation, anorexia, insomnia ■ Long half-life ■ Inhibits cytochrome P450 2D6; may raise blood levels of tricyclic antidepressants and other psychotrophic medications
Paroxetine (Paxil)	■ Short half-life; no active metabolites	■ Sedation, dry mouth ■ Inhibits P450 2D6
Sertraline (Zoloft)	■ Less P450 inhibition than fluoxetine and paroxetine	■ Loose stools, diarrhea ■ Dizziness
Tricyclics (TCAs) Desipramine (Norpramine) Nortriptyline (Pamelor, Aventyl)	■ Severe melancholic depression ■ History of favorable response in the past to TCAs	■ Anticholinergic: avoid with BPH and glaucoma; may cause postural hypotension ■ Quinidine-like properties; need to get baseline ECG; patients with bundle-branch block may progress to second-degree heart block ■ Other drugs in this family have stronger anticholinergic side effects and should be avoided in the elderly

Medication	Indication/ Advantages	Side Effects/ Precautions
Other Antidepressants		
Venlafaxine (*Effexor*)	■ Drug-resistant depression ■ Severe depression with contraindications to TCAs ■ Depression with anxiety or agitation ■ No significant anticholinergic effects	■ Nausea, HA, anorexia, nervousness, dizziness ■ Diastolic HTN (with high doses >275 mg)
Nefazodone (*Serzone*)		■ Increases levels of triazolam, alprazolam, ketoconazole, erythromycin; may result in prolonged QT interval due to P450 ■ Black box warning regarding hepatic failure
Trazodone (*Desyrel*)	■ Useful for insomnia ■ Depression with agitation	■ Increases levels of digoxin, phenytoin ■ Sedation, nausea, priapism
Mirtazapine (*Remeron*)	■ Stimulates appetite ■ Good for insomnia	■ Weight gain ■ Sedating ■ Rare agranulocytosis
Bupropion (*Wellbutrin*)	■ Patients with prominent apathy ■ OK for cardiac patients	■ May exacerbate pre-existing HTN ■ Contraindicated in seizure disorder ■ Anxiety, agitation, insomnia, weight loss

BPH indicates benign prostatic hyperplasia; ECG, electrocardiogram; SSRIs, selective serotonin reuptake inhibitors.

TABLE 8.39
Depression Scales

Cornell Scale for Depression in Dementia

- Developed to assess signs and symptoms of major depression in dementia
- Uses a semistructured interview with a qualified informant regarding the patient's behaviors in the week prior to the interview
- Patient observation/interview done after the informant interview; if disagreement between the results of the two interviews, the informant is reinterviewed for clarification
- Each of 19 items is scored from 0–2. Total scores above 10 indicate a probable major depressive episode. Total scores above 18 indicate a definite depressive episode
- See Table 8.40

Geriatric Depression Scale

- Self-reported measure to assess depressive symptoms in the elderly. Assesses symptoms during the preceding week
- Originally a 30-item, yes/no questionnaire; also available as a 15-question short form (1–4, 7–10, 12, 14, 15, 17, 21–23)
- Suitable for use in mild to moderate dementia, but not in advanced stages
- Score 1 point for each negative response to questions 1, 5, 7, 9, 15, 18, 21, 27, 29
- Score 1 point for each positive response to remaining questions
- Scores greater than 10 on original or 5 on short form suggest depression

TABLE 8.40

Cornell Scale for Depression in Dementia (CSDD)

Scoring System

a = unable to evaluate	1 = mild or intermittent
0= absent	2 = severe

Ratings should be based on symptoms and signs occurring during the week prior to interview. No score should be given if symptoms result from physical disability or illness.

	Item	Score
	A. Mood-Related Signs	
1.	Anxiety (anxious expression, rumination, worrying)	a 0 1 2
2.	Sadness (sad expression, sad voice, tearfulness)	a 0 1 2
3.	Lack of reactivity to pleasant events	a 0 1 2
4.	Irritability (easily annoyed, short-tempered)	a 0 1 2
	B. Behavioral Disturbance	
5.	Agitation (restlessness, handwringing, hair pulling)	a 0 1 2
6.	Retardation (slow movements, slow speech, slow reactions)	a 0 1 2
7.	Multiple physical complaints (score 0 if gastrointestinal symptoms only)	a 0 1 2
8.	Loss of interest; less involved in usual activities (score only if change occurred acutely, ie, in less than 1 month)	a 0 1 2
	C. Physical Signs	
9.	Appetite loss (eating less than usual)	a 0 1 2
10.	Weight loss (score 2 if greater than 5 lb in 1 month)	a 0 1 2
11.	Lack of energy; fatigues easily, unable to sustain activities (score only if change occurred acutely, ie, in less than 1 month)	a 0 1 2

TABLE 8.41

Geriatric Depression Scale*

Mood Assessment Scale

1.	Are you basically satisfied with your life?	Yes/No
2.	Have you dropped many of your activities and interests?	Yes/No
3.	Do you feel that your life is empty?	Yes/No
4.	Do you often get bored?	Yes/No
5.	Are you hopeful about the future?	Yes/No
6.	Are you bothered by thoughts you can't get out of your head?	Yes/No
7.	Are you in good spirits most of the time?	Yes/No
8.	Are you afraid that something bad is going to happen to you?	Yes/No
9.	Do you feel happy most if the time?	Yes/No
10.	Do you often feel helpless?	Yes/No
11.	Do you often get restless and fidgety?	Yes/No
12.	Do you prefer to stay at home, rather than going out and doing new things?	Yes/No
13.	Do you frequently worry about the future?	Yes/No
14.	Do you feel you have more problems with memory than most?	Yes/No
15.	Do you think it is wonderful to be alive now?	Yes/No
16.	Do you often feel downhearted and blue?	Yes/No
17.	Do you feel pretty worthless the way you are now?	Yes/No
18.	Do you worry a lot about the past?	Yes/No
19.	Do you find life very exciting?	Yes/No
20.	Is it hard for you to get started on new projects?	Yes/No
21.	Do you feel full of energy?	Yes/No
22.	Do you feel that your situation is hopeless?	Yes/No
23.	Do you think that most people are better off than you are?	Yes/No
24.	Do you frequently get upset over little things?	Yes/No
25.	Do you frequently feel like crying?	Yes/No
26.	Do you have trouble concentrating?	Yes/No
27.	Do you enjoy getting up in the morning?	Yes/No
28.	Do you prefer to avoid social gatherings?	Yes/No
29.	Is it easy for you to make decisions?	Yes/No
30.	Is your mind as clear as it used to be?	Yes/No

*See Table 8.39 for scoring and interpretation.

TABLE 8.42
Medicare Coverage of Supportive Services

Medicare Coverage of Skilled Nursing Care

Services Included

- Semiprivate room and meals
- Rehabilitation services
- Medications
- Nursing
- Use of appliances

Conditions That Must Be Met

- Follow within 30 days of a 3-day or longer hospital stay for a condition related to NH admission
- Care ordered by physician
- Care approved by Medicare intermediary

Medicare Coverage of Home Health

Services Included

- Part-time skilled nursing
- Physical therapy, speech therapy, occupational therapy
- Part-time home health aide
- Medical equipment if skilled nursing, PT, ST needed

Conditions That Must Be Met

- Be homebound and require intermittent (up to 21 days) skilled nursing, PT, ST
- Ordered by physician
- Care approved by Medicare intermediary

Medicare Coverage for Hospice Care

Services Included

- Inpatient and outpatient nursing
- Physician care
- Drugs
- Physical therapy, speech therapy, occupational therapy
- Homemaker
- Counseling
- Inpatient respite (5 days or less)
- Medical and social services

Continued

TABLE 8.42

Medicare Coverage of Supportive Services, cont'd

Conditions That Must Be Met

- Certified by physician as "terminally ill"
- Patient chooses hospice over standard Medicare benefits for terminal illness

PT indicates physical therapy; ST, speech therapy.

chapter 9

Cancer Care

William C. Crow, Jr, MD

IN THIS CHAPTER

- Most common sites: new cancer cases, deaths
- American Cancer Society guidelines for early detection: average-risk patients
- American Cancer Society guidelines for early detection of colon cancer: high-risk patients
- Detection of leukemia in children
- Detection of leukemia in adults
- Metastatic disease of unknown primary: general features
- Metastatic disease of unknown primary: common presentations
- Paraneoplastic syndromes
- Oncologic emergencies
- Commonly used chemotherapeutic agents
- Pain control: nonnarcotic, narcotics, adjuvant drugs
- Control of nausea and vomiting
- Frequency of emesis with various chemotherapeutic drugs
- Treatment of selected tumors (chemotherapy)
- Follow-up recommendations for common cancers

BOOKSHELF RECOMMENDATIONS

- Lenhard RE Jr, Osteen RT, Gansler T. *American Cancer Society Textbook of Clinical Oncology*. 3rd ed. Atlanta, GA: American Cancer Society; 2001.

FIGURE 9.1

Estimated New Cancer Cases

Top Five Leading Sites by Gender, US, 2002*

Men		Women	
Prostate	30%	Breast	31%
Lung and bronchus	14%	Lung and bronchus	12%
Colon and rectum	11%	Colon and rectum	12%
Urinary bladder	7%	Uterine corpus	6%
Melanoma of the skin	5%	Non-Hodgkin lymphoma	4%

*These percentages are updated regularly by the American Cancer Society. For additional information, visit www.cancer.org.

TABLE 9.1

American Cancer Society Guidelines for the Early Detection of Cancer

Cancer Site	Population	Test or Procedure	Frequency
Breast	Women, age 20+	Breast self-examination	Monthly, starting at age 20
		Clinical breast examination	Every 3 years, ages 20–39; annual, starting at age 40*
		Mammography	Annual, starting at age 40
Colorectal	Men and women, age 50+	Fecal occult blood test (FOBT) and flexible sigmoidoscopy[†]	Annual FOBT and flexible sigmoidoscopy every 5 years, starting at age 50
		(or)	
		Flexible sigmoidoscopy	Every 5 years, starting at age 50
		(or)	
		FOBT	Annual, starting at age 50
		(or)	
		Colonoscopy	Colonoscopy every 10 years, starting at age 50
		(or)	
		Double-contrast barium enema (DCBE)[†]	DCBE every 5 years, starting at age 50

Cancer Site	Population	Test or Procedure	Frequency
Prostate	Men, age 50+	Digital rectal examination and prostate specific antigen test	The prostate specific antigen test and the digital rectal examination should be offered annually, starting at age 50, for men who have a life expectancy of at least 10 years[‡] (begin at age 40 for African-American men)
Cervix	Women, age 18+	Pap test and pelvic examination	All women who are, or have been, sexually active, or have reached age 18 should have an annual Pap test and pelvic examination. After a woman has had 3 or more consecutive satisfactory normal annual examinations, the Pap test may be performed less frequently at the discretion of the physician
Cancer-related check-up	Men and women, age 20+	Examinations every 3 years from ages 20 to 39 and annually after age 40. The cancer-related check-up should include examination for cancers of the thyroid, testicles, ovaries, lymph nodes, oral cavity, and skin, as well as health counseling about tobacco, sun exposure, diet and nutrition, risk factors, sexual practices, and environmental and occupational exposures	

Adapted from Smith RA, von Eschenbach AC, Wender R, et al. American Cancer Society guidelines for the early detection of cancer: update of early detection guidelines for prostate, colorectal, and endometrial cancers. *CA Cancer J Clin*. 2001;51(1):38–75.

[*]Beginning at age 40, annual clinical breast examination should be performed prior to mammography.

[†]Flexible sigmoidoscopy together with FOBT is preferred compared with FOBT or flexible sigmoidoscopy alone.

[‡]Information should be provided to men about the benefits and limitations of testing.

TABLE 9.2

American Cancer Society Guidelines on Screening and Surveillance for the Early Detection of Colorectal Adenomas and Cancer: Women and Men at Increased Risk or at High Risk

Risk Category	Age to Begin	Recommendation	Comment
Increased Risk			
People with a single, small (<1 cm) adenoma	3–6 years after the initial polypectomy	Colonoscopy*	If the exam is normal, the patient can thereafter be screened as per average-risk guidelines
People with a large (1 cm +) adenoma, multiple adenomas, or adenomas with high-grade dysplasia or villous change	Within 3 years after the initial polypectomy	Colonoscopy*	If normal, repeat examination in 3 years; if normal then, the patient can thereafter be screened as per average-risk guidelines
Personal history of curative-intent resection of colorectal cancer	Within 1 year after cancer resection	Colonoscopy*	If normal, repeat examination in 3 years; if normal then, repeat examination every 5 years
Either colorectal cancer or adenomatous polyps, in any first-degree relative before age 60, or in two or more first-degree relatives at any age (if not a hereditary syndrome)	Age 40, or 10 years before the youngest case in the immediate family	Colonoscopy*	Every 5–10 years; colorectal cancer in relatives more distant than first-degree does not increase risk substantially above the average-risk group
High Risk			
Family history of familial adenomatous polyposis (FAP)	Puberty	Early surveillance with endoscopy, and counseling to consider genetic testing	If the genetic test is positive, colectomy is indicated; these patients are best referred to a center with experience in the management of FAP
Family history of hereditary non-polyposis colon cancer (HNPCC)	Age 21	Colonoscopy and counseling to consider genetic testing	If the genetic test is positive or if the patient has not had genetic testing, every 1–2 years until age 40, then annually; these patients are best referred to a center with experience in the management of HNPCC

Risk Category	Age to Begin	Recommendation	Comment
Inflammatory bowel disease; chronic ulcerative colitis; Crohn's disease	Cancer risk begins to be significant 8 years after the onset of pancolitis, or 12–15 years after the onset of left-sided colitis	Colonoscopy with biopsies for dysplasia	Every 1–2 years; these patients are best referred to a center with experience in the surveillance and management of inflammatory bowel disease

Adapted from Smith RA, von Eschenbach AC, Wender R, et al. American Cancer Society guidelines for the early detection of cancer: update of early detection guidelines for prostate, colorectal, and endometrial cancers. *CA Cancer J Clin.* 2001;51(1):38–75.

*If colonoscopy is unavailable, not feasible, or not desired by the patient, double-contrast barium enema alone, or the combination of flexible sigmoidoscopy and double-contrast barium enema, are acceptable alternative. Adding flexible sigmoidoscopy to DCBE may provide a more comprehensive diagnostic evaluation than DCBE alone in finding significant lesions. A supplementary DCBE may be needed if a colonoscopic exam fails to reach the cecum, and a supplementary colonoscopy may be needed if a DCBE identifies a possible lesion, or does not adequately visualize the entire colorectum.

TABLE 9.3

Common Presentations of Leukemia in Children

Disease	History	Physical	Laboratory
Acute Lymphoblastic Leukemia (75% of all cases in children; peak incidence: age 4)	Lethargy, irritability, anorexia, bone pain, arthralgias	Pallor, bleeding, petechiae, fever: 25%; splenomegaly: 60%; lymphadenopathy	Anemia, thrombocytopenia; WBC >10,000/mm^3 (50%), WBC > 50,000/mm^3 (20%); lymphoblasts in peripheral blood; bone marrow exam to confirm diagnosis
Acute Myeloid Leukemia (15%–20% of cases in children)	Fatigue	Pallor, easy bruising, petechiae, epistaxis, hepatomegaly, splenomegaly, lymphadenopathy	Profound anemia and thrombocytopenia; WBC normal, high, or low; bone marrow exam to confirm diagnosis
Juvenile Chronic Myelogenous Leukemia (children <2 years)	Skin lesions, shortness of breath	Eczema, xanthoma, café au lait spots, lymphadenopathy, massive hepatosplenomegaly	Anemia thrombocytopenia, leukocytosis; no Philadelphia chromosome; bone marrow diagnostic
Chronic Myelogenous Leukemia (3%–5% of cases in children)	Insidious onset, weight loss, anorexia, night sweats	Massive splenomegaly	WBC > 100,000/mm^3; ↑ platelet counts, ↑ Vitamin B_{12} level, ↑ uric acid level; leukocyte alkaline phosphatase ↓; Philadelphia chromosome diagnostic

WBC indicates white blood cell count.

TABLE 9.4

Common Presentations of Leukemia in Adults

Disease	History	Physical	Laboratory
Chronic Myelogenous Leukemia (20% of cases; median age at diagnosis: 45–50)	Fatigue, weight loss, early satiety, left upper quadrant fullness	Marked splenomegaly (60% of cases); lymphadenopathy uncommon	WBC 10,000–1,000,000/mm^3, ↑ platelet count in 50%, ↑ Vitamin B_{12}, leukocyte alkaline phosphatase; markedly ↓, ↑ uric acid; Philadelphia chromosome in bone marrow cells
Hairy Cell Leukemia (1%–2% of cases; median age: 50; 4:1 male)	Fatigue, weight loss, abdominal discomfort (splenomegaly)	Splenomegaly: 75%–80%; hepatomegaly: 33%; lymphadenopathy uncommon	Hb <10 in 67%; WBC <4000/mm^3; hairy cells; lymphocytes with cytoplasmic projections
Chronic Lymphocytic Leukemia (33% of cases; most patients >age 60; males 2:1 predominance)	Most asymptomatic	Enlarged lymph nodes (usually cervical) in 67% of patients; hepatomegaly in 10%; splenomegaly in 40%	WBC 40,000–150,000/mm^3
Acute Myelocytic Leukemia	Fatigue, headache	Not as much enlargement of lymph nodes, liver, and spleen as in acute lymphocytic leukemia; rubbery, fast growing masses in soft tissues (chloromas)	Auer rods (cytoplasmic inclusions that stain red with Wright-Giemsa stain), anemia, thrombocytopenia; bone marrow diagnostic
Acute Lymphocytic Leukemia	Fatigue, headache	Enlarged lymph nodes, liver, spleen; may involve testicles	Anemia, thrombocytopenia, bone marrow exam diagnostic

Hb indicates hemoglobin; WBC, white blood cell count.

TABLE 9.5

Metastatic Disease of Unknown Primary: General Features

Incidence	Types of Tumors found	Most Common Primary Sites	Basic Evaluation
2%–12% of patients	■ Adenocarcinoma: 40% ■ Undifferentiated carcinoma: 40% ■ Squamous carcinoma: 10% ■ Melanoma: <5% ■ Neuroblastoma: <5% ■ Neuroendocrine tumors: <5% ■ Other: <5%	■ Pancreas ■ Lung ■ Colon ■ Hepatobiliary organs	■ *Note:* It is more important to look for treatable disease than to investigate every possible unknown primary ■ History and physical exam ■ Breast and pelvic exam in women ■ Testicles and prostate exam in men ■ Chemistry screening panel ■ CBC ■ PSA (in men) ■ Chest x-ray ■ Abdominal and pelvic CT scan ■ Mammography in women ■ Additional studies based on suspicious findings

CBC indicates complete blood cell count; CT, computed tomography; PSA, prostate-specific antigen.

TABLE 9.6

Common Presentation of Metastatic Disease of Unknown Primary

Site of Presentation	Likely Primaries	Helpful Studies
Pulmonary nodules, pleural effusion, mediastinal masses	Lung, breast, lymphoma	Pulmonary nodule—usually open biopsy; pleural effusion—can do cytology; pleural biopsy
Bone metastases	Osteoblastic—prostate, small cell lung cancer, Hodgkin disease, osteolytic or mixed—breast	Direct biopsy of lesion, bone marrow biopsy, bone scan
Liver metastases	Adenocarcinomas from GI tract, breast cancer, lung cancer	Ultrasound, CT-guided needle biopsy
Ascites	Pancreas, stomach, colon; search for ovarian cancer in women as this can be treated	For ovarian cancer—pelvic ultrasound, CT, or MRI; serum tumor marker CA-125
High cervical lymphadenopathy	Nasopharyngeal or oropharyngeal cancer, lymphoma	Nasolaryngoscopy, CT, or MRI
Axillary adenopathy	Breast, lymphoma, small cell lung cancer	Breast exam, mammography; estrogen and progesterone receptor assays on nodal tissue obtained from the axilla; immunohistochemical study for lymphoma; if small cell histology is suggested—chest CT
Inguinal adenopathy	Lymphoma (Hodgkin or non-Hodgkin)	Pelvic and anorectal exam, testicular exam, pelvic sonogram; immunohistochemical and receptor studies of biopsied tissue

Continued

TABLE 9.6

Common Presentation of Metastatic Disease of Unknown Primary, cont'd

Site of Presentation	Likely Primaries	Helpful Studies
Retroperitoneal mass	Advanced stage lymphoma, prostate, germ cell, ovarian cancer	Look for more accessible site; examine peripheral nodes, prostate and testicles in men, pelvic organs in women; may do ultrasound of prostate or testes, or ovary in women; tumor markers = AFP, beta-HCG subunit, PSA
Brain	Breast, small cell lung cancer, lymphoma	If no other tissue available, consider brain biopsy

AFP indicates α-fetoprotein; CT, computed tomography; GI, gastrointestinal; MRI, magnetic resonance imaging; PSA, prostate-specific antigen.

TABLE 9.7

The Paraneoplastic Syndromes

Syndrome	Underlying Tumor	Evaluation
Cushing Syndrome	5% of patients with small cell lung cancer caused by ectopic production of ACTH	Usually don't look cushingoid—increased skin pigmentation, severe decrease in potassium; increased serum and urine ketosteroids; very poor prognosis
SIADH	Most commonly small cell lung cancer	Hyponatremia; inappropriately elevated urine osmolality; restrict free water; treat underlying tumor
Hypercalcemia	Squamous cell cancer of the head, neck, and lung; ovarian cancer, bladder cancer, hypernephroma	Requires direct testing for parathyroid hormone related protein (PTHRP); regular PTH assay will not help; check serum calcium; symptoms may not develop until the serum calcium is very high
Hyperthyroidism and acute thyrotoxicosis	Choriocarcinomas produce ectopic chorionic gonadotropin (functions like TSH)	Beta-blockers for symptoms, but main treatment is to treat the underlying tumor
Eaton-Lambert syndrome	Small cell lung cancer	Proximal muscle weakness of the limbs; unlike myasthenia gravis, the weakness tends to diminish with exercise
Subacute cerebellar degeneration	Small cell lung cancer, ovarian cancer, breast cancer	Patients may have ataxia, dysarthria, dysphagia, dementia
Hypertrophic pulmonary osteoarthopathy	Primary or metastatic lung tumor	Digital clubbing and tenderness along the distal long bones; x-ray shows elevated periosteum of long bones; bone scan shows increased uptake along cortical margins; pain relieved by removal of the tumor

ACTH indicates corticotropin; PTH, parathyroid hormone; SIADH, syndrome of inappropriate secretion of antidiuretic hormone; TSH, thyrotropin.

TABLE 9.8

Oncologic Emergencies

Emergency	Evaluation	Treatment
Fever and neutropenia	Bacterial infection following chemotherapy, neutrophil count <500/mm^3 probable sepsis; asplenic patient—any neutropenia must suspect sepsis	Must cover gram+, *Pseudomonas*, *Klebsiella*, gram− from the gut; broad-spectrum antibiotic (eg, Timentin + an aminoglycoside)
Thrombocytopenia	Spontaneous bleeding: platelet counts <10,000/mm^3; thrombocytopenic patient on chemotherapy—avoid aspirin and NSAID	May require platelet transfusion
Hypercoagulability	In patient with active disease, may be resistant to heparin and Coumadin	Consider vena cava filter; do not anticoagulate with primary brain tumor, CNS metastasis, spinal cord lesions
Disseminated intravascular coagulation	Seen with sepsis, acute leukemia, breast, lung, prostate, and pancreatic cancer; platelet count <100,000/mm^3; rapid ↓ in platelet count; prolonged INR and activated PTT; presence of fibrin degradation products; ↓ antithrombin III	Treat both underlying tumor and the DIC as soon as abnormal labs seen; heparin (300 to 500 U/h) or low-molecular-weight heparin; active bleeding: platelet concentrates and fresh frozen plasma
Hyperleukocytic syndrome	Patient with leukemia and WBC >100,000/mm^3, dyspnea, headaches, confusion, high blood viscosity, pseudohypoglycemia and pseudohyperkalemia (apparent very low blood sugar or very high potassium in the absence of mental changes or ECG abnormalities)	Leukopheresis
Hypercalcemia of malignancy	Most common life-threatening metabolic complication of cancer; may occur in absence of metastases; most common in multiple myeloma, breast cancer, squamous cell lung cancer	Rehydrate first with normal saline—IV furosemide; avoid thiazide diuretics; Calcitonin—↓ Ca^{+4} rapidly but effect short-lived; Pamidronate—sustained ↓ in Ca++ level
Hypercalcemia of malignancy vs primary hyperparathyroidism	**Malignancy** ■ Serum Ca++ ↑↑ ■ Cl level ↓ ■ PO_4 = ↑ or normal ■ HCO_3 = ↑ or normal alkaline phosphatase ↑	**Primary Hyperparathyroidism** ■ Serum Ca++ ↑ ■ Cl level ↑ ■ PO_4 = ↓ ■ HCO_3 ↓ ■ Alkaline phosphatase ↑

Emergency	Evaluation	Treatment
Tumor lysis syndrome	Occurs 6–72 hours after chemotherapy, ↑ risk with ↑ LDH, ↑ uric acid, ↑ creatinine; most commonly seen with high-grade lymphoma, leukemia with high WBC count, oat cell lung cancer	Prevention most important; pretreat with aggressive hydration and allopurinol before chemotherapy
SIADH	↓ serum Na+; inappropriately concentrated urine, most frequent in small cell lung cancer, metastatic lung disease, prostate cancer, pancreatic cancer	Na+ >125 mEq/L—fluid restriction; Na+ 120–125 mEq/L—normal saline + furosemide; Na+ <120 mEq/L—3% saline to ↑ Na+ no more than 1 mEq/L/h
Malignant pericardial tamponade	Seen in metastatic and primary lung cancer, breast cancer, leukemia and lymphoma, malignant melanoma. Heart may appear normal on chest x-ray, cardiac echo diagnostic	Surgery: pericardial window
Superior vena cava syndrome	Most common in lung cancer, lymphoma; patient may have swelling of face, neck vein distention; CT or MRI diagnostic	Elevate head of bed; supplemental oxygen; irradiation
Parenchymal brain metastasis	Most common in cancers of lung, breast, gastrointestinal, or genitourinary tracts, malignant melanoma. Headache and vomiting on wakening, MRI diagnostic	Emergency treatment with Dexamethasone
Malignant spinal cord compression	Most common in cancers of breast, lung, prostate, kidney, lymphomas, sarcomas, usually in thoracic spine, unremitting pain, worse on lying down, contrast-enhanced MRI diagnostic	Dexamethasone, radiotherapy, occasionally surgery

CNS indicates central nervous system; CT, computed tomography; DIC, disseminated intravascular coagulation; ECG, electrocardiogram; INR, international normalized ratio; LDH, lactate dehydrogenase; MRI, magnetic resonance imaging; NSAID, nonsteroidal anti-inflammatory drug; PTT, partial thromboplastin time; SIADH, syndrome of inappropriate secretion of antidiuretic hormone; WBC, white blood cell.

TABLE 9.9

Commonly Used Chemotherapeutic Agents

Drug	Class	Drug Interactions	Toxicity	Indications
Anagrelide (Agrylin)	Inhibit platelet aggregation	Sucralfate may decrease absorption	Hypotension, headache, palpitations	Essential thrombocytosis
Leucovorin calcium	Tetrahydrofolate derivative	↓ effectiveness and toxicity of methotrexate	Generally well tolerated	Rescue of high-dose methotrexate therapy; potentiate fluorouracil in GI malignancies
Leuprolide acetate (Leupron)	Gonadotropin-releasing hormone agonist	None reported	Hot flashes, impotence, ↑ LFTs, depression	Hormone-dependent advanced prostate cancer
Megestrol acetate (Megace)	Progestin	None noted	Menstrual changes, hot flashes	Breast and endometrial cancer, appetite stimulation
Melphalan (Alkeran)	Alkylating agent	None noted	Myelosuppression, nausea and vomiting	Multiple myeloma, ovarian cancer
Mercaptopurine	Antimetabolite	Allopurinol ↓ metabolism; must ↓ dose of mercaptopurine	Myelosuppression, nausea and vomiting	Acute lymphoblastic leukemia
Methotrexate	Antifolate antimetabolite	None reported	Myelosuppression, stomatitis, diarrhea	Acute leukemia, lymphoma, breast cancer, bladder cancer, squamous cell cancer, sarcomas
Asparaginase (Elspar)	Enzyme	None noted	Can have life-threatening hypersensitivity; anaphylaxis precautions; 2-unit test dose; coagulopathy, nausea, vomiting, ↑ LFTs	Acute lymphocytic leukemia also used in AML, CML, CLL, and non-Hodgkin lymphomas

Drug	Class	Drug Interactions	Toxicity	Indications
BCG	Vaccine	Immunosuppressive drugs	Dysuria, hematuria, fever	Intravesical instillation for noninvasive bladder tumors after removal of papillary tumors
Bicalutamide (Casodex)	Antiandrogen	↑ anticoagulant effect of warfarin	Hot flashes, ↓ libido, depression	Prostate cancer in combination with luteinizing hormone releasing hormone (LHRH) agonist agent
Bleomycin	Antibiotic	None noted	Pulmonary fibrosis, fever, rash	Germ cell tumors, Hodgkin disease
Carboplatin	Atypical alkylator	None reported	Myelosuppression; especially thrombocytopenia	Ovarian cancer, testicular cancer, squamous cell cancer of head and neck and cervix, lung cancer
Chlorambucil (Leukeran)	Alkylating agent	None noted	Myelosuppression	CLL, low-grade lymphomas
Cisplatin	Atypical alkylator	None noted	Nephrotoxicity, neurotoxicity, ototoxicity	Testicular and ovarian cancer, transitional cell carcinoma; used in many solid tumors and lymphoma
Cyclophosphamide (Cytoxan)	Alkylator	None reported	Myelosuppression, especially leukopenia; nausea and vomiting; hemorrhagic cystitis	Breast cancer, non-Hodgkin lymphoma, ovarian cancer, testicular cancer

Continued

TABLE 9.9

Commonly Used Chemotherapeutic Agents, cont'd

Drug	Class	Drug Interactions	Toxicity	Indications
Dacarbazine	Atypical alkylator		Myelosuppression, nausea and vomiting, fever	Malignant melanoma, Hodgkin disease
Dexamethasone (Decadron)	Steroid	Dilantin and Tegretol can ↑ metabolism and ↓ effectiveness	↑ WBC, ↑ BS, weight gain, adrenal suppression	Multiple myeloma, CLL, ALL, non-Hodgkin lymphoma; relieves symptoms of brain and spinal cord metastases
Doxorubicin (Adriamycin)	Antibiotic	None noted	Soft tissue vesicant, myelosuppression, cardiotoxicity	Breast cancer, adult sarcomas, pediatric solid tumors, Hodgkin disease, non-Hodgkin lymphoma, ovarian cancer
Erythropoietin (Epogen)	Growth factor for RBCs precursor	May temporarily ↓ effect of heparin, aluminum-containing antacids may ↓ effectiveness of Epogen	Hypertension, injection site pain, iron deficiency anemia—give supplemental iron	Symptomatic chemotherapy-induced anemia; anemia of chronic renal failure and HIV
Fluorouracil	Antimetabolite	None noted	Mucositis, diarrhea, some myelosuppression	Cancer of the colon, rectum, stomach, pancreas, breast
Gemcitabine (Gemzar)	Antimetabolite	None noted	Myelosuppression, nausea and vomiting, ↑ transaminases, fever during administration	Advanced pancreatic adenocarcinoma
Goserelin acetate (Zoladex)	LHRH	None noted	Hot flases, ↓ libido, impotence	Advanced prostate cancer

Drug	Class	Drug Interactions	Toxicity	Indications
Paclitaxel (Taxol)	Induces apoptosis in dividing cells	Cisplatin ↑ toxicity, Taxo may enhance the cardiotoxicity of doxorubicin	Mild vesicant, neutropenia, mucositis, peripheral neuropathy	Salvage therapy in ovarian and breast cancer
Pamidronate (Aredia)	Bisphosphonate inhibits bone resorption	None noted	↓ Ca++, ↓ potassium ↓ mg++. Generally well tolerated	Hypercalcemia of malignancy, pain relief from bone metastases in multiple myeloma, breast cancer, prostate cancer
Prednisone	Steroid	None noted	Indigestion, weight gain, adrenal suppression	Used in wide range of tumors
Procarbazine	Alkylating agent	MAO inhibitor; avoid fermented cheese, beer, wine, chocolate, TCAs	Myelosuppression, nausea and vomiting	Hodgkin disease; also non-Hodgkin lymphoma, multiple myeloma, brain tumors, melanoma, lung cancer
Tamoxifen (Nolvadex)	Antiestrogen	None noted	Hot flashes, rare venous thromboembolism	Breast cancer—primarily postmenopausal patients, estrogen receptor-positive tumors
Trastuzumab (Herceptin)	Monoclonal antibody	None noted	Fever, chills, nausea, vomiting; cardiotoxicity—do not use with doxorubicin	Her-2-neu overexpressing metastatic or locally advanced breast cancer

Continued

TABLE 9.9

Commonly Used Chemotherapeutic Agents, cont'd

Drug	Class	Drug Interactions	Toxicity	Indications
Vinblastine (Velban)	Vinca alkaloid	None noted	Soft-tissue vesicant; myelosuppression; some peripheral neuropathy	Hodgkin disease, non-Hodgkin lymphoma, germ cell tumor, breast cancer
Vincristine (Oncovin)	Vinca alkaloid	Asparaginase may ↓ hepatic metabolism	Vesicant, peripheral neuropathy	Hodgkin disease and other lymphoma, acute leukemia, rhabdomyosarcoma, neuroblastoma, Wilms tumor

AML indicates acute monocytic leukamia; CLL, chronic lymphocytic leukemia; CML, chronic myelogenous leukemia; GI, gastrointestinal; HIV, human immunodeficiency virus; MAC, monoamine oxidase, RBC, red blood cell count; TCA, tricyclic antidepressant; WBC, white blood cell count.

TABLE 9.10

Drugs Used in Treating Cancer Pain

Class	Drug Name	Dose Equivalents (mg) to 10 mg of Morphine (for the Narcotics)	Duration of Action (h)	Peak Effect (h)	Usual Oral Dose (mg)	Available Formulations	Comments
Non-narcotic	Aspirin	650	4–6	½–1½	650–975 every 4 h	Tablet, liquid, suppository	Anti-inflammatory effect, GI side effects limit use
	Acetaminophen	650	4–6	½–1½	650–975 every 4 h	Tablet, liquid, suppository	Lacks anti-inflammatory effect, better tolerated than aspirin
	Ibuprofen	400 mg	4–6	½–1½	200–800 mg every 4–6 h	Tablet, liquid	GI upset; renal impairment
Narcotic Agonists	Codeine	Oral = 200 IM = 130	4–6	1–1½	60 every 4 h	Tablet, liquid, injection	Most patients will not tolerate oral doses >90 mg every 4 hours, antitussive

Continued

TABLE 9.10

Drugs Used in Treating Cancer Pain, cont'd

Class	Drug Name	Dose Equivalents (mg) to 10 mg of Morphine (for the Narcotics)	Duration of Action (h)	Peak Effect (h)	Usual Oral Dose (mg)	Available Formulations	Comments
	Oxycodone	Oral = 30 IM = 15	3–5	1–1½	30 every 4 h	Tablet, liquid, injection	Antitussive, tolerated better than codeine by some patients
	Propoxyphene	Oral = 50	2–4	1–1½	50 every 4–6 h	Tablet	Usually in combination with nonopioid; may accumulate in renal failure; not recommended for long-term use
	Morphine	Oral = 30 IM = 10	3–4	½–1½	30 every 4 h	Tablet, liquid sustained release, suppository, injection	The "standard"

Class	Drug Name	Dose Equivalents (mg) to 10 mg of Morphine (for the Narcotics)	Duration of Action (h)	Peak Effect (h)	Usual Oral Dose (mg)	Available Formulations	Comments
	Methadone (Dolcphine)	Oral = 20 IM = 10	4–8	1–2	20 every 4 h	Tablet, injection	Can accumulate rapidly, somewhat more expensive than morphine
	Meperidine (Demerol)	Oral = 300 IM = 75	2–4	½–1	75–150 every 3 h	Tablet, injection	Most patients will not tolerate oral doses >150 mg; not recommended for cancer patients
	Hydromorphone (Dilaudid)	Oral = 8 IM = 2	4–6	½–1½	4–8 every 4 h	Tablet, liquid, suppository, injection	Good potency, large dose concentrated in small volume
	Levorphanol (Levo-Dromoran)	Oral = 4 IM = 2	4–8	½–1	2–4 every 6 h	Tablet, injection	Slightly longer-acting than morphine, lipophilic
	Oxymorphone (Numorphan)	IM = 1	4–6	½–1½	10 rectally every 4 h	Suppository and injection	No oral form available

Continued

TABLE 9.10

Drugs Used in Treating Cancer Pain, cont'd

Class	Drug Name	Dose Equivalents (mg) to 10 mg of Morphine (for the Narcotics)	Duration of Action (h)	Peak Effect (h)	Usual Oral Dose (mg)	Available Formulations	Comments
	Fentanyl transdermal patch (Duragesic)	100 μg/h= morphine 2 mg/h	48–72			Patch	Patches deliver 25, 50, 75, and 100 μg/h
Mixed Agonist/Antagonist	Pentazocine (Talwin)	Oral = 180 IM = 60	3–4	½–1	280 every 4 h	Tablet, injection	Only oral form available in combination with naloxone, aspirin, or acetaminophen; hallucinations in elderly, decreases narcotic effectiveness; not recommended

GI indicates gastrointestinal; IM, intramuscularly.

TABLE 9.11

Adjuvant Drugs for Cancer Pain

Generic Name	Dosage	Therapeutic Effects	Comments
Dexamethasone	4 mg po q 6 h	Improve appetite	Relief of pain from compression of spinal cord or ↑ intracranial pressure
Amitriptyline	Start with 10–25 mg q hs, ↑ to 75–100 mg q hrs	Potentiates opioid analgesia, elevates mood	Pain from postherpetic neuralgia, Pancoast tumor
Hydroxyzine	Start 25 mg tid, ↑ to 50–100 mg q 4–6 h	Potentiates opioid analgesia	Convulsions with >500 mg/d
Dextroamphetamine	2.5 mg po tid or 5 mg in the AM	Potentiates narcotic analgesia, elevates mood	For terminally ill patients with pain, depression, lethargy

TABLE 9.12

Antiemetic Agents to Treat Chemotherapy-Related Nausea and Vomiting

Generic Name	Brand Name	Mechanism of Action	Dose
Ondansetron	Zofran	5-HT3 receptor blockade	32 mg IV over 15 min or 0.15 mg/kg dose 30 min prior to chemotherapy and repeated at 4 and 8 h after first dose
Granisetron	Kytril	5-HT3 receptor blockade	IV: 10 mg/h IV over 5 minutes, 30 minutes prior to chemotherapy Oral: 1 mg po bid × 1 day; radiation-induced N and V: 2 mg po 1 hour before first radiation fraction each day
Dolasetron	Anzemet	5-HT3 receptor blockade	1.8 mg/kg up to 100 mg IV/po single dose
Metoclopramide	Reglan	Dopamine receptor blockade; 5-HT3 receptor blockade	1–3 mg/kg IV q 2 h × 2–4 doses
Dexamethasone	Decadron	Steroid; adjunctive agent for nausea and vomiting; mechanisms of action unknown	10–20 mg IV or po × 1 dose
Promethazine	Phenergan	Phenothiazine, dopamine receptor blockade	12.5–25 mg po/IM/IV q d—qid (adult dose)
Lorazepam	Ativan	Benzodiazepine, anxiolytic	1–2 mg IV q 4 h

TABLE 9.13

Frequency of Emesis With Selected Chemotherapeutic Agents

Frequency of Emesis	Agent
>90%	Cisplatin (high dose) Cyclophosphamide (high dose) Dacarbazine
60%–90%	Carboplatin Cisplatin (low dose) Cyclophosphamide (moderate dose) Doxorubicin (high dose) Methotrexate (high dose)
30%–60%	Cyclophosphamide (low dose) Doxorubicin (low dose) Methotrexate (moderate dose)
10%–30%	Docetaxel Fluorouracil Gemcitabine Methotrexate (low dose) Paclitaxel
<10%	Busulfan Bleomycin Chlorambucil (oral) Hydroxyurea Methotrexate (very low dose) Vinblastine Vincristine

TABLE 9.14
Cancer Chemotherapy

Cancer	Clinical Indication	Medical Regimen
Breast	Chemoprevention	Tamoxifen 20 mg po daily × 5 years
	Primary tumor >1 cm in diameter; patients with + lymph nodes	Adriamycin + Cytoxan regimen for 6 months. In estrogen receptor + patients, F/U with tamoxifen 20 mg bid
	Locally advanced disease	May need neoadjuvant chemotherapy to convert tumor to an operable size, postoperative chemotherapy
	Metastatic disease	Aggressive combination chemotherapy; endocrine therapy (tamoxifen, Megace, aromatase inhibitors); high-dose chemotherapy with stem cell support under investigation
Hodgkin Disease	Advanced stages, unfavorable histology	ABVD: Adriamycin, bleomycin, vinblastine, dacarbazine; 4-week cycle; minimum of 6 cycles
Non-Hodgkin Lymphoma	Chemotherapy treatment of choice for most patients	CHOP: Cytoxan, Adriamycin, Oncovin, prednisone. 3-week cycle, repeat for 6 cycles
Acute Lymphoblastic Leukemia	Adults	*Remission induction*: Vincristine, prednisone, asparaginase, and/or daunorubicin over 3–4 weeks *Consolidation*: High-dose methotrexate, Cytoxan, and cytarabine *Maintenance*: Daily mercaptopurine + weekly or biweekly methotrexate. Usually given for 2–3 years *CNS prophylaxis*: Intrathecal methotrexate alone or intrathecal methotrexate combined with craniospinal irradiation

Cancer	Clinical Indication	Medical Regimen
Acute Lymphoblastic Leukemia	Children	**Low-Risk Patients** *Remission Induction* (4–6 weeks): Vincristine IV weekly. Prednisone po daily, asparaginase IM biweekly. Intrathecal methotrexate, hydrocortisone, cytarabine (Ara-C) weekly × 6 during induction and then every 8 weeks for 2 years *Systemic Continuation Treatment*: Mercaptopurine po daily, methotrexate weekly po, IV, or IM for 2–3 years *Reinforcement*: Vincristine IV every 4 weeks, prednisone po × 7 days every 4 weeks for 2–3 years **High-Risk Patients** Require more intensive multidrug regimens
Acute Myelocytic Leukemia	Adults	*Remission induction*: An anthracycline (daunorubicin or idarubicin) + cytarabine *Consolidation*: Repeated cycles of high-dose cytarabine
Chronic Lymphocytic Leukemia	Adults	Do not treat asymptomatic early-stage disease *Indications for Treatment*: Fever, sweats, weight loss, fatigue, massive lymphadenopathy, hepatosplenomegaly, lymphocytosis >100,000/mm^3, advanced-stage disease.

Continued

TABLE 9.14
Cancer Chemotherapy, cont'd

Cancer	Clinical Indication	Medical Regimen
		Regimens: 1. Chlorambucil is the mainstay of treatment. It is usually given over 6–12 months. Prednisone is sometimes added 2. Fludarabine monophosphate has been used recently
Lung Cancer (Non–Small Cell)	Some controversy; usually given in relatively advanced disease (stage III A and beyond); combination therapy better than single agent	Cytoxan, Adriamycin, cisplatin (CAP); Bleomycin, etoposide, cisplatin (BEP); etoposide, cisplatin (EP); docetaxel, cisplatin (DOCP)
Lung Cancer (Small Cell)	Chemotherapy is the mainstay of treatment for all stages	**Examples of Regimens** Etoposide (VP-16), cisplatin, cytoxan, adriamycin, vincristine, etoposide (CAVE); etoposide, carboplatin
Testicular Cancer	High-stage seminomas (IIB, III)	Cisplatin, vinblastine, and bleomycin in combination
Testicular Cancer	Nonseminomas	Bleomycin, etoposide, and platinum

bid indicates twice daily; IM, intramuscularly; IV, intravenously; po, orally.

TABLE 9.15

Breast Cancer Follow-up*

	Months												Then Every 12 months
	3	6	9	12	15	18	21	24	30	36	42	48	
History													
Complete				•				•		•		•	•
Self-examination	•	•	•		•	•	•		•		•		
Lumps	•	•	•		•	•	•		•		•		
Pain	•	•	•		•	•	•		•		•		
Cough, dyspnea	•	•	•		•	•	•		•		•		
Weight loss, anorexia	•	•	•		•	•	•		•		•		
Physical													
Complete				•				•		•		•	•
Chest wall, axillae	•	•	•		•	•	•		•		•		
Remaining breast tissue	•	•	•		•	•	•		•		•		
Lymph nodes	•	•	•		•	•	•		•		•		
Abdomen, liver	•	•	•		•	•	•		•		•		
Skin, eyes (jaundice)	•	•	•		•	•	•		•		•		
Chest	•	•	•		•	•	•		•		•		
Bones	•	•	•		•	•	•		•		•		
Pelvis				•				•		•		•	

Continued

TABLE 9.15

Breast Cancer Follow-up, cont'd

	Months												Then Every
	3	6	9	12	15	18	21	24	30	36	42	48	12 months
Other													
Mammography		□		●		□		●		●		●	●
CBC				○				○		○		○	○
Serum calcium				○				○		○		○	○
Serum LDH				○				○		○		○	○
Serum alkaline phosphatase				○				○		○		○	○
Serum CEA				○				○		○		○	○
Serum phosphorus				○				○		○		○	○
Serum AST and ALT				○				○		○		○	○
Chest x-ray examiniation				○				○				○	Every other year
Bone scan		○		○									
Liver scan/ultrasonography				○									

Adapted from Fischer DS, Ungaro PC, Wilhelm MC. Cancer follow-up: how much is enough? *Patient Care.* 1992;26:201–224.

ALT indicates serum alanine aminotransferase; AST, serum aspartate aminotransferase; CBC, complete blood cell count; CEA, carcinoembryonic antigen; LDH, lactate dehydrogenase.

*With regard to frequency of follow-up visits, this table shows the minimum recommendation. Some of the consultants recommend shortening intervals between follow-up visits or tests.

Key:

● Recommended by all consultants

○ Not recommended by all consultants

□ If patient was treated with lumpectomy and radiotherapy

TABLE 9.16

Colon and Rectal Cancer Follow-up*

	First Year Months				Second-Fifth Year Months		Then Every 12 Months
	3	6	9	12	6	12	
History							
Complete				●		●	●
Weight loss, anorexia	●	●	●		●		
Bowel function (pain, change, blood)	●	●	●		●		
Abdominal pain	●	●	●		●		
Pruritus	●	●	●		●		
Dark urine	●	●	●		●		
Physical							
Complete				●		●	●
Abdomen, liver	●	●	●		●		
Stroma	●	●	●		●		
Rectum	●	●	●		●		
Lymph nodes	●	●	●		●		
Skin (jaundice)	●	●	●		●		
Other							
CBC	●	●	●	●	●	●	●
Fecal occult blood	○	●	○	○	●	●	●
Liver function		○		●	○	●	●
Serum CEA		●		●	In 2nd year only	●	●
Endoscopy: Sigmoidoscopy and barium enema (or)		●		●	In 2nd year only	●	●
Colonoscopy				●	Every other year after 3rd year		
Liver scan/ultrasonography				○		○	○
Chest x-ray examination				○		○	○

Adapted from Fischer DS, Ungaro PC, Wilhelm MC. Cancer follow-up: how much is enough? *Patient Care*. 1992;26:201–224.

CBC indicates complete blood cell count; CEA, carcinoembryonic antigen

*With regard to frequency of follow-up visits, this table shows the minimum recommendation. Some of the consultants recommend shortening intervals between follow-up visits or tests.

Key:

● Recommended by all consultants

○ Not recommended by all consultants

Liver function tests and serum CEA every 3 months for first 2–3 years. If complete colonoscopy not done at time of diagnosis, do at 6 months postoperatively. Otherwise, do colonoscopy at yearly intervals for first 2 years then every third year. At many institutions patients at great risk are candidates for regular computed tomographic imaging.

TABLE 9.17

Prostate Cancer Follow-up*

	Months							Then every 12 months
	3	6	9	12	16	20	24	
History								
Complete				●			●	●
Urinary symptoms	●	●	●		●	●		
Bone pain	●	●	●		●	●		
Cardiac symptoms	●	●	●		●	●		
Sexual problems	●	●	●		●	●		
Depression	●	●	●		●	●		
Radiation-induced problems	●	●	●		●	●		
Physical								
Complete				●			●	●
Prostatic bed, surgical field, meatus	●	●	●		●	●		
Rectum	●	●	●		●	●		
Lymph nodes	●	●	●		●	●		
Bladder	●	●	●		●	●		
Other								
Urinalysis	●	●	●	●	●	●	●	●
Prostate-specific antigen	○	●	○	●	○	○	●	●**
CBC		○		○			○	○
Chest x-ray examination/ ultrasound		○		●			●	●
Pelvic x-ray examination/ ultrasound		○		●			●	●
Bone scan				○				
BUN		○		○			○	○
Serum creatinine		○		○			○	○

Adapted from Fischer DS, Ungaro PC, Wilhelm MC. Cancer follow-up: how much is enough? *Patient Care.* 1992;26:201–224.

BUN indicates blood urea nitrogen; CBC, complete blood cell count.

*With regard to frequency of follow-up visits, this table shows the minimum recommendation. Some of the consultants recommend shortening intervals between follow-up visits or tests.

**Many experts recommend follow-up at 6-month intervals.

Key:

● Recommended by all consultants

○ Not recommended by all consultants

TABLE 9.18

Cervical Cancer Follow-up*

	First Year Months				Second-Fifth Year Months		Then Every 12 Months
	3	6	9	12	6	12	
History							
Complete				●		●	●
Vaginal bleeding, spotting, discharge	●	●	●		●		
Bone pain	●	●	●		●		
Leg edema	●	●	●		●		
Weight loss, anorexia	●	●	●		●		
Abdominal distention	●	●	●		●		
Bowel function	●	●	●		●		
Bladder function	●	●	●		●		
Physical							
Complete				●		●	●
Pelvis	●	●	●		●		
Rectum	●	●	●		●		
Abdomen	●	●	●		●		
Breasts	●	●	●		●		
Lymph nodes	●	●	●		●		
Colposcopy**	○	○	○		○	○	○
Other							
Urinalysis	●	●		●	●	●	●
Fecal occult blood	●	●		●	●	●	●
Pap smear		●	●	●	●	●	●
CBC		○		○	○	○	○
Serum CEA and CA 125				○		○	○
Chest x-ray examination				●		●	●
IVP				●		○	

Adapted from Fischer DS, Ungaro PC, Wilhelm MC. Cancer follow-up: how much is enough? *Patient Care.* 1992;26:201–224.

CBC indicates complete blood cell count; CEA, carcinoembryonic antigen; IVP, intravenous pyelogram.

*With regard to frequency of follow up visits, this table shows the minimum recommendation. Some of the consultants recommend shortening intervals between follow-up visits or tests.

**If cervix was not removed.

Key:

● Recommended by all consultants

○ Not recommended by all consultants

In follow-up of patients with cervical intraepithelial neoplasia, do colposcopy and cytology at the 3 month visit. Cervical cancer, see every 3-months the first year, every 3–4 months the second year, every 6 months next 3 years, then annually after 5 years. Pap smears at each visit. Annual chest film. Computed tomography or magnetic resonance imaging if patient has symptoms.

TABLE 9.19

Endometrial Cancer Follow-up*

	First Year Months				Second-Fifth Year Months		Then Every 12 Months
	3	6	9	12	6	12	
History							
Complete				●		●	●
Vaginal bleeding, spotting, discharge	●	●	●		●		
Pelvic pain	●	●	●		●		
Leg edema	●	●	●		●		
Weight loss, anorexia	●	●	●		●		
Abdominal distention, enlargement	●	●	●		●		
Estrogen supplementation	●	●	●		●		
Physical							
Complete				●		●	●
Pelvis	●	●	●		●		
Rectum	●	●	●		●		
Abdomen	●	●	●		●		
Breasts	●	●	●		●		
Lymph nodes	●	●	●		●		
Other							
Urinalysis	●	○		○	○	○	○
Fecal occult blood	●	●		●	●	●	●
Pap smear		●	●	●	●	●	●
CBC		○		○	○	○	○
Serum CEA and CA 125				○		○	○
Liver function studies				○	○	○	
Chest x-ray examination				●		●	●
IVP				○		○	

Adapted from Fischer DS, Ungaro PC, Wilhelm MC. Cancer follow-up: how much is enough? *Patient Care.* 1992;26:201–224.

CBC indicates complete blood cell count; CEA, carcinoembryonic antigen; IVP, intravenous pyelogram.

*With regard to frequency of follow-up visits, this table shows the minimum recommendation. Some of the consultants recommend shortening intervals between follow-up visits or tests.

Key:

● Recommended by all consultants

○ Not recommended by all consultants

Patients with stage I A, grade I cancer have physical and pelvic exam every 3 months for 2 years, then every 6 months for 3 years, then yearly.

TABLE 9.20

Hodgkin's Disease Follow-up*

	First Year Months			Second-Fifth Year Months		Then Every 12 Months
	1	3, 6, 9	12	4, 8	12	
History						
Complete			●		●	●
Weight loss, anorexia	●	●		●		
Fever	●	●		●		
Pruritus	●	●		●		
Pain (alcohol induced)	●	●		●		
Lumps	●	●		●		
Night sweats	●	●		●		
Respiratory symptoms	●	●		●		
Physical						
Complete			●		●	●
Lymph nodes	●	●		●		
Abdomen, liver, spleen	●	●		●		
Skin	●	●		●		
Oropharynx	●	●		●		
Chest	●	●		●		
Other						
CBC	●	●	●	●	●	●
Chest x-ray examination	●	●	●	●	●	●
Serum alkaline phosphatase	●		●		●	●
Serum LDH	●		●		●	●
Serum bilirubin	●		●		●	●
Serum AST	●		●		●	●
Urinalysis	●		●		●	●
ESR	○		○		○	○
Thyroid function		□	□			
Gallium scan			○			
Abdominal x-ray examination or CT scan		♦	♦		♦	♦

Adapted from Fischer DS, Ungaro PC, Wilhelm MC. Cancer follow-up: how much is enough? *Patient Care.* 1992;26:201–224.

AST indicates serum aspartate aminotransferase; CBC, complete blood cell count; CT, computed tomography; ESR, erythrocyte sedimentation rate; LDH, lactate dehydrogenase.

*With regard to frequency of follow-up visits, this table shows the minimum recommendation. Some of the consultants recommend shortening intervals between follow-up visits or tests.

Key:

● Recommended by all consultants

○ Not recommended by all consultants

□ At 6 months in first year, if patient received radiation therapy near thyroid gland

♦ At 6 months in first year, if patient had intra-abdominal Hodgkin disease

See at 3-month intervals × 2 years, 4–6 month intervals next 3 years, yearly after 5 years. Each visit: physical examination, complete blood cell count, erythrocyte sedimentation rate, alkaline phosphatase, liver function tests, chest x-ray if mediastinal disease was present. Periodic computed tomography scans may be indicated.

TABLE 9.21

Non-Hodgkin Lymphoma Follow-up*

	First Year Months			Second-Fifth Year Months		Then Every 12 Months
	1	3, 6, 9	12	4, 8	12	
History						
Complete			●		●	●
Weight loss, anorexia	●	●		●		
Fever	●	●		●		
Pain	●	●		●		
Lumps	●	●		●		
Night sweats	●	●		●		
Respiratory symptoms	●	●		●		
GI symptoms	●	●		●		
CNS symptoms	●	●		●		
Physical						
Complete			●		●	●
Lymph nodes	●	●		●		
Abdomen, liver, spleen	●	●		●		
Skin	●	●		●		
Oropharynx	●	●		●		
Chest	●	●		●		
Neurological examination	●	●		●		
Other						
CBC		●	●	●	●	●
Chest x-ray examination		●	●	●	●	●
Serum alkaline phosphatase	●		●		●	●
Serum LDH	●		●		●	●
Serum bilirubin	●		●		●	●
Serum AST	●		●		●	●
Urinalysis	●		●		●	●
Gallium scan			○			
Abdominal x-ray examination or CT scan		□	●		□	□

Adapted from Fischer DS, Ungavro PC, Wilhelm MC. Cancer follow-up: how much is enough? *Patient Care*. 1992;26:201–224.

AST indicates serum aspartate aminotransferase; CBC, complete blood cell count; CNS, central nervous system; CT, computed tomography; GI, gastrointestinal; LDH, lactate dehydrogenase.

*With regard to frequency of follow-up visits, this table shows the minimum recommendation. Some of the consultants recommend shortening intervals between follow-up visits or tests.

Key:

● Recommended by all consultants

○ Not recommended by all consultants

□ At 6 months in first year, if patient had diffuse large-cell lymphoma

chapter 10

Blood

William C. Crow, Jr, MD

IN THIS CHAPTER

- Differentiating platelet, coagulation, and vascular disorders
- Differential diagnosis of bleeding by mechanism
- Presumptive diagnosis of common bleeding disorders based on routine screening tests
- Primary hypercoagulable states (inherited)
- Secondary hypercoagulable states (acquired)
- Characteristics of coagulation factors
- Laboratory diagnosis of anemia
- Differential diagnosis of the hypochromic-microcytic states
- Characteristics of the thalassemias
- Normal microhematocrit values
- Normal leukocyte count in peripheral blood
- Normal leukocyte differential count in peripheral blood
- Serum immunoelectrophoretic patterns

BOOKSHELF RECOMMENDATIONS

- Lee G, Foerster J, Lukens J, Paraskevas F, Rodgers G. *Wintrobe's Clinical Hematology*. 10th ed. Philadelphia: Lippincott Williams & Wilkins; 1999.
- Lewis SM, Bain BJ, Bates I, eds. *Dacie and Lewis Practical Haematology*. 9th ed. New York: Churchill Livingstone; 2001.
- Hillman RS, Ault KA. *Hematology in Clinical Practice: A Guide to Diagnosis and Management*. New York: McGraw-Hill; 2002.

TABLE 10.1

Differentiating Platelet, Coagulation, and Vascular Disorders

Clinical Features	Platelet	Coagulation	Vascular
Onset	Immediate	Delayed	Immediate
Duration	Short	Prolonged	Variable
Precipitant	Trauma	Often spontaneous	Variable
Site	Skin, mucous membranes, GI tract	Joints, muscle, viscera	Skin, GI tract
Family history	Absent	Usually present	Usually absent
Drug-related	Often	Rarely	Sometimes
Sex predominance	Often female	Usually male	Usually female
Response to focal pressure	Usually effective	Ineffective	Effective
Platelet count	Normal, low, or excessive	Normal	Normal
Prothrombin time	Normal	Abnormal in cases of factor II, VII, IX, and X deficiency	Normal
Partial thromboplastin time	Normal	Abnormal with factor VIII or IX deficiency	Normal

GI indicates gastrointestinal.

TABLE 10.2

Differential Diagnosis of Bleeding by Mechanism

Qualitative Platelet Disorders	
Defective adhesion	Von Willebrand disease: high doses of semisynthetic penicillins and cephalosporins
Defective aggregation	Glazmann thrombasthenia; high doses of semisynthetic penicillins and cephalosporins
Defective activation	NSAIDs; dipyridamole; cardiopulmonary bypass
Defective acceleration	Factor V deficiency
Quantitative Platelet Disorders	
Thrombocytosis	Myeloproliferative disease
Thrombocytopenia	
Decreased production	Thiazides, alcohol, viral infection, marrow failure, megaloblastic anemia, myelophthisic process
Increased destruction	Quinidine, methyldopa, sulfonamides, phenytoin, barbiturates, lupus, infection, idiopathic thrombocytopenic purpura, chronic lymphocytic leukemia
Increased sequestration	Hypersplenism
Intrinsic Pathway Defects	
Factor VIII deficiency	Hemophilia A
Factor IX deficiency	Hemophilia B
Factor XI deficiency	Ashkenazi Jews
Extrinsic Pathway Defects	
Vitamin K-dependent factor deficiency	Poor diet, cholestasis, hepatocellular failure, coumarin, broad spectrum antibiotics
Vascular Defects	
Connective tissue fragility	Age, Cushing syndrome, scurvy, purpura simplex
Hereditary defect	Marfan syndrome, Rendu-Weber-Osler disease
Drug-induced	Procaine penicillin, sulfonamides, thiazides,quinine, iodides, coumarin

Continued

TABLE 10.2

Differential Diagnosis of Bleeding by Mechanism, cont'd

Paraproteinemia	Myeloma, macroglobulinemia, cyroglobulinemia
Connective tissue disease	Lupus, rheumatoid arthritis, Sjogren's syndrome
Multiple Defects	
Uremia	
Chronic hepatocellular failure	
Disseminated intravascular coagulation	
HIV infection	

HIV indicates human immunodefiency virus; NSAIDs, nonsteroidal anti-inflammatory drugs.

TABLE 10.3

Presumptive Diagnosis of Common Bleeding Disorders Based on Routine Screening Tests

Presumptive Problem	Platelet Count	Bleeding Time	Prothrombin Time (PT)	Partial Thromboplastin Time (PTT)	Thrombin Time (TT)	Miscellaneous
Thrombocytopenia	↓	N, ↑	N	N	N	
Platelet function defect or vascular cefect	N	↑	N	N	N	
Von Willebrand disease	N	↑	N	↑	N	↓ VIII_{cr}, ↓ VIII_{ag}, ↓ VIII_{VWF}
Extrinsic pathway defect (VII)	N	N	↑	N	N	
Intrinsic pathway defect (VIII, IX, XI, XII, prekallikrein, high-molecular-weight kininogen, inhibitor)	N	N	N	↑	N	
Common pathway or multiple pathway defects, excluding fibrinogen	N	N	↑	↑	N	

Continued

TABLE 10.3

Presumptive Diagnosis of Common Bleeding Disorders Based on Routine Screening Tests, cont'd

Presumptive Problem	Platelet Count	Bleeding Time	Prothrombin Time (PT)	Partial Thromboplastin Time (PTT)	Thrombin Time (TT)	Miscellaneous
Fibrinogen deficiency or dysfunction, vitamin K deficiency, liver disease, primary fibrinolysis	N	N	↑	↑	↑	High levels of fibrin (ogen) degradation products (FDP)
Disseminated intravascular coagulation	↓	N, ↑	↑	↑	↑	High levels of FDP
Factor XIII deficiency	N	N	N	N	N	Positive clot solubility

Adapted from Blacklow RS, ed. *MacBryde's Signs and Symptoms: Applied Pathologic Physiology and Clinical Interpretation*. 6th ed. Philadelphia: Lippincott Williams & Wilkins; 1983:551.

N indicates normal; , ↓ decreased; , ↑ increased.

TABLE 10.4

Primary Hypercoagulable States (Inherited)

Condition	Genetics	Incidence	Clinical Features	Diagnosis	Treatment
Antithrombin III deficiency	Autosomal dominant	Asymptomatic heterozygous 1:350, symptomatic 1:2000 to 1:5000	In 2.5% of patients with recurrent thrombosis and/or <45 years old. Thrombosis complicates pregnancy or puerperium in 30%–45% of Patients	Test after *off* anticoagulation for at least 2 weeks	Unfractionated or low-molecular-weight heparin → Coumadin. INR 2.0–3.0 for at least 3 months. Two or more events; life-long anticoagulation. After one event if thrombosis is unusual or life-long threatening site
Protein C deficiency	Autosomal dominant	1:200 to 1:500	In 3%–4% of patients with venous thromboembolism. Homozygotes may have neonatal purpura fulminans. Heterozygotes may have warfarin-induced skin necrosis. Complicates pregnancy in 10%–20%	As above	As above
Protein S deficiency		2%–3% of patients with venous thromboembolism	Complicates pregnancy in 10%–20%	As above	As above

Continued

TABLE 10.4

Primary Hypercoagulable States (Inherited), cont'd

Condition	Genetics	Incidence	Clinical Features	Diagnosis	Treatment
Activated protein C Resistance (factor V Leiden)	Heterozygosity ↑ risk 5–10 X Homozygosity ↑ risk of thrombosis 50–100 X	3%–7% of whites. 10%–64% of patients with venous thromboembolism	Complicates pregnancy in 30%	As above	Heparin in pregnancy. Avoid coumadin in pregnant patient
Prothrombin gene mutation		6%–18% of patients with venous thromboembolism			
Hyperhomocyst-einemia	Heterozygous most common	0.3%–1.4%	Risk factor for both arterial and venous thrombosis. Risk of stroke, MI, peripheral arterial disease	Measure total plasma homocysteine after an overnight fast	Unclear whether anti-coagulation helpful. Supplementing with 1 mg folate, 100 mg pyridoxine, and 0.4 mg cobalamin may help prevent thrombosis

INR indicates international normalized ratio; MI, myocardial infraction.

TABLE 10.5

Secondary Hypercoagulable States (Acquired)

Condition	Mechanism	Clinical Features	Diagnosis	Treatment
Malignancy—most commonly pancreatic, adenocarcinoma of GI tract or lung, ovary	Malignant tissues elaborate procoagulant substances that initiate chronic DIC	DVT, pulmonary embolism. Trousseau syndrome (migrating superficial thrombophlebitis of upper and lower extremities), nonbacterial thrombotic endocarditis		May be difficult to anticoagulate. Sometimes requires continuous heparin infusion, vena cava filter
Myeloproliferative disorders and paroxysmal, nocturnal, hemoglobinuria	Polycythemia vera (↑ blood viscosity). Essential thrombocythemia, CML, myelofibrosis and myeloid metaplasia, paroxysmal nocturnal hemoglobinuria	DVT, pulmonary embolism, hepatic vein thrombosis (Budd-Chiari syndrome) associated with myeloproliferative disorders and paroxysmal nocturnal hemoglobinuria		Usual anticoagulation for myeloproliferative disorders and paroxysmal nocturnal hemoglobinuria. In polycythemia, ↓ Hct to normal range. In essential thrombocythemia, ↓ platelet count with chemotherapy
Antiphospholipid antibody syndrome	Damage to vessel wall	2/3 venous events 1/3 arterial events CVAs, nonbacterial endocarditis, spontaneous abortions	Any combination of anticardiolipin antibodies, lupus anticoagulant, biologic false-+ VDRL	Presence of lupus anticoagulant prolongs activated PTT at baseline and makes monitoring difficult. Low-molecular weight-heparin

Continued

TABLE 10.5

Secondary Hypercoagulable States (Acquired), cont'd

Condition	Mechanism	Clinical Features	Diagnosis	Treatment
				preferred. Then long-term Coumadin to maintain INR at 3.0
Pregnancy and oral contraceptives	↑ Thrombin generation, platelet activation	Special vulnerability to thrombosis in the puerperium. DVT and pulmonary embolism most common complications	Usual studies for DVT and PE	Unfractionated or low-molecular-weight heparin. Avoid Coumadin in pregnancy
Postoperative state and trauma	↓ venous blood flow in the lower extremities. Activation of coagulation system by release of tissue factor from injured tissue	General surgery: 20%–25% DVT. 2% of these have PE. Hip surgery and knee reconstruction = DVTs in 45%–70% without prophylaxis, PE in as many as 20% of patients after hip surgery. DVT in over 50% of major trauma patients (may be asymptomatic)	Usual studies	As above

CML indicates chronic myelogenous leukemia; CVAs, cerebrovascular accidents; DIC, disseminated intravascular coagulation; DVT, deep vein thrombosis; GI, gastrointestinal; INR, international normalized ratio; Hct; hematocrit; PTT, partial thromboplastin time.

TABLE 10.6

Characteristics of Coagulation Factors

Factor	Descriptive Name	Source	Approximate Half-life (h)	Function
I	Fibrinogen	Liver	120	Substrate for fibrin clot (CP)
II	Prothrombin	Liver; VKD	60	Serine protease (CP)
V	Proaccelerin, labile factor	Liver	12–36	Cofactor (CP)
VII	Serum prothrombin conversion accelerator, proconvertin	Liver; VKD	6	? Serine protease (EP)
VIII	Antihemophilic factor or globin	Endothelial cells and ? elsewhere	12	Cofactor (IP)
IX	Plasma thromboplastin component; Christmas factor	Liver; VKD	24	Serine protease (IP)
X	Stuart-Prower factor	Liver; VKD	36	Serine protease (CP)
XI	Plasma thromboplastin antecedent	? Liver	40–84	Serine protease (IP)
XII	Hageman factor	? Liver	50	Serine protease, contact activation (IP)
XIII	Fibrin stabilizing factor	? Liver	96–180	Transglutaminase (CP)
Prekallikrein	Fletcher factor	? Liver	?	Serine protease, contact activation (IP)
High-molecular-weight kininogen	Fitzgerald factor; Flaujeac or Williams factor	? Liver	?	Cofactor, contact activation (IP)

Adapted from Blacklow RS, ed. *MacBryde's Signs and Symptoms: Applied Pathologic Physiology and Clinical Interpretation.* 6th ed. Philadelphia: Lippincott, Williams & Wilkins; 1983:539.

VKD indicates Vitamin K-dependent; CP, common pathway; EP, extrinsic pathway; IP, intrinsic pathway.

FIGURE 10.1

Laboratory Diagnosis of Anemia

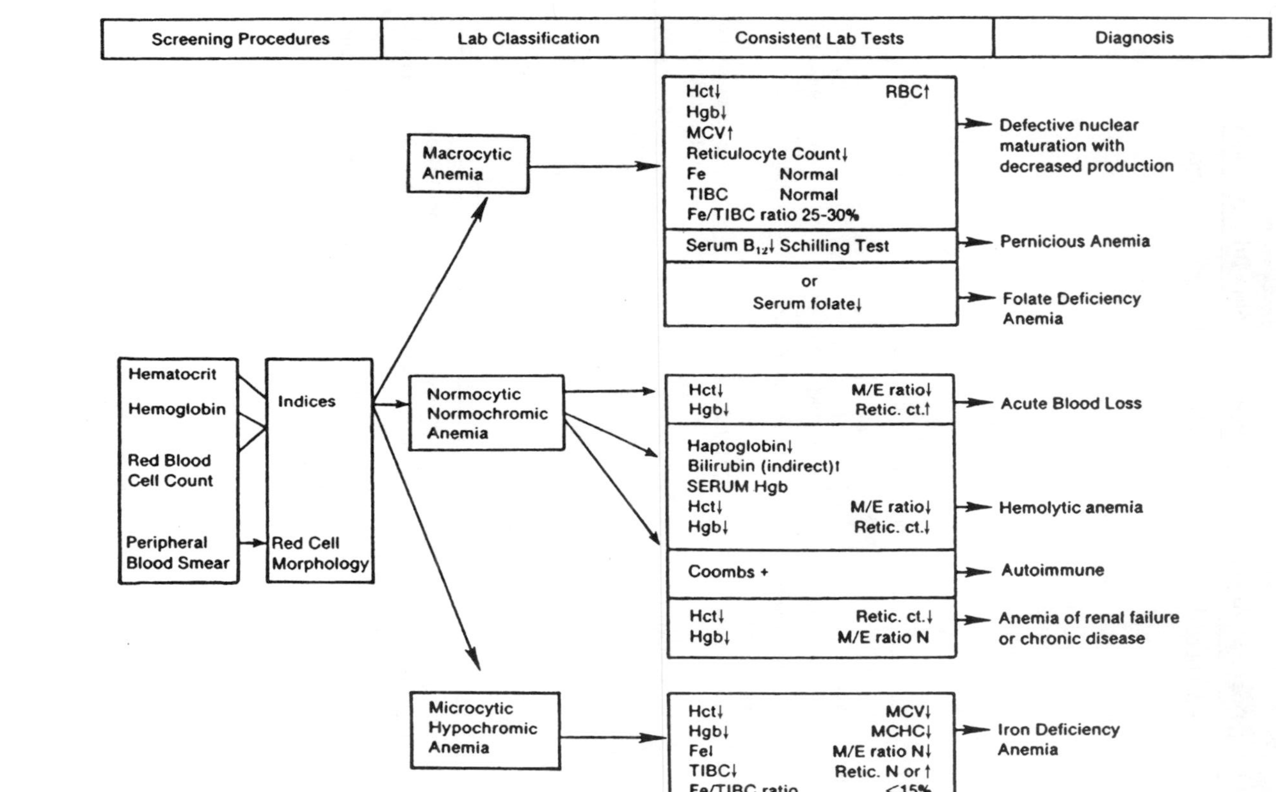

Reproduced with permission from Bolinger AM, Korman NR. Anemia. In: Young LY, Koda-Kimble MA, eds. *Applied Therapeutics: The Clinical Use of Drugs*. 4th ed. Vancouver, Wash: Applied Therapeutics; 1988:1053.

TABLE 10.7

Differential Diagnosis of the Hypochromic-Microcytic States

Blood Parameter	Deficiency	Transferrin Defect	Defect in Iron Utilization	Defect in Iron Reutilization
Peripheral blood				
Microcytosis (*M*) vs hypochromia (*H*)	M > H	M > H	M > H	M < H
Polychromatophilic targeted cells	Absent	Absent	Present	Absent
Stippled red cells	Absent	Absent	Present	Absent
RDW	Increased	Increased	Increased	Normal
Serum Iron				
Iron-binding capacity	↑ : ↓	↓ : ↓	↑ : Normal	↓ : ↓
Percent saturation of transferrin	<10%	0	>50%	>10%
Serum Ferritin (normal 30–300 ng/mL)	<12	(No data available)	>400	30–400
Bone Marrow				
Erythrocyte-granulocyte ratio (normal 1:3 to 1:5)	1:1–1:2	1:1–1:2	1:1–5:1	1:1–1:2
Marrow iron	Absent	Present	Increased	Present
Ringed sideroblasts	Absent	Absent	Present	Absent

Adapted from Berkow R, Fletcher AJ, eds. Hematology and oncology. In: *The Merck Manual of Diagnosis and Therapy.* 16th ed. Rahway, NJ: Merck & Co; 1992:1149, and Frenkel EP. *Houston Med.* 1976;6(11).

RDW indicates red blood cell volume distribution width, expressing the degree of anisocytosis (ie, variation in cell size).

TABLE 10.8

Characteristics of the Thalassemias

Category	Anemia	MCV	Percent H_8A_2	Percent H_8F
β Thalassemia				
Heterozygous	Mild	↓	↑	Variable
Homozygous	Severe	↓	Variable	↑ up to 90%
βδ Thalassemia				
Heterozygous	Mild	↓	N or ↓	>5%
Homozygous	Moderate-severe	↓	Absent	100%
α Thalassemia				
Single gene defect	None	N-↓	N	N
Double gene defect	Mild	↓	N-↓	<5%
Triple gene defect	Modere	↓	N-↓ (Hb H or Bart's Hb present)	Variable

Adapted from Berkow R, Fletcher AJ, eds. Hematology and oncology. In: *The Merck Manual*. 15th ed. Rahway, NJ: Merck & Co; 1987:1123.

TABLE 10.9

Normal Microhematocrit Values

Age	Average Normal	Minimal Normal
Children of Both Sexes		
At birth	56.6	51.0
First day	56.1	50.5
End of first week	52.7	47.5
End of second week	49.6	44.7
End of third week	46.6	42.0
End of fourth week	44.6	40.0
End of second month	38.9	35.1
End of fourth month	36.5	32.9
End of sixth month	36.2	32.6
End of eighth month	35.8	32.3
End of tenth month	35.5	32.0
End of first year	35.2	31.7
End of second year	35.5	32.0
End of fourth year	37.1	33.4
End of sixth year	37.9	34.2
End of eighth year	38.9	35.1
End of twelfth year	39.6	35.7
Men		
End of fourteenth year	44	39.6
End of eighteenth year	47	42.3
18–50 years	47	42.3
50–60 years	45	40.5
60–70 years	43	38.7
70–80 years	40	36.0
Nonpregnant Women		
14–50 years	42	36
50–80 years	40	36
Pregnant Women		
End of fourth month	42	30
End of fifth month	40	30
End of sixth month	37	30
End of seventh month	37	30
End of eighth month	39	30
End of ninth month	40	30

Table courtesy M. Strumia, MD.

TABLE 10.10

Normal Leukocyte Count in Peripheral Blood

Age	Leukocyte Count (Cells/mm^3)	
	Average	**95% Range***
Birth	18,100	9000–30,000
12 hours	22,800	13,000–38,000
24 hours	18,900	9400–34,000
1 week	12,200	5000–21,000
2 weeks	11,400	5000–20,000
4 weeks	10,800	5000–19,500
2 months	11,000	5500–18,000
4 months	11,500	6000–17,500
6 months	11,900	6000–17,500
8 months	12,200	6000–17,500
10 months	12,000	6000–17,500
12 months	11,400	6000–17,500
2 years	10,600	6000–17,000
4 years	9100	5500–15,500
6 years	8500	5000–14,500
8 years	8300	4500–13,500
10 years	8100	4500–13,500
12 years	8000	4500–13,500
14 years	7900	4500–13,000
16 years	7800	4500–13,000
18 years	7700	4500–12,500
20 years	7500	4500–11,500
21 years	7400	4500–11,000

Adapted from Albritton EC. *Standard Values in Blood.* Philadelphia: WB Saunders; 1952:50–51.

*Average value ± 2 SDs.

TABLE 10.11

Normal Leukocyte Differential Count in Peripheral Blood*

Age	Segmented Neutrophils		Band Neutrophils		Eosinophils		Basophils		Lymphocytes		Monocytes	
	%	No/mm^3	%	No/mm^3	%	No/mm^3	%	No/mm^3	%	No/mm^3	%	No/mm^3
At birth	52	9400	9.1	1650	2.2	400	0.6	100	31 ± 5	5500	5.8	1050
12 hours	58	13,200	10.2	2330	2.0	450	0.4	100	24	5500	5.3	1200
24 hours	52	9800	9.2	1750	2.4	450	0.5	100	31	5800	5.8	1100
1 week	39	4700	6.8	830	4.1	500	0.4	50	41	5000	9.1	1100
2 weeks	34	3900	5.5	630	3.1	350	0.4	50	48	5500	8.8	1000
4 weeks	30	3300	4.5	490	2.8	300	0.5	50	56 ± 15	6000	6.5	700
2 months	30	3300	4.4	490	2.7	300	0.5	50	57	6300	5.9	650
4 months	29	3300	3.9	450	2.6	300	0.4	50	59	6800	5.2	600
6 months	28	3300	3.8	450	2.5	300	0.4	50	61	7300	4.8	580
8 months	27	3300	3.3	410	2.5	300	0.4	50	62	7600	4.7	580
10 months	27	3200	3.3	400	2.5	300	0.4	50	63	7500	4.6	550
12 months	28	3200	3.1	350	2.6	300	0.4	50	61	7000	4.8	550
2 years	30	3200	3.0	320	2.6	280	0.5	50	59	6300	5.0	530
4 years	39	3500	3.0	270	2.8	250	0.6	50	50 ± 15	4500	5.0	450
6 years	48	4000	3.0	250	2.7	230	0.6	50	42	3500	4.7	400
8 years	50	4100	3.0	250	2.4	200	0.6	50	39	3300	4.2	350
10 years	51	4200	3.0	240	2.4	200	0.5	40	38 ± 10	3100	4.3	350
12 years	52	4200	3.0	240	2.5	200	0.5	40	38	3000	4.4	350
14 years	53	4200	3.0	240	2.5	200	0.5	40	37	2900	4.7	380

Continued

TABLE 10.11

Normal Leukocyte Differential Count in Peripheral Blood, cont'd

	Segmented Neutrophils		Band Neutrophils		Eosinophils		Basophils		Lymphocytes		Monocytes	
Age	**%**	**No/mm³**	**%**	**No/mm³**	**%**	**No/mm³**	**%**	**No/mm³**	**%**	**No/mm³**	**%**	**No/mm³**
16 years	54	4200	3.0	230	2.6	200	0.5	40	35 ± 10	2800	5.1	400
18 years	54	4200	3.0	230	2.6	200	0.5	40	35	2700	5.2	400
20 years	56	4200	3.0	230	2.7	200	0.5	40	33	2500	5.0	380
21 years	56	4200	3.0	220	2.7	200	0.5	40	34 ± 10	2500	4.0	300

Adapted from Albritton EC. *Standard Values in Blood.* Philadelphia: WB Saunders; 1952:50–51.

*Average values based on the average normal leukocyte counts in Table 10.10.

FIGURE 10.2

Serum Immunoelectrophoretic Patterns

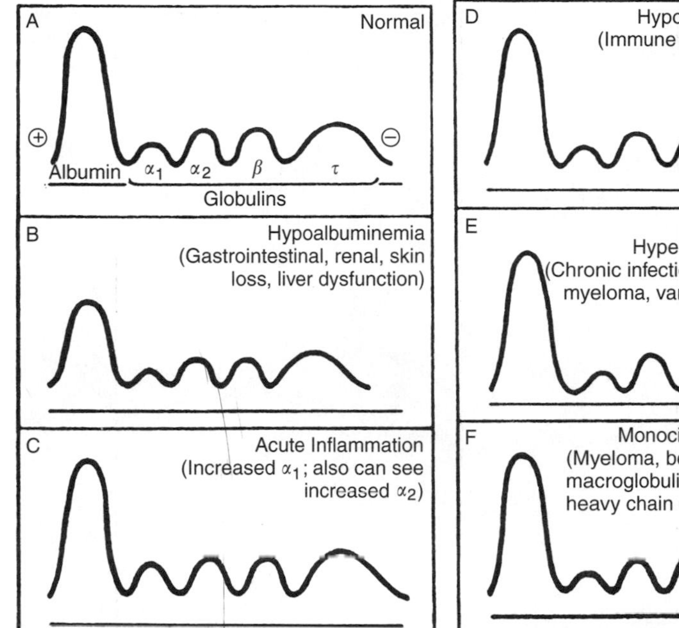

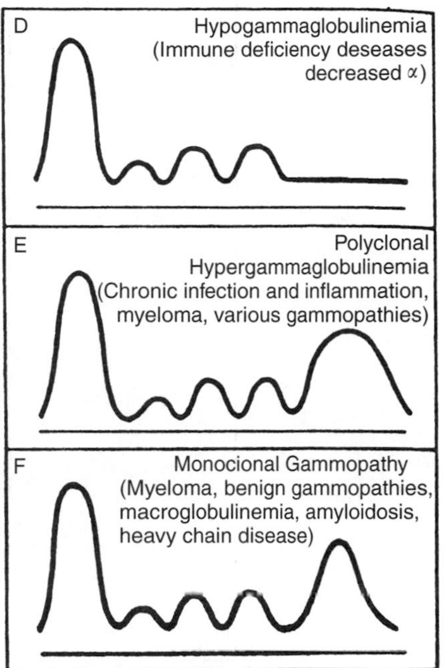

Reproduced with permission from Goodwin JS. Clinical assessment of the immune system: Which tests? When? In: Goodwin JS, ed. *Mediguide to Inflammatory Diseases*. Vol 1, No. 2. New York: Dellacorte; 1983:2.

chapter 11

Endocrine Disorders

David S. Gregory, MD

IN THIS CHAPTER

- Diabetes mellitus diagnostic tree
- Treatment preparations: insulin
- Treatment preparations: oral
- Initial insulin dosage
- Diabetic ketoacidosis decision tree
- Preoperative and postoperative management of diabetes mellitus
- Hypoglycemia therapy in diabetes
- Diabetes complication prevention, diagnosis, and therapy
- Hypoglycemia decision tree
- Thyroid function tests
- Thyroid tests affected by drugs
- Thyroid disease decision tree
- Hyperthyroidism management tree
- Hypothyroidism management tree
- Adrenal excess decision tree
- Adrenal insufficiency decision tree
- Adrenal insufficiency management
- Perioperative steroid replacement
- Hyperparathyroidism decision tree
- Hypoparathyroidism decision tree
- Galactorrhea decision tree

BOOKSHELF RECOMMENDATIONS

- Wilson JD, Foster DW, eds. *Williams Textbook of Endocrinology*. 9th ed. Philadelphia, PA: WB Saunders; 1998.
- *Washington Manual of Medical Therapeutics*. 30th ed. St Louis, MO: Washington University School of Medicine, Department of Medicine; 2001.

FIGURE 11.1

Diabetes Mellitus Diagnostic Tree

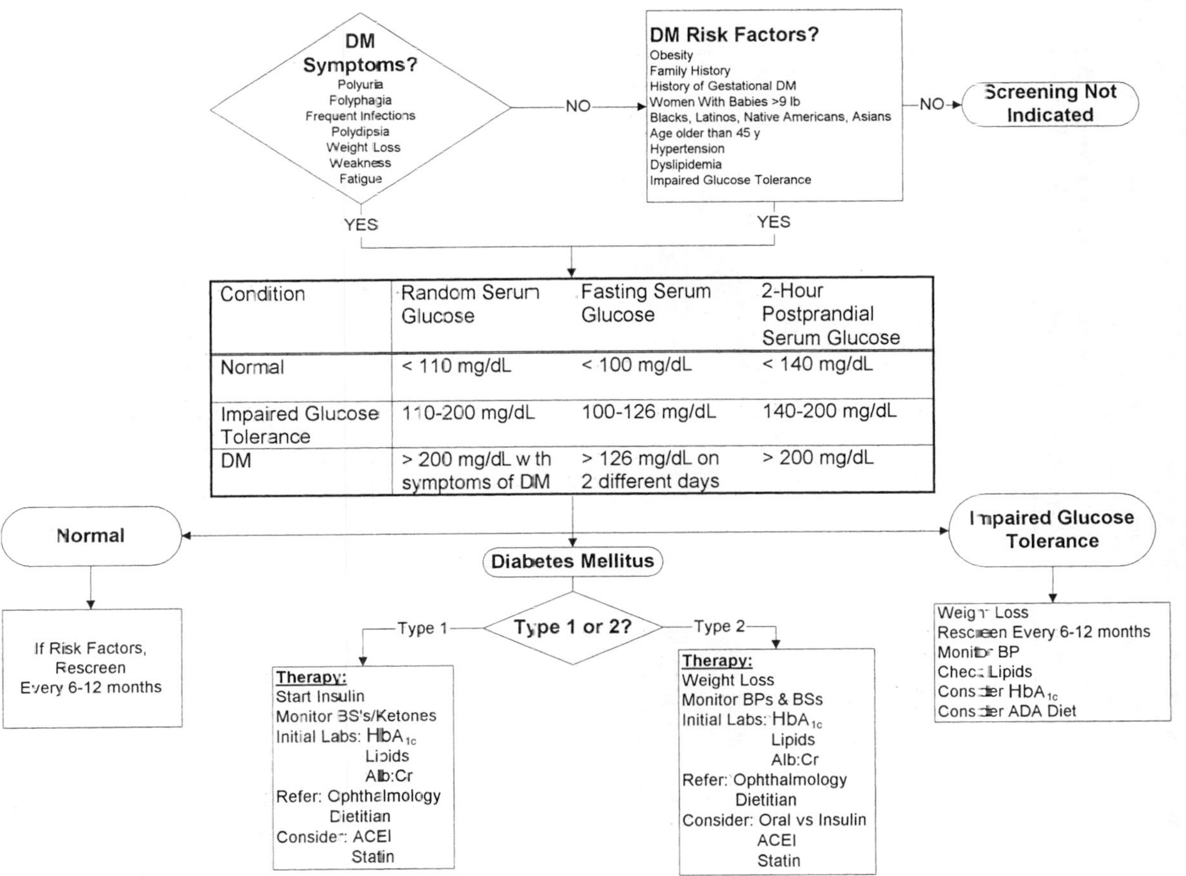

Condition	Random Serum Glucose	Fasting Serum Glucose	2-Hour Postprandial Serum Glucose
Normal	< 110 mg/dL	< 100 mg/dL	< 140 mg/dL
Impaired Glucose Tolerance	110-200 mg/dL	100-126 mg/dL	140-200 mg/dL
DM	> 200 mg/dL with symptoms of DM	> 126 mg/dL on 2 different days	> 200 mg/dL

TABLE 11.1

Treatment Preparations: Insulin

Type	Source	Onset (Hours)	Peak Effect (Hours)	Duration (Hours)
Rapid Acting				
Lispro (SC only)—Humalog	Human	<¼–½	½–1½	3–5
Regular (SC or IV)				
Humulin R	Human	½–1	2–4	4–12
Novolin	Human	½–1	2–5	8
Intermediate Acting (SC only)				
NPH (isophane)				
Humulin N	Human	1–2	6–12	18–24
Iletin NPH II	Porcine	1–2	6–12	18–24
Lente (zinc)				
Iletin Lente II	Porcine	1–3	6–14	18–24
Mixtures (SC only)				
"Premixed"				
Humulin 70/30 (70% Humulin N/ 30% Humulin R)	Human	½–1	4–6	24
Humalog 75/25 (75% Lispro protamine/ 25% Lispro)	Human	<¼–½	½–4	24
Long Acting (SC only)				
Do not mix!				
Ultralente	Human	2–4	10–16	19–48
Glargine (Lantus)	Human	1–1½	No true peak	11–24+

IV indicates intravenous; SC, subcutaneous.

TABLE 11.2

Treatment Preparations: Oral

Type	Contraindications	Use With Caution With	Dosing
Biguanide			
Metformin (Glucophage)	Hypersensitivity Metabolic acidosis Renal insufficiency (Cr > 1.5 mg/dL in males) (Cr > 1.4 mg/dL in female) CHF Radiocontrast Lactation	Surgery Acute illnesses Liver disease Cardiogenic shock Pancreatitis Hypoxia Alcohol abuse Elderly Pregnancy—class B	*Initial:* 500 mg bid or 850 mg/day *Increase by:* 500 mg per wk or 850 mg every other wk to 500–850 mg TID *Maximum Dose:* 2550 mg/day
Sulfonylureas			
Glimepiride (Amaryl)	DKA Hypersensitivity Lactation	Sulfa allergy G-6-PD deficiency Pregnancy—Class C	1–8 mg with first meal of each day
Glipizide (Glucotrol XL)	IDDM monotherapy DKA Hypersensitivity Lactation	Sulfa allergy G-6-PD deficiency Pregnancy—Class C	5–20 mg 30 minutes before first meal of each day
Glyburide (DiaBeta, Micronase)	IDDM monotherapy DKA Hypersensitivity Lactation	Sulfa allergy G-6-PD deficiency Pregnancy—Class C	2.5–10 mg with first meal of each day or 2.5–10 mg bid
Thiazolidinediones			
Pioglitazone (Actose)	IDDM monotherapy Hypersensitivity NYHA class III/IV Lactation	Impaired liver function CHF HTN Pregnancy—Class C	15–45 mg/day (30 mg/day maximum with other orals)
Rosiglitazone (Avandia)	IDDM monotherapy Hypersensitivity NYHA class III/IV Lactation	Impaired liver function CHF HTN Pregnancy—Class C	4–8 mg/day or 2–4 mg bid (4 mg/day maximum with sulfonylureas)
α-Glucosidase inhibitors			
Acarbose (Precose) Miglitol (Glyset)	DKA Hypersensitivity Inflammatory bowel disease Colonic ulceration Partial bowel obstruction Lactation Renal failure (Cr > 2.0 mg/dL)	Liver disease Renal insufficiency Pregnancy—Class B	*Initial:* 25 mg/day/tid *Increase By:* 25 mg/day every 2–3 mo *Maximum dose:* 50 mg tid (<60 kg) 100 mg tid (>60 kg)

Continued

TABLE 11.2

Treatment Preparations: Oral, cont'd

Type	Contraindications	Use With Caution With	Dosing
Combinations Glyburide/metformin (Glucovance)	See both drugs	See both drugs	*Initial therapy:* *Start:* 1.25/250 mg/day or bid *Increase by:* 1.25 mg/250 mg/day every 2 wk *Previous glyburide or metformin alone:* *Start:* 2.5 mg/500 mg or 5 mg/500 mg bid (starting dose not greater than previous monotherapy dose) Maximum Dose: 20 mg/2000 mg/day

bid indicates twice daily; CHF, congestive heart failure; IDDM, insulin-dependent diabetes mellitus; tid, three times daily.

TABLE 11.3

Initial Insulin Dosage

If Insulin Is Only Diabetes Treatment:

- Typical Daily Dose = 0.5–1.0 Units/Lean Body kg

If Insulin Is Used With Other Diabetes Treatments:

- Typical Daily Dose ≤ 0.5 Units/Lean Body kg

Conventional Regimen "Rule of Thirds"	Multidose Regimen	Insulin Pump Regimen
■ Before breakfast—2/3 daily dosage —2/3 Intermediate acting (4/9 daily dosage) —1/3 Rapid acting (2/9 daily dosage) ■ Before dinner—1/3 daily dosage —2/3 Intermediate acting (2/9 daily dosage) —1/3 Rapid acting (1/9 daily dosage)	■ 40%–50% daily dose via long or intermediate acting daily or bid ■ 50%–60% daily dose via rapid-acting insulin with each meal (each dose estimated from carbohydrate intake)	■ 50% daily dose via long acting ■ 50% daily dose via preprandial rapid-acting insulin doses via pump (each dose estimated from carbohydrate intake)

Sliding Scale

- Rapid-acting insulin alone in hospitalized patients, depending on bedside blood glucose results, will not achieve satisfactory control
- Intermediate-acting insulin, based on one of the above regimens, provides better results

Requirements Regardless of Regimen

- Blood glucose checks—initially QAC & QHS to determine if adjustments are needed
- Education regarding symptoms & treatment of hypoglycemia

FIGURE 11.2

Diabetic Ketoacidosis Decision Tree

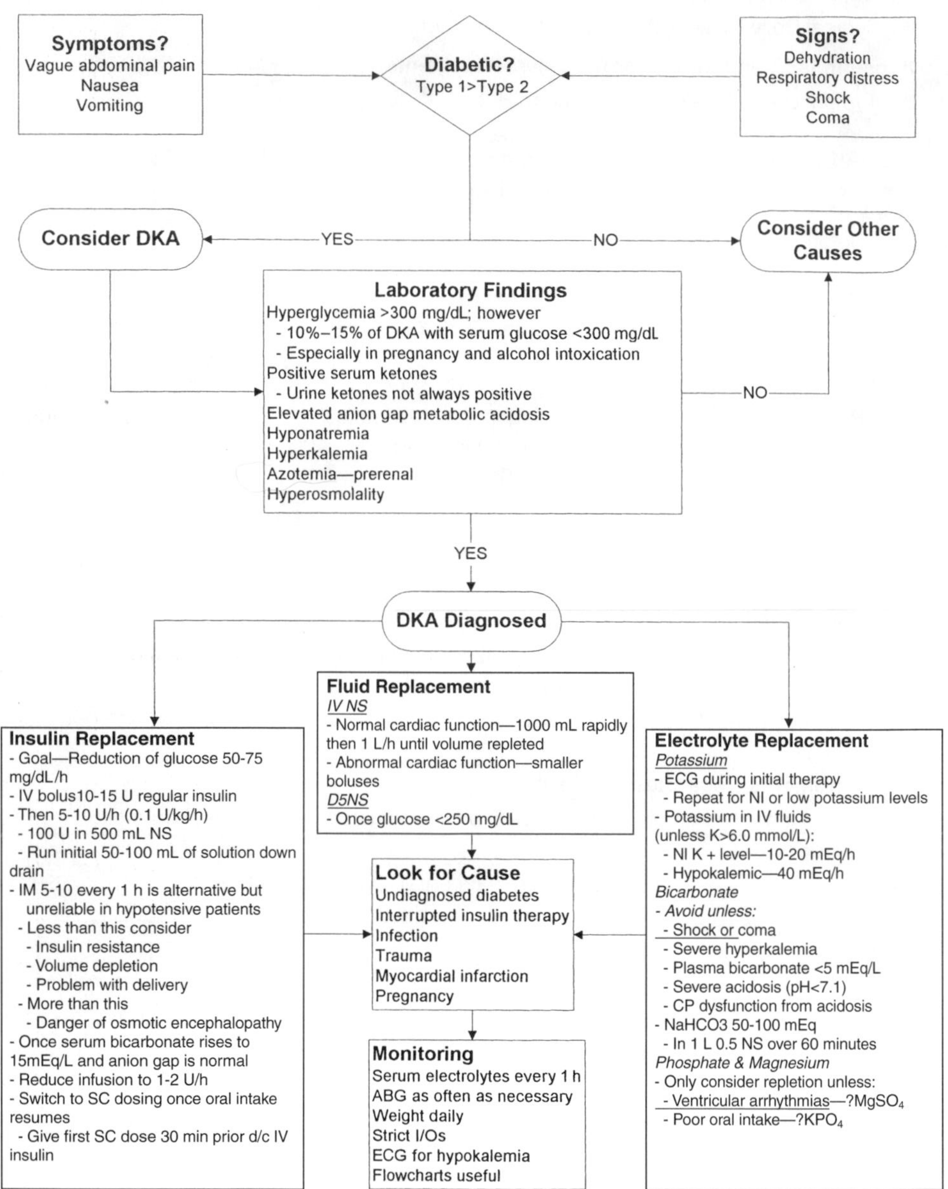

FIGURE 11.3

Pre- and Post-Operative Management of Diabetes Mellitus

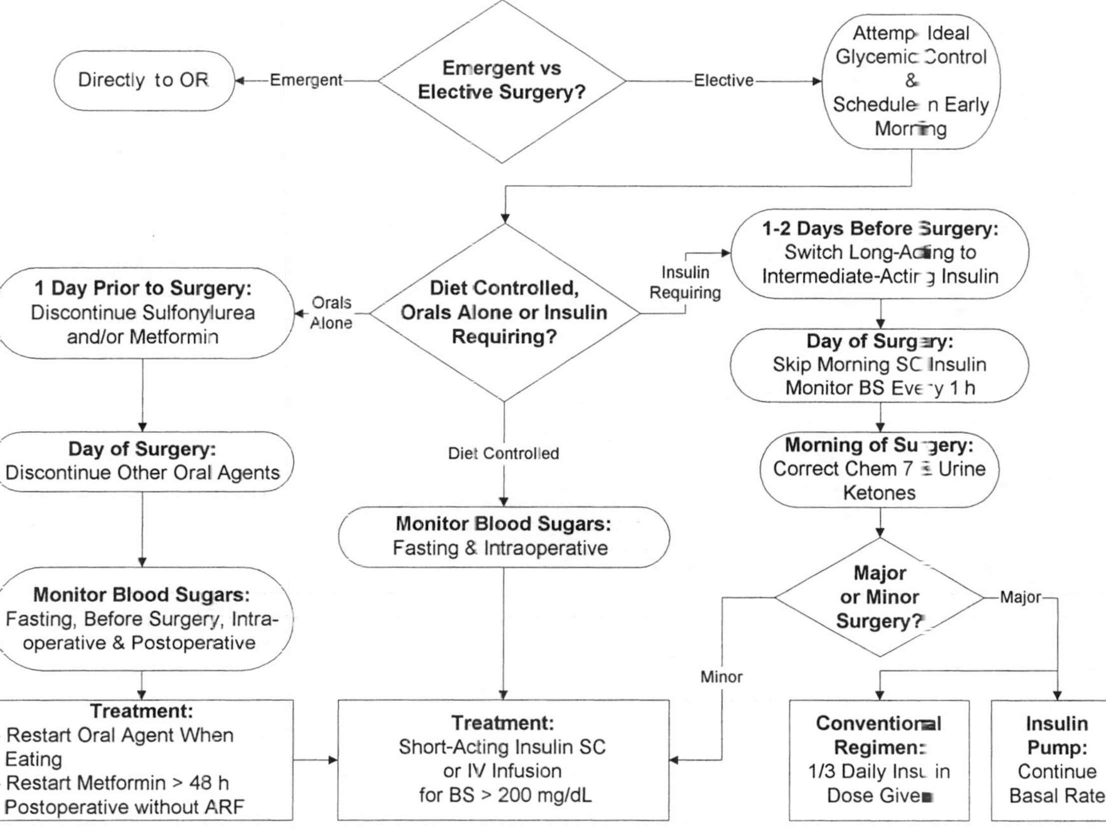

FIGURE 11.4

Hypoglycemia Therapy in Diabetes

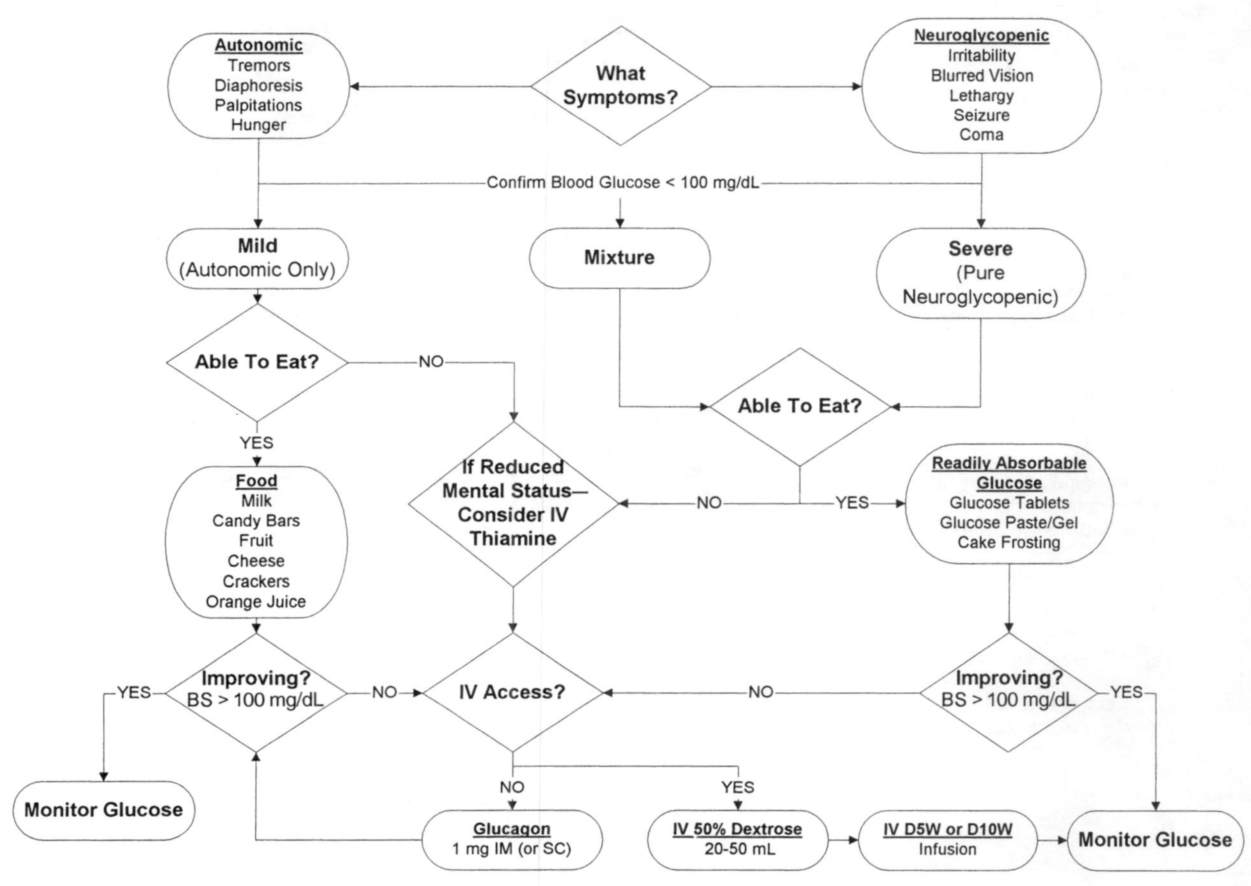

TABLE 11.4

Diabetes Complication Prevention, Diagnosis, and Therapy

Complication	Screening	Prevention	Diagnosis	Therapy
Overall	■ HbA_{1C}, every 3–6 months ■ Physician examination, every 3–6 months	■ Optimized, long-term glycemic control is the best prevention!	■ Have high suspicion!	■ Weight loss ■ Oral or insulin Tx ■ Control BP ■ Control lipids
Nephrologic				
■ Renal failure	■ 24-h urine protein quantitation or ■ Albumin:creatinine	ACE inhibitor: ■ If BP > 130/80 mm Hg ■ Or if microalbuminuria	■ 24-h creatinine clearance	■ ACE inhibitor
Sensorineural				
■ Peripheral neuropathy	■ Monitor sensation in feet, annually (vibration/microfilament)	■ Optimized glycemic control only	■ Nerve conduction velocities (NCVs)	■ TCA, Tegretol, capsaicin, Neurontin
Gastrointestinal				
■ Gastroparesis	Monitor for symptoms of: ■ Early satiety, nausea, vomiting	■ Optimized glycemic control only	■ Barium swallow/^{99m}Tc meal	■ Metaclopramide, erythromycin
■ Diabetic diarrhea	■ Nocturnal diarrhea with incontinence	■ Optimized glycemic control only	■ Clinical symptoms only	■ Clonidine
Genitourinary				
■ Erectile dysfunction	■ Monitor for symptoms	■ Optimized glycemic control only	■ Penile tumescence	■ Sildenafil, vacuum devices, implants

Continued

TABLE 11.4

Diabetes Complication Prevention, Diagnosis, and Therapy, cont'd

Complication	Screening	Prevention	Diagnosis	Therapy
Ophthalmologic				
■ Retinal hemorrhage	■ Dilated funduscopy, annually	■ Education concerning symptoms	■ Fluorescein angiography	■ Laser surgery
■ Cataracts	■ Monitor for cloudy vision	■ Education concerning symptoms	■ Slit-lamp exam	■ Phacoemulsification
Infectious				
■ Diabetic foot	■ Foot examination, biannually	■ Education regarding foot care	■ Physical exam	■ Antibiotics/amputation
■ Pneumonia	■ Quit smoking	■ Pneumococcal and flu vaccine	■ Physical/chest x-ray	■ Antibiotics
■ Teeth	■ Dental examinations, biannually	■ Regular brushing and flossing	■ Dental examination	■ Antibiotics/extraction
Vascular				
■ Stroke and PVD	■ Carotid and peripheral pulse exam, annually	■ Consider aspirin prophylaxis ■ Control lipids and BP	■ Stroke: clinical ■ PVD: ABI/ arteriography	■ Disease specific
Cardiac				
■ Myocardial infarction	■ Monitor symptoms during exertion	■ Disease specific	■ ECG/enzymes	■ Disease specific
■ Dizziness	■ Orthostatic blood pressures	■ Optimized glycemic control only	■ Valsalva ECG	■ Fludrocortisone, salt

FIGURE 11.5

Hypoglycemia Decision Tree

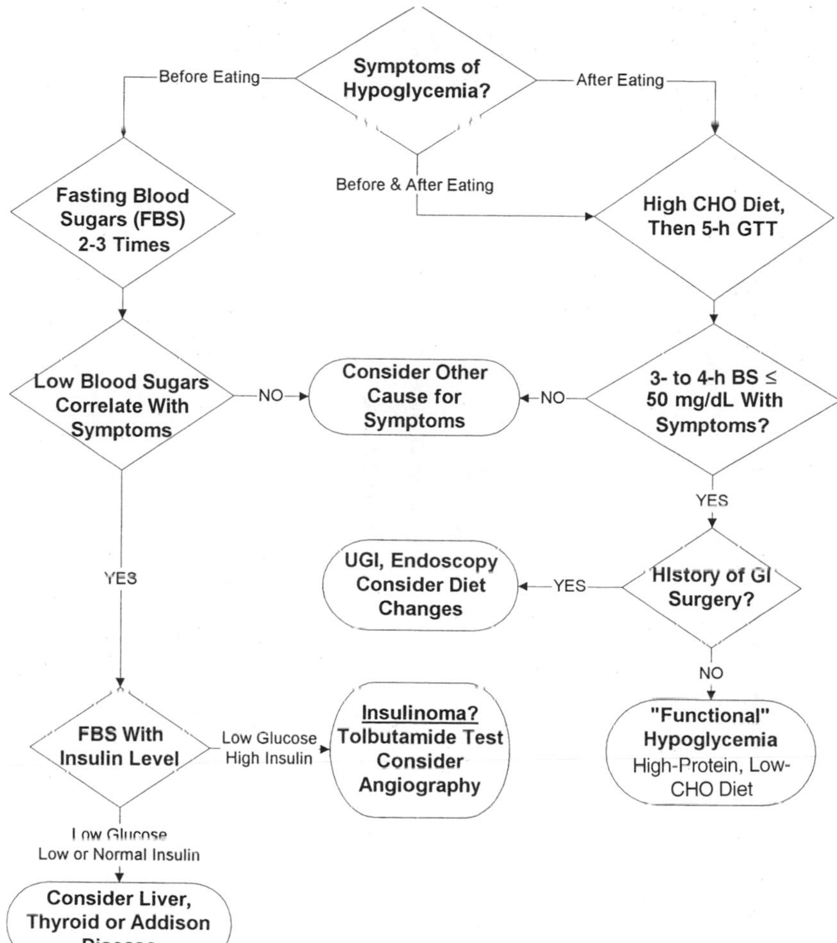

TABLE 11.5
Thyroid Function Tests

Test	Substance Measured	Normal Values	Indication	Comment
Serum T_4	Total thyroid hormone (99.97% bound)	5–12 ng/dL	Screening for thyroid disease	Affected by TBG
Free T_4	Unbound thyroid hormone	2 ng/dL	Confirmation of questionable case	Not very precise
T_3 Uptake	Relative saturation of thyroid binding proteins	25%–35%	Combined with T_4 to give thyroid index	Indirect measure of TBG
Free T_4 Index (FT_4I)	Calculated product of T_3 uptake and T_4	1–4 ng/dL	Screening for thyroid disease	
Serum T_3	Triiodothyronine concentration	115–190 ng/dL	Evaluation of hyperthyroidism	Confused with T_3 uptake
Serum TSH	Total thyroid-stimulating hormone	2–11 μU/mL	Most useful screen for primary hypothyroidism	Use high-sensitivity test
TRH	Capacity of pituitary to respond to thyrotropin-releasing hormone (TRH)	Raises TSH	Resolve borderline cases	If no rise in TSH, hyperthyroid state exists

T_3 indicates triiodothyronine; T_4, thyroxine; TRH, throtropin-releasing hormone; TSH, thyrotropin.

TABLE 11.6

Thyroid Tests Affected by Drugs

Test	Effect	Drug
Free T_4	Decreased	■ Dilantin ■ Lithium ■ Depakene ■ High-dose Salicylate ■ High-dose Glucocorticoid ■ Desipramine ■ Amiodarone
	Increased	■ Amiodarone ■ Propranolol ■ Amphetamine ■ Heroin ■ Methadone ■ PCP ■ Fluorouracil ■ Perphenazine
TSH	Increased	■ Lithium ■ Amiodarone ■ Amphetamines
	Decreased	■ Interleukin-2 ■ Alpha-interferon ■ Amiodarone

PCP indicates Phenyclidine; T_4, thyroxine; TSH, thyrotropin.

FIGURE 11.6

Thyroid Disease Decision Tree

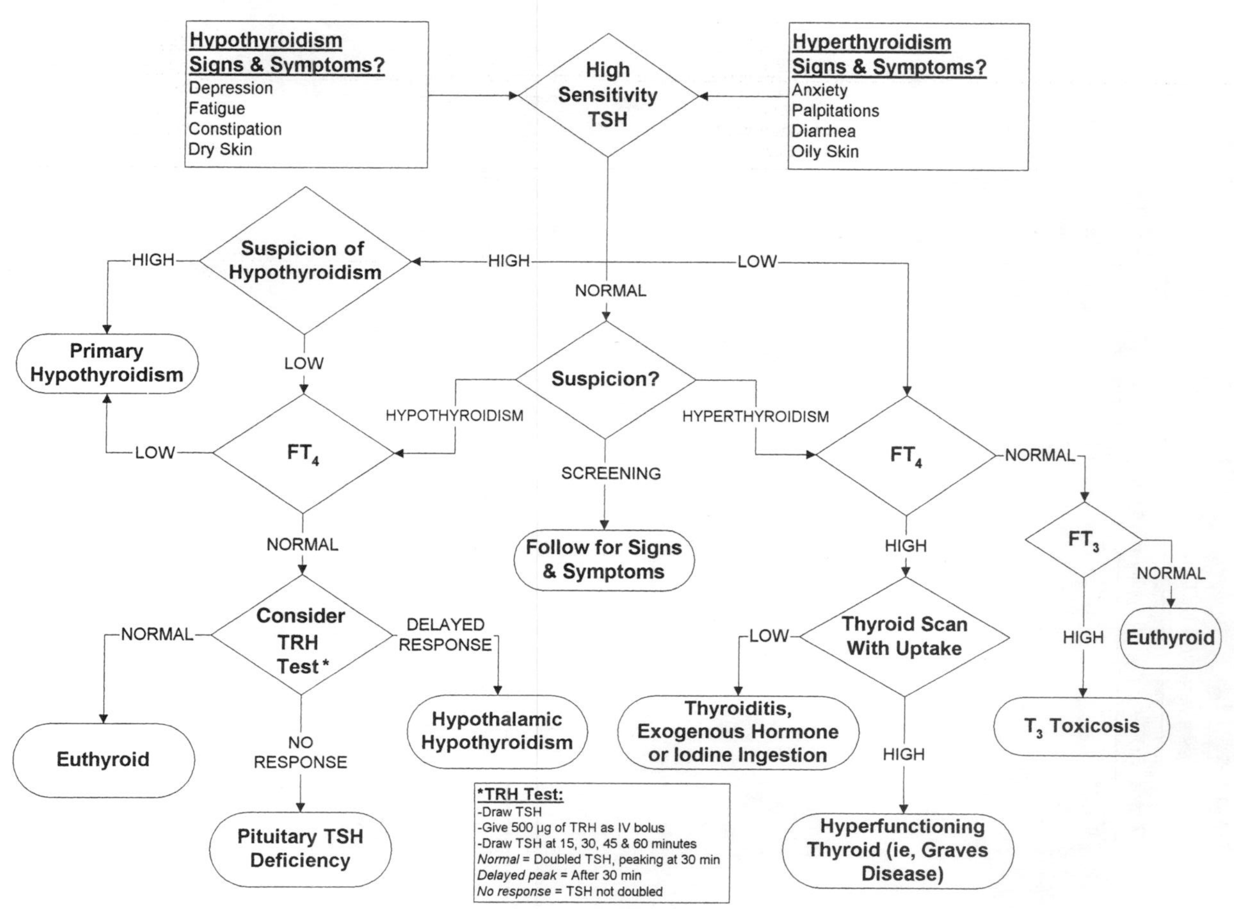

FIGURE 11.7

Hyperthyroidism Management Tree

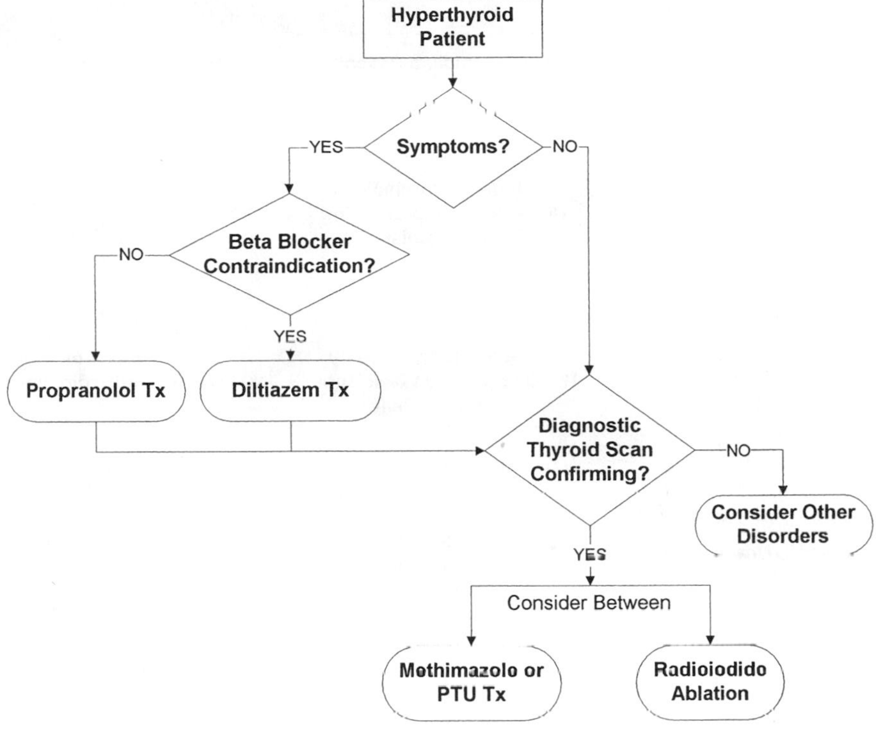

FIGURE 11.8

Hypothyroidism Management Tree

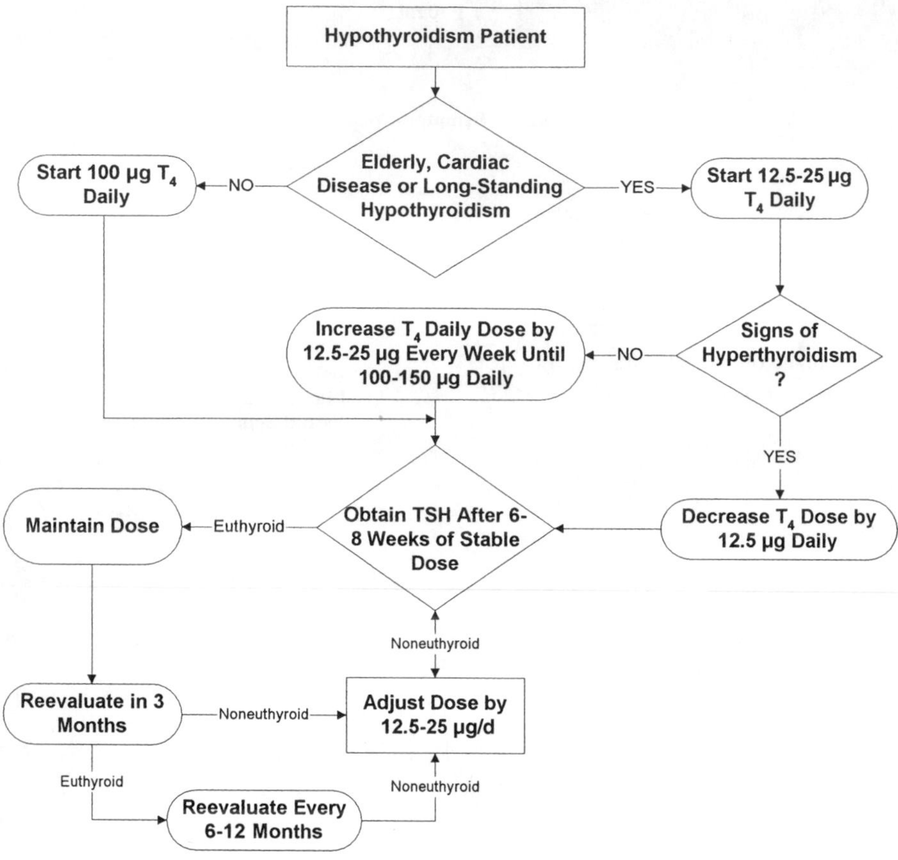

FIGURE 11.9

Adrenal Excess Decision Tree

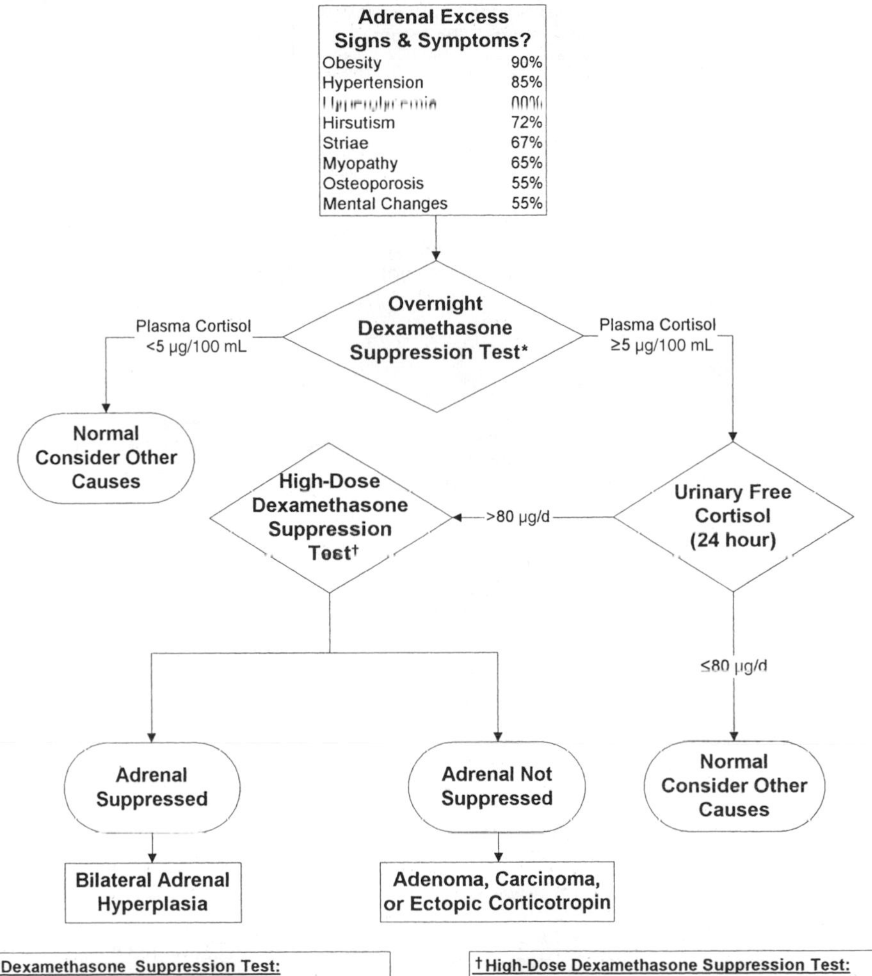

***Dexamethasone Suppression Test:**
- Give dexamethasone 1 mg and sedative at bedtime
- Ensure undisturbed sleep
- Draw fasting cortisol in AM

†High-Dose Dexamethasone Suppression Test:
- Collect Baseline 24-h urinary cortisol and creatinine
- Measure plasma cortisol at 8 AM and 8 PM
- Give dexamethasone 2 mg orally every 6 h for 2 days, while collecting 24-h urinary cortisol and creatinine
- Measure plasma cortisol at 8 AM after 48 hours of dexamethasone

FIGURE 11.10

Adrenal Insufficiency Decision Tree

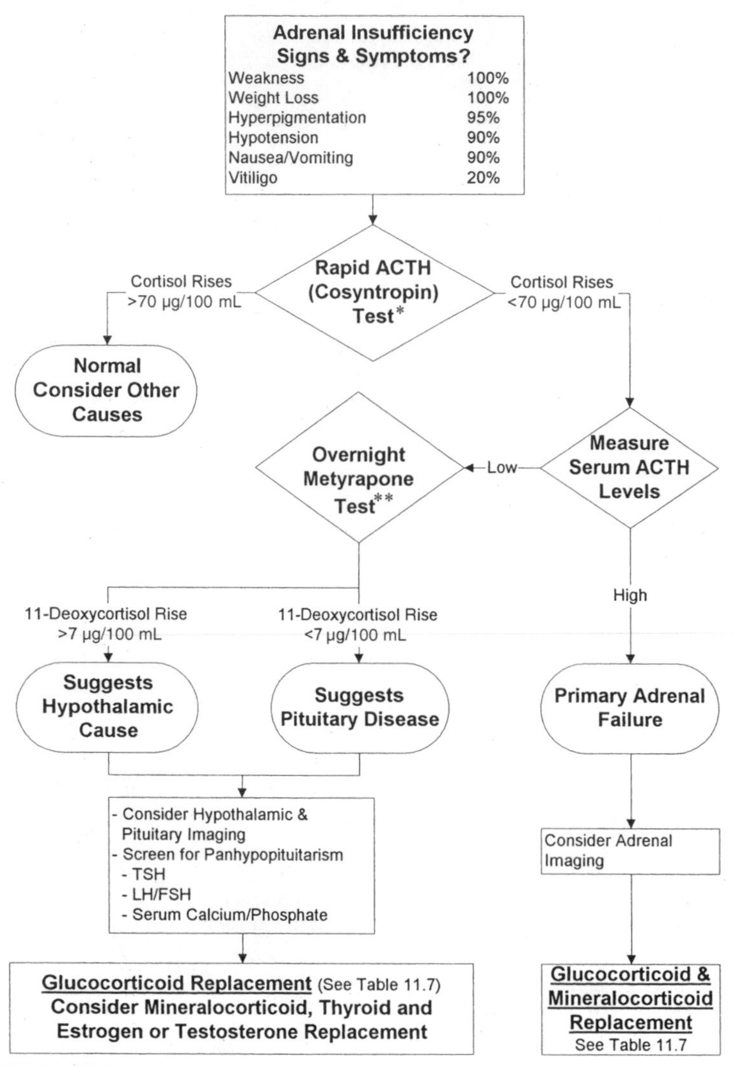

***Rapid ACTH (Cosyntropin) Test:**
- Measure baseline plasma cortisol
- Give cosyntropin 250 μg
- Obtain plasma cortisol at 30 and 60 minutes after injection

****Overnight Metyrapone Test:**
- Give metyrapone 3 g orally at bedtime with food
- Measure plasma 11-deoxycortisol at 7 AM

TABLE 11.7

Adrenal Insufficiency Management

Situation	Therapy	Monitor	Patient Education
Maintenance Therapy			
Glucocorticoid replacement	Dexamethasone 0.25–0.75 mg qhs *or* Prednisone 2.5–7.5 mg qhs *or* Hydrocortisone 15–20 mg qAM and 5–10 mg each early afternoon	Clinical symptoms and morning plasma ACTH	Life threatening MedicAlert bracelet; emergency medical information card; dexamethasone (4 mg/1 mL saline) in prefilled syringes
Mineralocorticoid replacement	Fludrocortisone 0.05–0.2 mg/d *and* Liberal salt intake	Orthostatic BP/pulses; edema; serum potassium; plasma renin activity	Contact physician if edema or dizziness occurs
Minor Febrile Illness or Stress	Increase glucocorticoid dose 2–3 times usual dose during illness; no change in fludrocortisone	Contact physician if worsens or lasts more than 3 days	Outpatient, local anesthesia procedures; need no extra dosing
Acute/Severe Stress or Trauma	Patient injects Dexamethasone 4 mg IM (if available) *or* Provider injects Hydrocortisone 50 mg IV Q8h *and* Boluses with D5NS IV until Normotensive	BP/pulse; mental status	Life threatening MedicAlert bracelet Emergency medical information card See physician immediately

TABLE 11.8

Perioperative Steroid Replacement

Day	IV Hydrocortisone	IM Hydrocortisone	Oral Hydrocortisone	Fludrocortisone
Operative Day	300 mg, plus	50 mg preoperative and 50 mg postoperative	—	—
Postoperative Day	200 mg, plus	50 mg q12 h		
1	150 mg, plus	50 mg q12 h	—	—
2	100 mg, plus	50 mg q12 h	—	—
3	—	50 mg q12 h, plus	25 mg q6 h	—
4	—	25 mg q12 h, plus	25 mg q6 h	—
5	—	25 mg, plus	25 mg q6 h	0.05–0.2 mg*
6	—	—	25 mg q6 h	0.05–0.2 mg*
7	—	—	25 mg q8 h	0.05–0.2 mg*
8–10	—	—	25 mg q12 h	0.05–0.2 mg*
11–20	—	—	20 mg @ 8 AM	0.05–0.2 mg*
>20	—	—	10 mg @ 4 PM	0.05–0.2 mg*

Adapted from Tuck M. Adrenal disease. In: Hershman JM, ed. *Management of endocrine disorders*. Philadelphia: Lea & Febiger; 1980.

*Adjust Fludrocortisone depending on blood pressure, body weight, and serum electrolytes.

FIGURE 11.11

Hyperparathyroidism Decision Tree

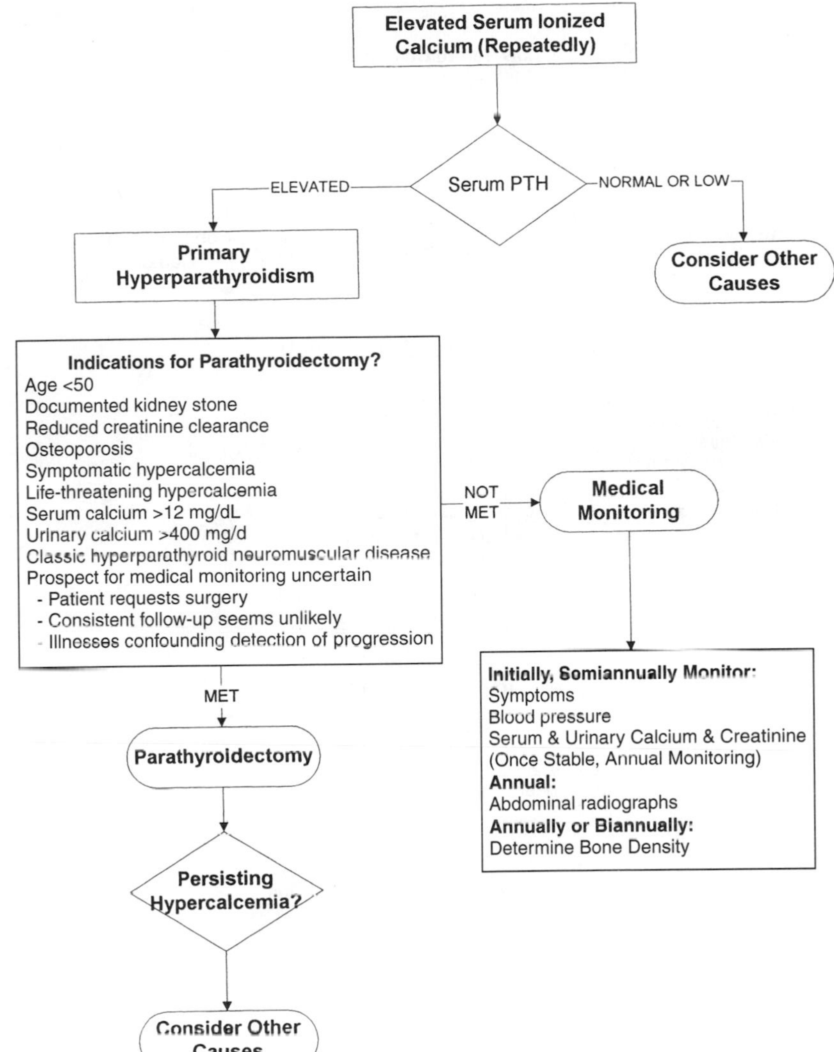

FIGURE 11.12

Hypoparathyroidism Decision Tree

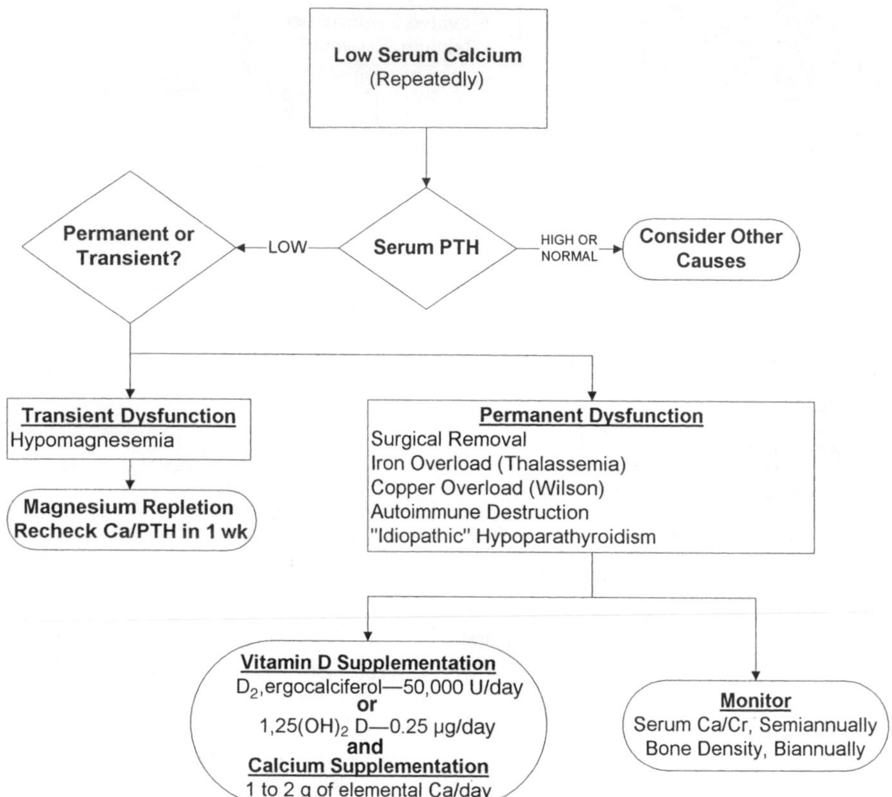

FIGURE 11.13

Galactorrhea Decision Tree

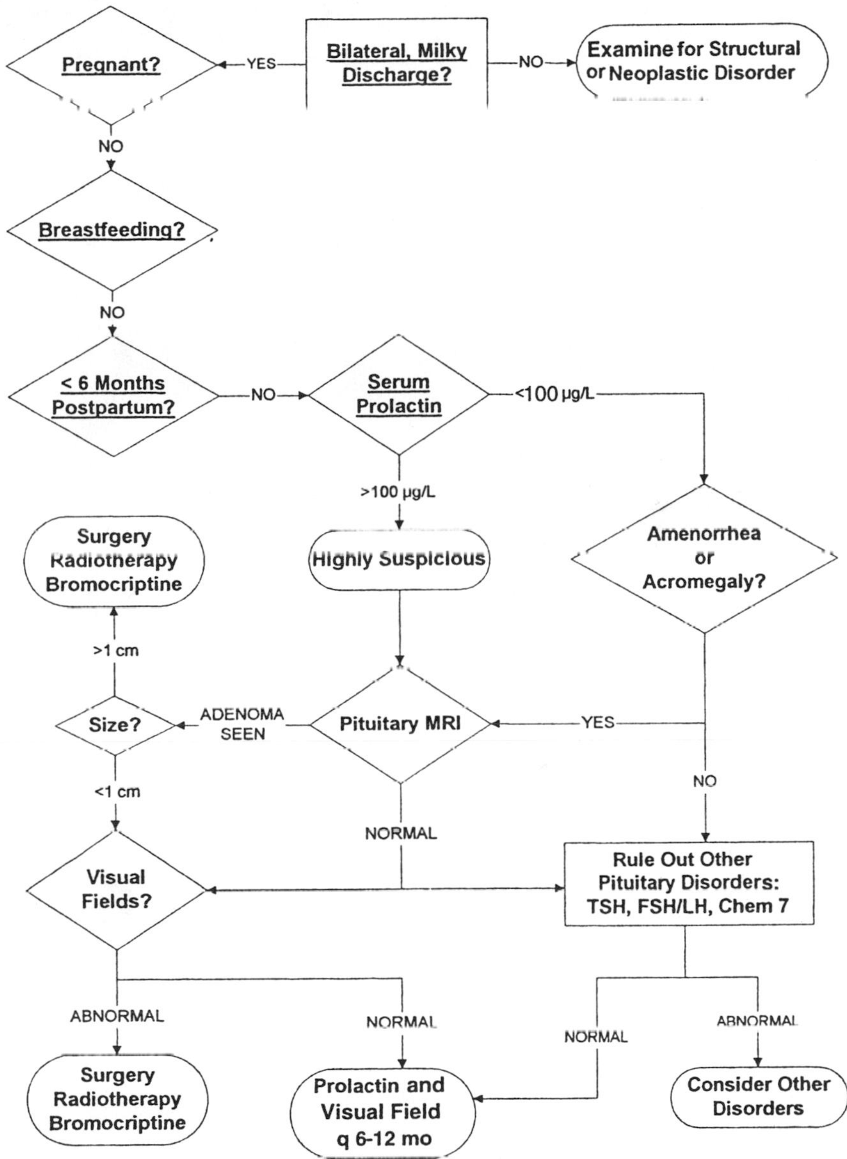

chapter 12

The Nervous System

John A. Vaughn, MD

IN THIS CHAPTER

- Neurological development
- Normal adult anatomy and physiology
- Seizure disorders
- Classification of seizure disorders
- Electroencephalogram findings according to seizure type
- Management of first seizure
- Medications for seizure treatment
- Pediatric considerations
- Primary and secondary headache syndromes
- Red flags in the evaluation of acute headaches
- Medications for headache treatment
- Intervertebral disk disease
- Vertebral disk anatomy
- Cervical and lumbar disk disease
- Location of pain, reflex, and motor abnormality according to level of nerve root involvement
- Common peripheral nerve lesions
- Neuroimaging and electromyography in the evaluation of intervertebral disk disease
- Medications for neuropathic pain
- Bell palsy
- Vertigo
- Differential diagnosis of central and peripheral vertigo
- Evaluation of cranial nerve VIII disorders
- Cerebrovascular disease

- National Stroke Association recommendations for prevention of a first stroke
- Asymptomatic carotid artery disease
- Management of symptomatic carotid artery disease
- Acute ischemic stroke
- Dementia
- Alzheimer dementia: diagnostic criteria
- Vascular dementia: diagnostic criteria
- Medications for the treatment of Alzheimer dementia
- Parkinson disease
- Drugs commonly used for the treatment of Parkinson disease
- Neurodiagnostic tools
- Preferred initial imaging study by clinical presentation
- Lumbar puncture technique
- Normal cerebrospinal fluid values
- Selected disorders and associated cerebrospinal fluid studies
- Alternative therapies for disorders of the nervous system
- Online resources

BOOKSHELF RECOMMENDATIONS

- American Psychiatric Association. *Diagnostic and Statistical Manual of Mental Disorders: DSM-IV*. 4th ed. Washington, DC: American Psychiatric Association; 1994.
- Behrman RE, ed. *Nelson Textbook of Pediatrics*. 16th ed. Philadelphia, PA: WB Saunders; 2000.
- Brant WE, Helms CA, eds. *Fundamentals of Diagnostic Radiology*. 2nd ed. Philadelphia, PA: Lippincott Williams & Wilkins; 1999.
- Duthie EH, Katz PR, eds. *Practice of Geriatrics*. 3rd ed. Philadelphia, PA: WB Saunders; 1998.
- Goetz CG, ed. *Textbook of Clinical Neurology*. Philadelphia, PA: WB Saunders; 1999.
- Rakel RE, Bope ET, eds. *Conn's Current Therapy 2001*. 53rd ed. Philadelphia, PA: WB Saunders; 2001.
- Tasman A, Kay J, Lieberman JA, eds. *Psychiatry*. 1st ed. Philadelphia, PA: WB Saunders Company; 1997.
- Weinstock MB, Neides DM, eds. *The Resident's Guide to Ambulatory Care—Frequently Encountered and Commonly Confused Clinical Conditions*. 4th ed. Columbus, Ohio: Anadem Publishing; 2000.

NEUROLOGICAL DEVELOPMENT

TABLE 12.1

The Developing Child

Age	Language	Gross Motor	Fine Motor	Social
Newborn	Crying	Lacks control of muscle groups	No skill	Fixes on objects; startles easily
1 Month	Cooing; single vowel sounds	Lifts chin briefly	No skill	Indefinite stare at surroundings
2 Months	Cooing; single vowel sounds	Lifts head up 45°	Hand to mouth	Social smile
4 Months	Laughs; squeals	**Rolls over**; head up 90° (prone)	Two hand reach and grasp	Follows 180°; recognizes bottle
6 Months	Monosyllable babbling	**Sits alone without support**	Reaches for dropped toy; palmar grasp	Talks to mirror image and plays peek-a-boo
9 Months	Single syllables; responds to NO	Crawls, pulls to stand; "cruises"	**Thumb-finger (pincer) grasp**	Stranger anxiety; shout for attention
12 Months	**First word**; uses "mama," "dada" correctly	**Walks alone**; pivots to pick up objects	Fine pincer grasp; learns to use cup	Takes toys off table to play on floor
15 Months	4–6 words	Stands without support	Builds tower of two blocks	Points to and vocalizes wants

Continued

TABLE 12.1

The Developing Child, cont'd

Age	Language	Gross Motor	Fine Motor	Social
18 Months	**Two words together**; knows 6–10 words	Walks up steps; kicks ball	Turns pages two at a time; scribbles	Performs simple tasks; hugs doll
2 Years	50 words; **2- to 3-word sentences**	Walks down steps; overhand throw	Copy vertical line; turns doorknob	"MINE"; dry at night
3 Years	Knows full name; 4-word sentences	Jumps from bottom step; rides tricycle	Zips and unzips; copy circle	**Toilet trained**; **dresses with help**
4 Years	5-word sentences; sings songs	Hops on one foot; running jump	Laces shoes; buttons clothes	Separates from parents; bathes self
5 Years	Counts to 10; asks "why"	Skips; balances on one foot	May tie shoelaces	Dresses/undresses without help

TABLE 12.2
Timing of Pediatric Reflexes

Reflex	Onset	Duration
Palmar grasp	7 months	2–3 months
Rooting	8 months	Less prominent after 1 month
Moro	7–8 months	5–6 months
Tonic neck	35 weeks	6–7 months
Parachute	7–8 months	Remains throughout life

Adapted from Behrman RE, Kliegman R, Jenson HB, eds. *Nelson Textbook of Pediatrics.* 16th ed. Philadelphia: WB Saunders; 2000.

DEFINITIONS OF REFLEXES

Palmar grasp: The normal infant will grasp an object placed in the palm and will reinforce the grasp if an attempt is made to withdraw the object.
Rooting: Touching the corner of a normal infant's mouth will cause the bottom lip to lower on the same side and the tongue to move towards the stimulated side.
Moro: Elicited by startling the infant: allowing the infant's head to fall back suddenly, making a sudden loud noise or disturbing the exam table. The arms are symmetrically abducted and extended and the thumbs are flexed. This is followed by flexion and adduction of the upper extremities.
Tonic neck: While in the supine position, passive rotation of the head causes an extension of the extremities on the side of the body to which the face is pointing and a corresponding flexure of the extremities on the opposite side (the "fencing position").
Parachute: The infant is quickly rotated in the forward direction as if falling forward. The infant spontaneously extends the upper extremities as a protective mechanism. This reflex appears before the onset of walking.

ABNORMAL NEUROLOGICAL DEVELOPMENT

Evaluation always begins with a thorough history and physical examination. Particular attention should be placed on family and birth history. The physical exam should focus on the neurological exam as well as growth parameters: length and weight percentile and head circumference. There are no standard laboratory and radiography guidelines in the work-up of developmental delay. These tests are done on an individual basis, usually under the direction of a pediatric neurologist or a pediatric developmental specialist.

In the management of abnormal neurological development, a multidisciplinary approach is used. This involves the family, family physician, pediatric neurologist or a pediatric developmental specialist, physical and speech therapists, and special education teachers.

NORMAL ADULT ANATOMY AND PHYSIOLOGY

FIGURE 12.1

Spinal Nerve and Dermatome Chart

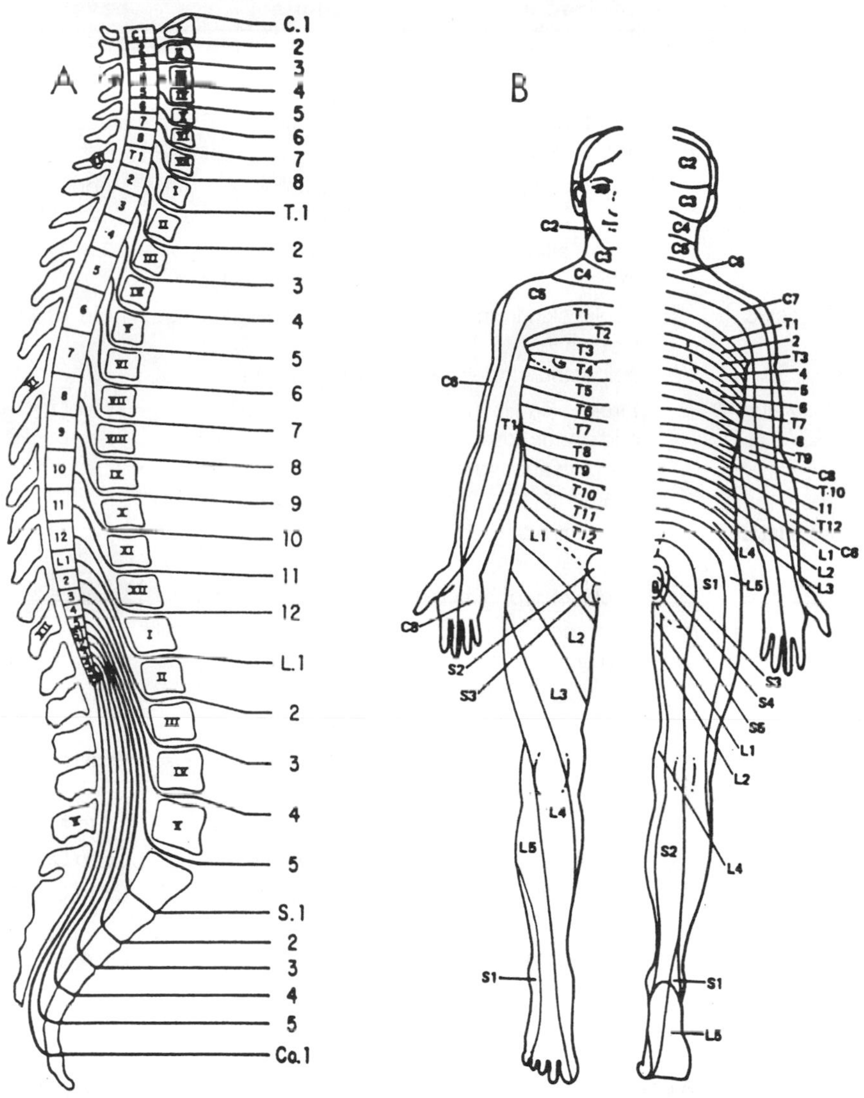

TABLE 12.3

Normal Reflexes

Reflex	Elicited by	Response	Segmental Level
Corneal	Touch cornea with cotton wisp	Contraction, orbicularis oculi	Pons
Pharyngeal	Touch posterior wall of pharynx	Contraction of pharynx	Medulla
Palatal	Touch soft palate	Elevation of palate	Medulla
Scapular	Stroke interscapular skin	Contraction of scapular muscles	C5 to T2
Epigastric	Stroke skin from nipples to epigastrium	Epigastrium "dimples" toward stroke	T7 to T9
Abdominal	Stroke skin along and under costal margins and inguinal ligaments	Contraction of abdominal muscles in quadrant stimulated	T8 to T12
Cremasteric	Stroke medial surface of upper thigh	Elevation of testicle, same side	L1 to L2
Gluteal	Stroke skin of buttock	Contraction of glutei	L4 to L5
Bulbocavernous	Pinch dorsum of glans	Contraction of bulbous urethra	S3 to S4
Anal	Prick perianal skin	Contraction of rectal sphincter	S5
Jaw Jerk	Tap mandible, mouth open	Jaw closes	Pons
Triceps	Tap triceps tendon	Elbow extends	C7 to T1
Biceps	Tap biceps tendon	Elbow flexes	C5 to C6
Radial	Tap styloid process of radius	Supinator longus contracts	C5 to C6
Knee	Tap patellar tendon	Knee extends	L3 to L4
Ankle	Tap Achilles tendon	Ankle extends	S1 to S3

Adapted from Mancall EL. *Alpers and Mancall's Essentials of the Neurologic Examination*. 2nd ed. Philadelphia, PA: FA Davis Co; 1981:23, 25.

TABLE 12.4

Effects of Autonomic Stimulation on Selected Body Organs

Organ	Sympathetic Effects	Parasympathetic Effects
Eye		
Pupil	Dilation	Contraction
Ciliary process	None	Excitation
Gastrointestinal glands	Inhibition or no effect	Copious, serous, or watery secretion and enzymes
Salivary gland	Thick, viscous secretion	Serous or water secretion
Sweat glands	Copious secretion	None
Heart	Increase in rate and force of contraction	Decrease in rate and force of contraction
Lungs	Constricts blood vessels, dilates bronchi	Constricts bronchi
Gastrointestinal	Inhibits peristalsis, stimulates sphincters	Stimulates peristalsis, inhibits sphincters
Liver	Release of glucose	None
Genitalia	Ejaculation, orgasm	Erection, lubrication
Blood vessels	Constricts abdominal muscles, constricts or dilates other smooth muscles, depending on receptors in tissue	None
Bladder	Uncertain	Stimulates smooth muscle for emptying, contracts detrusor, relaxes internal sphincter

Adapted from Chaplin JP, Demers A. *Primer of Neurology and Neurophysiology*. New York: John Wiley & Sons; 1978:97.

SEIZURE DISORDERS

TABLE 12.5

Classification of Seizure Disorders

Focal (Partial)	
Simple	Characterized by motor, sensory, autonomic, or psychic symptoms during which **consciousness is preserved**. Most common causes include mesial temporal sclerosis, congenital malformation, neoplasm, CNS infection, head trauma, and cerebrovascular disease. Less than one third are associated with EEG changes.
Complex	Characterized by an **alteration of consciousness**. Often begin with a motionless stare or arrest of activity followed by automatisms, eye movements, and speech disturbances. Causes are the same as simple partial but the pathology usually encompasses a larger area of the cerebral cortex. Over two thirds are associated with EEG changes.
Generalized	
Tonic/clonic	**Most common type of seizure in children, adolescents, and adults**. Characterized by a prodromal stage that may last minutes to days. The tonic phase consists of flexion of the trunk, upward deviation of the eyes, and a contraction of the abdominal muscles causing a forced expiration and vocalization, followed by a period of generalized extension lasting 10 to 15 seconds. The clonic phase consists of tonic contractions alternating with periods of atonia until there is a final generalized tonic spasm. Causes include idiopathic seizures, hyponatremia, hypoglycemia, alcohol withdrawal, and various drugs (tricyclic antidepressants, antipsychotics, anticholinergics, antihistamines, methylxanthines, antibiotics, and barbiturate and benzodiazepine withdrawal.
Absence	**Typical** absence seizures involve a sudden cessation of activity and unresponsiveness accompanied by rhythmic blinking, automatisms, and staring. They last less than 10 seconds, involve no aura or postictal state, and are usually precipitated by hyperventilation and/or photic stimulation. Short bursts of behavioral changes occur. **Atypical** absence seizures last longer than 10 seconds, begin and end more gradually, have a less noticeable alteration of consciousness, and are rarely provoked by hyperventilation or photic stimulation.
Myoclonic	Bilateral, synchronous and rapid muscular contractions during which consciousness is preserved.
Atonic	Abrupt loss of postural tone lasting 1 to 2 seconds that may be preceded by myoclonic jerks. Consciousness is usually impaired with rapid recovery. Patients usually experience a minor postictal state.

CNS indicates central nervous system; EEG, electroencephalogram.

TABLE 12.6

EEG Findings According to Seizure Type

Seizure Type	EEG Findings
Simple focal	Paroxysmal depolarization shift (synchronous burst of action potentials)
Complex focal	Interictal: focal or lateralized sharp waves, spikes and slow waves Ictal: Rhythmic sinusoidal activity or repetitive spike discharges
Tonic/clonic	Interictal: normal background activity with bilaterally synchronous and symmetrical spikes, polyspikes, or spike-wave complexes
Typical absence	Interictal: generalized 3.0-Hz spike-wave complexes with normal background activity
Atypical absence	0.5- to 2.5-Hz slow spike-wave complexes with abnormal background activity
Myoclonic	Generalized polyspikes or spike-wave complexes
Atonic	Ictal: polyspike-wave or spike-wave discharges

EEG indicates electroencephalogram.

MANAGEMENT OF FIRST SEIZURE

Rule out toxic, metabolic, infectious, vascular, and traumatic causes based upon presentation. All patients with an idiopathic seizure should undergo magnetic resonance imaging and electroencephalography (EEG).

Recurrence rates vary from 27%–71%, with 80% of recurrences occurring within 2 years (most within 6 months). Predictors of recurrence include evidence of neurological abnormality on exam or diagnostic studies, EEG abnormalities, and partial seizure. The risk of recurrence increases with the number of abnormalities present.

Treatment should be continued for 1–2 years and then gradually withdrawn, since most recurrences occur within this time period. Driving restriction should be implemented according to individual state laws (most states require 3–12 months of restriction).

TABLE 12.7

Guidelines for Seizure Medications in Adults

Drug	Indication	Starting Dose (mg/d)	Maintenance Dose (mg/d)	Doses/Day	Target Plasma Concentration (μg/mL)	Side Effects
Phenobarbital	Generalized Complex partial Status epilepticus	60	60–240	1–2	10–40	Alters mood, aggression, insomnia, Dupuytren syndrome
Phenytoin (Dilantin)	Generalized Complex partial Status epilepticus	200 po 3–5 mg/kg 10–15 mg/kg IV for status	200–600	1–3	10–20	Gum hypertrophy, acne, ataxia, tremor, nystagmus
Diazepam (Valium)	Status epilepticus	5–10 mg IV	NA	NA	NA	Sedation
Lorazepam (Activan)	Status epilepticus	4–8 mg IV	NA	NA	NA	Sedation
Carbamazepine (Tegretol)	Generalized Complex partial	200	400–1200	2–4	6–12	Morbilliform rash, agranulocytosis
Ethosuximide (Zarontin)	Absence (Petit mal)	500	500–2000	1–2	40–100	Nausea, vomiting, lethargy, dizziness, ataxia
Valproic acid (Depakene)	Generalized Partial absence	500	500–3000	1–2	50–100	Hepatotoxicity, pancreatitis, thrombocytopenia, tremor, weight gain

Drug	Indication	Starting Dose (mg/d)	Maintenance Dose (mg/d)	Doses/Day	Target Plasma Concentration (μg/mL)	Side Effects
Felbamate (Felbatol)	Generalized Complex partial	1200	1200–3600	3–4	NA	Life-threatening aplastic anemia and liver toxicity, requires weekly blood tests
Lamotrigine (Lamictal)	Generalized Complex partial	50	300–500	2	NA	Life-threatening skin rash, tremor, headache, nausea
Gabapentin (Neurontin)	Generalized Complex partial	300	900–1800	3	NA	Somnolence, ataxia, fatigue
Primidone (Mysoline)	Generalized Complex partial Myoclonic	250	250–1500	1–2	5–12	Fatigue, rash, agranulocytosis, lupus-like syndrome
Clonazepam (Klonopin)	Myoclonic Status epilepticus	1	2–8	1–2	NA	Aggression, hyperkinesia
Tiagabine (Gabitril)	Complex Partial	4	32–56	2–4	NA	Impaired concentration, speech problems, somnolence
Oxcarbazepine (Trileptal)	Partial	600	600–2400	2	NA	Somnolence, dizziness, diplopia, fatigue, hyponatremia

IV indicates intravenously; NA, not applicable; po, orally.

TABLE 12.8

Guidelines for Seizure Medications in Children

Drug	Indication	Starting Dose (mg/d)	Maintenance Dose (mg/kg/d)	Doses/Day	Target Plasma Concentration (µg/mL)	Side Effects
Phenobarbitol	Generalized Complex partial Status epilepticus	4	4–8	1–2	10–40	Alters mood, aggression, insomnia, Dupuytren syndrome
Phenytoin (Dilantin)	Generalized Complex partial Status epilepticus	5	5–15	1–2	10–20	Gum hypertrophy, acne, ataxia, tremor, nystagmus
Diazepam (Valium)	Status epilepticus	0.2–0.5 mg/kg/dose IV q 15–30 min Max total dose <5 years: 5 mg; >5 years:10 mg Rectal doses: 0.5 mg/kg/dose, repeat 0.25 mg/kg/dose in 10 min prn	NA	NA	NA	Sedation
Lorazepam (Ativan)	Status epilepticus	0.05–0.1 mg/kg/dose IV over 2–5 min; max 4 mg/dose	NA	NA	NA	Sedation

Drug	Indication	Starting Dose (mg/d)	Maintenance Dose (mg/kg/d)	Doses/Day	Target Plasma Concentration (μg/mL)	Side Effects
Carbamazepine (Tegretol)	Generalized Complex partial	5 (not to exceed 100 mg/d)	10–25	2–4	6–12	Morbilliform rash, lethargy, agranulocytosis
Ethosuximide (Zarontin)	Absence (Petit mal)	10	15–30	1–2	40–100	Nausea, vomiting, lethargy, dizziness, ataxia
Valproic acid (Depakene)	Generalized Partial Absence	10	15–40	1–3	50–100	Hepatotoxicity, pancreatitis, thrombocytopenia, tremor, weight gain
Felbamate (Felbatol)	Generalized Complex partial	15	15–45	3–4	NA	Life-threatening aplastic anemia and liver toxicity; requires weekly blood tests
Primidone (Mysoline)	Generalized Complex partial Myoclonic	10	20–30	1–2	5–12	Fatigue, rash, agranulocytosis, lupus-like syndrome
Clonazepam (Klonopin)	Myoclonic Infantile spasm Status epilepticus	0.025	0.025–0.1	2–3	NA	Aggression, hyperkinesia
Lamotrigine (Lamictal)	Adjunct for Generalized Partial complex	2 (no valproic acid) 0.2 (with valproic acid)	5–15	2	NA	Life-threatening skin rash, tremor, headache, nausea

IV indicates intravenously; NA, not applicable; prn, when necessary.

FEBRILE SEIZURES IN CHILDREN

Febrile seizures occur in 2%–5% of children during a sudden rise in temperature early in the course of an illness. 30% of patients experience a single recurrence. The age of onset ranges from 3 months to 5 years with a peak incidence from 18 to 24 months. The risk of recurrence is highest in children younger than 1 year of age and those with complicated seizures. 2% to 9% of children who suffer a febrile seizure will develop afebrile seizures.

Simple febrile seizures are responsible for 80% to 90% of cases. They involve generalized convulsions lasting less than 15 minutes. Laboratory testing, electroencephalography (EEG), and neuroimaging studies are not indicated. Anticonvulsants are not recommended because they don't reduce the risk of recurrence and are associated with a high incidence of side effects. The mainstay of management is parental reassurance. Parents should receive instruction on temperature control (antipyretics, sponge bathing) and first aid.

Complex febrile seizures exceed 15 minutes in duration, occur more than once in a 24-hour period, or show focal motor manifestations. Patients have a higher rate of subsequent epilepsy and should undergo a neuroimaging study to rule out structural lesions.

INFANTILE SPASMS

Infantile spasms are brief symmetric contractions of the neck, trunk, and extremities. The usual age at onset is between 4 and 8 months. They are NOT caused by immunizations. EEG demonstrates high-voltage, bilaterally asynchronous, slow-wave activity—*hypsarrhythmia*.

Cryptogenic infantile spasms are present in infants with a normal pregnancy and birth history, developmental milestones, and neurologic examination. Head computed tomography and magnetic resonance imaging scans are normal. They represent 10%–20% of infantile spasms and are associated with a good prognosis.

Symptomatic infantile spasms are directly related to a specific prenatal, perinatal, or postnatal factor. Causes include hypoxic-ischemic encephalopathy, congenital infections, inborn errors of metabolism, prematurity, central nervous system infections, and head trauma. They are associated with a poor prognosis; 80%–90% are associated with mental retardation.

WORKUP FOR A FIRST AFEBRILE SEIZURE IN A HEALTHY CHILD

Fasting glucose, calcium, magnesium, and serum electrolyte levels should be obtained.

An electroencephalogram (EEG) with activation procedures—hyperventilation, photic stimulation, and sleep deprivation—should also be obtained. A normal EEG does not rule out the diagnosis of epilepsy because the interictal recording is normal in approximately 40% of patients. The activation procedures greatly increase the sensitivity of the EEG.

Neuroimaging (computed tomography and magnetic resonance imaging [MRI]) should be reserved for patients with a suspected intracranial lesion based on history or abnormal neurologic finding. Routine use of these procedures in patients with a first afebrile seizure and normal exam has a negligible yield. **Indications for an MRI** include complex partial seizures, focal neurologic signs during or after the seizure, seizures of increasing frequency or severity, changing seizure pattern, evidence of increased intracranial pressure or trauma, and a first seizure in all adolescents.

HEADACHE

TABLE 12.9

Primary Headache Syndromes: Diagnostic Criteria

Tension	At least 10 headache episodes fulfilling criteria 1 through 3; less than 180 days per year with such headaches. 1. Headache lasting from 30 minutes to 7 days. 2. At least two of the following pain characteristics: a. Pressing or tightening (nonpulsating) quality b. Mild or moderate intensity c. Bilateral location d. No aggravation by routine physical activity 3. Both of the following: a. No nausea or vomiting (anorexia may occur) b. No photophobia and phonophobia, or only one is present
Migraine Without Aura	At least five attacks fulfilling criteria 1 through 3: 1. Headache lasting 4 to 72 hours (untreated or unsuccessfully treated) 2. At least two of the following pain characteristics: a. Unilateral location b. Pulsating quality c. Moderate or severe intensity d. Aggravation by physical activity 3. During headache, at least one of the following: a. Nausea and/or vomiting b. Photophobia and phonophobia
Migraine With Aura	At least two attacks with at least three of the following characteristics: 1. One or more fully reversible aura symptoms indicating focal cerebrocortical and/or brainstem dysfunction 2. At least one aura symptom develops gradually over more than 4 minutes, or two or more symptoms occur in succession 3. No aura symptom lasts more than 60 minutes; if more than one aura symptom is present, accepted duration is proportionally increased 4. Headache follows aura, with a free interval of less than 60 minutes (headache may also begin before or simultaneously with aura)

Cluster	At least five attacks fulfilling criteria 1 through 3: 1. Severe unilateral orbital, supraorbital and/or temporal pain lasting 15 to 180 minutes (untreated). 2. Headache associated with at least one of the following signs on the pain side: conjunctival injection, lacrimation, nasal congestion, rhinorrhea, forehead and facial sweating, miosis, ptosis, eyelid edema 3. Frequency of attacks: one every other day to eight per day
Other Primary Headache Syndromes	1. Mixed (migraine/tension) 2. Rebound (ie, caffeine) 3. Neuralgias 4. Paroxysmal hemicrania 5. Headache associated with cough, exertion, sexual activity, cold

TABLE 12.10

Secondary Headache Syndromes

Traumatic	Acute posttraumatic headache, epidural/subdural hematoma
Infectious	Meningitis, sinusitis, viral or bacterial systemic infection
Vascular	Acute CVA, subarachnoid hemorrhage, AV malformation
Temporal arteritis	Patients over 50 years old with jaw claudication, unitemporal pain, and visual symptoms.
Nonvascular intracranial disorder	Mass lesion (tumor, abscess), post–lumbar puncture (low CSF pressure)
Pseudotumor cerebri	Usually occurs in obese, young females and is associated with papilledema, visual loss, and elevated CSF pressure
Metabolic	Sleep apnea (hypoxia and hypercapnia associated with morning headache), hypoglycemia, dialysis
Other	Substance abuse or withdrawal, disorder of facial or cranial structures

AV indicates atrioventricular; CVA, cerebrovascular accident; CSF, cerebrospinal fluid.

TABLE 12.11

Red Flags in the Evaluation of Acute Headaches

Red Flag	Differential Diagnosis	Possible Workup
New headache in patient 50 years of age or older	Temporal arteritis, mass lesion	Erythocyte sedimentation rate, neuroimaging
Sudden onset	Subarachnoid hemorrhage, pituitary apoplexy, vascular malformation, mass lesion	Neuroimaging; lumbar puncture (if neuroimaging is negative)
Increasing in frequency and severity	Mass lesion, subdural hematoma, medication overuse	Neuroimaging, drug screen
New-onset headache in an immuno-compromised patient	Meningitis (chronic or carcinomatous), brain abscess (including toxoplasmosis), metastasis	Neuroimaging; lumbar puncture (if neuroimaging is negative)
Accompanied by signs of systemic illness (fever, stiff neck, rash)	Meningitis, encephalitis, Lyme disease, systemic infection, collagen vascular disease	Neuroimaging, lumbar puncture, serology
Focal neurologic signs or symptoms	Mass lesion, vascular malformation, stroke, collagen vascular disease	Neuroimaging, collagen vascular evaluation (including antiphospholipid antibodies)
Papilledema	Mass lesion, pseudotumor cerebri, meningitis	Neuroimaging, lumbar puncture
History of head trauma	Intracranial hemorrhage, posttraumatic headache	Neuroimaging of brain, skull, and, possibly, cervical spine

Adapted from Clinch CR. Evaluation of acute headaches in adults. *Am Fam Physician.* 2001; 63(4):685–692.

DIAGNOSTIC TESTING IN THE EVALUATION OF HEADACHE

The US Headache Consortium guidelines on the use of neuroimaging state that neuroimaging should be considered in patients with nonacute headache with an abnormal finding on the neurologic examination. It is not usually warranted in patients with headache and a normal neurologic examination.

Computed tomographic (CT) scan is the imaging method of choice for acute headache. It is greater than 90% sensitive for the detection of acute subarachnoid hemorrhage and is also sensitive enough to detect other intracranial pathology that may cause acute headache (ie, acute hydrocephalus, enlarging mass). Magnetic resonance imaging is more sensitive than CT scanning in identifying intracranial (especially posterior fossa) pathology but the US headache consortium guidelines state that this superior sensitivity is of little clinical importance in the evaluation of nonacute headache.

TABLE 12.12

Drugs for the Treatment of a Migraine Headache

Drug	Dosage (Per Event)	Side Effects
Triptans		
Sumatriptan (Imitrex)	6-mg injection SC; 100-mg tablet orally; 5- or 20-mg spray intranasally Maximum 2 injections, 3 tablets or 40 mg intranasally/24-h period	*Serious*: transient increase in blood pressure, exacerbation of angina *Common*: tingling, flushing, transient nausea
Rizatriptan (Maxalt)	5- or 10-mg tablet or wafer (Maxalt-MLT) every 2 hours. Maximum 30 mg/ 24-h period	*Serious*: tachycardia or bradycardia *Common*: elevated BP, chest pain, dizziness, throat tightness, myalgias, sweating
Zolmitriptan (Zomig)	2.5 or 5 mg tablet. Maximum 200 mg/ 24-h period	*Serious*: dysrhythmias, coronary vasospasm, MI, hypertensive crisis *Common*: Similar to Rizatriptan, also flushing
Naratriptan (Amerge)	1- or 2.5-mg tablet. Maximum 200 mg/ 24-h period	Same as Rizatriptan
Almotriptan (Axert)	6.25- or 12.5-mg tablet. Maximum 25 mg/ 24-h period	Same as Rizatriptan
Ergotamines		
Ergotamine/caffeine (Cafergot)	1- or 2-mg tablet. Maximum 6 mg/24-h period	Nausea, vomiting, abdominal pain, diarrhea
Dihydroergotamine (DHE 45)	1 mg SC injection. Maximum 2 doses/ 24-h period	Same as Cafergot
Dihydroergotamine (Migranal)	1 spray (0.5 mg) in each nostril. Maximum 6 sprays (3 mg)/24-h period or 8 sprays (4 mg)/wk	*Serious*: coronary vasospasm, MI, peripheral ischemia, hypertension *Common*: Nausea, weakness, numbness, myalgias, chest pain, edema

Drug	Dosage (Per Event)	Side Effects
Other		
NSAIDs	According to individual agent	GI upset, GI hemorrhage
Narcotics	According to individual agent	Drowsiness, GI upset, constipation, addiction potential
Isometheptene 65 mg/ dichloralphenazone 100 mg/acetaminophen 325 mg (Midrin)	2 capsules. Maximum 5/12-h period	Drowsiness, dizziness, nausea

BP indicates blood pressure; GI, gastrointestinal; MI, myocardial infarction; NSAID, nonsteroidal anti-inflammatory drug.

TABLE 12.13

Drugs for the Prevention of a Migraine Headache

Drug	Daily Dose	Side Effects
Amytriptyline	10–150 mg	Weight gain, somnolence, dry mouth, arrythmias, urinary retention
Diltiazem (Cardizem, Tiazac, Dilacor, Cartia)	90–270 mg	Arrythmias, CHF, hypotension, GI upset, edema, rash. Use caution in hepatic or renal dysfunction
Divalproex sodium (Depakote)	500–750 mg (may be divided)	Nausea, fatigue, weight gain, hair loss, tremor, liver toxicity, fetal malformation
Divalproex ER	500 mg	See above
Methysergide	2–8 mg	Muscle cramps, insomnia, tissue fibrosis
Nifedipine	30 mg	Headache, tachycardia, depression
NSAIDs	Per individual medication	Dyspepsia, gastritis, GI bleeding
Propranolol	40–320 mg 60–320 mg (long acting)	Fatigue, bradycardia, bronchospasm
Verapamil	280–320 mg	Headache, bradycardia, weight gain, constipation, depression

CHF indicates congestive heart failure; GI, gastrointestinal; NSAID, nonsteroidal anti-inflammatory drug.

INTERVERTEBRAL DISK DISEASE

The intervertebral disk is composed of a central nucleus pulposus surrounded by the annulus fibrosus. Herniation is the rupture of the annulus with displacement of the central nucleus. The peak incidence of symptomatic degenerative disk disease is in people 30 to 50 years old. The most common site of cervical disk herniation is the C6–C7 level, while the most common site of lumbar disk herniation is the L5–S1 level.

TABLE 12.14

Location of Pain and Reflex Abnormality According to Level of Cervical Nerve Root Involvement

Level	Action	Pain Sensation	Reflex Abnormality
C5	Shoulder abduction (15–90°) Elbow flexion Shoulder abduction (0–15°) Humerus external rotation	Lateral shoulder Lateral upper arm Lateral epicondyle	Biceps
C6	Elbow flexion in semipronation Pronation Radial wrist extension	Posterior shoulder Lateral forearm Thumb and index finger	Brachioradialis
C7	Elbow extension Radial wrist extension Finger extension	Posterior shoulder Medial forearm Index and middle fingers	Triceps
C8	Thumb flexion Finger flexion	Interscapular medial forearm Little finger	Finger flexors
T1	Finger abduction Little finger abduction	Medial forearm Medial epicondyle	None

Adapted from Goetz CG, ed. *Textbook of Clinical Neurology*. Philadelphia, PA: WB Saunders; 1999.

TABLE 12.15

Location of Pain and Motor Deficits According to Level of Lumbar Nerve Root Involvement

Level	Pain Sensation	Motor Deficit
T12–L1	Inguinal region and medial thigh	None
L1–2	Anterior and medial upper thigh	Quadriceps (slight); slightly diminished suprapatellar reflex
L2–3	Anterolateral thigh	Quadriceps; diminished patellar or suprapatellar reflex
L3–4	Posterolateral thigh and anterior tibia	Quadriceps; diminished patellar reflex
L4–5	Dorsum of foot	Extensor of big toe and foot
L5–S1	Lateral aspect of foot	Diminished or absent Achilles reflex

Adapted from Humphreys SC, Eck JC. Clinical evaluation and treatment options for herniated lumbar disc. *Am Fam Physician*. 1999;59:575–582.

TABLE 12.16
Common Peripheral Nerve Lesions

Syndrome	Nerve	History	Physical Exam
Carpal tunnel	Median nerve at wrist	Intermittent hand pain or paresthesias especially at night; weak grip, decreased fine motor skills	Decreased thumb adduction, thenar atrophy, decreased sensation of first, second, thrid digits. Positive Phalen and Tinel signs
Cubital tunnel	Ulnar nerve at elbow	Elbow pain, hand weakness, numbness of ulnar side of hand	Decreased finger abduction, decreased thumb adduction, atrophy of intrinsic hand muscles (if severe), claw hand (if severe), decreased sensation of digits 4 (ulnar side) and 5, positive Tinel sign at elbow
Meralgia paresthetica	Lateral femoral cutaneous nerve	Numbness/pain of lateral thigh (more common in obesity, pregnancy)	Usually no motor deficit, increased light touch and pinprick response over lateral thigh
Tarsal tunnel	Posterior tibial nerve	Burning/tingling of ankle and sole, increased with ambulation	Usually no motor deficit, decreased sensation on plantar foot, positive Tinel sign of nerve

Adapted from McKnight JT, Adcock BB. Paresthesias: a practical diagnostic approach. *Am Fam Physician.* 1997;56:2253–2260.

EVALUATION OF INTERVERTEBRAL DISK DISEASE

Neuroimaging is usually not indicated unless the patient fails to show improvement after 4–6 weeks of conservative therapy. **Magnetic resonance imaging (MRI)** is preferred in most cases; it allows visualization of multiple levels in multiple planes and the high contrast of epidural fat and cerebrospinal fluid allows visualization of subtle compression. **Computed tomography with myelography** can visualize the entire length of the spine and best defines the root sleeves. It also provides the best visualization of lateral pathology and small osteophytes and is indicated if MRI is nondiagnostic.

Electromyography (EMG) can be used to evaluate both motor and sensory nerves. It can determine the presence and extent of a peripheral neuropathy, distinguish between axonal loss and demyelination, localize lesions, and distinguish between a polyneuropathy and mononeuropathy. EMG is useful in following the course of peripheral nerve disease and recognizing subclinical polyneuropathies.

MANAGEMENT OF INTERVERTEBRAL DISK DISEASE

Conservative measures should be used initially. They include rest in a comfortable position, early remobilization, exercises and oral analgesics for pain as needed. In addition, environmental measures are often very useful. These may include ice, heat, massage, ultrasound, transcutaneous electrical nerve stimulation (TENS), acupuncture, exercise, and traction.

There are clear and well-defined indications for surgery. These are acute myelopathy, cauda equina syndrome (hypotonic bladder and rectal sphincters with perineal pain and anesthesia in a "saddle distribution"), severe or progressive motor deficits, intractable pain, and failure of conservative therapy for 6 to 12 weeks.

NEUROPATHIC PAIN

Neuropathic pain is associated with many peripheral neuropathies, including diabetic, uremic, and human immunodeficiency virus- and alcohol-associated neuropathy. It can be described as burning, stinging, needle-like, or stabbing.

TABLE 12.17

Drugs for the Treatment of Neuropathic Pain

Medication	Dose
1st Line	
Tricyclic antidepressants	10–25 mg to 100–150 mg po qhs
Gabapentin (Neurontin)	300 mg po tid to 6000 mg po divided into 3–5 doses daily
Carbamazepine (Tegretol)	200 mg po bid to 400 mg po tid-qid (follow levels if taking more than 600 mg per day)
2nd Line	
Tramadol (Ultram)	50 mg po bid to 100 mg po qid
Mexilitine (Mexitil)	200 mg po qd to 300 mg po tid
Phenytoin (Dilantin)	200 mg po qhs to 200 mg po qid (follow levels on high doses)
Topical agents	
Capsaicin 0.075% (Zostrix)	Apply tid-qid
Salicylate 10%–15%	Apply tid-qid
Menthol 16%/Camphor 3%	Apply qid
Ketoprofen compounds	Apply bid-qid
Carbamazepine 5%/lidocaine 5%	Apply bid-qid

Adapted from Rakel RE, Bope ET. *Conn's Current Therapy 2001*. 53rd ed. Philadelphia, PA: WB Saunders; 2001.

bid indicates twice daily; po, orally; qd, once daily; qid, four times daily; tid, three times daily.

BELL PALSY

Bell palsy is an acute paralysis of cranial nerve VII (facial nerve). There are 20 new cases/10,000 population annually with an equal incidence in men and women and an equal involvement of left and right facial nerves. It is thought to be caused by a herpesvirus infection. Clinical signs and symptoms include acute, unilateral weakness or paralysis of the face, a viral prodrome (60%), numbness or pain of the ear, tongue, or face (50%), and decreased tear and saliva production in the involved side (10%).

Evaluation includes a physical exam to rule out cerebrovascular, infectious, neoplastic, or traumatic causes of facial nerve paralysis. It is important to document involvement of all facial nerve branches, a normal otoscopic examination, the absence of skin vesicles or blisters (zoster) and the absence of parotid gland mass. Neuroimaging is not indicated.

Eighty-four percent of patients will completely recover within 3 weeks without medication. The great majority of the remainder will improve within 3 to 6 months, while approximately 15% have residual weakness. By 6 months all patients should demonstrate some improvement. Patients with poor recovery by 3 months may require surgical decompression of the facial nerve. An electromyogram should be obtained and referral made to an ear, nose, and throat surgeon who performs middle cranial fossa surgery. Treatment with prednisone (1 mg/kg/day tapered over 7–14 days) and Famvir (500 mg orally three times daily for 10 days) has been shown to hasten recovery if started within 4 days of symptom onset and should be implemented in patients with no contraindications. It is absolutely critical to maintain good eye lubrication until the patient recovers. Ophthalmic lubricating solution during the day and ointment at night should be used along with an eye patch to enhance moisture retention.

VERTIGO

Vertigo is defined as the sensation that the environment is rotating around an individual.

TABLE 12.18

Peripheral Vertigo (75% of Patients With Vertigo)

	Clinical Signs and Symptoms	Treatment
Benign positional vertigo (BPV)	BPV is responsible for 20% of all patients with vertigo and is caused by dislodged calcium carbonate crystals floating within the semicircular canals. Symptoms are brief because dizziness occurs only while the debris shifts position. Vertigo is precipitated by movement and may be elicited by the **Dix-Hallpike maneuver**. In this maneuver, the patient sits and then is moved backward rapidly to the supine position so that the head is hanging off the end of the table. If no dizziness or nystagmus is appreciated after 20 seconds, the maneuver is repeated with the head turned 45° to the right, and (after another 20 seconds) to the left	Positional maneuvers are the most effective treatment for BPV. Vestibular suppressants may also be beneficial
Meniere disease	The patient presents with tinnitus, sensation of fullness in one ear, fluctuating hearing changes and episodic vertigo. Tinnitus is constant but becomes louder during an acute episode. The diagnosis is usually made based on history, but audiometry that reveals a fluctuating low-tone sensorineural hearing loss is confirmatory. After the diagnosis is made, FTA-Abs, ANA, CBC and fasting blood glucose should be drawn to identify treatable causes.	Vestibular suppressants and antiemetics Salt reduction is helpful in reducing the frequency and intensity of episodes. Patients may be prescribed a low-salt-diet and/or a salt-wasting diuretic (Ie, HCTZ)
Vestibular neuronitis	This condition is thought to be caused by viral infections involving the vestibular portion of cranial nerve VIII. The patient presents with vertigo, nausea, and malaise usually lasting 2–3 days, with less intense symptoms persisting for 1–2 weeks. 10% of patients may take up to 2 months for improvement. Hearing is *not* impaired.	Vestibular suppressants and antiemetics Vestibular exercises

Continued

TABLE 12.18

Peripheral Vertigo (75% of Patients With Vertigo), cont'd

	Clinical Signs and Symptoms	Treatment
Labyrinthitis	Vestibular neuronitis *with hearing abnormalities*	
Acoustic neuroma	Typically a person 40 years or older with mild vertigo accompanied by an asymmetrical (sensorineural) hearing loss. Physical exam (including other cranial nerves) is otherwise completely normal. MRI will confirm the diagnosis. An audiogram should be obtained within 6 months if the patient notes minor hearing loss. Most lesions remain stable over many years and surgery is not necessary.	If hearing loss worsens, an MRI should be obatined. If the tumor is small and/or the patient refuses surgery, periodic hearing evaluations should be performed and the MRI should be repeated yearly. If there is a change in hearing, the MRI should be repeated more frequently. Gamma knife treatment is available for poor surgical candidates.

ANA indicates antinuclear antibody; CBC, complete blood cell count; FTA-Abs, flourescent treponemal antibody absorption test; MRI, magnetic resonance imaging.

TABLE 12.19

Central Vertigo (25% of Patients With Vertigo)

Stroke and TIA	Responsible for 33% of central vertigo
Vertebrobasilar migraines	Responsible for 15% of central vertigo
Vertebrobasilar insufficiency	
Multiple sclerosis	
Temporal lobe epilepsy	
CNS neoplasm, infection, or trauma	
Ototoxic medications (should be avoided or discontinued in patients with vertigo if possible)	■ Streptomycin, tobramycin, vancomycin, kanamycin, neomycin, amikacin, dactinomycin ■ Diuretics: furosemide, bumetanide, ethacrynic acid ■ Quinine ■ Aspirin and other salicylates ■ Chemotherapeutic agents

CNS indicates central nervous system; TIA, transient ischemic attack.

TABLE 12.20

Useful Studies in the Evaluation of CN VIII Disorders

Syndrome	Neuroimaging	Electro-physiology	Fluid and Tissue Analysis	Other Tests
Peripheral hearing loss	Usually normal MRI, CT	BAER ECOG MLR	NA	Audiogram abnormal
CPA syndrome (acoustic neuroma)	Lesion in CPA: MRI, CT	BAER	CSF	Audiogram abnormal
Central vertigo	MRI, CT for suspected brainstem or cerebellar lesion	BAER	CSF Blood	ENG Rotatory chair test
Benign peripheral vertigo: BPV	Normal	Normal	NA	ENG
Meniere disease	Normal	BAER ECOG	NA	Audiogram ENG
Vestibular neuritis	MRI may show enhancement of vestibular nerve	NA	NA	ENG

Adapted from Goetz CG, ed. *Textbook of Clinical Neurology.* Philadelphia: WB Saunders; 1999.

BAER indicates brain stem auditory evoked responses; CSF, cerebrospinal fluid; CT, computed tomography; ECOG, electrocochleography; ENG, electronystagmography; MLR, middle latency response; MRI, magnetic resonance imaging.

TABLE 12.21

Vestibular Suppressants

Drug	Dose	Adverse Reactions
Meclizine (Antivert, Bonine)	12.5–50 mg po q 4–6 hours	Sedation, use carefully in BPH and glaucoma
Lorazepam (Ativan)	0.5 mg po bid	Mild sedation, dependency
Clonazepam (Klonopin)	0.5 mg po bid	Mild sedation, dependency
Scopolamine (Transderm-Scop)	0.5 mg patch q 3 days	Topical allergy, use carefully in glaucoma, dysrhythmias, BPH
Dimenhydrinate (Dramamine)	50 mg po q 4–6 h	Sedation, use carefully in BPH and glaucoma
Diazepam (Valium)	2–10 mg po, IM, or IV given as 1 dose	Sedation, dependency, respiratory depression, use carefully in glaucoma

Adapted from Goetz CG, ed. *Textbook of Clinical Neurology*. Philadelphia: WB Saunders; 1999.
bid indicates twice daily; BPH, benign prostatic hyperplasia; IM, intramuscularly; IV, intravenously; po, orally.

CEREBROVASCULAR DISEASE

TABLE 12.22

Cerebrovascular Disease

Definitions	A neurologic deficit due to cerebral ischemia is defined as a **stroke** if it lasts greater than 24 hours, and a **transient ischemic attack (TIA)** if it lasts less than 24 hours
Epidemiology	The annual incidence is estimated at 731,000 cases. There are 4 million stroke survivors; it is the major cause of serious disability in adults. 80% of strokes are ischemic, while 20% are thromboembolic
Risk factors	Age, hypertension, diabetes, hypercholesterolemia, carotid artery stenosis, history of TIA, atrial fibrillation, smoking, and sedentary lifestyle

TABLE 12.23

National Stroke Association Summary Recommendations for Prevention of a First Stroke

Condition	Recommendation
Hypertension	The Sixth Report of the Joint National Committee on Prevention, Detection, Evaluation, and Treatment of High Blood Pressure recommendations for lifestyle modification, initiation of specific therapy, and multidisciplinary management strategies
Myocardial infarction	Aspirin therapy if previous myocardial infarction (MI) or warfarin at an international normalized ratio of 2–3 in patients with atrial fibrillation, left ventricular thrombus, or significant left ventricular dysfunction, and statin agents after MI in patients with normal to high lipid levels.
Atrial fibrillation*	Patients >75 years old with or without risk factors should be treated with warfarin; patients aged 65–75 years with risk factors should be treated with warfarin and those without risk factors should be treated with warfarin or aspirin; patients <65 years old with risk factors should be treated with warfarin, those without risk factors should be treated with aspirin.
Diabetes mellitus	American Diabetes Association recommends for control of diabetes to reduce microvascular complications (further studies are needed to determine if aggressive glycemic control lowers the risk of stroke)
Lipid levels	Statin agents in patients with high cholesterol and coronary heart disease and National Cholesterol Education Program guideline principles for dietary and pharmacologic management of patients with hyperlipidemia or atherosclerotic disease
Asymptomatic carotid artery disease†	Carotid endarterectomy for asymptomatic carotid stenosis ≥60% (but <100%) when surgical morbidity and mortality is <3%
Lifestyle factors	Modification of smoking, alcohol consumption, physical activity, and diet according to published guidelines

*Risk factors include previous transient ischemic attack, systemic embolism or stroke, hypertension, and left ventricular dysfunction. Efforts to improve patient and practitioner awareness regarding the benefits and risks of warfarin will serve as a first step toward increasing appropriate usage. The warfarin international normalized ratio goal is 2.0 to 3.0 with a target value of 2.5.

†The asymptomatic carotid artery stenosis cut point of at least 60% should be replicated in other studies.

SCREENING FOR ASYMPTOMATIC CAROTID ARTERY DISEASE

There is insufficient evidence to recommend for or against screening with either physical examination or carotid ultrasound. Men who are over 60, have risk factors for stroke, and are good surgical candidates are most likely to benefit.

Venous Doppler ultrasonography is noninvasive and may be used for initial screening. Cerebral angiography is used for the precise measurement of the degree of stenosis. These tests are used for the evaluation of symptomatic carotid artery disease as well.

TABLE 12.24

Management of Asymptomatic Carotid Artery Disease

Surgical	Carotid endarterectomy (CEA) is indicated for asymptomatic lesions *of at least 60% stenosis* with a local surgical risk of less than 3%.
Medical	Aspirin 81–325 mg po qd
	For people unable to take aspirin:
	Clopidogrel (Plavix) 75 mg po qd (or)
	Ticlopidine (Ticlid) 250 mg po bid (or)
	Extended-release dipyridamole (Persantine) 200 mg and aspirin 25 mg po bid

bid indicates twice daily; po, orally; qd, once daily.

TABLE 12.25

Management of Symptomatic Carotid Artery Disease

	Medical	Surgical (CEA)
Cardioembolic (ie, AFIB)	Anticoagulation with warfarin (Coumadin) to a goal INR of 2.0–3.0 Aspirin 81–325 mg po qd for patients who cannot take warfarin	NA
Atherothrombotic	See Table 12.24	**70%–99% stenosis:** proven benefit in good surgical candidates who have had ≥1 TIA within the last 2 years **50%–69% stenosis:** less benefit than for higher degree of stenosis, *but patients with a recent TIA do have a reduced stroke rate.* <**50% stenosis:** no benefit from CEA

INR indicates international normalized ratio; po, orally; qd, once daily; TIA, transient ischemic attack.

TABLE 12.26

Evaluation of an Acute Ischemic Stroke

History	Precise establishment of time of symptom onset is very important in guiding therapy. Preceding TIA symptoms are more likely to be associated with an ischemic stroke whereas headache more often occurs with hemorrhagic and embolic stroke
Physical	*Neurologic*: may help to localize the lesion site *Cardiovascular*: assess heart rhythm, murmurs, blood pressure, carotid bruits *Mental Status*: loss of consciousness or confusion should prompt consideration of other diagnoses
Laboratory	CBC, glucose, PT, PTT, lipid profile, and serum VDRL. ESR (in the elderly) to exclude giant cell arteritis. In young patients, antiphospholipid antibodies to identify immune-related disease processes predisposing to stroke and tests for platelet viscosity, function, and collagen vascular diseases (protein C, protein S, antithrombin III, factor V Leiden mutation) may be indicated
Differential	Hypoglycemia, migraine headaches, seizures, brain mass, hemorrhagic stroke

CBC indicates complete blood cell count; ESR, erythrocyte sedimentation ratio; PT, prothrombin time; PTT, partial thromboplastin time; TIA, transient ischemic attack.

TABLE 12.27

Imaging Studies for Acute Ischemic Stroke

Cardiac	12-lead EKG may be obtained to exclude MI and dysrhythmias. Cardiac echo is useful to evaluate for a cardiogenic source of emboli. **Cardiac imaging is very low yield in patients with no history or physical evidence of cardiac disease**
Vascular	In addition to cerebral angiography and venous Doppler ultrasonography, MR angiography is valuable for identifying lesions of extra-cranial carotid circulation.
Cerebral	**CT without contrast is the best initial imaging study**. It can identify other conditions that may mimic a stroke, such as neoplasm, abscess, and subdural or epidural hemorrhage. Contrast enhancement allows greater detection of subacute infarcts. The drawbacks to CT are that the infarct may not be seen for 24–48 hours and posterior fossa and cortical infarcts may not be seen due to bone artifact. In these situations, MRI should be obtained.

CT indicates computed tomography; EKG, electrocardiogram; MI, myocardial infarction; MR, magnetic resonance; MRI, magnetic resonance imaging.

TABLE 12.28

Medical Management of Acute Ischemic Stroke

Aspirin	A dose of 160–325 mg po qd is recommended for patients not receiving tPA, IV heparin, or warfarin. Aspirin should be started within 48 hours of onset and may be used safely in combination with subcutaneous heparin.
Heparin	There is no conclusive evidence either for or against the use of heparin in the treatment of acute stroke. 3–5 days of IV heparin is an option for cardioembolic stroke, large-artery atherosclerotic-ischemic stroke, and progressing thromboembolic stroke. There is a small risk of cerebral hemorrhage with the use of heparin. Use of a standardized sliding scale based on weight and PTT measurements should be used; a bolus is NOT recommended at the initiation of therapy. A brain CT should be done prior to initiation of IV heparin to exclude hemorrhage and estimate the size of the infarction.

CT indicates computed tomography; IV, intravenously; po, orally; PTT, partial thromboplastin time; qd, once daily; tPA, tissue-type plasminogen activator.

TABLE 12.29

Poststroke Rehabilitation

Acute care setting	Prophylaxis for deep venous thrombosis in patients with limited mobility Swallowing assessment before starting oral intake Prevention of decubiti ulcers and pressure sores Fall risk assessment Treatment of urinary incontinence or retention Minimizing indwelling catheter use Mobilization as soon as possible
Rehabilitation facility	Patient and caregiver education Evaluation and treatment of persistent urinary incontinence Bowel management programs for patients with constipation or fecal incontinence Physical therapy directed at improving functional performance Detection and treatment of depression
Community residence	Working to minimize the stress of caregiving on both the patient and caregivers Facilitation of patient reintegration into family and social roles and valued activities Fall prevention emphasizing environmental risk factors Prevention of stroke recurrence and complications

DEMENTIA

Dementia is defined as a generalized and sustained decline in intellectual functioning. In the evaluation of dementia, a thorough history and physical examination should be performed to rule out metabolic, infectious, iatrogenic, or toxic causes. The Mini-Mental State Examination is the cornerstone of diagnosis and monitoring of disease progression. In addition, **routine laboratory analysis in all patients should include** urinalysis with microscopy, complete blood cell count, complete metabolic panel (including thyroid and liver function tests), vitamin B_{12} and folate levels, and rapid plasma reagin–VDRL test.

TABLE 12.30

The Mini-Mental State Examination

	Maximum Score
Orientation	
1. What is the year, season, day, month, date?	5
2. Where are we (state, country, town, hospital, floor)?	5
Registration	
3. Name three objects, then have the patient name them. Give one point per each correct answer; repeat until all three are named (record number of tries).	3
Attention/Calculation	
4. Begin with 100 and serially subtract seven until stopped. Stop patient after five correct responses, or ask patient to spell "world" backward.	5
Recall	
5. Ask patient to name the three objects named earlier. Give one point per correct answer.	3
Language	
6. Have patient identify a pencil (pen) and watch.	2
7. Ask patient to repeat "no ifs, ands, or buts."	1
8. Have patient follow a three-step command, for example, "Take the paper in your right hand, fold it in half, and put it on the floor."	3
9. Have the patient read this statement and obey it: "Close your eyes."	1
10. Ask the patient to write a sentence.	1
11. Have patient copy a design.	1
	Total*: 30

Adapted from Folstein MF, Folstein SE, McHugh PR. Mini-mental state: a practical method for grading the cognitive state of patients for the clinician. *J Psychiatr Res.* 1975;12(3):189–198.

*Significant cognitive impariment ≤23.

TABLE 12.31

Diagnostic Criteria for Dementia of the Alzheimer Type

Diagnostic Criteria for Dementia of the Alzheimer Type

A. The development of multiple cognitive deficits manifested by both
   (1) Memory impairment (impaired ability to learn new information or to recall previously learned information)
   (2) One (or more) of the following cognitive disturbances:
      (a) aphasia (language disturbance)
      (b) apraxia (impaired ability to carry out motor activities despite intact motor function)
      (c) agnosia (failure to recognize or identify objects despite intact sensory function)
      (d) disturbance in executive functioning (ie, planning, organizing, sequencing, abstracting)

B. The cognitive defects in criteria A1 and A2 each cause significant impairment in social or occupational functioning and represent a significant decline from a previous level of functioning

C. The course is characterized by gradual onset and continuing cognitive decline

D. The cognitive defects in criteria A1 and A2 are not due to any of the following:
   (1) Other central nervous system conditions that cause progressive deficits in memory and cognition (eg, cerebrovascular disease, Parkinson disease, Huntington disease, subdural hematoma, normal-pressure hydrocephalus, brain tumor)

Code based on type of onset and predominant features:

With Early Onset: if onset at age 65 years or below

290.11 With Delirium: if delirium is superimposed on the dementia

290.12 With Delusions: if delusions are the predominant feature

290.13 With Depressed Mood: if depressed mood (including presentations that meet full symptom criteria for a major depressive episode) is the predominant feature. A separate diagnosis of mood disorder due to a general medical condition is not given

290.10 Uncomplicated: if none of the above predominates in the current clinical presentation

With Late Onset: if onset is after age 65 years

290.3 With Delirium: if delirium is superimposed on the dementia

290.20 With Delusions: if delusions are the predominant feature

290.21 With Depressed Mood: if depressed mood (including presentations that meet full symptom criteria for a major depressive episode) is the predominant feature. A separate diagnosis of mood disorder due to a general medical condition is not given

290.0 Uncomplicated: if none of the above predominates in the current clinical presentation

Specify if:

With Behavioral Disturbance

Coding note: Also code 331.0 Alzheimer disease on axis III

Adapted from The American Psychiatric Association. *Diagnostic and Statistical Manual of Mental Disorders*. 4th ed. Text rev. Washington DC: American Psychiatric Association; 2000.

TABLE 12.32

Diagnostic Criteria for Vascular Dementia

Diagnostic Criteria for 290.4x Vascular Dementia

A. The development of multiple cognitive deficits manifested by both
   (1) Memory impairment (impaired ability to learn new information or to recall previously learned information)
   (2) One (or more) of the following cognitive disturbances:
      (a) aphasia (language disturbance)
      (b) apraxia (impaired ability to carry out motor activities despite intact motor function)
      (c) agnosia (failure to recognize or identify objects despite intact sensory function)
      (d) disturbance in executive functioning (ie, planning, organizing, sequencing, abstracting)

B. The cognitive deficits in criteria A1 and A2 each cause significant impairment in social or occupational functioning and represent a significant decline from a previous level of functioning

C. Focal neurological signs and symptoms (eg, exaggeration of deep tendon reflexes, extensor plantar response, pseudobulbar palsy, gait abnormalities, weakness of an extremity) or laboratory evidence indicative of cerebrovascular disease (eg, multiple infarctions involving cortex and underlying white matter) that are judged to be etiologically related to the disturbance

D. The deficits do not occur exclusively during the course of a delirium

Code based on predominant features:

290.41 With Delirium: if delirium is superimposed on the dementia

290.42 With Delusions: if delusions are the predominant feature

290.43 With Depressed Mood: if depressed mood (including presentations that meet full symptom criteria for a major depressive episode) is the predominant feature. A separate diagnosis of mood disorder due to a general medical condition is not given

290.40 Uncomplicated: if none of the above predominates in the current clinical presentation

Specify if:

With Behavioral Disturbance

Coding notes: Also code cerebrovascular condition on axis III

Adapted from The American Psychiatric Association. *Diagnostic and Statistical Manual of Mental Disorders.* 4th ed. Text rev. Washington, DC: American Psychiatric Association; 2000.

TABLE 12.33

Comparison of Alzheimer and Vascular Dementia

	Alzheimer	Vascular
Epidemiology	The most common cause of dementia (55%–65% of all cases) Prevalence doubles with every 5 years of age between the ages of 65 and 85 years. Affects women 3 times as often as men	The second most common cause of dementia (10% of all cases) although the incidence has decreased due to better standards of care, improved diagnostic techniques, and lifestyle changes. It affects men twice as much as women
Risk factors	Age Gender Family history: Risk is 4 times greater if a 1st-degree relative has the disease Down syndrome History of head trauma Risk is 2 times greater Low level of education: An uneducated person older than 75 years is 2 times as likely to develop Alzheimer than someone with 8 years of education	Identical to those of coronary artery disease: Hypercholesterolemia, smoking, hypertension, diabetes, obesity, sedentary lifestyle, and family history of CVA or CAD
Evaluation	Neuroimaging and laboratory evaluation are only useful to rule out other causes of dementia Confirmatory diagnosis can only be made with a postmortem examination of the brain	Differentiated from Alzheimer on the basis of the early appearance of neurological signs and radiographic evidence of cerebral ischemia. MRI (without contrast) will show evidence of prior infarcts
Treatment	See Table 12.34	Primary and secondary prevention of cerebrovascular disease is the mainstay of treatment. Anticoagulation and platelet inhibition (see section on CVAs) are useful for treating ongoing TIAs or for preventing further CVAs, but there is no medical treatment available to improve mental functioning after a CVA

CAD indicates coronary artery disease; CVA, cerebrovascular accident; MRI, magnetic resonance imaging; TIA, transient ischemic attack.

TABLE 12.34

Medications for the Treatment of Alzheimer Disease

Drug (Trade Name)	Initial Dose	Maintenance Dose	Side Effects
Cholinesterase Inhibitors			
Tacrine (Cognex)	10 mg qid	40–160 mg/d	Headache, dizziness, nausea, vomiting, diarrhea, elevated LFTs
Donepezil (Aricept)	5 mg qhs	5–10 mg/d	Headache, nausea, diarrhea
Rivastigmine (Exelon)	1.5 mg bid	6–12 mg/d in 2 divided doses	Nausea, vomiting, abdominal pain, loss of appetite, dizziness, headache
Galantamine (Reminyl)	4 mg bid	16–24 mg/d in 2 divided doses	Dizziness, headache, nausea, vomiting
Miscellaneous			
Selegiline (Eldepryl)	NA	5 mg bid	Nausea, dizziness, abdominal pain, confusion
Ginkgo biloba	NA	120–240 mg/d in 2–3 divided doses	Mild GI upset, headache, dizziness, palpitations, bleeding
Vitamin E	NA	400 IU/d	Rare: nausea, diarrhea, cramps, fatigue, headache

bid indicates twice daily; GI, gastrointestinal; NA, not applicable; qid, four times daily.

TABLE 12.35

Functional Assessment in Patients With Dementia*

Activities of daily living (ADLs)	*Personal self-care* Feeding, bathing, toileting *Mobility* Ability to move from bed to a chair or standing position, ability to walk (with or without assistive devices) or use a wheelchair Continence Frequency of urinary and fecal incontinence
Instrumental activities of daily living (IADLs)	*Within the home* Cooking, housecleaning, laundry, management of bank accounts, ability to use the telephone, management of medications *Outside the home* Shopping, ability to use necessary transportation

*Patients should be evaluated for their level of dependence on others for both ADLs and IADLs.

PARKINSON DISEASE

TABLE 12.36

Clinical Signs and Symptoms*

Resting tremor	Usually asymmetrical early in the clinical course but becomes bilateral in later stages. It involves limbs, hand ("pill-rolling" tremor), jaw, face, and tongue
Rigidity	An attempt to passively move a patient's limb may reveal "cogwheel" rigidity in which the limb will "lock" intermittently during the passive range of motion
Bradykinesia	Slowing of activities of daily living, masked facies, dysarthria and drooling. Patients may also demonstrate micrographia (slow and small handwriting)
Postural instability	Occurs in the more advanced stages of the disease. Patients walk with small steps in a shuffling gait. They may also demonstrate festination (a tendency to fall forward or backward while attempting to right oneself by taking rapid steps)

*The presence of the signs and symptoms in this table along with a good clinical response to empiric levodopa or dopamine agonists is sufficient to make the diagnosis. Magnetic resonance imaging may be performed to rule out other diagnoses (stroke, intoxications, or other degenerative disorders).

TABLE 12.37

Drugs Commonly Used for Parkinson Disease

Drug	Availability	Frequency and Administration	Comments
Dopamine Precursor			
Levodopa/ carbidopa (Sinemet)	10/100-, 25/100-, 25/250-, and 50/200- (as Sinemet CR) mg tablets	tid (bid for Sinemet CR)	Less effective as disease progresses; "on-off effect"; dose-related dyskinesias, anorexia, nausea, hypotension, mental status changes. Taper gradually on discontinuance
COMT Inhibitors			**Adjuncts to Carbidopa/ Levodopa**
Entacapone (Comtan)	200-mg tablet	Up to 8 times daily	Use with caution in patients with hypotension or liver dysfunction
Tolcapone (Tasmar)	100-mg tablet 200-mg tablet	tid	Orthostatic hypotension diarrhea, hallucinations may occur. Use with caution in renal or hepatic dysfunction
Dopamine Agonists			
Bromocriptine (Parlodel)	1.25-mg tablets	qd for 3 days, then increase up to 15–30 mg qd-bid with meals	Dopamine antagonist; adjunctive treatment with levodopa
Pergolide (Permax)	0.05-mg tablets	qd for 3 days, then increase up to 1.5–3.0 mg qd-tid	Same as bromocriptine
Ropirinole (Requip)	0.25-, 0.5-, 1-, 2-, 5-mg tablets	tid	Titrate dose in weekly increments. Syncope with bradycardia, hypotension, and GI effects may occur

Drug	Availability	Frequency and Administration	Comments
Pramipexole (Mirapex)	0.125-, 0.25-, 0.5-, 1-, 1.25-, 1.5-mg tablets	tid	Titrate dose gradually. Postural hypotension, dizziness, somnolence, nausea, and constipation may occur. Caution in patients with renal dysfunction and preexisting dyskinesias
Anticholinergics			
Trihexyphenidyl (Artane)	2- and 5-mg tablets; 0.4-mg/mL elixir; 5-mg sustained release capsules	tid: tablets and elixir qd-bid: Sustained release capsules	Additive to other agents. Side effects include dry mouth, constipation, urinary retention, glaucoma exacerbation, impaired mental status
Benztropine mesylate (Cogentin)	0.5-, 1-, and 2-mg tablets; 1-mg/mL injectable	bid	Same as trihexyphenidyl. May help control tremor only
Monoamine Oxidase Inhibitor			
Selegiline (Eldepryl)	5-mg tablets	bid	Side effects include nausea and orthostasis. Interaction with Prozac and Demerol
Other			
Amantadine	100-mg capsules	bid-tid (reduce with renal impairment)	Initial dose is 100 mg daily. Used to treat early disease or as an adjunct to main therapy. Initial effect reached in 48 hours. Half-life is 2–4 hours

bid indicates twice daily; GI, gastrointestinal; qd, once daily; tid, three times daily.

NEURODIAGNOSTIC TOOLS

TABLE 12.38

Preferred Initial Imaging Study by Clinical Presentation

Clinical Presentation	CT Without Contrast	CT With Contrast	MRI Without Contrast	MRI With Contrast
Trauma	**XX**			
Stroke	**XX**			
Seizure	**a**	**a**	**a**	**XX**
Infection	**a**	**a**	**a**	**XX**
Cancer	**a**	**a**	**a**	**XX**
Acute headache	**XX**			
Chronic headache			**XX**	
Dementia			**XX**	
Coma	**XX**			

Adapted from Brant WE, Helms CA. *Fundamentals of Diagnostic Radiology*. 2nd ed. Philadelphia, PA: Lippincott Williams & Wilkins; 1999.

XX indicates best study to obtain; a, acceptable in certain situations.

TABLE 12.39

Lumbar Puncture Technique

1. Place patient on side on a firm mattress or padded examination table.
2. Flex patient with thighs on abdomen and neck moderately flexed.
3. Palpitate L4 spinous process at level of iliac crest. Needle should be inserted into interspace either above (L3–L4) or below (L4–L5) this landmark.
4. Clean skin if necessary with soap and water.
5. Swab an area from the puncture site with an 8- to 10-inch radius with Merthiolate, iodine, or povidone-iodine solution.
6. Drape sterile towels over area, leaving an opening at the puncture site.
7. Use sterile gloves and inject 1–2 mL of local anesthetic (eg, 1% Xylocaine) about 2 cm into the interspace.
8. Use a 20-gauge spinal needle with stylet, in the midline, angulated 5–15° cephalad; advance slowly.
9. If needle meets bone, withdraw partially and redirect.
10. Withdraw stylet every 2–3 mm to see if CSF appears; usually a slight "click" will be felt on entering the subdural space.
11. When this occurs, advance the needle 2–3 mm more, and withdraw the stylet.
12. Determine opening pressure with manometer.
13. Withdraw 1 mL in each of four tubes, and send first tube for cultures and gram stain, second for WBC and RBC, third for glucose and protein, and fourth for other indicated studies (eg, viral titers or cultures, india ink prep, fungal cultures, VDRL, rickettsial titers, or cytologies).
14. Use same procedure for infant, except use a 22-gauge, 1½-inch spinal needle; have assistant hold patient in sitting position and obtain approximately 0.5 mL per tube.
15. If tap is bloody, centrifuge 1–2 mL. If supernatant is clear, the tap is probably traumatic; if it is xanthochromic, the blood was probably present before the tap.

CSF indicates cerebrospinal fluid; RBC, red blood cell count; WBC, white blood cell count.

TABLE 12.40

Normal CSF Values

Substance	Normal CSF Value
Protein (g/dL)	0.028 (28 mg/dL)
Glucose (mg/dL)	50 to 80
pH	7.3
Opening pressure	10–20 cm H_2O
WBC	0–5 cells/mm^3
RBC	0 cells/mm^3
Color	Clear, colorless
Differential	Mononuclear cells

Adapted from Goetz CG, ed. *Textbook of Clinical Neurology*. Philadelphia, PA: WB Saunders; 1999.

CSF indicates cerebrospinal fluid; RBC, red blood cell count; WBC, white blood cell count.

TABLE 12.41

Selected Disorders and Associated CSF Studies

Disorder	Expected Results	Comments
Meningitis (purulent)	↑ protein, ↓ glucose, ↑ CSF PMNs, (+) gram stain and culture, ↑ opening pressure	(+) cryptococcal antigen and india ink in cryptococcal meningitis
	↑ lactic acid	Mononuclear cells possible in partially treated bacterial meningitis
Meningitis (aseptic)	↑ protein, normal glucose, ↑ CSF WBC (10 to 1000 mononuclear cells/mm^3)	PMNs possible in early aseptic meningitis
Subarachnoid hemorrhage	↑ ↑ protein, ↓ glucose, ↑ ↑ RBC, ↑ WBC, xanthochromia	Protein is normal or significantly ↓, glucose is normal or slightly ↑
Multiple sclerosis	↑ protein, mildly ↑ WBC, normal glucose, oligoclonal bands, myelin basic protein, ↑ IgG index	Abnormal CSF in 90% of cases; Protein and cell counts normal in 2/3 of cases
Pseudotumor cerebri	↑ protein, normal cell counts, ↑ opening pressure (250 to 600 mm H_2O)	CSF removal may be therapeutic in some cases

Adapted from Goetz CG, ed. *Textbook of Clinical Neurology*. Philadelphia: WB Saunders; 1999.
CSF indicates cerebrospinal fluid; RBC, red blood cell count; WBC, white blood cell count.

TABLE 12.42

Alternative Therapies That Are Possibly Effective for Disorders of the Nervous System

	Dose	Drug Interactions	Adverse Effects	Contraindications
Seizures in Children				
Medium chain triglycerides (MCT)	60% of caloric intake is from MCT	None known	GI upset, irritability, and essential fatty acid deficiency	Cirrhosis, diabetes, mechanical ventilation
Headache				
Magnesium (cluster and migraine)	1 g IV	Nifedipine, fluoroquinolones, muscle relaxants, diuretics	Urticaria	Elderly, heart block, renal disease, malabsorption syndromes
Melatonin (cluster prevention)	10 mg po qhs. People should not drive for 4 to 5 hours after dose	Procardia XL, immuno-suppressants	Depression, drowsiness, dizziness, fatigue, abdominal cramps, reduced alertness	Cancer, cerebral palsy, hypertension, depression, liver disease, seizures

	Dose	Drug Interactions	Adverse Effects	Contraindications
Olive oil (migraine prevention in adolescents)	Preparations containing 1382 mg of oleic acid qd	May potentiate antihypertensives	Hypoglycemia in diabetics, biliary colic	Gallstones
Peppermint oil (tension)	10% peppermint oil in ethanol solution applied topically to forehead and temples, q 15–30 min	H_2 blockers and antacids can decrease the effect of peppermint oil	Skin irritation and contact dermatitis	Achlorhydria
Chasteberry	20–40 mg po qd	Oral contraceptives, antipsychotics	GI upset, nausea, urticaria, rash, acne, and metrorrhagia	In vitro fertilization
Feverfew (migraine prevention)	50–100 mg po qhs	Anticoagulants, NSAIDs may reduce feverfew effectiveness	None known	

Continued

TABLE 12.42

Alternative Therapies That Are Possibly Effective for Disorders of the Nervous System, cont'd

	Dose	Drug Interactions	Adverse Effects	Contraindications
Neuropathic Pain				
Magnesium	500–1000 mg IV q 4 h	Nifedipine, fluoroquinolones, muscle relaxants, diuretics	Urticaria	Elderly, heart block, renal disease, malabsorption syndromes
Vertigo				
Ginkgo leaf	120–160 mg divided tid	Anticoagulants, MAOIs, trazodone, thiazide diuretics, interferes with cytochrome P450	GI upset, headache, dizziness, palpitations, constipation, allergic skin reactions	Bleeding disorders, diabetes, infertility, seizures
Cerebrovascular Disease				
Mesoglycan	100–144 mg po qd	May increase bleeding risk in people on anticoagulants	GI upset, headache, diarrhea, local cutaneous reactions	Bleeding disorders
Vinpocetine	5–10 mg po tid	May potentiate anticoagulants and anti-hypertensives	GI upset, facial flushing, hypotension, headache, sleep disturbances	Bleeding disorders

	Dose	Drug Interactions	Adverse Effects	Contraindications
Dementia				
Ginkgo leaf	120–240 mg divided TID	Anticoagulants, MAOIs, trazodone, thiazide diuretics, interferes with cytochrome P450	GI upset, headache, dizziness, palpitations, constipation, allergic skin reactions	Bleeding disorders, diabetes, infertility, seizures
Acetyl-L-carnitine	1500–4000 mg qd	None known	Nausea and vomiting, agitation	None known
Huperzine A	50–200 μg bid	Anticholinergics, acetylcholinesterase inhibitors	Nausea, sweating, blurred vision, hyperactivity, anorexia, bradycardia, fasciculations	Asthma, PUD, seizures
Parkinson				
Phenylalanine	200–500 mg per day	MAOIs, levodopa, neuroleptics	Birth defects, exacerbates tremor in patients on levodopa	Schizophrenia, hypertension, stroke

Adapted from Natural Medicines Comprehensive Database; www.naturalcatabase.com. Copyright 1995–2001, Therapeutic Research, Stockton, CA.

bid indicates twice daily; GI, gastrointestinal; IV, intravenously; MAOI, monoamine oxidase inhibitor; NSAID, nonsteroidal anti-inflammatory drug; po, orally; qd, once daily; tid, three times daily.

FURTHER EDUCATION

TABLE 12.43

Online Resources

Internet	www.mdconsult.com
	www.webmd.com
	www.aafp.org
	www.ama-assn.org
	www.stroke.org
	www.mayohealth.org
	www.naturaldatabase.com
Personal Digital Assistants	www.epocrates.com
	www.journaltogo.com
	www.handheldmed.com
	www.pdamd.com
	www.palm.com

chapter 13

The Heart and Vascular System

Mrunal Shah, MD

IN THIS CHAPTER

- Overview statement
- Evaluation of the heart
- Hypertension
- Hyperlipidemia
- Coronary heart disease
- Bacterial endocarditis
- Peripheral vascular disease
- Advanced cardiac life support
- Other cardiac conditions

BOOKSHELF RECOMMENDATIONS

- Braunwald E, Zipes DP, Libby P, eds. *Heart Disease: A Textbook of Cardiovascular Medicine*. 6th ed. Philadelphia, PA: WB Saunders Company; 2001.
- Cummins RO. *ACLS Provider Manual*. Dallas, TX: American Heart Association; 2001.
- Alpert JS, Dalen JE, Rahimtoola SH, eds. *Valvular Heart Disease*. 3rd ed. Philadelphia, PA: Lippincott Williams & Wilkins; 2000.
- Kaplan NM, Lieberman E, Neal W. *Kaplan's Clinical Hypertension*. 8th ed. Philadelphia, PA: Lippincott Williams & Wilkins; 2002.
- Siberry GK, Iannone R, Childs B. *The Harriet Lane Handbook: A Manual for Pediatric House Officers*. 15th ed. St Louis, MO: Mosby, Inc; 2000.

EVALUATION OF THE HEART

FIGURE 13.1

Heart Sounds and Murmurs

Normal Splitting

Wide Splitting
Right Bundle Branch Block

Pulmonic Stenosis

Atrial Septal Defect

Mitral Regurgitation
or
Ventricular Septal Defect

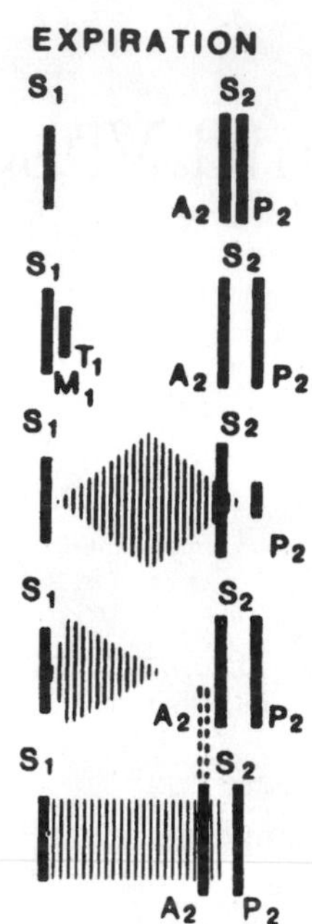

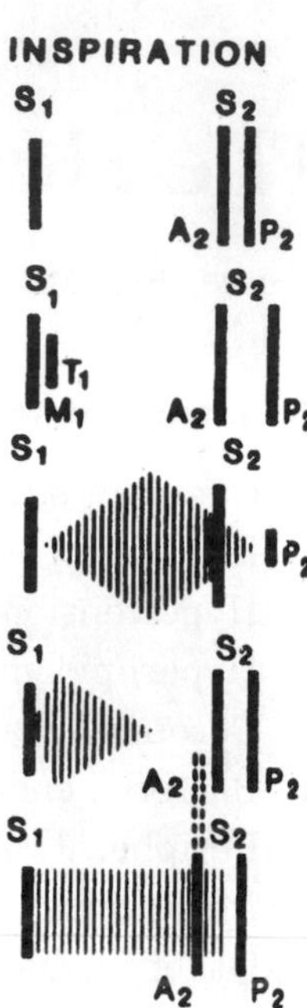

FIGURE 13.2

Extra Heart Sounds*

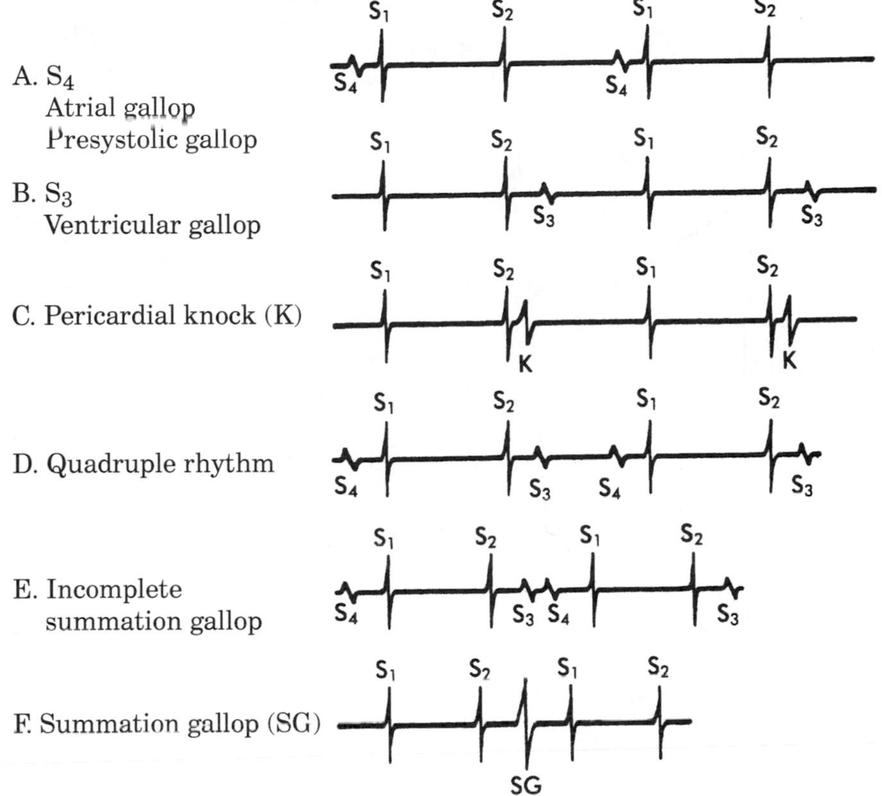

Reproduced with permission from the American Heart Association. (*Examination of the heart, Part IV: Auscultation of the heart*; 1990.)

*Diastolic filling sounds. (**A**) Fourth heart sound (S_4) occurs in presystole and is frequently called atrial or presystolic gallop. (**B**) Third heart sound (S_3) occurs during rapid phase of ventricular filling. It is normal and commonly heard in children and young adults, disappearing with increasing age. In middle age, it is called *pathological S_3*, or *ventricular gallop*, and indicates ventricular dysfunction or atrioventricular valve incompetence. (**C**) In constrictive pericarditis, sound in early diastole (K) is earlier, louder, and higher pitched than usual pathological S_3. (**D**) Quadruple rhythm results if both S_4 and S_3 are present. (**E**) At faster heart rates, these sounds occurring in rapid succession may give the illusion of mid-diastolic rumble. (**F**) When the heart rate is sufficiently fast, two rapid phases of ventricular filling reinforce each other and loud summation gallop (SG) may appear; this may be louder than either S_3 or S_4 alone.

FIGURE 13.3

Composite Image of Cardiac Physiology

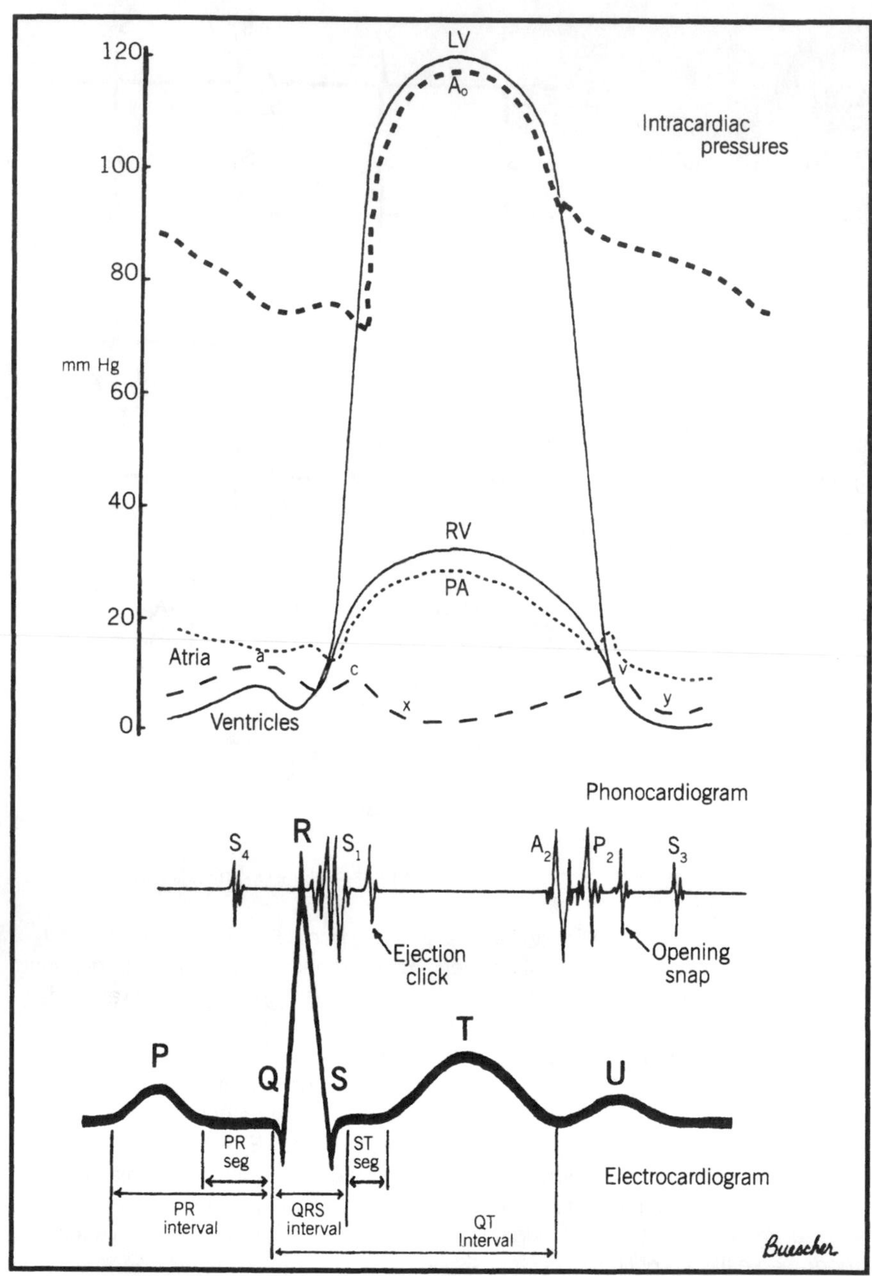

Reproduced with permission from Elsevier Science. (Siberry GK, Iannone R, Childs B. *The Harriet Lane Handbook: A Manual for Pediatric House Officers*. 15th ed. St. Louis: Mosby, Inc; 2000.)

TABLE 13.1

Grading Heart Murmers

Grading of Murmurs (classification of Freeman and Levine)
Grade 1: Murmur very difficult to hear and not immediately apparent
Grade 2: Faintest murmur immediately heard
Grade 3: Intermediate intensity
Grade 4: Intermediate intensity with thrill
Grade 5: Loudest murmur heard with rim of stethoscope touching skin
Grade 6: Murmur audible with stethoscope removed from chest wall

Nonorganic (innocent)
Systolic: Usually heard at the pulmonic area, second left interspace or at the left border of the sternum or in the mitral area. It is not transmitted and is unaccompanied by hypertrophy of the heart or any other evidence of abnormality. It is usually heard only in the sitting position and changes with position.

Organic
Mitral regurgitation: Systolic; maximum intensity at apex, transmitted to axilla, heard behind at angle of scapula. Accentuation of pulmonic second sound.

Aortic stenosis: Systolic; maximum intensity at right second interspace close to sternum. Transmitted upward into great vessels of the neck.

Aortic regurgitation: Diastolic; replaces or follows the second sound. Maximum intensity at second right interspace, radiating to third and downward.

Mitral stenosis: Presystolic; running into snapping first sound. Heart in mitral area. Not transmitted. Usually accompanied by a thrill along left margin of heart area.

TABLE 13.2

Heart Murmurs and Maneuvers to Differentiate Them

Maneuver	AS	IHSS	MR	MVP
Isometric—squeeze hands	Decrease	Decrease	Increase	No change
Valsalva—causes decreased ventricular filling	Decrease	Increase	Decrease	Increase
Squatting—increases venous return and arteriolar resistance	No change	Decrease	Increase	Decrease
Standing—decreases heart size	Increase	Increase	Decrease	Increase
Amyl nitrite—decrease in left ventricular volume and pressure	Increase	Increase	Decrease	Increase

IHSS indicates idiopathic hypertrophic subaortic stenosis.

TABLE 13.3

Evaluation of Murmurs

Physical, Roentgenographic, or Electrocardiographic Feature	Mitral Regurgitation	Ventricular Septal Defect	Tricuspid Regurgitation	Aortic Stenosis
Systolic murmur	Harsh and pansystolic	Harsh and pansystolic	Pansystolic	Ejection, crescendo-decrescendo
Primary location of murmur	Apex	Left sternal border	Left sternal border	Base of heart; occasionally apical
Radiation of murmur	Axilla; occasionally base and neck	Left precordium		Carotids
Thrill	Occasionally present at apex	Usually present at left sternal border	Rare	Occasionally present at base
Murmur with inspiration	No change	No change	Increases	No change
Valsalva maneuver	May increase	Increases or no change	No change	Decreases
Venous pressure	Often normal	Slightly elevated with prominent A and V waves	Elevated, with very prominent V waves	Usually normal
Pulsatile liver	No	No	Yes	No
Pulmonary component of S_2	Normal; occasionally increased	Normal or loud; usually delayed	Usually increased	Normal
Apical impulse	Hyperkinetic; occasionally heaving	Hyperkinetic	Weak or normal	Forceful and sustained
Electrocardiogram	Left ventricular hypertrophy; left atrial hypertrophy	Biventricular hypertrophy (Katz-Wachtel phenomenon)	Right ventricular hypertrophy; occasional right atrial hypertrophy	Left ventricular hypertrophy with associated ST-T changes
Chest roentgenogram	Moderately enlarged, marked left atrial enlargement	Enlarged left and right ventricle	Enlarged right ventricle	Often normal heart size or left ventricular hypertrophy

Adapted from Haffajee CI: Chronic mitral regurgitation. In: Dalen JS. *Valvular Heart Disease*. 2nd ed. Boston: Little, Brown and Company; 1987:141.

ELECTROCARDIOGRAPHY

TABLE 13.4

Electrical Events

Evaluate each electrical component of the electrocardiogram using the following tables of normal values.

P Wave

Upright in I, II, and aV_F
Inverted in III, aV_R
Amplitude should not exceed 2 or 3 mm

PR Interval

Becomes shorter as the rate rises

Age	Average Interval
1 year	0.11 seconds
6 years	0.13 seconds
12 years	0.14 seconds
Adult	0.12–0.20 seconds

QRS Complex

Normal: 0.04–0.10 second
Normal variant or conduction delay: 0.10–0.12 second
Right or left bundle-branch block: 0.12 second

If the QRS is greater than 0.12 second and occurs before the expected sinus beat, the following may be helpful in diagnosis:

Feature	RBBB Morphology	QRS	Direction of Initial 0.02 second of QRS
Ventricular ectopy	60%–70%	Monophasic in V1 or triphasic R > R	Different from normal beats
Supraventricular beat with aberrancy	90%	Triphasic R < R	Same as normal beat

RBBB indicates right bundle-branch block.

TABLE 13.5

Drugs That Will Affect the ECG

Drug	Effect	Toxicity
Disopyramide	Prolonged QT Widened QRS	AV block Ventricular dysrhythmia
Quinidine	Prolonged QT Widened QRS	Intraventricular block Ventricular dysrhythmia
Procainamide	Prolonged QT Widened QRS	Intraventricular block Ventricular dysrhythmia
Digitalis	Depression of ST segment	PVCs, PAT, AV block 1, 2, 3
Tricyclic antidepresants	Prolonged conduction time	Dysrhythmia, tachycardia
Encainide	Widened QRS Unchanged or prolonged QT	Ventricular dysrhythmia AV block
Flecainide	Widened QRS Prolonged PR Unchanged or prolonged QT	Ventricular dysrhythmia First-degree AV block Intraventricular block
Amiodarone	Prolonged PR Prolonged QT	Ventricular dysrhythmia SA node dysfunction AV block Intraventricular block

ECG indicates electrocardiogram; AV, atrioventricular; PVCs, premature ventricular contractions; PAT, paroxysmal atrial tachycardia; and SA, sinoatrial.

PR PROLONGATION

A PR prolongation is a delay or interruption in conduction between the atria and ventricles. First-degree atrioventricular (AV) block has a PR interval of greater than 0.20 second.

FIGURE 13.4

Causes of PR Prolongation

<table>
<tr><td colspan="3">Second- or third-degree AV block (atrial rate greater than ventricular rate)</td></tr>
<tr><td colspan="3">Does PR interval vary?</td></tr>
<tr><td colspan="2">YES</td><td>NO</td></tr>
<tr><td colspan="2">Does R-R length vary?</td><td rowspan="2">Second-degree block
■ 2:1 block
or
■ Mobitz II</td></tr>
<tr><td>YES

Second-degree block
■ Mobitz I (Wenkebach)</td><td>NO

Third-degree block
■ Junctional rate 40–60 narrow complexes
■ Ventricular rate 20–40 wide complexes</td></tr>
</table>

TABLE 13.6
QRS Derangements

Right Bundle-Branch Block (RBBB)
QRS > 0.12 second
V_1: Late intrinsicoid, M-shaped QRS
V_6: Early intrinsicoid
I: Wide S wave

Incomplete RBBB
Same as above except QRS < 0.12 second

Left Bundle-Branch Block (LBBB)
QRS > 0.12 second
V_1: Early intrinsicoid
V_2: Late intrinsicoid, no Q wave
I: Monophasic R

Left Anterior Hemiblock
Normal QRS duration
Left axis deviation
Small Q in I, and R in III

Left Posterior Hemiblock
Normal QRS duration
Right axis deviation
Small R in I and Q in III
No evidence of right ventricular hypertrophy

Right and Left Bundle-Branch Block Are Associated With the Following:
Coronary artery disease
Hypertensive cardiovascular disease
Rheumatic heart disease
Cardiomyopathy
Myocarditis
Nonspecific fibrosis
Trauma

RBBB Only	LBBB Only
Congenital heart disease	Aortic valvular disease
Pulmonary embolism	Short left main coronary artery
Cor pulmonale	

AXIS DEVIATION

FIGURE 13.5

Calculation of Axis Deviation

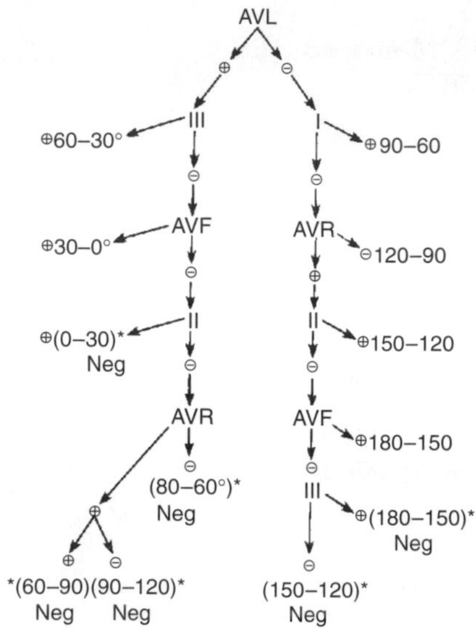

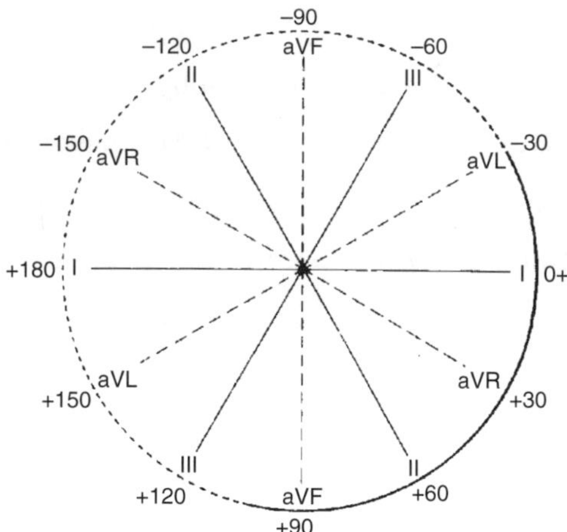

TABLE 13.7

Method to Calculate Axis Deviation

To determine the axis, proceed through the vector flow sheet shown in Figure 13.5, looking at each QRS complex on the electrocardiogram (ECG) to decide if it is positive or negative. Start with the QRS in aV_L. Work through each QRS in the limb of the flowsheet until a range is identified, then go to the axis diagram in Figure 13.5 to find the area of the range you have determined.

Look at each lead on the ECG bounding that range to determine which has the QRS of greatest magnitude. The vector is in the direction closest to that lead.

Example:
Range: −60 to −90
aV_F's QRS is greater in magnitude than III's → vector is −90.

Interpretation of axis
−30 to +90: Normal axis
−30 to −90: Left axis deviation
+90 to +180: Right axis deviation
−90 to +180: Marked right axis deviation

ST AND T WAVE CHANGES

FIGURE 13.6

Common ST Changes

ST-T CHANGES

A Normal

B Early Repolarization

C Epicardial Injury

D Subendocardial Injury

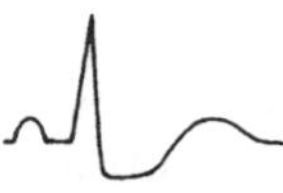

E Digitalis

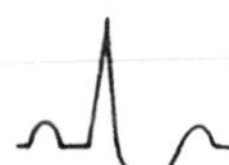

F Hypokalemia Quinidine, Cerebral Hemorrhage

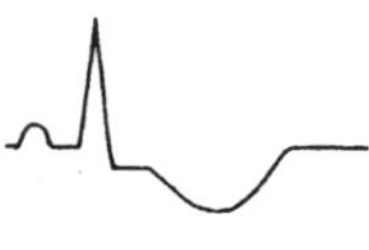

G Strain

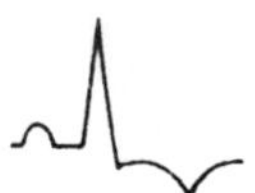

FIGURE 13.7

Progression of ST Changes in Ischemia

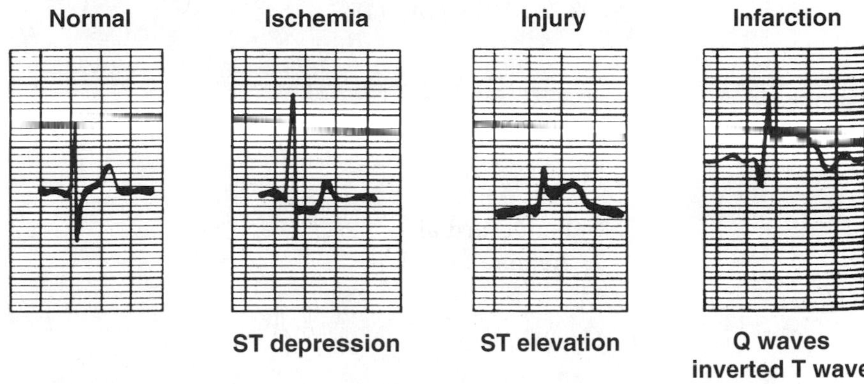

FIGURE 13.8

T Wave Changes

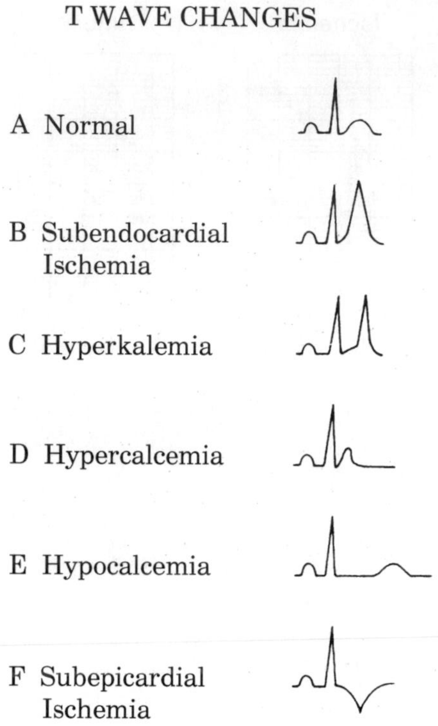

T WAVE CHANGES

A Normal

B Subendocardial Ischemia

C Hyperkalemia

D Hypercalcemia

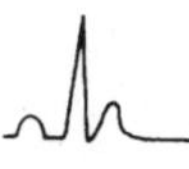

E Hypocalcemia

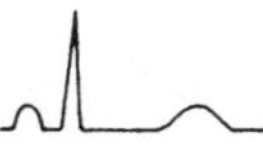

F Subepicardial Ischemia

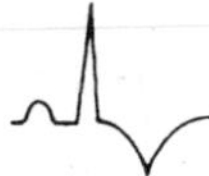

TABLE 13.8

Localization of Disease

Area of Ischemia	ECG Changes	Coronary Artery
Anteroseptal	V_1–V_4	LAD
Anterior	V_3–V_5	Prox LAD
Inferior wall	II, III, aV_F	Right 80%, Left circ 20%
Inferior wall with posterior involvement	II, III, aV_F and R in V_1	Left circ
Apical	V_2–V_5 and II, III, aV_F	Distal LAD
Lateral wall	V_5, V_6	Nondominant circ

ECG indicates electrocardiogram; LAD, left anterior descending.

HYPERTENSION

TABLE 13.9
Hypertension

Staging				
Category	**Systolic**	**Diastolic**	**Follow-up**	**Treat**
Optimal	<120 and	<80	2–5 years	
Normal	<130 and	<85	In 2 years	
High-normal	130–139 or	85–89	In 1 year	If high risk
Hypertension				
Stage 1	140–159 or	90–99	2 months	If high risk
Stage 2	160–179 or	100–109	1 month	Any risk
Stage 3	>180 or	>110	1 week	Any risk

Diagnostic Dilemmas	
White-coat hypertension	A common clinical dilemma faced by clinicians is the "white-coat"syndrome. Many patients, as many as 30%, will have normal ambulatory blood pressure readings, but still have consistently elevated readings while in the office. Although long-term data are unclear, over a 5- to 10-year interval, very little if any cardiovascular damage is found.
Isolated systolic hypertension in the elderly	The tendency of physicians in treating the elderly is to avoid therapy unless necessary. The systolic pressure is more closely associated with morbidity and mortality than the diastolic pressure. Therefore, treatment should be aggressive with isolated systolic hypertension. The goals are the same of <140/<90 mm Hg. However, it is acceptable to watch blood pressures of <160 mm Hg while titrating doses. Always consider secondary causes of hypertension if they truly present after 60 years of age.
Treatment options	Treatment should always include lifestyle modification, regardless of level of hypertension. This includes a decreased sodium, low-fat diet, increased cardiovascular exercise (30–40 minutes a day, >4 days/week), daily aspirin, and regular ambulatory checks of blood pressure. The decision to start medications depends on the level of hypertension and the number/type of risk factors. An individual with diabetes, heart disease, renal disease, or vascular disease should be treated even without hypertension. See below for recommendations. The individual with stage 2 or 3 hypertension needs medications regardless of risk factors. The following table gives recommendations for antihypertensive choice based on various patient profiles/characteristics.

TABLE 13.10

Secondary Causes of Hypertension

Causes	Screening Test
Coarctation	PA and lateral chest x-ray
Cushing syndrome	Plasma control after 1 mg dexamethasone suppression
Drugs Amphetamines, cocaine, oral contraceptives, estrogens, steroid or thyroid excess	Blood and/or urine screens
Increased intracranial pressure	CT scan of the head
Pheochromocytoma	Urine metanephrine or VMA clonidine suppression test
Primary aldosteronism Conn sydrome Idiopathic hyperaldosteronism	Serum potassium Stimulated plasma renin activity Urine potassium
Renovascular disease Renal parenchymal disease Chronic pyelonephritis Congenital renal disease Diabetic nephropathy Glomerulonephritis Gout Interstitial nephrophathy Obstructive uropathy Polycystic disease Renin-secreting tumors Vasculitis	Screening tests, different for each disease Consider imaging studies (U/S, IVP, CT, biopsy)
Renovascular hypertension	IVP Suppressed or stimulated plasma renin activity

PA indicates posteroanterior; CT, computed tomography; VMA, vanillylmandelic acid; U/S, unltrasound; IVP, intravenous pyelography.

TABLE 13.11

The Relationship of Renin and Aldosterone in Disease

Disease	Renin	Aldosterone	Diagnosis
Low renin state	Low	Low	Diabetes, renal insufficiency, fluid overload, and normal sodium
Pseudohypo-aldosteronism	Very high	Very high	Salt wasting with acidosis, hyperkalemia in infants
Gordon syndrome	Reduced	Reduced	Hyperkalemia, acidosis in the absence of renal insufficiency
Pseudohyper-aldosteronism	Elevated	Elevated	Licorice ingestion
Renovascular hypertension	Elevated or normal	Elevated or normal	Abnormal IVP, renal vein renins differ
Primary aldosteronism	None	Elevated	Hyperkalemia, hypertension
Renal tumor/cyst	Elevated	Elevated	Abnormal IVP or ultrasound

Adapted from Stein JH, ed. *Internal Medicine*. 4th ed. St. Louis: Mosby, Inc; 1994.

IVP indicates intravenous pyelogram.

TABLE 13.12

Patient Type and Antihypertensive Choice

Characteristic	Preferred Agent	Drugs to Avoid
African Americans	Monotherapy with diuretic or CCB	?β-blockers
Age <50	α-blocker, β-blocker, ACEI	Diuretic
Age >65	Thiazide, CCB, ACEI	Central α-agonist
Asthma/COPD	α-blocker, CCB, clonidine	β-blocker and ?ACEI
BPH	α-blocker	
Bradycardia, SSS	ACEI, ARB	β-blocker, central CCB
CAD	β-blocker, CCB, ACEI	Direct vasodilator
Caucasian	β-blocker, diuretic	
CHF	ACEI, diuretic, hydralazine, carvedilol, nitrates	CCB
Chronic liver disease	Diuretic, α-blocker, clonidine	β-blocker, methyldopa
Depression	α-blocker, ACEI, CCB	Reserpine, β-blocker
DM	ACEI, α-blocker, CCB	Caution with β-blocker, diuretic
Erectile dysfunction	α-blocker, ACEI, CCB	β-blocker, diuretic
Glaucoma	β-blocker, clonidine, diuretic	
Gout	α-blocker, ACEI, CCB	Diuretic, β-blocker
Hyperlipidemia	α-blocker, ACEI, CCB	Diuretic, β-blocker
Isolated systolic HTN	Diuretic, DHPCCB	β-blocker, vasodilator
Migraine HA	β-blocker, CCB	Vasodilator
Obesity	α-blocker, ACEI, CCB	β-blocker, diuretic
Osteoporosis	Thiazide diuretic	Loop diuretic
Physically active	α-blocker, ACEI, CCB	β-blocker
Pregnancy	Methyldopa, labetalol, hydralazine	β-blocker, diuretic, reserpine, ACEI
PVD	ACEI, CCB, α-blocker	β-blocker
Renal insufficiency	Loop diuretic, ACEI, CCB	Thiazide, K+sparing diuretic, possibly ACEI
TIA/CVA	ACEI, CCB	Central α-agonist

α-Blocker indicates alpha receptor blocking agent; ACEI, angiotensin-converting enzyme inhibitor; β-blocker, beta receptor blocking agent; CCB, calcium-channel blocking agent; DHPCCB, dihydropyridine calcium-channel blocking agent; COPD, chronic obstructive pulmonary disease; BPH, benign prostatic hypertrophy; SSS, sick sinus syndrome; ARB, angiotensin II receptor blocker; CAD, coronary artery disease; DM, diabetes mellitus; HTN, hypertension; HA, headache; PVD, peripheral vascular disease; TIA, transient ischemic attack; CVA, cerebrovascular accident.

FIGURE 13.9

JNC VI Hypertension Treatment Algorithm

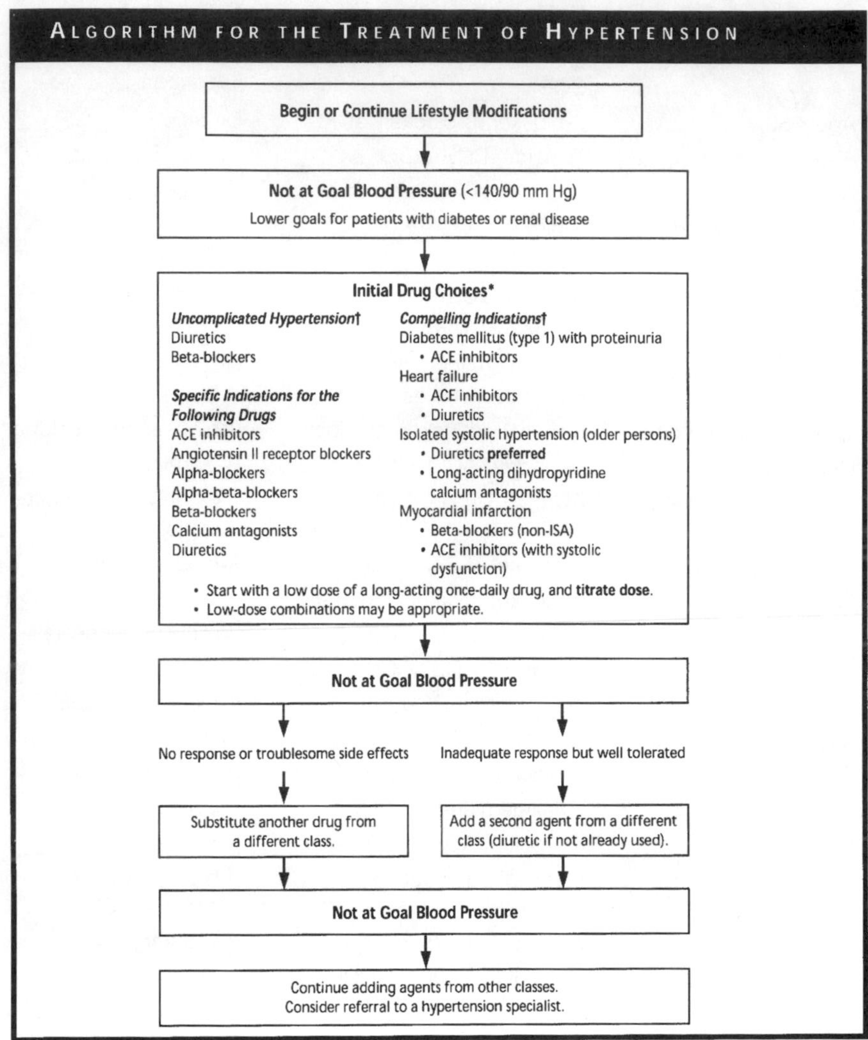

*Unless contraindicated. ACE indicates angiotensin-converting enzyme; ISA, intrinsic sympathomimetic activity.

†Based on randomized controlled trials.

TABLE 13.13

Beta Blockers

Generic Name	Trade Name	Dosage Range (mg/day)	Dosage Frequency	Ave Cost*	Comments
Nonselective Agents					β_1 selective agents
Nadolol	Corgard	20–240†	qd	$27	will inhibit β_2 in higher doses
Propranolol	Inderal	80–240†	bid	$8	All may aggravate asthma COPD, and CHF
Propranolol (long-acting)	Inderal LA	60–240†	qd	$68	Avoid using in insulin dependent diabetics;
Timolol	Blocadren	20–40†	bid	$12	all will block hypoglycemic symptoms
Cardioselective Agents					
Atenolol	Tenormin	25–100†	qd	$3	Reduce dose over 1–2 wks when discontinuing
Metoprolol	Lopressor	50–200†	bid	$10	
Metoprolol (long-acting)	Toprol XL	50–200†	qd	$37	No clear advantage for agents with ISA activity, and these are not cardioprotective after MI
Betaxolol	Kerlone	5–40	qd	$31	
Bisoprolol	Zebeta	5–20†	qd	$34	
Intrinsic Sympathomimetic Agents (ISA)					
Carteolol	Cartrol	2.5–10†	qd	$40	Increase incidence of bradycardia and conduction disturbances when used with verapamil and diltiazem.
Acebutolol	Sectral	400–1200†	bid	$52	
Pindolol	Visken	10–60†	bid	$28	

qd indicates daily; bid, twice daily; COPD, chronic obstructive pulmonary disease; CHF, congestive heart failure; ISA, intrinsic sympathomimetic activity; MI, myocardial infarction.

*Average cost for one month of therapy based on recommended dosage range.

†Dosage reductions are required in renal impairment and elderly.

TABLE 13.14

Calcium-Channel Blockers

Generic Name	Trade Name	Dosage Range (mg/d)	Dosage Frequency	Ave Cost*	Comments
Diltiazem	Cardizem	90–360	tid	$15	Verapamil and diltiazem may reduce heart rate and can cause heart block
Diltiazem (long-acting)	Cardizem CD, Tiazac, Cardizem SR, Diltia XT	120–360	qd	$41	
Verapamil	Calan, Isoptin	80–240	tid	$12	
Verapamil (long-acting)	Tarka, Calan SR, Verelan	120–360	qd	$28	
Dihyropyridines					Dihyropyridines are more potent vasodilators and can cause more dizziness, headache, flushing, peripheral edema, and tachycardia
Amlodipine	Norvasc	2.5–10	qd	$48	
Felodipine	Plendil	5–20	qd	$46	
Isradipine	DynaCirc	2.5–10	bid	$29	
Isradipine (long-acting)	DynaCirc CR	2.5–10	qd	$55	
Nicardipine	Cardene	20–40	tid	$25	
Nicardipine (long-acting)	Cardene SR	30–60	bid	$69	
Nifedipine	Procardia, Adalat	30–90	tid	$10	
Nifedipine (long-acting)	Procardia XL, Adalat CC	30–90	qd	$48	

tid indicates three times daily; qd, daily; bid, twice daily.

*Average cost for 1 month of therapy based on recommended dosage range.

TABLE 13.15

Angiotensin Converting Enzyme Inhibitors (ACEI)

Generic Name	Trade Name	Dosage Range (mg/d)	Dosage Frequency	Ave Cost*	Comments
Benazepril	Lotensin	10–40†	qd–bid	$20	Diuretic dosages should be reduced or DC before starting ACEI to prevent hypotension May cause hyperkalemia in patients with renal impairment or those taking K sparing agents Can cause ARF in patients with renal artery stenosis Contraindicated in renal artery stenosis and pregnancy S/E include rash, taste disturbances, hypotension, neutropenia, angioedema, and cough
Captopril	Capoten	25–450†	bid–tid	$15	
Enalapril	Vasotec	2.5–40†	qd–bid	$32	
Fosinopril	Monopril	10–40	qd	$28	
Lisinopril	Prinivil, Zestril	5–40†	qd–bid	$31	
Quinapril	Accupril	10–80†	qd–bid	$45	
Ramipril	Altace	2.5–20†	qd	$45	

qd indicates daily; bid, twice daily; tid, three times daily; DC, discontinued; ARF, acute renal failure; S/E, side effects.

*Average cost for one month of therapy based on recommended dosage range.
†Dosage reductions are required in renal impairment and elderly.

TABLE 13.16

Angiotensin Receptor Blockers (ARBs)

Generic Name	Trade Name	Dosage Range (mg/d)	Dosage Frequency	Ave Cost*	Comments
Candesartan	Atacand	8–32	qd	$47	Contraindicated in renal stenosis, biliary obstruction and pregnancy
Eprosartan	Teveten	400–800	qd	$36	Can cause hyperkalemia, especially when given with K supplements and diuretics
Irbesartan	Avapro	150–300	qd	$45	S/E of edema, URI, ↓ BUN/SCr, tachycardia,
Losartan	Cozaar	50–100†	qd	$47	and cough
Telmisartan	Micardis	40–80	qd	$40	
Valsartan	Diovan	80–160	qd	$43	

qd indicates daily; S/E, side effects; URI, upper respiratory infection; BUN, blood urea nitrogen; SCr, serum creatinine.

*Average cost for one month of therapy based on recommended dosage range.

†Dosage reductions are required in renal impairment and elderly.

HYPERLIPIDEMIA

TABLE 13.17

ATP III Classification of Cholesterol

LDL Cholesterol: Primary Target (mg/dL)	
<100	Optimal
100–129	Near optimal/above optimal
130–159	Borderline high
160–189	High
>190	Very high
Total Cholesterol (mg/dL)	
<200	Desirable
200–239	Borderline high
>240	High
HDL Cholesterol (mg/dL)	
<40	Low
>60	High
Triglycerides (mg/dL)	
<150	Normal
150–199	Borderline high
200–499	High
>500	Very high

Adapted with permission from NIH,NHLBI, NCEP Executive Summary, May 2001, Publication 01-3305.

LDL indicates low-density lipoprotein; HDL, high-density lipoprotein.

TABLE 13.18

Major Risk Factors That Modify LDL Goals

Cigarette smoking
Hypertension (BP > 140/90 mm Hg or on medication)
Low HDL cholesterol (<40)
Family history of premature CHD (First degree male <55 years old; first degree female <65 years old)
Age (men > 45 yo; women >55 years old)
An HDL >60 mm/dL counts as a "negative" risk factor, and removes one from the total count

Adapted with permissoin from NIH, NHLBI, NCEP Executive Summary, May 2001, Publication 01-3305.

LDL indicates low-density lipoprotein; BP, blood pressure; HDL, high-density lipoprotein; CHD, coronary heart disease.

TABLE 13.19

LDL Goals and Cutpoint for Therapy

Risk Category	LDL Goal (mg/dL)	LDL Level to Treat (mg/dL)
CHD or equivalents ▪ DM, AAA, CVA, TIA, PVD ▪ Metabolic syndrome	<100	>130
2+ risk factors	<130	>160
0–1 risk factors	<160	>190

Adapted with permission from NIH,NHLBI, NCEP Executive Summary, May 2001, Publication 01-3305.

LDL indicates low-density lipoprotein; CHD, coronary heart disease; DM, diabetes mellitus; AAA, abdominal aoritic aneurysm; CVA, cerebrovascular accident; TIA, transient ischemic attack; PVD, peripheral vascular disease.

TREATMENT OPTIONS

As with most other conditions, patients should always be on an aggressive diet and exercise routine for at least 3 months. The decision to start therapy is not without concern of side effects. The evidence is so compelling that it is difficult not to start therapy. Choosing the right drug is mostly dependent on reaching a goal LDL. However, goals for therapy can include reducing triglycerides, raising HDL, or all of the above. Tolerability becomes the last factor. Underlying hepatic disease may force the use of nicotinic derivatives or bile acid sequestrants. The following table reviews the treatment options taken from National Cholesterol Education Program tables.

TABLE 13.20

Drugs Affecting Lipid Metabolism

Drug Class	Agent's Generic Name (Brand Name)	Daily Doses	Lipid Lipoprotein Effects	Side Effects	Cautions
HMG CoA reductase inhibitors (statins)	Lovastatin (Mevacor) Pravastatin (Pravachol) Simvastatin (Zocor) Fluvastatin (Lescol) Atorvastatin (Lipitor)	20–80 mg 20–40 mg 20–80 mg 20–80 mg 10–80 mg	LDL ↓ 18%–55% HDL ↑ 5%–15% TG ↓ 7%–30%	Myopathy Increased liver enzymes	*Absolute*: Active or chronic liver disease *Relative*: Concomitant use of certain drugs*
Bile acid sequestrants	Cholestyramine (LoCHOLEST, Prevalite, Questran, LoCHOLEST light, Questran light) Colestipol (Colestid) Colesevelam (Welchol)	4–16 g 5–20 g 2.6–3.8 g	LDL ↓ 15%–30% HDL ↑ 3%–5% TG No change or increase	Gastrointestinal distress Constipation Decreased absorption of other drugs	*Absolute*: Dysbetalipoproteinemia TG >400 mg/dL *Relative*: TG >200 mg/dL

Continued

TABLE 13.20

Drugs Affecting Lipid Metabolism, cont'd

Drug Class	Agent's Generic Name (Brand Name)	Daily Doses	Lipid Lipoprotein Effects	Side Effects	Cautions
Nicotinic acid	Immediate release or crystalline (Niacor) Extended release (Niaspan)	1.5–3 g 1–2 g	LDL ↓ 5%–25% HDL ↑ 15%–35% TG ↓ 20%–50%	Flushing Hyperglycemia Hyperuricemia (or gout) Upper GI distress Hepatotoxicity	*Absolute*: Chronic liver disease Severe gout *Relative*: Diabetes Hyperuricemia Peptic ulcer disease
	Sustained release (various)	1–2 g			
Fibric acids	Gemfibrozil (Lopid, others) Fenofibrate (Tricor)	600 mg bid 160 mg	LDL ↓ 5%–20% *(may be increased in patients with high TG)* HDL ↑ 10%–20% TG ↓ 20%–50%	Dyspepsia Gallstones Myopathy	*Absolute*: Severe renal disease Severe hepatic disease

Adapted with permission from NCEP guidelines 2001, ATP III.

HMG CoA indicates hydroxymethyl glutaryl coenzyme A; LDL, low-density lipoprotein; HDL, high-density lipoprotein; TG, triglyceride; bid, twice daily; GI, gastrointestinal.

*Cyclosporine, macrolide antibiotics, various anti-fungal agents, and cytochrome P-450 inhibitors (fibrates and niacin should be used with appropriate caution).

CORONARY ARTERY DISEASE

TABLE 13.21

Risk Factors for Coronary Artery Disease

Male
Age >45 in men, >55 in women
Hypertension, controlled or uncontrolled
Hyperlipidemia, hypertriglyceridemia
Significant family history of premature heart disease
(First degree relative M < 55 or F < 65)
Diabetes mellitus
Obesity
Smoking history

TABLE 13.22

Characterization of Chest Pain

Typical	Atypical
Substernal chest discomfort	Sharp, dull, or other chest pain
Tightness, heaviness, or crushing	Radiation to back, abdomen, face
Radiates to left arm/shoulder and jaw/teeth	Fleeting or lasting hours/days
Lasts 10–20 minutes	Nonexertional
Exertional in onset, responds to rest	Isolated shortness of breath
Shortness of breath	Fatigue, malaise
Nausea	Palpitations
Diaphoresis	Tearing pain, acutely severe radiating to the back (think of dissection)
	Pleuritic chest pain (think of pulmonary embolism)
	Cough, dyspnea, fevers (think of pneumonia)

STRESS TESTING

TABLE 13.23

Cardiac Function Testing Modalities

Studies	Situation
Stress ECG	Intermediate pretest probability Not at extremes of age With 1 or 2 risk factors Nondiabetic Not at high or low risk for CHD No underlying ECG abnormalities (ST, T, or Q)
Stress perfusion scans	High pretest probability Diabetic Multiple risk factors Need for anatomy or flow states Postintervention risk stratification ECG abnormalities at rest Typical chest pain without risk factors
Catheterization	Typical chest pain and significant risk factors High pretest probability Known CAD Failed stress test Unstable angina

ECG indicates electrocardiogram; CHD, coronary heart disease; CAD, coronary artery disease.

MANAGING AMBULATORY ANGINA

TABLE 13.24

Nitrates Commonly Used for Angina Treatment

Preparation	Dosage	Onset (min)	Duration
Sublingual nitroglycerin	0.3–0.6 mg prn	2–5	10–30 min
Aerosol nitroglycerin	0.4 mg prn	2–5	10–30 min
Oral isosorbide dinitrate	5–40 mg tid	30–60	4–6 h
Oral isosorbide mononitrate	10–20 mg bid	30–60	6–8 h
Oral isosorbide mononitrate-SR	30–120 mg/d	30–60	12–18 h
2% Nitroglycerin ointment	0.5–2.0 in tid	20–60	3–8 h
Transdermal nitroglycerin patches	5–15 mg/d	>60	12 h

Adapted from Department of Medicine, Washington University School of Medicine. *Washington Manual of Medical Therapeutics*. 30th ed. Philadelphia: Lippincott Williams & Wilkins; 2001.

SR indicates sustained-release preparation; prn, as needed, tid, three times daily; bid, twice daily.

TABLE 13.25
Diagnosis of Acute Myocardial Infarction

History	Typical chest pain High pretest probability
ECG Changes In contiguous leads	ST segment elevation or depression T wave inversion New LBBB (left bundle-branch block) New Q wave New-onset dysrhythmia (afib, VT, VF, etc)
Cardiac Markers In order of detectability	Troponin T Troponin I CPK (MB) AST (SGOT) LDH
Imaging	CXR with CHF Abnormal echo, thallium or MIBI scans Consider primary left heart catheterization
Differential Diagnosis	Thoracic aneurysm Pericarditis Pneumonia Pulmonary embolus Pneumothorax Trauma

ECG indicates electrocardiogram; afib, atrial fibrillation; VT, ventricular tachycardia; VF, ventricular fibrillation; CPK (MB), creatine phosphokinase (MB fraction); AST, aspartate aminotransferase; SGOT, serum glutamic oxaloacetic transaminase; LDH, lactate dehydrogenase; CXR, chest x-ray; CHF, congestive heart failure; MIBI, technetium Tc 99m sestamibi.

FIGURE 13.10

Enzyme Levels after Myocardial Infarction

Plot of the appearance of cardiac markers in blood vs time after onset of symptoms. Peak A, early release of myoglobin or CK-MB isoforms after AMI; peak B, cardiac troponin after AMI; peak C, CK-MB after AMI; peak D, cardiac troponin after unstable angina. Data are plotted on a relative scale, where 1.0 is set at the AMI cutoff concentration.

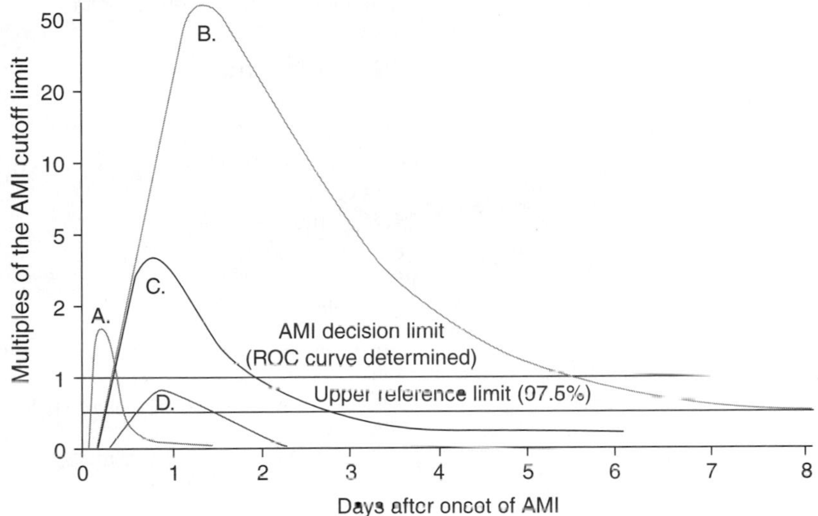

Reproduced with permission from the American Association for Clinical Chemistry. (Wu AH, Apple FS, Gibler WB, et al. National Academy of Clinical Biochemistry Standards of Laboratory Practice: recommendations for the use of cardiac markers in coronary artery diseases. *Clin Chem.* 1999;45(7):1104–1121.)

TABLE 13.26

Management of Acute Myocardial Infarction

Airway Admit	Monitor for adequate airway, consider intubation
Breathing	Immediately begin O_2 by nasal cannula or face mask if available
Circulation	Initiate IV access Consider blood for severe anemia
Drugs	Morphine 1–4 mg IV NTG SL or IV drip
Extra complications Monitor for and treat	PVC CHF Dysrhythmias (VT, VF) Heart block Papillary muscle dysfunction Ventricular aneurysm VSD Pericarditis

IV indicates intravenous; NTG, nitroglycerin; SL, sublingual; PVC, premature ventricular contraction; CHF, congestive heart failure; VT, ventricular tachycardia; VF, ventricular fibrillation; VSD, ventricular septal defect.

AMBULATORY MANAGEMENT OF CONGESTIVE HEART FAILURE

TABLE 13.27

Medications in Congestive Heart Failure

Medication	Support
Digoxin	Moderate, no change in outcomes
Furosemide	Moderate
Spironolactone	Moderate
Angiotensin-converting enzyme inhibitors	Moderate to extensive
Angiotensin II receptor blockers	Moderate (growing extensive)
Beta-blockers (including carvedilol)	Moderate
Calcium-channel blockers	Avoid except amlodipine
Conenzyme Q10	Minimal
Low-sodium diets	Minimal
Home health	Moderate

BACTERIAL ENDOCARDITIS

TABLE 13.28

Conditions for Consideration

DO Require Prophylaxis	DO NOT Require Prophylaxis
Prosthetic valves	MVP without regurgitation*
Previous bacterial endocarditis	Secundum ASD
Complex cyanotic congenital heart disease	Surgically repaired ASD, VSD, PDA
Most other congenital heart malformations	Previous CABG
Rheumatic heart disease	Functional or innocent murmurs
Hypertrophic cardiomyopathy	Previous Kawasaki disease without valvular dysfunction
MVP with regurgitation and/or thickening	Previous RHD without valvular dysfunction
	Cardiac pacemakers

Adapted with permission from the American Heart Association; 1997.

MVP indicates mitral valve prolapse; ASD, atrial septal defect; VSD, ventricular septal defect; PDA, patent ductus arteriosus; CABG, coronary artery bypass graft; RHD, rheumatic heart disease.

*Controversial and should be used with clinical judgement.

TABLE 13.29

Procedures for Consideration

DO Require Prophylaxis	DO NOT Require Prophylaxis
Dental Procedures	**Dental Procedures**
Dental extractions	Restorative dentistry
Surgery, root planning, etc	Local anesthetics
Implants	Intracanal endodontic treatment
Subgingival implants	Suture removal
Cleanings where bleeding is expected	Placement of removable appliances
	Oral impressions
	Fluoride treatments
	Oral radiographs
	Shedding of primary teeth
Medical Procedures	**Medical Procedures**
Tonsillectomy and adenoidectomy	Intubation
Operations that involve mucosa	Flexible bronchoscopy
Rigid bronchoscopy	Tympanostomy tubes
Sclerotherapy for esophageal varices	TEE (optional in high risk)
Esophageal stricture dilation	Endoscopy (optional in high risk)
ERCP	Vaginal hysterectomy (optional in HR)
Biliary tract surgery	Vaginal delivery (optional in HR)
Prostatic surgery	Cesarean section
Cystoscopy	Urethral catheterization
Urethral dilation	D&C
	Therapeutic abortion
	Sterilization procedures
	IUD
	Cardiac catheterization including PTCA

ERCP indicates endoscopic retrograde cholangiopancreatography; TEE, transesophageal echocardiography; HR, high risk; D&C, dilation and curettage; IUD, intrauterine device; PTCA, percutaneous transluminal coronary angiography.

TABLE 13.30

Prophylactic Regimens

Situation	Agent	Regimen
Standard	Amoxicillin	Adults: 2.0 g; children: 50 mg/kg orally 1 h before procedure
Allergic to penicillin	Clindamycin	Adults: 600 mg; children: 20 mg/kg orally 1 h before procedure
	Cephalexin Cefadroxil	Adults: 2.0 g; children: 50 mg/kg orally 1 h before procedure
	Azithromycin Clarithromycin	Adults: 500 mg; children: 15 mg/kg orally 1 h before procedure
Unable to take orals	Ampicillin	Adults: 2.0 g intramuscularly (IM) or intravenously (IV); children: 50 mg/kg IM or IV within 30 min before procedure
Unable to take orals AND allergic to penicillin	Clindamycin	Adults: 600 mg; children: 20 mg/kg IV within 30 min before procedure
	Cefazolin	Adults: 1.0 g; children: 25 mg/kg IM or IV within 30 min before procedure

PERIPHERAL VASCULAR DISEASE

TABLE 13.31

Peripheral Vascular Disease

History	Risk factors Rest pain in the forefoot Nonhealing foot ulcer Gangrene	
	Intermittent claudications	Severe, achy extremity pain with exertion, relieved with rest
Physical exam	Inspection for ulcers, hair loss, atrophy Femoral bruit, iliac bruit Pulse exam is diminished or absent	
Diagnostic testing	Ankle-Brachial Index (ABI)	Ratio of systolic pressure of upper:lower extremities Normal is 0.9–1.3
	Treadmill test (repeat ABI before and after) MRI with MR angiography	
Treatment	Euglycemia Smoking cessation Treatment of risk factors Regular exercise routine	
	Trental (pentoxifylline)	Increased RBC flexibility, inhibited platelet aggregation, reduced fibrinogen levels. Little supporting evidence
	Pletal (cilostazol)	Phosphodiesterase inhibitor increasing cAMP, inhibiting platelet aggregation and causing vasodilation. Significant supporting evidence. Contraindicated in CHF
	Vascular surgery	Severe, resistant disease or limb-threatening disease

MRI indicates magnetic resonance imaging; MR, magnetic resonance; RBC, red blood cell; cAMP, cyclic adenosine monophosphate; CHF, congestive heart failure.

ADVANCED CARDIAC LIFE SUPPORT PROTOCOLS

The following algorithms were obtained from the 2001 AHA/ACC ACLS course materials. It includes the most up-to-date information and medications.

FIGURE 13.11

Comprehensive ECC Algorithm

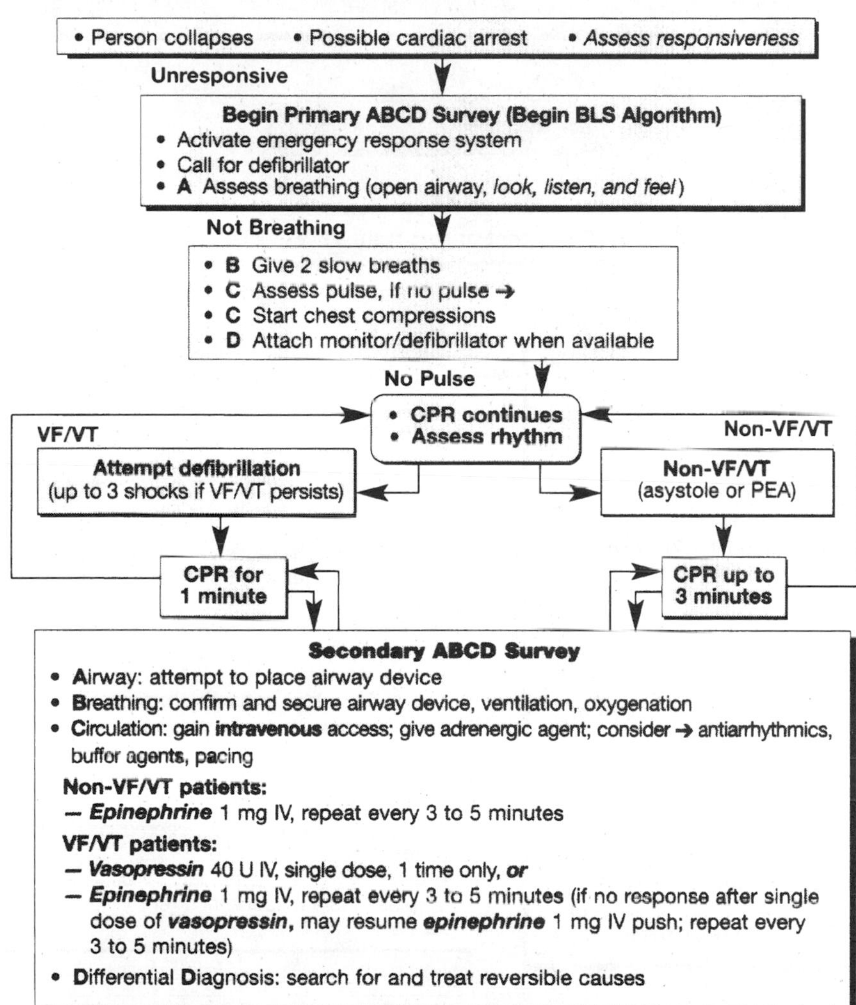

Reproduced with permission from 2001 AHA/ACC ACLS Protocols.

FIGURE 13.12

Ventricular Fibrillation/Pulseless Ventricular Tachycardia (VF/VT) Algorithm

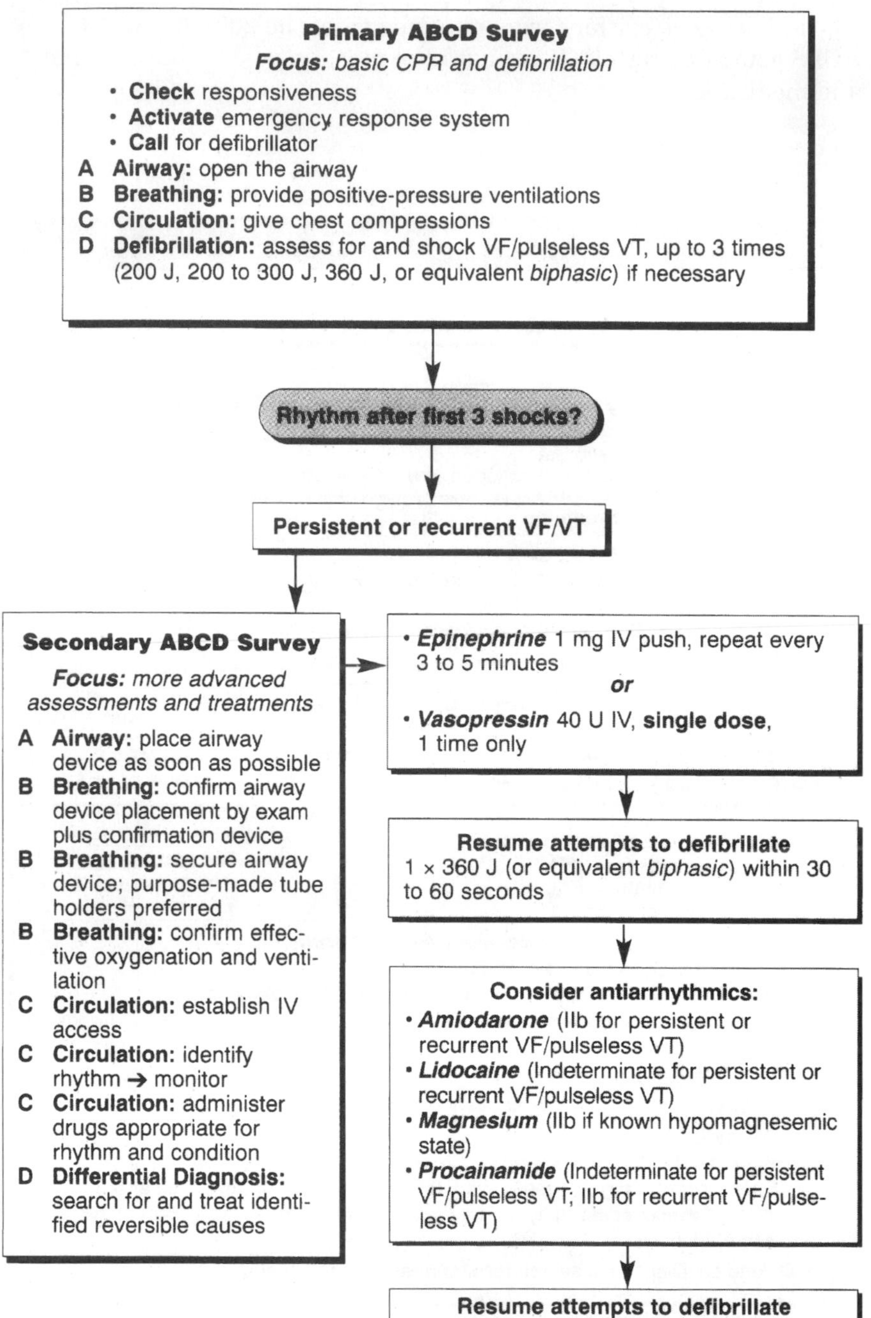

Reproduced with permission from 2001 AHA/ACC ACLS Protocols.

FIGURE 13.13

Pulseless Electrical Activity Algorithm

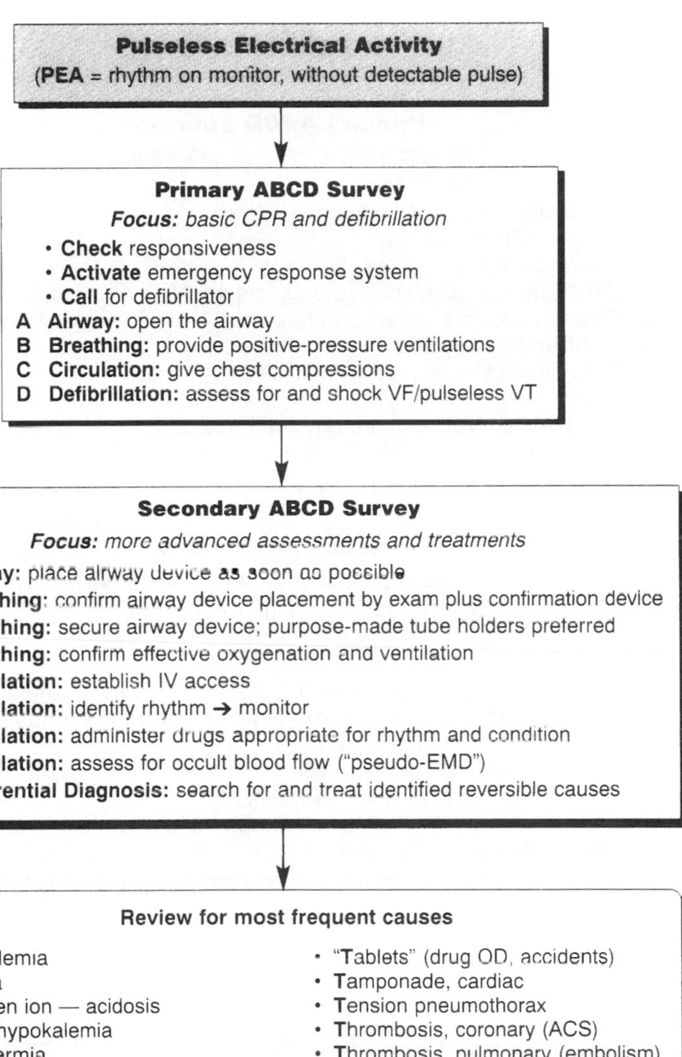

Reproduced with permission from 2001 AHA/ACC ACLS Protocols.

FIGURE 13.14

Asystole: The Silent Heart Algorithm

Asystole: The Silent Heart Algorithm

Asystole

Primary ABCD Survey

Focus: *basic CPR and defibrillation*

- **Check** responsiveness
- **Activate** emergency response system
- **Call** for defibrillator

A **Airway:** open the airway
B **Breathing:** provide positive-pressure ventilations
C **Circulation:** give chest compressions
C **Confirm** true asystole
D **Defibrillation:** assess for VF/pulseless VT; shock if indicated

Rapid scene survey: is there any evidence that personnel should ***not*** attempt resuscitation (eg, DNAR order, signs of death)?

Secondary ABCD Survey

Focus: *more advanced assessments and treatments*

A **Airway:** place airway device as soon as possible
B **Breathing:** confirm airway device placement by exam plus confirmation device
B **Breathing:** secure airway device; purpose-made tube holders preferred
B **Breathing:** confirm effective oxygenation and ventilation
C **Circulation:** confirm true asystole
C **Circulation:** establish IV access
C **Circulation:** identify rhythm → monitor
C **Circulation:** give medications appropriate for rhythm and condition
D **Differential Diagnosis:** search for and treat identified reversible causes

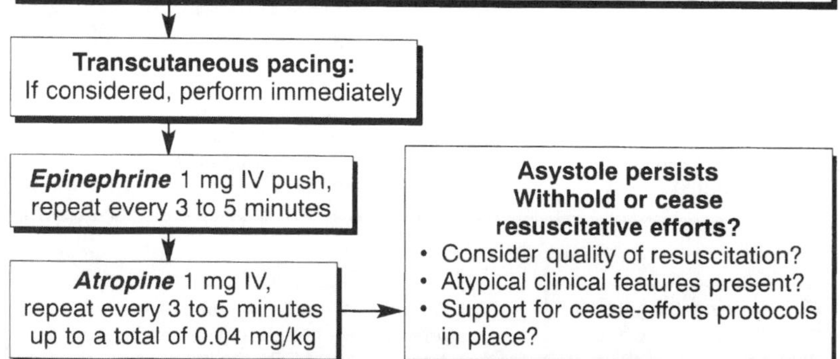

Reproduced with permission from 2001 AHA/ACC ACLS Protocols.

FIGURE 13.15

Bradycardia Algorithm (Patient Not in Cardiac Arrest)

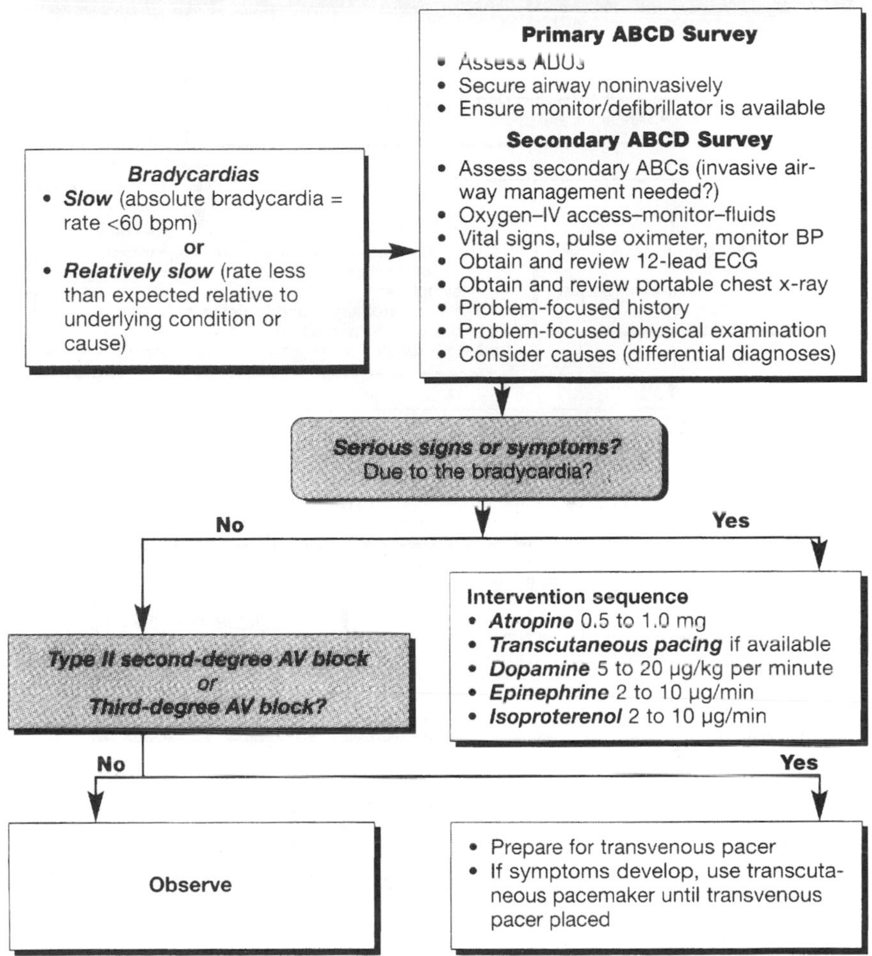

Reproduced with permission from 2001 AHA/ACC ACLS Protocols.

FIGURE 13.16

The Tachycardias: Overview Algorithm

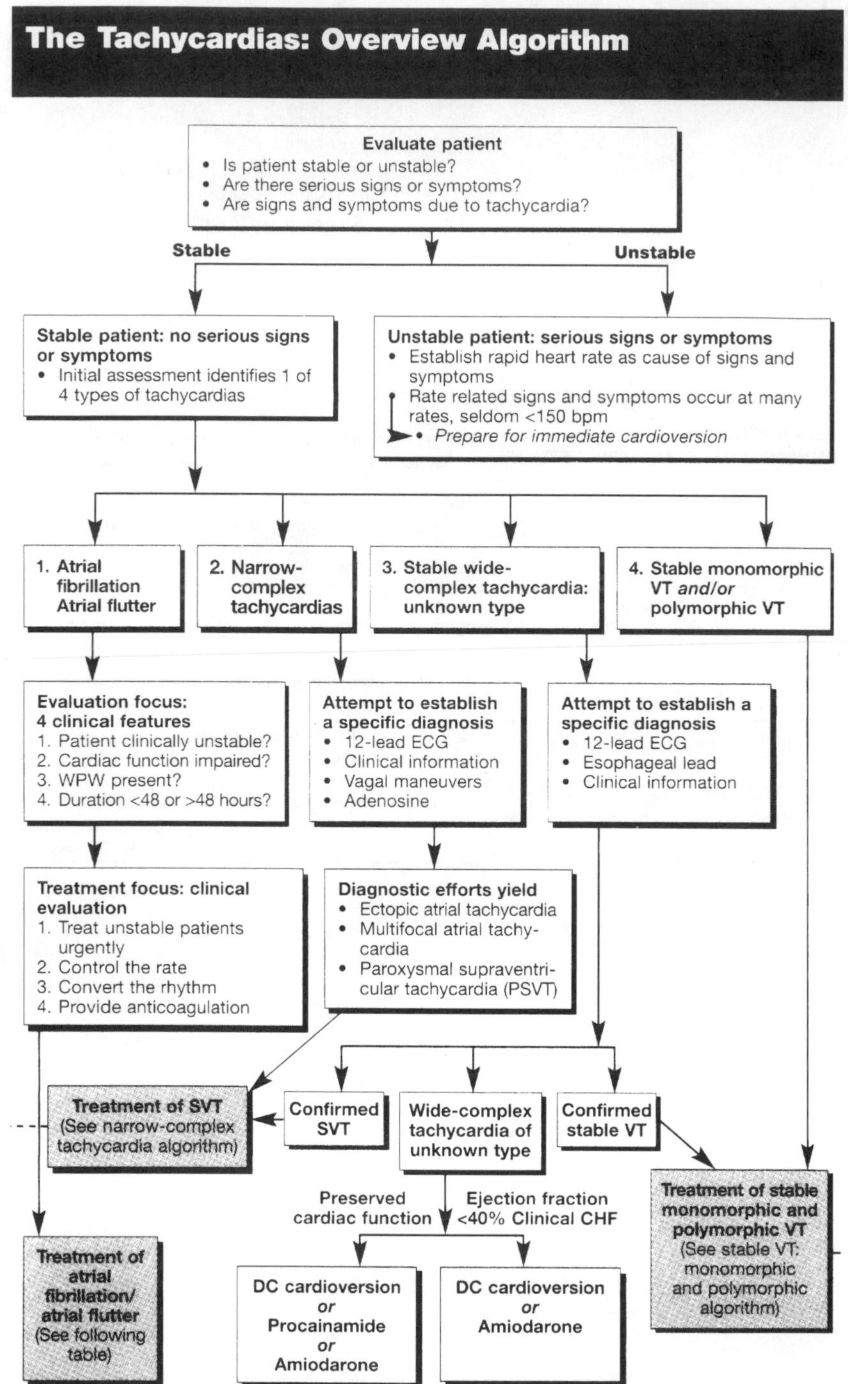

Reproduced with permission from 2001 AHA/ACC ACLS Protocols.

FIGURE 13.17

Narrow-Complex Tachycardia

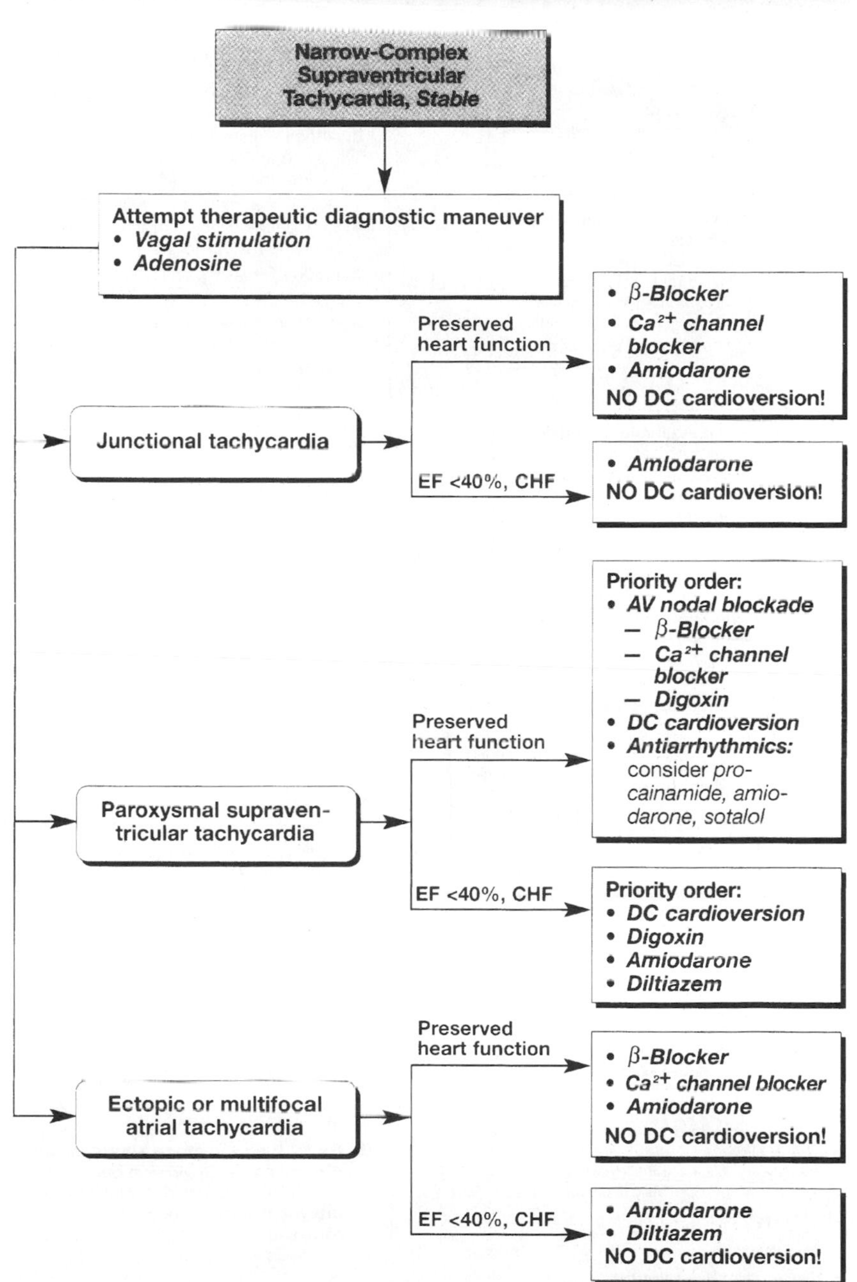

Reproduced with permission from 2001 AHA/ACC ACLS Protocols.

FIGURE 13.18

Electrical Cardioversion Algorithm

Electrical Cardioversion Algorithm

Tachycardia
With serious signs and symptoms related to the tachycardia

↓

If ventricular rate is >150 bpm, prepare for **immediate *cardioversion*.** May give brief trial of medications based on specific arrhythmias. Immediate cardioversion is generally not needed if heart rate is ≤150 bpm.

↓

Have available at bedside
- Oxygen saturation monitor
- Suction device
- IV line
- Intubation equipment

↓

Premedicate whenever possible

↓

Synchronized cardioversion
- Ventricular tachycardia
- Paroxysmal supraventricular tachycardia
- Atrial fibrillation
- Atrial flutter

100 J, 200 J, 300 J, 360 J monophasic energy dose (or clinically equivalent biphasic energy dose)

Notes:

1. Effective regimens have included a sedative (eg, ***diazepam, midazolam, barbiturates, etomidate, ketamine, methohexital)*** with or without an analgesic agent (eg, ***fentanyl, morphine, meperidine).*** Many experts recommend anesthesia if service is readily available.
2. Both monophasic and biphasic waveforms are acceptable if documented as clinically equivalent to reports of monophasic shock success.
3. Note possible need to resynchronize after each cardioversion.
4. If delays in synchronization occur and clinical condition is critical, go immediately to unsynchronized shocks.
5. Treat polymorphic ventricular tachycardia (irregular form and rate) like ventricular fibrillation: see ventricular fibrillation/pulseless ventricular tachycardia algorithm.
6. Paroxysmal supraventricular tachycardia and atrial flutter often respond to lower energy levels (start with 50 J).

Steps for Synchronized Cardioversion

1. Consider sedation.
2. Turn on defibrillator (monophasic or biphasic).
3. Attach monitor leads to the patient ("white to right, red to ribs, what's left over to the left shoulder") and ensure proper display of the patient's rhythm.
4. Engage the synchronization mode by pressing the "sync" control button.
5. Look for markers on R waves indicating sync mode.
6. If necessary, adjust monitor gain until sync markers occur with each R wave.
7. Select appropriate energy level.
8. Position conductor pads on patient (or apply gel to paddles).
9. Position paddle on patient (sternum-apex).
10. Announce to team members: *"Charging defibrillator—stand clear!"*
11. Press "charge" button on apex paddle (right hand).
12. When the defibrillator is charged, begin the final clearing chant. State firmly in a forceful voice the following chant before each shock:
    - *"I am going to shock on three. One, I'm clear."* (Check to make sure you are clear of contact with the patient, the stretcher, and the equipment.)
    - *"Two, you are clear."* (Make a visual check to ensure that no one continues to touch the patient or stretcher. In particular, do not forget about the person providing ventilations. That person's hands should not be touching the ventilatory adjuncts, including the tracheal tube!)
    - *"Three, everybody's clear."* (Check yourself one more time before pressing the "shock" buttons.)
13. Apply 25 lb pressure on both paddles.
14. Press the "discharge" buttons simultaneously.
15. Check the monitor. If tachycardia persists, increase the joules according to the electrical cardioversion algorithm.
16. **Reset the sync mode after each synchronized cardioversion because most defibrillators default back to unsynchronized mode.** This default allows an immediate shock if the cardioversion produces VF.

Steps for Synchronized Cardioversion

1. Consider sedation.
2. Turn on defibrillator (monophasic or biphasic).
3. Attach monitor leads to the patient ("white to right, red to ribs, what's left over to the left shoulder") and ensure proper display of the patient's rhythm.
4. Engage the synchronization mode by pressing the "sync" control button.
5. Look for markers on R waves indicating sync mode.
6. If necessary, adjust monitor gain until sync markers occur with each R wave.
7. Select appropriate energy level.
8. Position conductor pads on patient (or apply gel to paddles).
9. Position paddle on patient (sternum-apex).
10. Announce to team members: "Charging defibrillator—stand clear!"
11. Press "charge" button on apex paddle (right hand).
12. When the defibrillator is charged, begin the final clearing chant. State firmly in a forceful voice the following chant before each shock:
    - "I am going to shock on three. One, I'm clear." (Check to make sure you are clear of contact with the patient, the stretcher, and the equipment.)
    - "Two, you are clear." (Make a visual check to ensure that no one continues to touch the patient or stretcher. In particular, do not forget about the person providing ventilations. That person's hands should not be touching the ventilatory adjuncts, including the tracheal tube.)
    - "Three, everybody's clear." (Check yourself one more time before pressing the "shock" buttons.)
13. Apply 25 lb pressure on both paddles.
14. Press the "discharge" buttons simultaneously.
15. Check the monitor. If tachycardia persists, increase the joules according to the electrical cardioversion algorithm.
16. Reset the sync mode after each synchronized cardioversion because most defibrillators default back to unsynchronized mode. This default allows an immediate shock if the cardioversion produces ventricular fibrillation.

FIGURE 13.19

Stable Ventricular Tachycardia

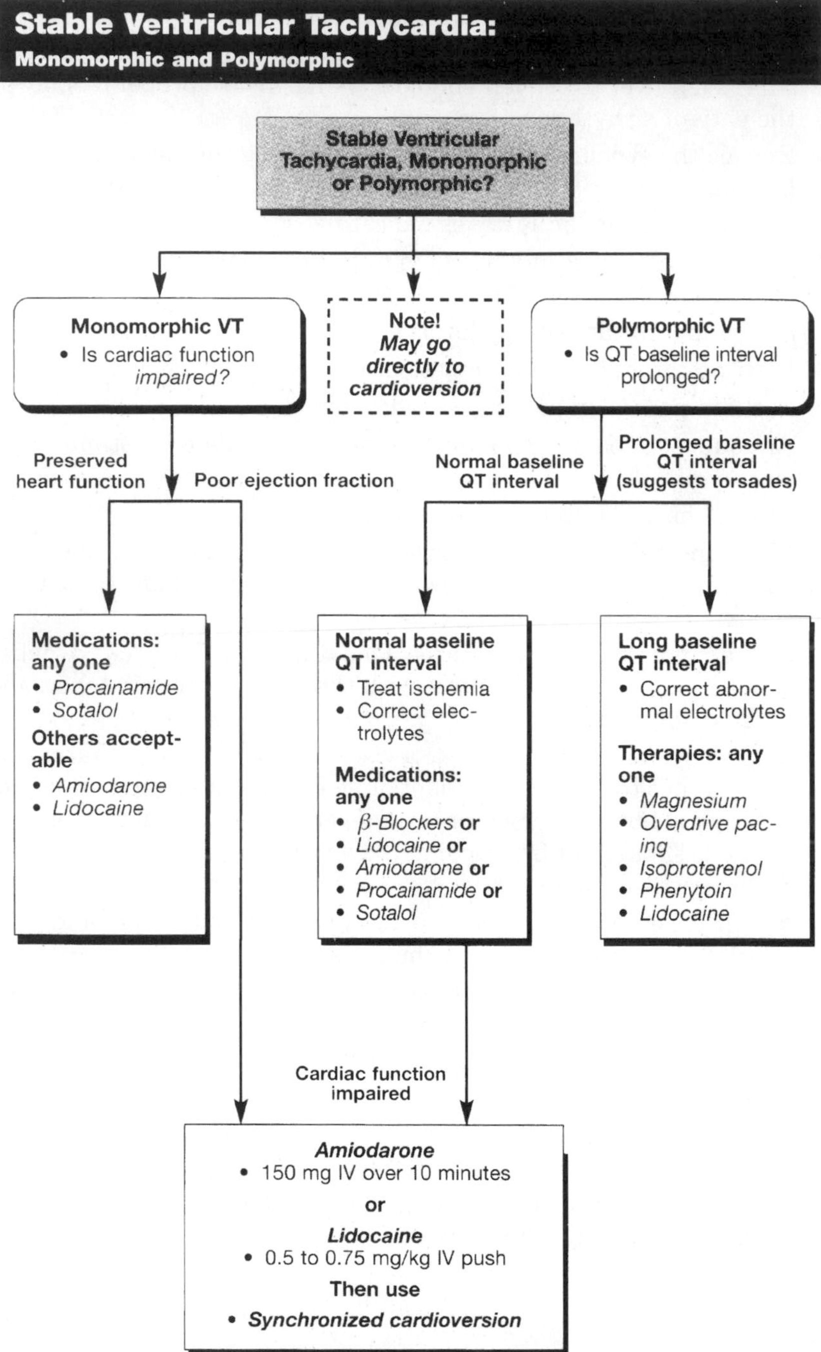

Reproduced with permission from 2001 AHA/ACC ACLS Protocols.

FIGURE 13.20

Ischemic Chest Pain Algorithm*

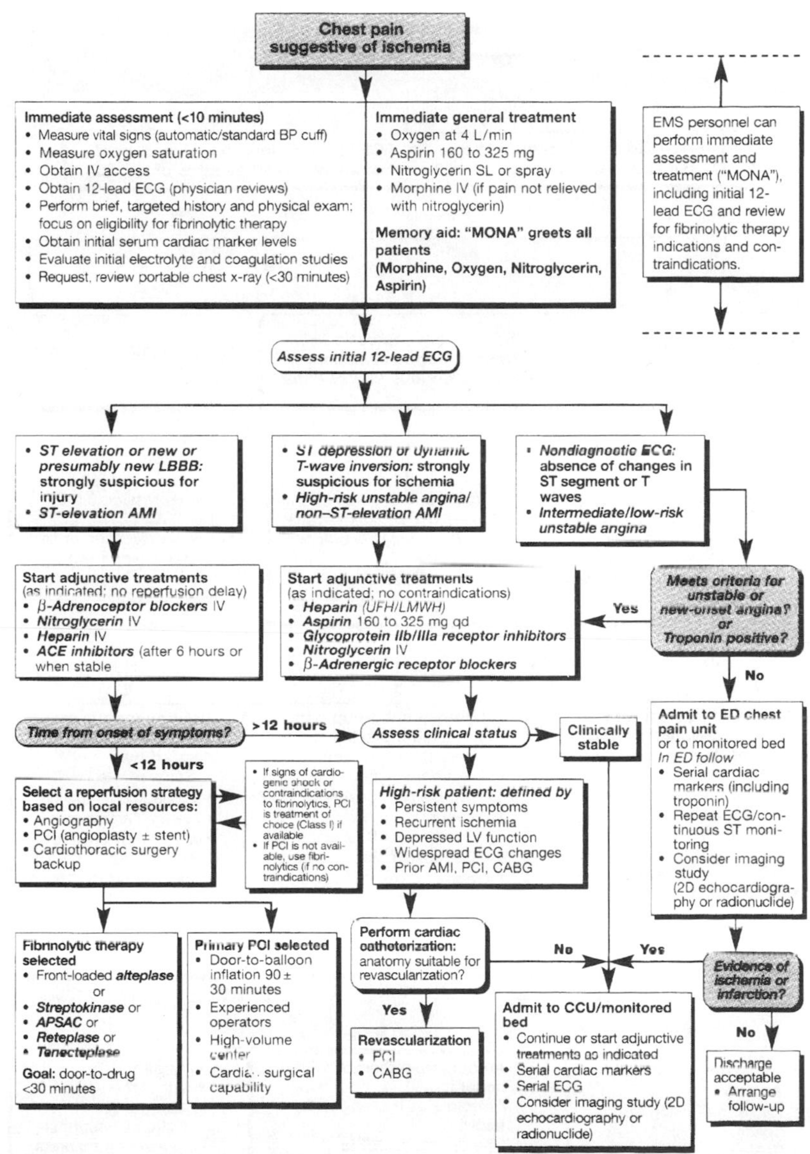

Reproduced with permission from 2001 AHA/ACC ACLS Protocols.

*This algorithm provides general guidelines that may not apply to all patients. Carefully consider proper indications and contraindications.

FIGURE 13.21
Acute Coronary Syndromes

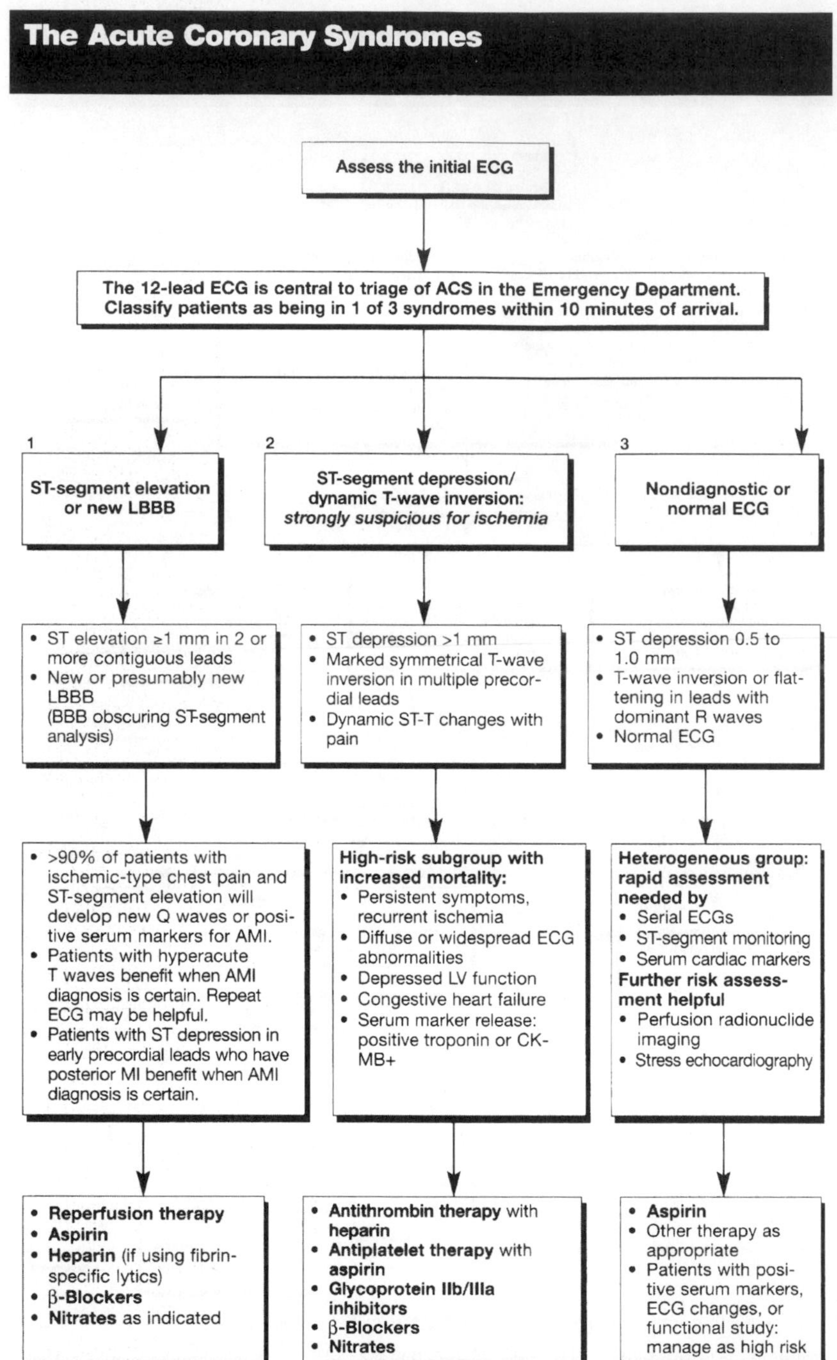

Reproduced with permission from 2001 AHA/ACC ACLS Protocols.

FIGURE 13.22

Algorithm for Suspected Stroke

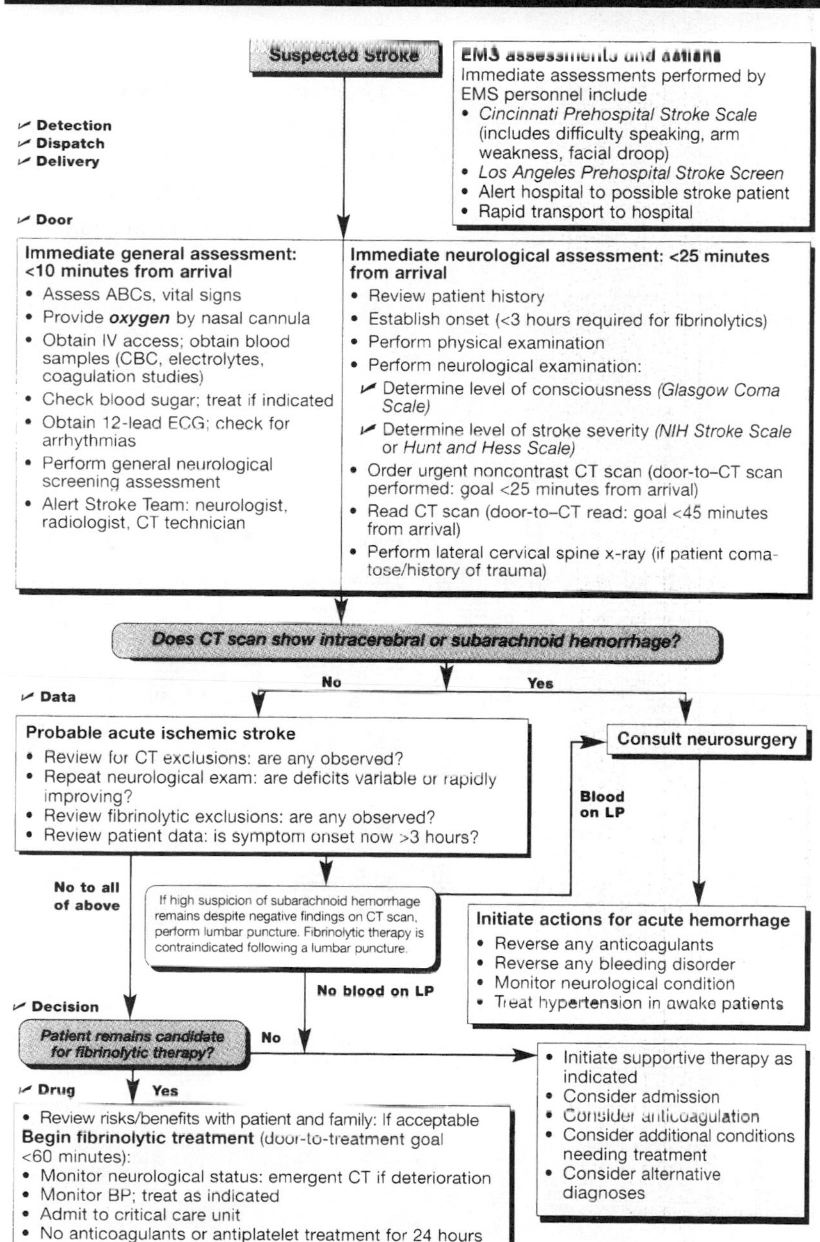

Reproduced with permission from 2001 AHA/ACC ACLS Protocols.

OTHER CARDIAC CONDITIONS

TABLE 13.32
Acute Pericarditis

Signs	Pericardial friction rub: may be three-component rub Pericardial effusion: best diagnosed with echocardiogram Pulsus paradoxus: ECG changes: ST elevation in all leads except aVr and only rarely in V_1
Treatment	Watch for effusion and tamponade Consider anti-inflammatory drugs

ECG indicates electrocardiogram.

FIGURE 13.23
Electrocardiogram Changes in Acute Pericarditis

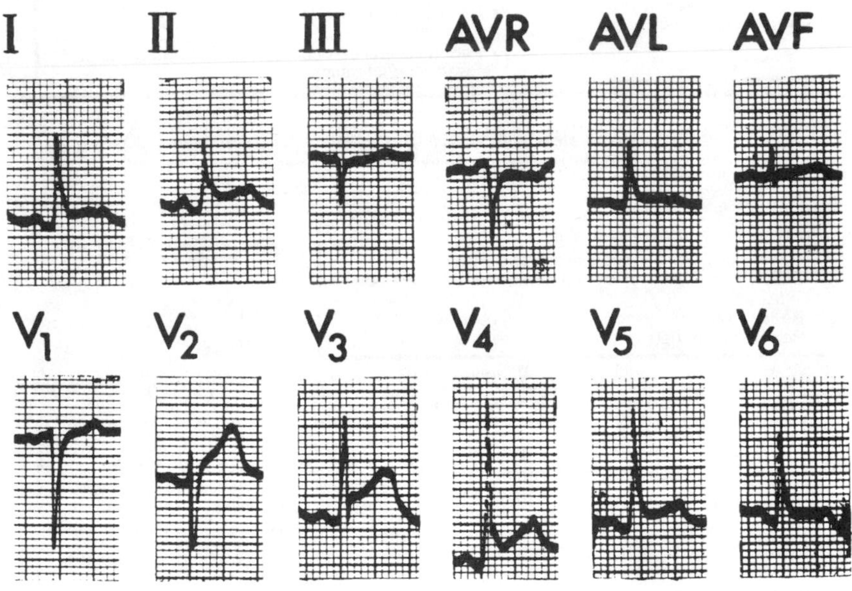

TABLE 13.33

Cardiomyopathy

Either primary myocardial disease or secondary to systemic disease, causing poor function of heart muscle.

Congestive	**Signs** Congestive heart failure, arrhythmias, cardiac chamber dilation, mitral and tricuspid valve regurgitation **Treatment** Bed rest, digitalis, diuretics, afterload and preload reduction, consider anticoagulation
Restrictive	**Signs** Dependent edema, elevated jugular venous pulse, ascites, enlarged heart, enlarged liver, ECG changes **Treatment** Transvenous biopsy, treat CHF
Hypertrophic (idiopathic hypertrophic subaortic stenosis [IHSS])	**Signs** Hypertrophy of left ventricle, murmur, diastolic dysfunction and CHF **Treatment** Beta-blockers, surgical excision of hypertrophy, avoid ionotropes and limit exercise

ECG indicates electrocardiogram; CHF, congestive heart failure.

FIGURE 13.24

Workup and Management of Syncope

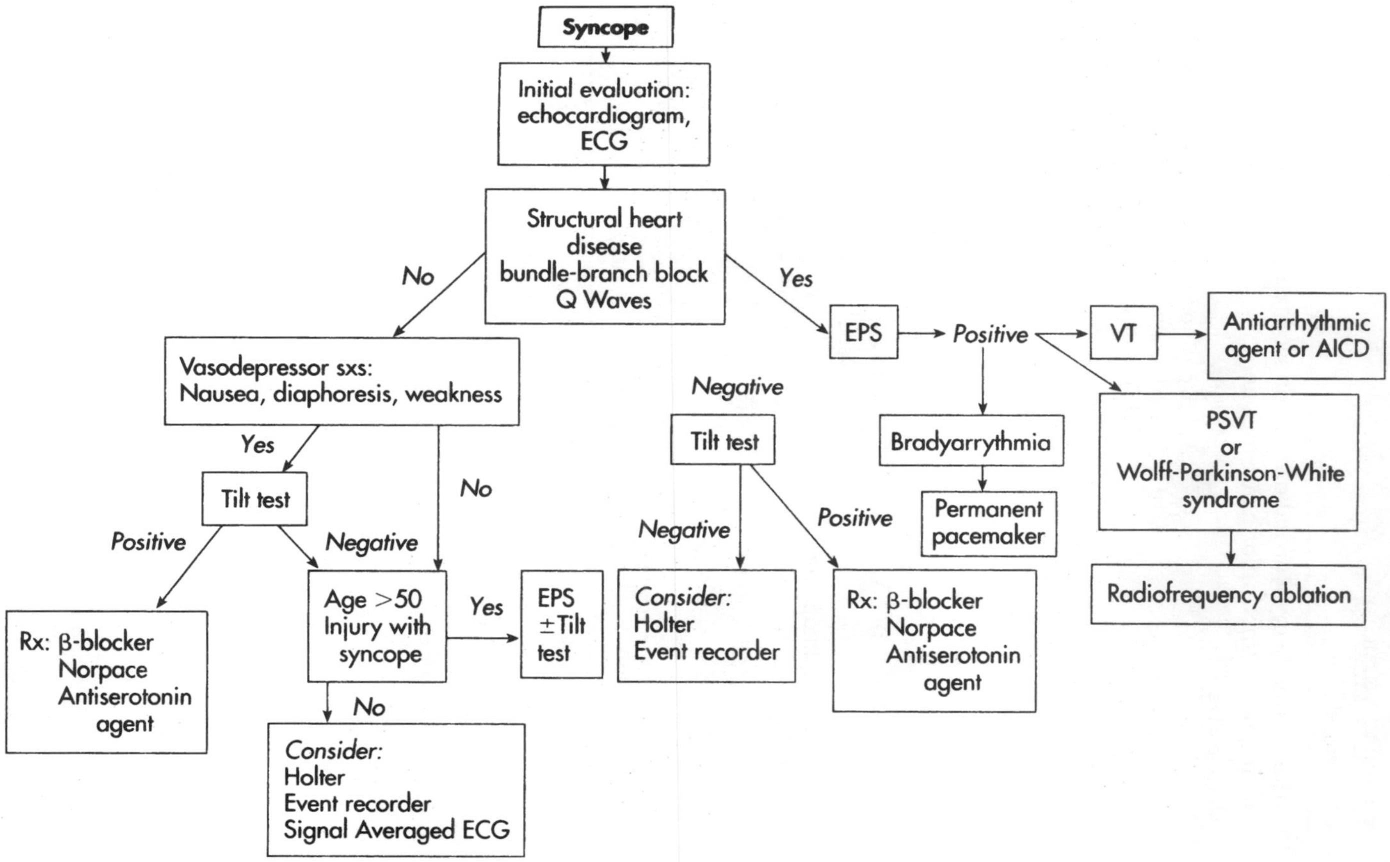

Syncope

Initial evaluation: echocardiogram, ECG

Structural heart disease
bundle-branch block
Q Waves

No

Vasodepressor sxs:
Nausea, diaphoresis, weakness

Yes

Tilt test

Positive

Rx: β-blocker
Norpace
Antiserotonin agent

Negative

Age >50
Injury with syncope

Yes

EPS ±Tilt test

No

Consider:
Holter
Event recorder
Signal Averaged ECG

No

Yes

EPS

Positive

VT

Antiarrhythmic agent or AICD

PSVT
or
Wolff-Parkinson-White syndrome

Radiofrequency ablation

Bradyarrythmia

Permanent pacemaker

Negative

Tilt test

Negative

Consider:
Holter
Event recorder

Positive

Rx: β-blocker
Norpace
Antiserotonin agent

DYSRHYTHMIAS

FIGURE 13.25

Normal Sinus Rhythm

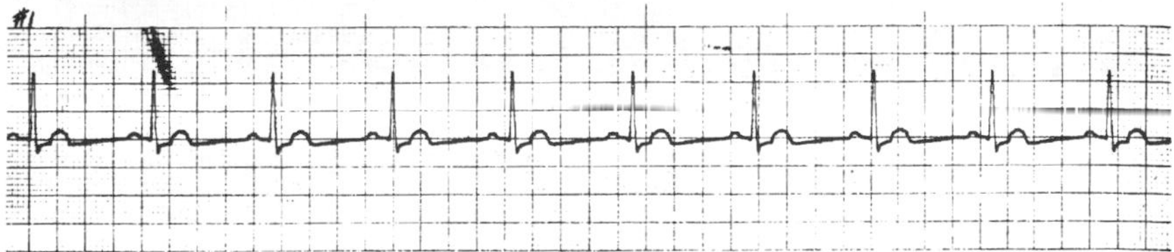

Criteria
Rate: 60–100 beats/min
Rhythm: Regular
P waves: Upright in leads I, II, aV_F

FIGURE 13.26

Sinus Bradycardia

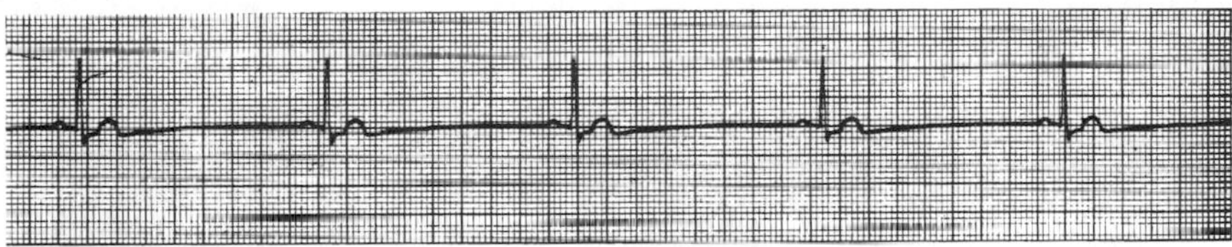

Criteria
Rate: <60 beats/min
Rhythm: Regular
P waves: Upright in leads I, II, aV_F

FIGURE 13.27

Sinus Tachycardia

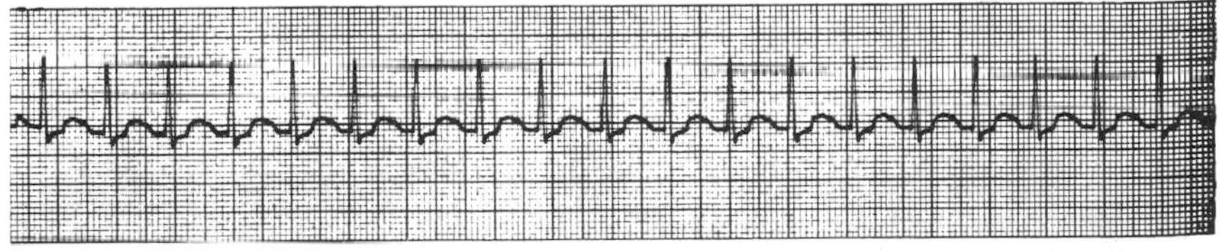

Criteria
Rate: >100 beats/min
Rhythm: Regular
P waves: Upright in leads I, II, aV_F

FIGURE 13.28

Premature Atrial Contractions

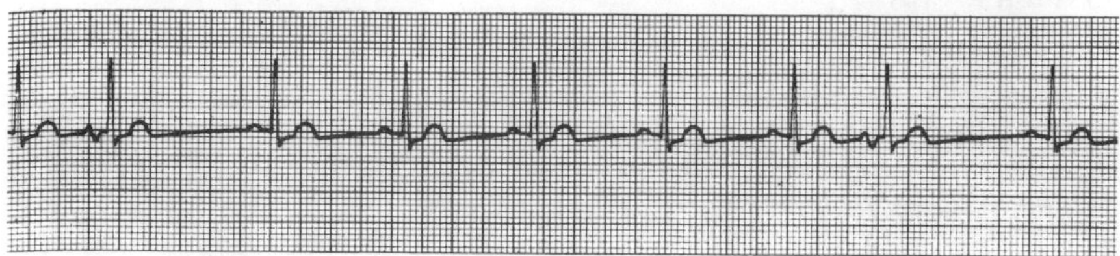

Criteria

Rhythm: Irregular

P waves: Differ in morphology because they are from different foci. PP interval varies.

PR interval: Normal or prolonged

QRS: Normal or prolonged

FIGURE 13.29

Paroxysmal Atrial Tachycardia

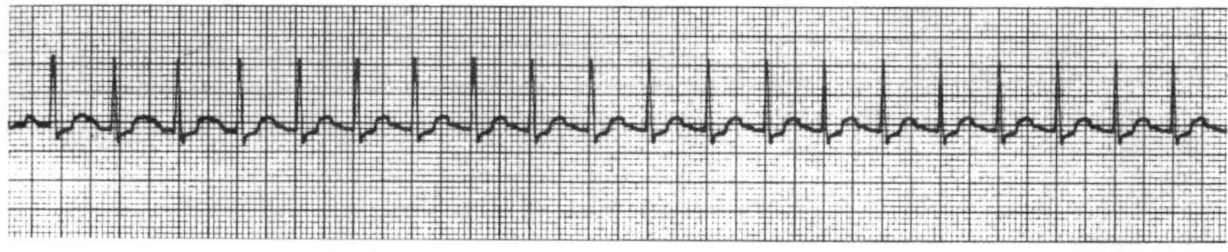

Criteria

Rate: 160–220 beats/min

Rhythm: Atrial, regular; ventricular, may have block (2:1, 3:1, or 4:1)

P waves: Hard to see; different from sinus P waves

PR interval: Normal or prolonged

QRS: Normal or prolonged

FIGURE 13.30

Atrial Flutter

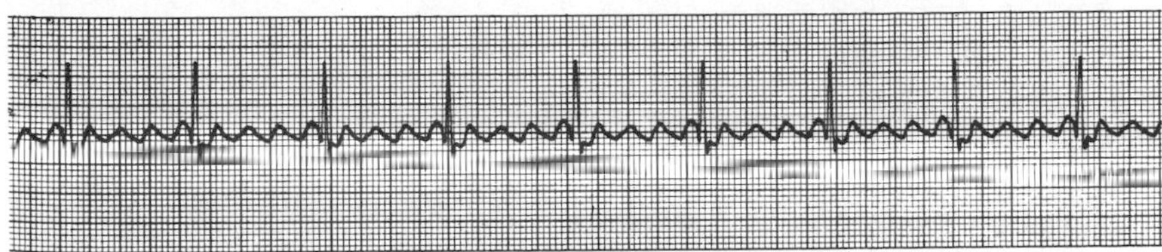

Criteria

Rate: Usually 300 beats/min (range, 220–350 beats/min)
Rhythm: Atrial, regular; ventricular, varying block (2:1, 3:1)
P waves: Sawtooth pattern seen in I, II, aV_F
PR interval: Regular
QRS: Usually normal, perhaps aberrant

FIGURE 13.31

Atrial Fibrillation

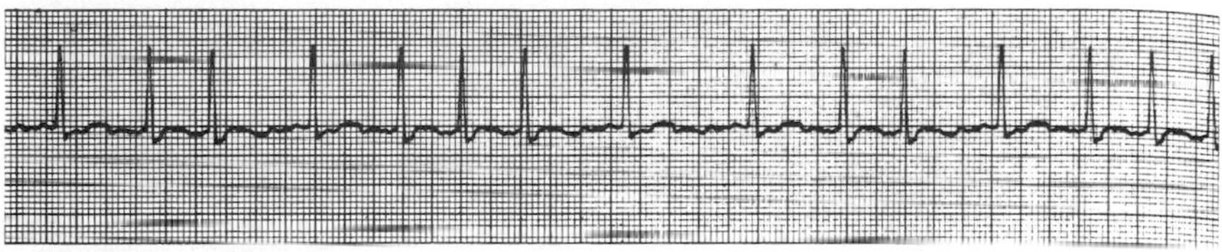

Criteria

Rate: Atrial, 400–700 beats/min; ventricular, 160–180 beats/min
Rhythm: Irregular
P waves: No P waves
QRS: Usually normal, perhaps aberrant

FIGURE 13.32

Premature Junctional Complexes

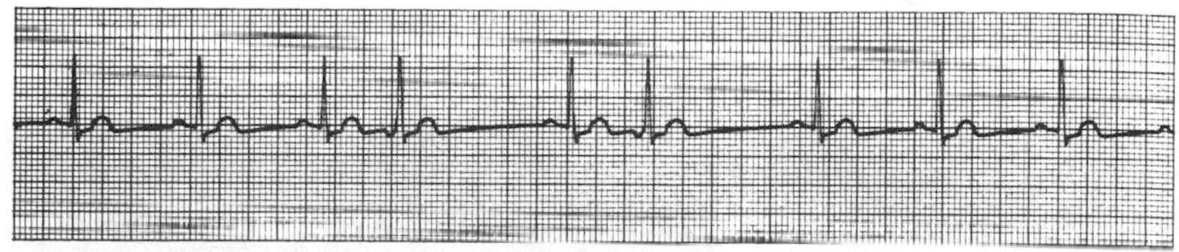

Criteria

Rhythm: Irregular
P waves: Negative in leads I, II, aV_F
PR interval: If P wave is before the QRS, the PR interval is less than 0.12 second; PR interval may be prolonged or show complete block
QRS: Normal or widened

FIGURE 13.33

Junctional Escape Complexes

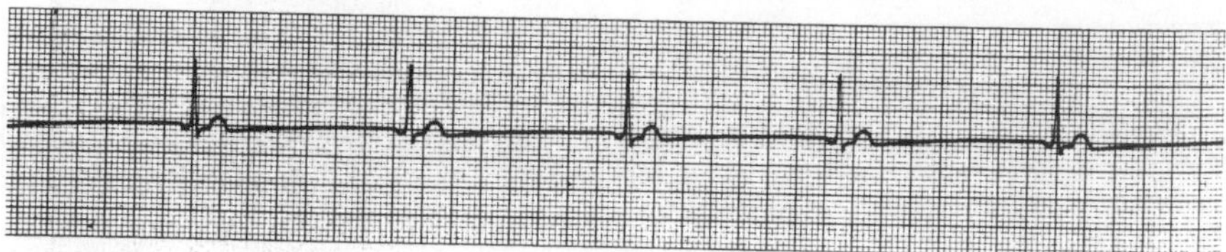

Criteria

Rate: 40–60 beats/min
Rhythm: Complexes may or may not occur regularly
P waves: Negative in leads II, III, aV_F; may precede, coincide with, or follow QRS
PR interval: Variable
QRS: Normal

FIGURE 13.34

Premature Ventricular Complexes

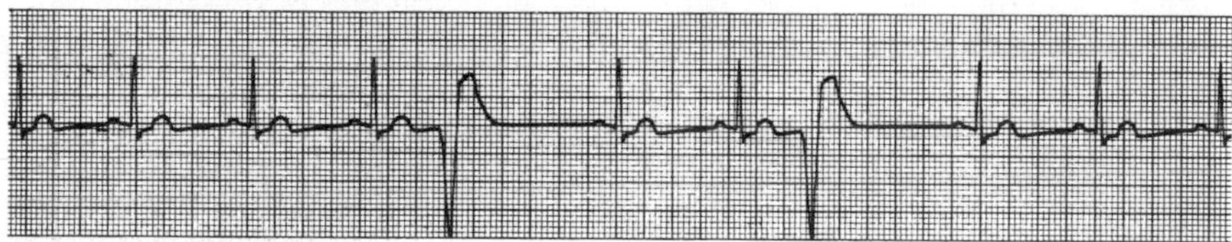

Criteria

Rhythm: Irregular
P waves: Often hidden by QRS of premature ventricular contraction
QRS: >0.12 second; bizarre morphology
ST segment and T waves: Opposite in polarity to the QRS
Full compensatory pause

FIGURE 13.35

Ventricular Tachycardia

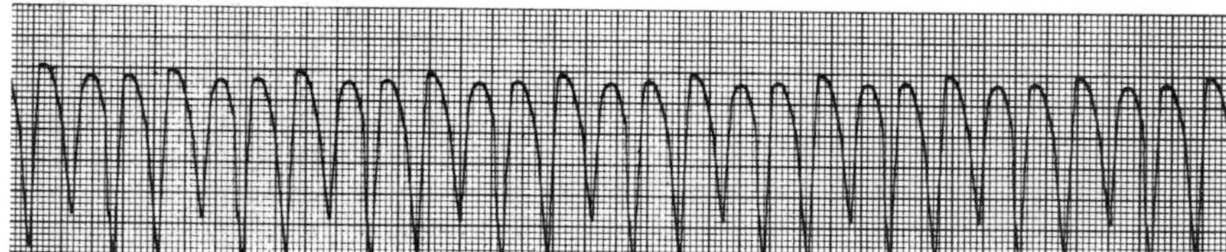

Criteria

Rate: >100–220 beats/min
Rhythm: Usually regular
P waves: May not be seen
QRS: Wide
ST segment and T wave: Opposite in polarity to the QRS

FIGURE 13.36

Ventricular Fibrillation

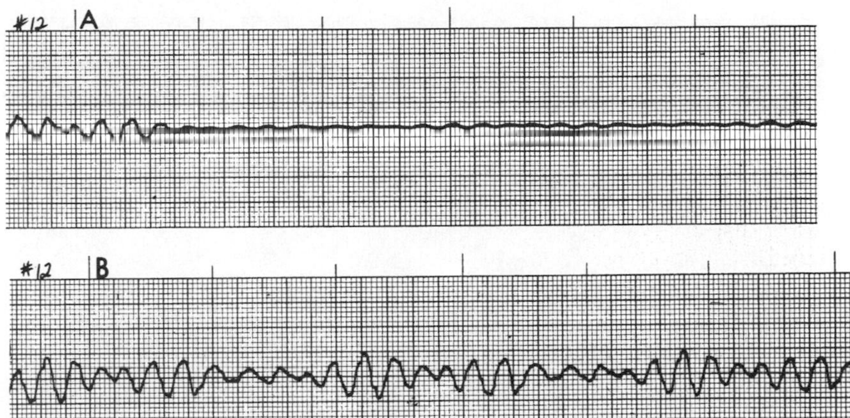

Criteria

Rate: Very rapid, cannot count
Rhythm: Irregular
P waves: QRS, ST segment, or T wave

FIGURE 13.37

First-Degree Atrioventricular (AV) Block

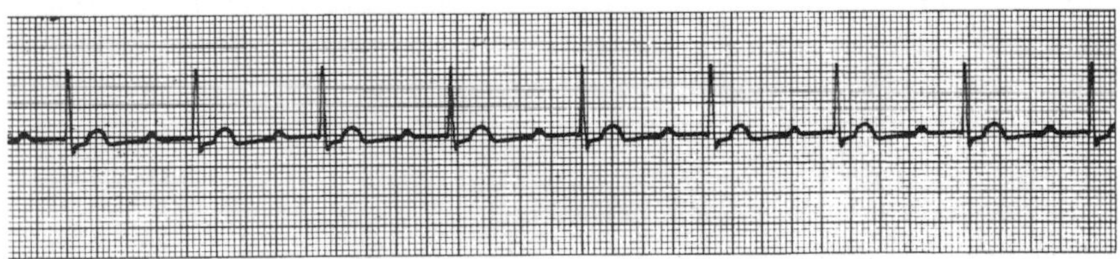

Criteria

Rhythm: Regular
P waves: Followed by QRS
PR interval: >0.20 second

FIGURE 13.38

Second-Degree Atrioventricular (AV) Block (Mobitz Type I, Wenchebach)

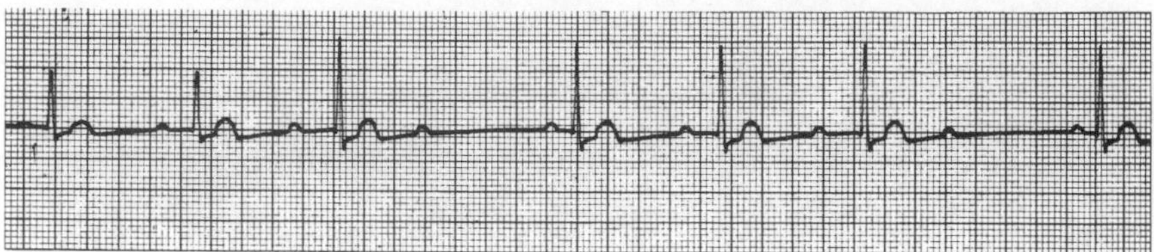

Criteria

Rate: Atrial, normal; ventricular, less than atrial
Rhythm: Atrial, regular; ventricular, irregular; progressive shortening of PR interval until QRS is dropped
P waves: Normal
PR interval: Progressive increase until one P wave is blocked
QRS: Normal

FIGURE 13.39

Mobitz Type II

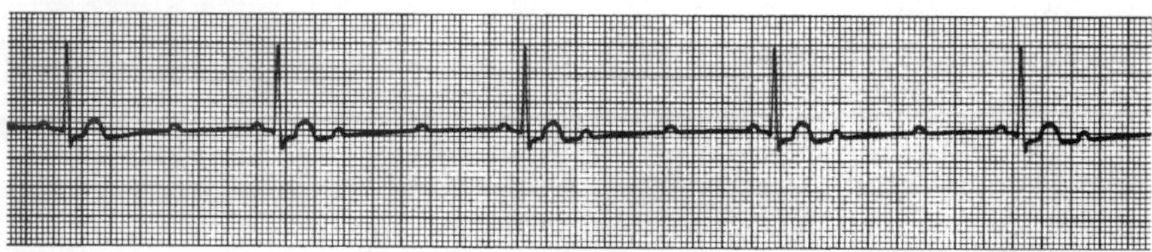

Criteria

Rate: Atrial, normal; ventricular, less than atrial
Rhythm: Atrial, regular; ventricular, regular or irregular with pauses at nonconducted beats
P waves: Normal except for blocked one
PR interval: Normal or prolonged
QRS: Normal or wide

FIGURE 13.40

Third-Degree Atrioventricular (AV) Block

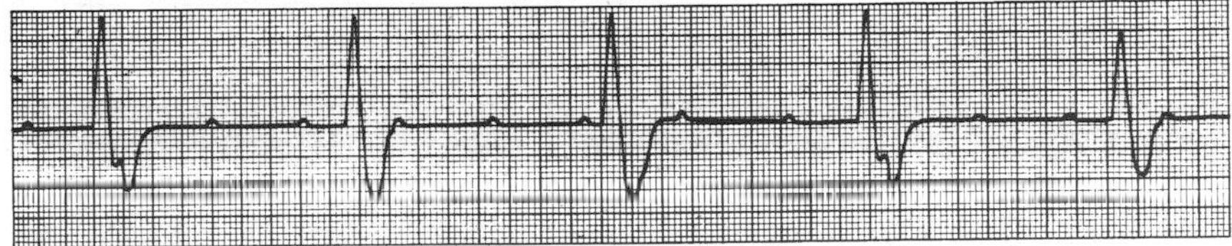

Criteria

Rate: Atria and ventricles at different rates; ventricles slower than atria
Rhythm: Atria, usually regular; ventricular, regular
P waves: Normal
PR interval: Varies
QRS: Normal or wide
PR interval: Progressive increase until on P wave is blocked
QRS: Normal

FIGURE 13.41

Wolff-Parkinson-White (WPW) Syndrome

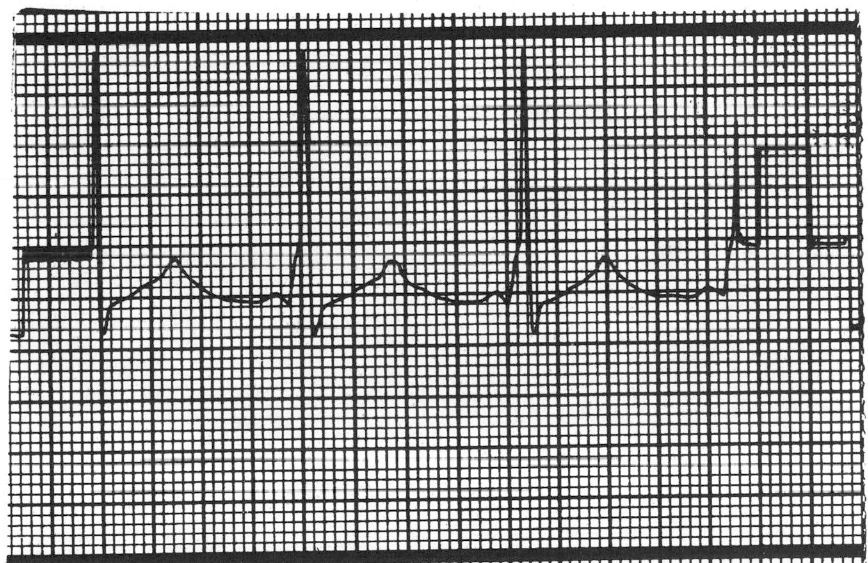

Criteria

PR: 0.12 second
QRS: 0.11 second
Delta wave
These changes may be intermittent

FIGURE 13.42

Torsades de Pointes

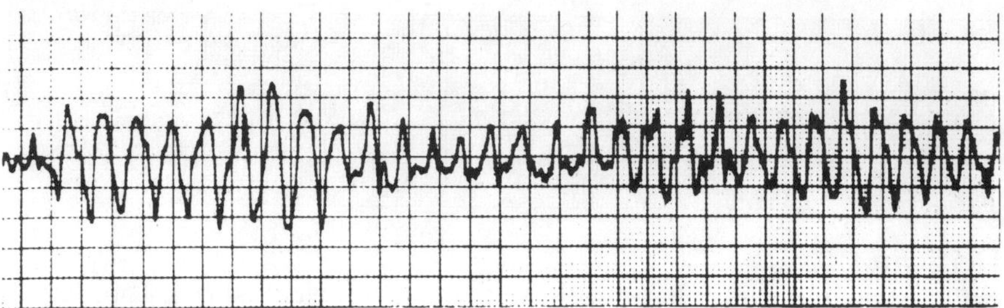

Torsades de Pointes is a ventricular dysrhythmia resulting from QT interval prolongation. Causes of this include severe bradycardia and drug effects (group IA antidysrhythmics).

chapter 14

The Respiratory System

Dean G. Gianakos, MD

IN THIS CHAPTER

- Pulmonary function tests
- Peak expiratory flow tables
- Asthma management
- Treatment of pneumonia
- Guide to smoking cessation
- Treatment of venous thromboembolic disease
- Evaluation of sleep complaints
- Common radiographic findings
- Management of latent tuberculosis infection
- Evaluation of pleural fluid
- Indications for long-term oxygen therapy
- Arterial blood gas interpretation
- Chronic obstructive pulmonary disease management
- Management of acute respiratory failure
- Weaning from mechanical ventilator
- Chest tube insertion
- Orotracheal intubation
- Thoracentesis

BOOKSHELF RECOMMENDATIONS

- *MKSAP 12, Pulmonary Medicine*. Philadelphia, PA: American College of Physicians–American Society of Internal Medicine; 2001.
- Goroll AH, Mulley AG, May LA. *Primary Care Medicine: Office Evaluation and Management of the Adult Patient*. 4th ed. Philadelphia, PA: Lippincott Williams & Wilkins; 2000.
- Ahya SH, Flood K, Paranjothi S, Lee H, eds. *The Washington Manual of Medical Therapeutics*. 30th ed. Philadelphia, PA: Lippincott Williams & Wilkins; 2001.

TABLE 14.1

Pulmonary Function Tests: Use and Interpretation

1. **Spirometry**
   - Use to diagnose airflow obstruction (ie, asthma, COPD, cystic fibrosis)
   - FEV_1/FVC ratio <0.70 indicates airflow obstruction
   - An FEV_1 increase of 12% (or 200 cc) after bronchodilator administration suggests airflow obstruction, despite a normal FEV_1/FVC ratio
2. **Lung volumes**
   - Order when suspect a restrictive lung defect (ie, interstitial lung disease)
   - Total lung capacity <80% predicted value indicates restriction
   - A reduced FVC during spirometry suggests a restrictive defect, but lung volumes necessary to confirm
3. **DLCO (diffusing capacity)**
   - Order when considering pulmonary vascular disease or interstitial lung disease (reduced in both of these conditions)
   - Often reduced in COPD
   - May be increased in asthma
4. **Flow volume loops**
   - Consider use in diagnosis of upper airway obstruction (tumor, vocal cord dysfunction)

COPD indicates chronic obstructive pulmonary disease; FEV_1, forced expiratory volume in 1 second; FVC, forced vital capacity.

TABLE 14.2A

Predicted Average Peak Expiratory Flow for Normal Males*

(Liters per minute)

Age	Height (in)				
	60	65	70	75	80
20	554	602	649	693	740
25	543	590	636	679	725
30	532	577	622	664	710
35	521	565	609	651	695
40	509	552	596	636	680
45	498	540	583	622	665
50	486	527	569	607	649
55	475	515	556	593	634
60	463	502	542	578	618
65	452	490	529	564	603
70	440	477	515	550	587

TABLE 14.2B

Predicted Average Peak Expiratory Flow for Normal Females*

(Liters per minute)

Age	Height (in)				
	60	65	70	75	80
20	390	423	460	496	529
25	385	418	454	490	523
30	380	413	448	483	516
35	375	408	442	476	509
40	370	402	436	470	502
45	365	397	430	464	495
50	360	391	424	457	488
55	355	386	418	454	482
60	350	380	412	445	475
65	345	375	406	439	468
70	340	369	400	432	461

TABLE 14.2C

Predicted Average Peak Expiratory Flow for Normal Children and Adolescents*
(Liters per minute)

Height (in)	Males and Females	Height (in)	Males and Females
43	147	56	320
44	160	57	334
45	173	58	347
46	187	59	360
47	200	60	373
48	214	61	387
49	227	62	400
50	240	63	413
51	254	64	427
52	267	65	440
53	280	66	454
54	293	67	467
55	307		

Tables 14.2A, B, and C adapted from Executive Summary: Guidelines for the Diagnosis and Management of Asthma, NIH Publication No. 91-3042A, June 1991, National Heart, Lung, and Blood Institute, National Institutes of health, Bethesda, Md.

*These tables are average and are based on tests with a large number of people. An individual's Peak expiratory flow rate (PEFR) may vary widely. Further, many individuals' PEFR values are consistently higher or lower than the average values. It is recommended that PEFR objectives for therapy be based upon each individual's "personal best," which is established after a period of PEFR monitoring while the individual is under effective treatment.

TABLE 14.3

Differential Diagnostic Possibilities for Asthma

Infants and Children

Upper airway diseases

- Allergic rhinitis and sinusitis

Obstruction involving large airways

- Foreign body in trachea or bronchus
- Vocal cord dysfunction
- Vascular rings or laryngeal webs
- Laryngotracheomalacia, tracheal stenosis, or bronchostenosis
- Enlarged lymph nodes or tumor

Obstructions involving small airways

- Viral bronchiolitis or obliterative bronchiolitis
- Cystic fibrosis
- Bronchopulmonary dysplasia
- Heart disease

Other causes

- Recurrent cough not due to asthma
- Aspiration from swallowing mechanism dysfunction or gastroesophageal reflux

Adults

- Chronic obstructive pulmonary disease (chronic bronchitis or emphysema)
- Congestive heart failure
- Pulmonary emboli
- Laryngeal dysfunction
- Mechanical obstruction of the airways (benign and malignant tumors)
- Pulmonary infiltration with eosinophilia
- Cough secondary to drugs (angiotensin-converting enzyme [ACE] inhibitors)
- Vocal cord dysfunction

Adapted from the National Institutes of Health, National Heart, Lung, and Blood Institute. (Expert Panel Report 2, Guidelines for the Diagnosis and Management of Asthma; NIH Publication No.97-4051, April 1997, National Institutes of Health, National Heart, Lung, and Blood Institute, Bethesda, Md.)

TABLE 14.4

Assessment Questions for Environmental and Other Factors That Can Make Asthma Worse*

Inhalant Allergens

Does the patient have symptoms year round? (If yes, ask the following questions. If no, see next set of questions.)

- Does the patient keep pets indoors? What type?
- Does the patient have moisture in any room of his or her home (eg, basement)? (Suggests house dust mites, molds)
- Does the patient have mold visible in any part of his or her home? (Suggests molds)
- Has the patient seen cockroaches in his or her home in the past month? (Suggests significant cockroach exposure)
- Assume exposure to house dust mites unless patient lives in semiarid region. However, if a patient living in a semiarid region uses a swamp cooler, exposure to house dust mites must still be assumed.

Do symptoms get worse at certain times of the year? (If yes, ask when symptoms occur.)

- Early spring? (Trees)
- Late spring? (Grasses)
- Late summer to autumn? (Weeds)
- Summer and fall? (*Alternaria*, *Cladosporium*)

Tobacco Smoke

- Does the patient smoke?
- Does anyone smoke at home or work?
- Does anyone smoke at the child's daycare?

Indoor/Outdoor Pollutants and Irritants

- Is a wood-burning stove or fireplace used in the patient's home?
- Are there unvented stoves or heaters in the patient's home?
- Does the patient have contact with other smells or fumes from perfumes, cleaning agents, or sprays?

Workplace Exposures

- Does the patient cough or wheeze during the week, but not on weekends when away from work?
- Do the patient's eyes and nasal passages get irritated soon after arriving at work?
- Do coworkers have similar symptoms?
- What substances are used in the patient's worksite? (Assess for sensitizers)

Continued

TABLE 14.4

Assessment Questions for Environmental and Other Factors That Can Make Asthma Worse*, cont'd

Rhinitis

- Does the patient have constant or seasonal nasal congestion and/or postnasal drip?

Gastroesophageal Reflux

- Does the patient have heartburn?
- Does food sometimes come up the patient's throat?
- Has the patient had coughing, wheezing, or shortness of breath at night in the past 4 weeks?
- Does the infant vomit followed by cough or have wheezy cough at night? Are symptoms worse after feeding?

Sulfite Sensitivity

- Does the patient have wheezing, coughing, or shortness of breath after eating shrimp, dried fruit, or processed potatoes or after drinking beer or wine?

Medication Sensitivities and Contraindications

- What medication does the patient use now (prescription and nonprescription)?
- Does the patient use eyedrops? What type?
- Does the patient use any medications that contain beta-blockers?
- Does the patient ever take aspirin or other nonsteroidal anti-inflammatory drugs?
- Has the patient ever had symptoms of asthma after taking any of these medications?

Adapted from the National Institutes of Health, National Heart, Lung, and Blood Institute. (Expert Panel Report 2, Guidelines for the Diagnosis and Management of Asthma; N:H Publication No.97-4051, April 1997, National Institutes of Health, National Heart, Lung, and Blood Institute, Bethesda, Md.)

*These questions are examples and do not represent a standardized assessment or diagnostic instrument. The validity and reliability of these questions have not been assessed.

TABLE 14.5

Control Measures for Environmental Factors That Make Asthma Worse

Allergens. Reduce or eliminate exposure to the allergen(s) the patient is sensitive to, including:

- **Animal dander**: Remove animal from the house or, at a minimum, keep the animal out of the patient's bedroom and seal or cover with filter air ducts that lead to the bedroom.
- **House dust mites**:
  —Essential: Encase mattress in an allergen-impermeable cover; encase pillow in an allergen-impermeable cover or wash it weekly; wash sheets and blankets on the patient's bed in hot water weekly (water temperature of $\geq$130°F is necessary for killing mites).
  —Desirable: Reduce indoor humidity to less than 50%; remove carpets from bedroom; avoid sleeping or lying on upholstered furniture; remove carpets that are laid on concrete.
- **Cockroaches**: Use poison bait or traps to control. Do not leave food or garbage exposed.
- **Pollens (from trees, grass, or weeds) and outdoor molds**: To avoid exposure, adults should stay indoors with windows closed during the season in which they have problems with outdoor allergens, especially during the afternoon.

Tobacco Smoke. Advise patients and others in the home who smoke to stop smoking or to smoke outside the home. Discuss ways to reduce exposure to other sources of tobacco smoke, such as from daycare providers and the workplace.

Indoor/Outdoor Pollutants and Irritants. Discuss ways to reduce exposures to the following:

- Wood-burning stoves or fireplaces
- Unvented stoves or heaters
- Other irritants (eg, perfumes, cleaning agents, sprays)

Adapted from the National Institutes of Health, National Heart, Lung, and Blood Institute. (Highlights on the expert Panel Report 2: Guidelines for the Diagnosis and Management of Asthma. NIH Publication No.97-4051A, May 1997, National Institutes of Health, National Heart, Lung, and Blood Institute, Bethesda, Md.)

TABLE 14.6

Stepwise Approach for Managing Asthma in Adults and Children Older Than 5 Years

Goals of Asthma Treatment

- Prevent chronic and troublesome symptoms (eg, coughing or breathlessness in the night, in the early morning, or after exertion)
- Maintain (near) "normal" pulmonary function
- Maintain normal activity levels (including exercise and other physical activity)
- Prevent recurrent exacerbations of asthma and minimize the need for emergency department visits or hospitalizations
- Provide optimal pharmacotherapy with minimal or no adverse effects
- Meet patient's and families' expectation of and satisfaction with asthma care

Classification of Severity: Clinical Features Before Treatment*

	Symptoms†	Nighttime Symptoms	Lung Function
Step 4 Severe persistent	■ Continual symptoms ■ Limited physical activity ■ Frequent exacerbations	Frequent	FEV_1 or PEF ≤60% predicted PEF variability >30%
Step 3 Moderate persistent	■ Daily symptoms ■ Daily use of inhaled short-acting β_2-agonist ■ Exacerbations affect activity ■ Exacerbations ≥2 times a week; may last days	>1 time a week	FEV_1 or PEF >60% and ≤80% predicted PEF variability >30%
Step 2 Mild persistent	■ Symptoms >2 times a week but <1 time a day ■ Exacerbations may affect activity	>2 times a month	FEV_1 or PEF ≥80% predicted PEF variability 20%–30%
Step 1 Mild intermittent	■ Symptoms ≤2 times a week ■ Asymptomatic and normal PEF between exacerbations	≤2 times a month	FEV_1 or PEF ≥80% predicted PEF variability <20%

	Symptoms[‡]	Nighttime Symptoms	Lung Function
	■ Exacerbations brief (from a few hours to a few days); intensity may vary		

Adapted from the National Institutes of Health, National Heart, Lung, and Blood Institute. (Highlights on the expert Panel Report 2: Guidelines for the Diagnosis and Management of Asthma. N:H Publication No.97-4051A, May 1997, National Institutes of Health, National Heart, Lung, and Blood Institute, Bethesda, Md.)

*The presence of one of the features of severity is sufficient to place a patient in that category. An individual should be assigned to the most severe grade in which any feature occurs. The characteristics noted in this table are general overlap because asthma is highly variable. Furthermore, an individual's classification may change over time.

[†]Patients at any level of severity can have mild, moderate, or severe exacerbations. Some patients with intermittent asthma experience severe and life-threatening exacerbations separated by long periods of normal lung function and no symptoms.

TABLE 14.7

Stepwise Approach for Managing Asthma in Adults and Children Older Than 5 Years

	Long-term Control	Quick Relief	Education
Step 4 **Severe persistent**	Daily medications: ■ **Anti-inflammatory**: **inhaled corticosteroid (high dose)** AND ■ Long-acting bronchodilator: either **long-acting β_2-agonist**, sustained-release theophyline, or long-acting β_2-agonist tablets AND ■ Corticosteroid tablets or syrup long term (2 mg/kg/d, generally do not exceed 60 mg per day)	■ Short-acting bronchodilator: **inhaled β_2-agonists** as needed for symptoms ■ Intensity of treatment will depend on severity of exacerbations; see component 3: Managing exacerbations ■ Use of short-acting inhaled β_2-agonists on a daily basis, or increasing use, indicates the need for additional long-term control therapy.	Steps 2 and 3 actions plus: ■ Refer to individual education/counseling
Step 3 **Moderate persistent**	Daily medication: ■ Either **Anti-inflammatory**: **inhaled corticosteroid (medium dose)** OR **Inhaled corticosteroid (low-medium dose)** and add long-acting bronchodilator, especially for nighttime		Step 1 actions plus: ■ Teach self-monitoring ■ Refer to group education if available ■ Review and update self-management plan

	Long-term Control	Quick Relief	Education
	symptoms: either **long-acting inhaled β_2-agonist**, sustained-release theophylline, or long-acting β_2-agonist tablets. ■ If needed **Anti-inflammatory**: **inhaled corticosteroid (medium-high dose)** AND **Long-acting bronchodilator**, especially for nighttime symptoms; either **long-acting inhaled β_2-agonist**, sustained-release theophylline, or long-acting β_2-agonist tablets		
Step 2 Mild persistent	One daily medication: ■ **Anti-inflammatory**: either **inhaled corticosteroid** (low doses) or **cromolyn or nedocromil** (children usually begin with a trial of cromolyn or nedocromil) ■ Sustained-release theophylline to serum concentration of 5–15 μg/mL is	■ Short-acting bronchodilator: **inhaled β_2-agonists** as needed for symptoms ■ Intensity of treatment will depend on severity of exacerbation; see component 3: Managing exacerbations ■ Use of a short-acting inhaled β_2-agonist on	Step 1 actions plus: ■ Teach self-monitoring ■ Refer to group education if available ■ Review and update self-management plan

Continued

TABLE 14.7

Stepwise Approach for Managing Asthma in Adults and Children Older Than 5 Years, cont'd

	Long-Term Control	Quick Relief	Education
	an alternative, but not preferred, therapy. Zafirlukast or zileuton may also be considered for patients ≥12 years of age, although their position in therapy is not fully established	a daily basis, or increasing use, indicates the need for additional long-term-control therapy	
Step 1 Mild Intermittent	No daily medication needed	■ Short-acting bronchodilator: **inhaled β_2-agonist** as needed for symptoms. ■ Intensity of treatment will depend on severity of exacerbation; see component 3 managing exacerbations. ■ Use of short-acting inhaled β_2-agonist more than 2 times a week may indicate the need to initiate long-term control therapy	■ Teach basic facts about asthma ■ Teach inhaler/spacer/holding chamber technique ■ Discuss role of medications ■ Develop self-management plan ■ Develop action plan for when and how to take rescue action, especially for patients with a history of severe exacerbations ■ Discuss appropriate environmental control measures to avoid exposure to known allergens and irritants (see component 4)

Adapted from the National Institutes of Health, National Heart, Lung, and Blood Institute. (Expert Panel Report 2, Guidelines for the diagnosis and Management of Asthma; N:H Publication No.97-4051, April 1997, National Institutes of Health, National Heart, Lung, and Blood Institute, Bethesda, Md.)

Step Down:
Review treatment every 1 to 6 months; a gradual stepwise reduction in treatment may be possible.

Step Up:
If control is not maintained, consider step up. First, review patient medication technique, adherence, and environmental control (avoidance of allergens or other factors that contribute to asthma severity).

Notes

- The stepwise approach presents general guidelines to assist clinical decision making; it is not intended to be a specific prescription. Asthma is highly variable; clinicians should tailor specific medication plans to the needs and circumstances of individual patients.
- Gain control as quickly as possible; then decrease treatment to the least medication necessary to maintain control. Gaining control may be accomplished by either starting treatment at the step most appropriate to the initial severity of the condition or starting at a higher level of therapy (eg, a course of systemic corticosteroids or higher dose of inhaled corticosteroids).
- A rescue course of systemic corticosteroids may be needed at any time and at any step.
- Some patients with intermittent asthma experience severe and life-threatening exacerbations separated by long periods of normal lung function and no symptoms. This may be especially common with exacerbations provoked by respiratory infections. A short course of systemic corticosteroids is recommended.
- At each step, patients should control their environment to avoid or control factors that make their asthma worse (eg, allergens, irritants); this requires specific diagnosis and education.
- Referral to an asthma specialist for consultation or comanagement is *recommended* if there are difficulties achieving or maintaining control of asthma or if the patient requires step 4 care. Referral may be *considered* if the patient requires step 3 care. (See also component 1: initial assessment and diagnosis.)

TABLE 14.8

Some Inhaled Drugs for Maintainance Treatment of Chronic Asthma

Drug	Formation	Adult Dosage	Pediatric Dosage*	Cost†
β_2-adrenergic, long-acting	Metered-dose inhaler	2 puffs q12 h	1–2 puffs q12 h	$73.00
Salmetrol-*Servent*‡	(21 μg/puff)			
(Serevent Diskus)	Dry-powder inhaler (50 μg/inhalation)	1 inhalation q12 h	1 inhalation q12 h	$76.20
Corticosteroids				
Beclomethasone dipropionate	Meter-dose inhaler			
(Vanceril)	(42 μg/puff)	4–8 puffs bid	2–4 puffs bid	$52.63
(Vanceril Double-Strength)	(84 μg/puff)	2–4 puffs bid	1–2 puffs bid	$53.33
(QVAR‡)	(40 μg/puff)	2–4 puffs bid	1–2 puffs bid	$49.58
	(80 μg/puff)	1–2 puffs bid	1 puff bid	$31.22
Budesonide *(Pulmicort Turbuhaler)*	Dry-powder inhaler (200 μg/inhalation)	1–2 inhalation bid	1–2 inhalations bid	$37.16
Flunisolide *(Aerobid)*	Metered-dose inhaler (250 μg/puff)	2–4 puffs bid	2 puff bid	$80.41
Fluticasone propionate *(Flovent‡)*	Metered-dose inhaler (44,110 or 220 μg/inhalation)	2–4 puffs bid	1–2 puffs bid	$49.30
(Flovent Rotadisk)	Dry-powder inhaler (50,100 or 250 μg/inhalation)	1 inhalation bid (100 μg/inhalation)	1 inhalation bid (50 μg/inhalation)	$51.76
Triamcinolone acetonide *(Azmacort)*	Metered-dose inhaler (100 μg/puff)	2 puffs tid-qid or 4 puffs bid	1–2 puffs tid-qid or 2–4 puffs bid	$44.87

Drug	Formation	Adult Dosage	Pediatric Dosage*	Cost†
Corticosteroid/ long-acting β_2-adrenergic agonist combination				
Fluticasone/salmeterol (*Advair Diskus*‡)	Dry-powder inhaler (100, 250, or 500 μg/50 mg per inhalation)	1 inhalation q12 h		$103.94

Adapted from The Medical Letter, Vol. 43 (Issue1102), April 16, 2001.

*For children weighing less than 40 kg.

†Cost is based on 30 days' treatment with the lowest recommended adult dosage, according to AWP listings in *Drug Topics Red Book Update* April 2001. Fluticasone/salmeterol cost is based on AWP listing in *First DataBank NDDF*, April 6, 2001.

‡Not approved by the Food and Drug Administration for use in children less than 12 years old.

FIGURE 14.1

Management of Asthma Exacerbations: Emergency Department and Hospital-Based Care

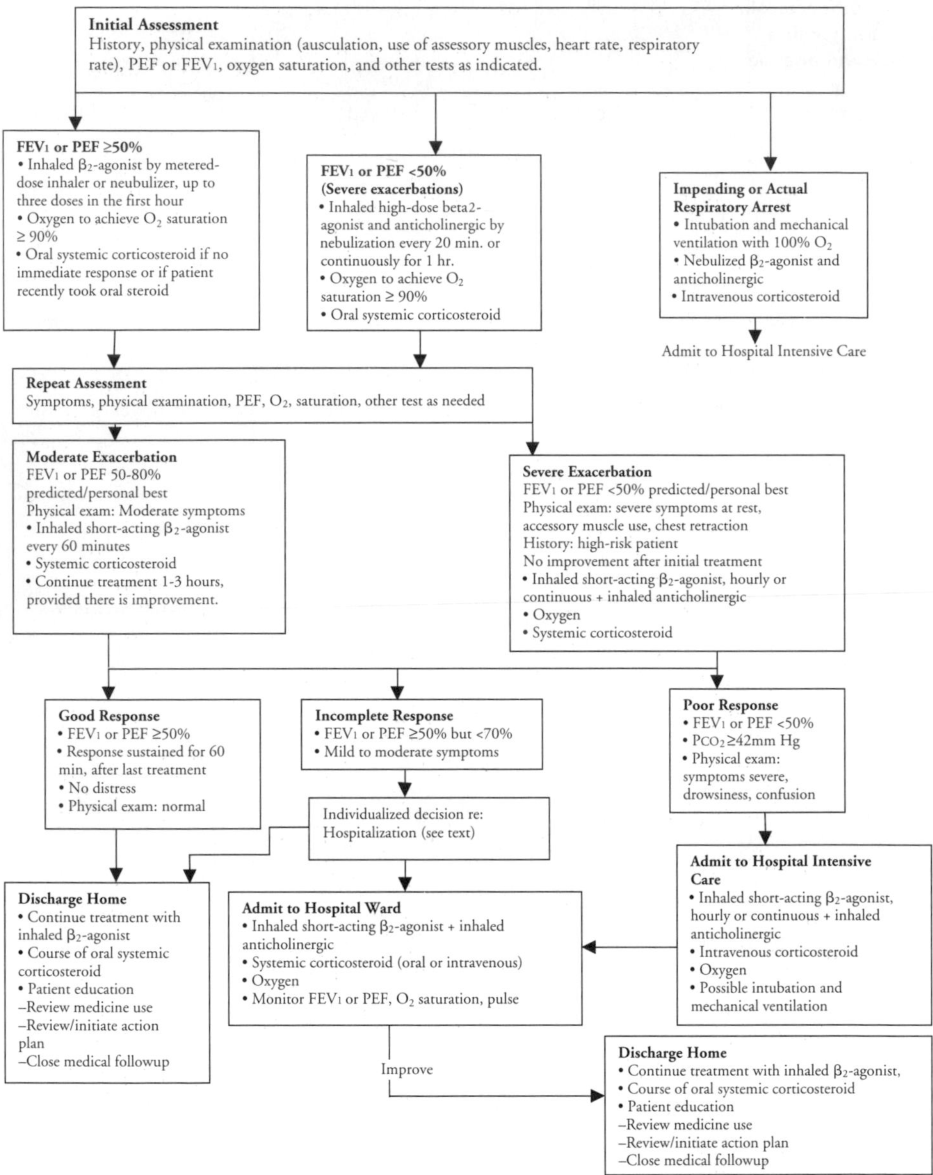

Reproduced with permission from the National Institutes of Health, National Heart, Lung, and Blood Institute. (Highlights on the expert Panel Report 2: Guidelines for the Diagnosis and Management of Asthma. N:H Publication No.97-4051A, May 1997, National Institutes of Health, National Heart, Lung, and Blood Institute, Bethesda, Md.)

TABLE 14.9

Treatment of Community-Acquired Pneumonia

Outpatients, No Cardiopulmonary Disease, No Modifying Factors*†

Organisms	Therapy
Streptococcus pneumoniae	Advanced generation macrolide:
Mycoplasma pneumoniae	Azithromycin or clarithromycin‡
Chlamydia pneumoniae (alone or as mixed infection)	OR
	Doxycycline§
Haemophilus influenzae	
Respiratory viruses	
Miscellaneous	
Legionella spp	
Mycobacterium tuberculosis	
Endemic fungi	

Adapted from Niederman MS, Mandell LA, Anzueto A, et al. Guidelines for the management of adults with community acquired pneumonia: diagnosis, assessment of therapy, antimicrobial therapy and prevention. *Am J Respir Crit Care Med.* 2001;163(7):1730–1754.

*Excludes patients at risk for human immunodeficiency virus.

†In roughly 50%–90% of the cases no etiology was identified.

‡Erythomycin is not active against *H influenzae* and the advance generation macrolides azithromycin and clarithromycin are better tolerated.

§Many isolates of *S pneumoniae* are resistant to tetracycline, and it should be used only if the patient is allergic to or intolerant of macrolides.

Outpatients, with Cardiopulmonary Disease, and/or Other Modifying Factors*†

Organisms	Therapy‡
Streptococcus pneumoniae (including DRSP)	β-Lactum (oral cefpodoxime, cefuroxime, high-dose amoxicillin, amoxicillin/clavulanate; or parenteral ceftriaxone followed by oral cefpodoxime)
Mycoplasma pneumoniae	PLUS
Chlamydia pneumoniae	Macrolide or doxycycline§
Mixed infection (bacteria plus a typical pathogen or virus)	OR
Haemophilus influenzae	Antipneumococcal fluoroquinolone (used alone)‖
Enteric gram-negatives	
Respiratory viruses	
Miscellaneous	
Moraxella catarrhalis, Legionella spp, aspiration (anaerobes), *Mycobacterium tuberculosis*, endemic fungi	

Adapted from Niederman MS, Mandell LA, Anzueto A, et al. Guidelines for the management of adults with community acquired pneumonia: diagnosis, assessment of therapy, antimicrobial therapy and prevention. *Am J Respir Crit Care Med.* 2001;163(7):1730–1754.

DRSP indicates drug-resistant *S pneumoniae.*

*Excludes patients at risk for human immunodeficiency virus.

†In roughly 50%–90% of the cases no etiology was identified.

‡In no particular order.

§High-dose amoxicillin is 1 g every 8 h; if a macrolide is used, erythomycin does not provide coverage of *H. influenzae*, and thus when amoxicillin is used, the addition of doxycycline or of an advanced-generation macrolide is required to provide adequate coverage of *H influenzae.*

‖See text for agents.

Inpatients, Not in ICU*†

Organisms	Therapy‡
a. Cardiopulmonary Disease and/or Modifying Factors (Including Being From a Nursing Home)	
Streptococcus pneumoniae (including DRSP) *Haemophilus influenzae* *Mycoplasma pneumoniae* *Chlamydia pneumoniae* Mixed infection (bacteria plus atypical pathogen) Enteric gram-negatives Aspiration (anaerobes) Viruses *Legionella* spp Miscellaneous *Mycobacterium tuberculosis*, endemic fungi, *Pneumocystis carinii*	Intravenous β-lactam§ (cefotaxime, ceftriaxone, ampicillin/sulbactam, high-dose ampicillin) PLUS Intravenous or oral macrolide or doxycycline‖ OR Intravenous antipneumococcal fluoroquinolone alone
b. No Cardiopulmonary Disease, No Modifying Factors	
S pneumoniae *H influenzae* *M pneumoniae* *C pneumoniae* Mixed infection (bacteria plus atypical pathogen) Viruses *Legionella* spp Miscellaneous *M tuberculosis*, endemic fungi, *P carinii*	Intravenous azithromycin alone If macrolide allergic or intolerant: Doxycycline and a β-lactam OR Monotherapy with an antipneumococcal fluoroquinolone

Adapted from Niederman MS, Mandell LA, Anzueto A, et al. Guidelines for the management of adults with community acquired pneumonia: diagnosis, assessment of therapy, antimicrobial therapy and prevention. *Am J Respir Crit Care Med.* 2001;163(7):1730–1754.

DRSP indicates drug-resistant *S pneumoniae*; ICU, intensive care unit.

*Excludes patients at risk for human immunodeficiency virus.

†In roughly one third to one half of the cases no etiology was identified.

‡In no particular order.

§Antipseudomonal agents such as cefepime, piperacillin/tazobactam, imipenem, and meropenem are generally active against DRSP, but not recommended for routine use in this population that does not have risk factors for *P aeruginosa*.

||Use of doxycycline or an advanced-generation macrolide (azithromycin or clarithromycin) will provide adequate coverage if the selected β-lactam is susceptible to bacterial β-lactamases (see text).

ICU-Admitted Patients*†

Organisms	Therapy*‡
a. No Risks for *Pseudomonas aeruginosa*	
Streptococcus pneumoniae (including DRSP) *Legionella* spp *Hemophilus influenzae* Enteric gram-bacilli *Staphylococcus aureus* *Mycoplasma pneumoniae* Respiratory viruses Miscellaneous *Chlamydia pneumoniae* *Mycobacterium tuberculosis*, endemic fungi	Intravenous β-lactam (cefotaxime, ceftriaxone)§ *plus either* Intravenous macrolide (azithromycin) OR Intravenous fluoroquinolone
b. Risks for *Pseudomonas aeruginosa*	
All of the above pathogens plus *P aeruginosa*	Selected intravenous antipseudomonal β-lactam (cefepime, imipenem, meropenem, piperacillin/tazabactam)|| *plus* intravenous antipseudomonal quinolone (ciprofloxacin) OR Selected intravenous antipseudomonal β-lactam (cefepime, imipenem, meropenem, piperacillin|| tazabactam) *plus* intravenous aminoglycoside PLUS EITHER intravenous macrolide (azithromycin) OR intravenous nonpseudomonal fluoroquinolone

Adapted from Niederman MS, Mandell LA, Anzueto A, et al. Guidelines for the management of adults with community acquired pneumonia: diagnosis, assessment of therapy, antimicrobial therapy and prevention. *Am J Respir Crit Care Med*. 2001;163(7):1730–1754.

DRSP indicates drug-resistant *S pneumoniae*; ICU, intensive care unit.

*Excludes patients at risk for human immunodeficiency virus.

†In roughly one third to one half of the cases no etiology was identified.

‡In no particular order.

§Antipseudomonal agents such as cefephime, piperacillin/tazobactam, imipenem, and meropenem are generally active against DRSP, but not recommended for routine use in this population that does not have risk factors for *P aeruginosa*. Combination therapy required.

||If β-lactam allergic, replace the listed β-lactam with aztreonam and combine with aminoglycoside and an antipneumococcal fluoroquinolone as listed.

TABLE 14.10

Suggestions for the Clinical Use of Pharmacotherapies for Smoking Cessation*

Pharmacotherapy	Precautions/ Contraindications	Side Effects	Dosage	Duration	Availability	Cost/day†
First-Line Pharmacotherapies (Approved for Use for Smoking Cessation by the FDA)						
Bupropion SR	History of seizure History of eating disorder	Insomnia Dry mouth	150 mg every morning for 3 days, then 150 mg twice daily (begin treatment 1–2 weeks pre-quit)	7–12 weeks, maintenance up to 6 months	Zyban (prescription only)	$3.33
Nicotine gum		Mouth soreness Dyspepsia	1–24 cigs/day: 2 mg gum (up to 24 pcs/day); 25+cigs/day: 4 mg gum (up to 24 pcs/day)	Up to 12 weeks	Nicorette, Nicorette Mint (OTC only)	$6.25 for 10, 2-mg pieces $6.87 for 10, 4-mg pieces

Continued

TABLE 14.10

Suggestions for the Clinical Use of Pharmacotherapies for Smoking Cessation*, cont'd

Pharmacotherapy	Precautions/Contraindications	Side Effects	Dosage	Duration	Availability	Cost/day†
Nicotine inhaler		Local irritation of mouth and throat	6–16 cartridges/day	Up to 6 months	Nicotrol Inhaler (prescription only)	$10.94 for 10 cartridges
Nicotine nasal spray		Nasal irritation	8–40 doses/day	3–6 months	Nicotrol NS (prescription only)	$5.40 for 12 doses
Nicotine patch		Local skin reaction Insomnia	21 mg/24 hours 14 mg/24 hours 7 mg/24 hours	4 weeks Then 2 weeks Then 2 weeks	Nicoderm CQ (OTC only), generic patches (prescription and OTC)	Brand name patches $4.00–4.50‡
			15 mg/16 hours	8 weeks	Nicotrol (OTC only)	

Adapted from the US Department of Health and Human Services (*Treating Tobacco Use and Dependence*, Washington, DC: US Department of Health and Human Services, Public Health Service; October 2000).

FDA indicates Food and Drug Administration; OTC, over the counter.

*The information contained within this table is not comprehensive. Please see package insert for additional information.

†Prices based on retail prices of medication purchased at a national chain pharmacy, located in Madison, Wisconsin, April 2000.

‡Generic brands of the patch recently became available and may be less expensive.

TABLE 14.11

Common Elements of Practical Counseling for Smoking Cessation

Practical Counseling (Problem Solving/Skills Training) Treatment Component	Examples
Recognize danger situations—Identify events, internal states, or activities that increase the risk of smoking or relapse.	■ Negative affect ■ Being around other smokers ■ Experiencing urges ■ Being under pressure
Develop coping skills—Identify and practice coping or problem-solving skills. Typically, these skills are intended to cope with danger situations.	■ Learning to anticipate temptation ■ Learning cognitive strategies that will reduce negative moods ■ Accomplishing lifestyle changes that reduce stress, improve quality of life, or produce pleasure ■ Learning cognitive and behavioral activities to cope with smoking urges (eg, distracting attention)
Provide basic information—Provide basic information about smoking and successful quitting.	■ Any smoking (even a single puff) increases the likelihood of full relapse ■ Withdrawal typically peaks within 1–3 weeks after quitting ■ Withdrawal symptoms include negative mood, urges to smoke, and difficulty concentrating ■ The addictive nature of smoking

Adapted from the US Department of Health and Human Services (*Treating Tobacco Use and Dependence*, Washington, DC: US Department of Health and Human Services, Public Health Service; October 2000).

TABLE 14.12

The Use of Low-Molecular-Weight Heparin (LMWH) in the Treatment of Venous Thromboembolic Disease

1. If diagnosis suspected, check for contraindications to LMWH, and get baseline PTT, PT, and CBC.
2. If no contraindications, begin LMWH. Enoxaparin sodium 1 mg/kg SC q 12 h. Single dose should not exceed 180 mg (or use tinzaparin sodium, 175 anti-Xa IU/kg SC daily).
3. If deep venous thrombosis or pulmonary embolus confirmed by imaging study, continue LMWH and start warfarin therapy at 5 mg/day on day 1.
4. Check platelet count between days 3 and 5.
5. Stop LMWH on day 4 or 5, as long as INR > 2.
6. Continue warafin for $\geqslant$3 months. Goal: INR 2.5; 2.0–3.0 range.
7. If patient has recurrent disease or continuing risk factor (cancer, coagulation disorder), consider treating for $\geqslant$12 months.

Adapted from the Sixth ACCP Consensus Conference on Antithrombotic Therapy: Quick Reference Guide for Clinicians, 2001, p 17–19.

CBC indicates complete blood cell count; INR, international normalized ratio; PT, prothrombin time; PTT, partial thromboplastin time.

FIGURE 14.2

Sleep Disorders

Daytime Somnolence	Insomnia
Sleep apnea	Stress
Narcolepsy	Travel
Depression	Acute/chronic illness
Medications	Restless leg syndrome
Restless leg syndrome	Medications
Poor sleep	Depression
Other	Alcohol
	Other

Sleep Disorder	Diagnosis	Treatment
Sleep apnea	▪ Nocturnal gasping, large neck ▪ Overnight sleep study	▪ CPAP ▪ Dental appliances ▪ Surgery ▪ Avoid alcohol
Narcolepsy	▪ Cataplexy, sleep paralysis, hypnogogic hallucinations ▪ Overnight sleep study, multiple sleep latency test	▪ Exercise ▪ Scheduled naps ▪ Methylphenidate ▪ Modafinil ▪ Other
Restless leg syndrome	▪ Motor restlessness (particularly at night), relieved with activity ▪ Overnight sleep study	▪ Dopaminergic agents: Levodopa Pramipexole ▪ Avoid caffeine and antidepressants ▪ Other

CPAP indicates continuous positive airway pressure.

TABLE 14.13

Common Radiographic Findings

Hilar Adenopathy

- Sarcoidosis
- Lymphoma
- Carcinoma
- Tuberculosis
- Fungal: coccidioidomycosis, histoplasmosis

Intersititial Infiltrates

- Idiopathic pulmonary fibrosis
- Viral pneumonia
- *Mycoplasma* pneumonia, *Pneumocystis carinii* pneumonia
- Drug induced (ie, nitrofurantoin)
- Lymphangitic carcinomatosis
- Connective tissue disease (ie, rheumatoid arthritis, systematic lupus erythematosus)
- Sarcoidosis
- Congestive heart failure
- Occupational (ie, silicosis, asbestosis)
- Other

Lung Nodules

- Bronchogenic carcinoma, metastatic tumor
- Fungal or mycobacterial granuloma
- Carcinoid
- Hamartoma (benign)
- Rheumatoid nodule
- Pneumonia
- Atelectasis
- Infarction
- Other

TABLE 14.14

Criteria for Tuberculin Positivity, by Risk Group

Reactions ⩾15 mm of Induration Are Considered Positive in Persons With No Risk Factors for TB

Reaction ⩾5 mm of Induration	Reaction ⩾10 mm of Induration
Human immunodeficiency virus (HIV)–positive persons	Recent immigrants (ie, within the last 5 years) from high-prevalence countries
Recent contacts of tuberculosis (TB) case patients	Injection drug users
Fibrotic changes on chest radiograph consistent with prior TB	Residents and employees plus one of the following high-risk congregate settings: prisons and jails, nursing homes and other long-term care facilities for the elderly, hospitals and other health care facilities, residential facilities for patients with acquired immunodeficiency syndrome (AIDS), and homeless shelters
Patients with organ transplants and other immunosuppressed patients (receiving the equivalent of ⩾15 mg/d of predisone for 1 month or more)	Mycobacteriology laboratory personnel Persons with the following clinical conditions that place them at high risk: silicosis, diabetes mellitus, chronic renal failure, some hematologic disorders (eg, leukemias and lymphomas), other specific malignancies (eg, carcinoma of the head or neck and lung), weight loss of ⩾10% of ideal body weight, gastrectomy, and jejunoileal bypass
	Children younger than 4 years or infants, children, and adolescents exposed to adults at high risk

Adapted from the American Thoracic Society (Targeted tuberculin testing and treatment of latent tuberculosis infection. *Am J Respir Crit Care Med.* 2000; 161(4 pt 2):S221–247).

Risk of TB patients treated with corticosteroids increases with higher dose and longer duration. For persons who are otherwise at low risk and are tested at the start of employment, a reaction of ⩾15 mm of induration is considered positive. (Adapted with permission from the Centers for Disease Control and Prevention. Screening for tuberculosis and tuberculosis infection in high-risk populations: recommendations of the Advisory Council for the Elimination of Tuberculosis. *Morb Mortal Wkly Rep.* 1995;44[No. RR-1]:19–34.)

TABLE 14.15

Changes From Prior Recommendations on Tuberculin Testing and Treatment of Latent Tuberculosis Infection (LTBI)

Tuberculin Testing

- Emphasis on target tuberculin testing among person at high risk for recent LTBI or with clinical conditions that increase the risk for tuberculosis (TB), regardless of age; testing is discouraged among persons at lower risk
- For patients with organ transplants and other immunosuppressed patients (eg, persons receiving the equivalent of ≥15 mg/d of predisone for 1 month or more), 5 mm of induration rather than 10 mm of induration as a cut-off level for tuberculin positivity
- A tuberculin skin test conversion is defined as an increase of ≥10 mm of induration within a 2-y period, regardless of age

Treatment of Latent Tuberculosis Infection

- For human immunodeficiency virus (HIV)–negative person, isoniazid given for 9 months is preferred over 6-month regimens
- For HIV-positive persons and those with fibrotic lesions on chest x-ray consistent with previous TB, isoniazid should be given for 9 months instead of 12 months
- For HIV-negative and HIV-positive persons, rifampin and pyrazinamide should be given for 2 months
- For HIV-negative and HIV-positive persons, rifampin should be given for 4 months

Clinical and Laboratory Monitoring

- Routine baseline and follow-up laboratory monitoring can be eliminated in most person with LTBI, except for those with HIV infection, pregnant women (or those in the immediate postpartum period), and persons with chronic liver disease or those who drink alcohol regularly
- Emphasis on clinical monitoring for signs and symptoms of possible adverse effects, with prompt evaluation and changes in treatment, as indicated

Treatment of Latent TB Infections

Drugs	Duration (mo)	Interval	Rating (Evidence)	
			HIV$^-$	HIV$^+$
Isoniazid	9	Daily	A (II)	A (II)
		Twice weekly	B (II)	B (II)
Isoniazid	6	Daily	B (I)	C (I)
		Twice weekly	B (II)	C (I)
Rifampin-	2	Daily	B (II)	A (I)
pyrazinamide	2–3	Twice weekly	C (II)	C (I)
Rifampin	4	Daily	B (II)	B (III)

Adapted from the American Thoracic Society (Targeted tuberculin testing and treatment of latent tuberculosis infection. *Am J Respir Crit Care Med.* 2000;161 (4 pt 2): S221–247).

A indicates preferred; B, acceptable alternative; C, offer when A and B cannot be given.

I indicates randomized clinical trial data; II, data from clinical trials that are not randomized or were conducted in other populations; III, expert opinion.

TABLE 14.16

Evaluation of Pleural Fluid

Exudate	Common Causes
Protein >2.9 g/dL	Pneumonia
Fluid/serum protein ratio >0.5	Pancreatitis
Fluid/serum LDH ratio >0.6	Malignancy
Fluid cholesterol >45 mg/dL	Connective tissue disease
Fluid LDH >2/3 upper limit of normal for serum LDH	Pulmonary emboli

Transudate	Common Causes
Protein <3.0 g/dL	CHF
Fluid/serum protein ratio <0.5	Nephrotic
Fluid/serum LDH ratio <0.6	Liver disease
Fluid LDH <2/3 upper limit of normal for serum LDH	Low albumin conditions

CHF indicates congestive heart failure; LDH, lactate dehydrogenase.

TABLE 14.17

Indications for Long-term Oxygen Therapy

Absolute:

- Pa_{O_2} ≤55 mm Hg or Sa_{O_2} ≤88%

In Presence of Cor Pulmonale:

- Pa_{O_2} 55–59 mm Hg or Sa_{O_2} ≥89%
- ECG evidence of "P" pulmonale, hematocrit >55%, congestive heart failure

Only Specific Situations:

- Pa_{O_2} ≥60 mm Hg or Sa_{O_2} ≥90%
- With lung disease and other clinical needs, such as sleep apnea with nocturnal desaturation not corrected by CPAP
- If the patient meets criteria at rest, O_2 should also be prescribed during sleep and exercise, appropriately titrated
- If the patient is normoxemic at rest but desaturates during exercise or sleep (Pa_{O_2} ≤55 mm Hg), O_2 should be prescribed for these indications
- Also consider nasal CPAP or BiPAP

Adapted from the American Thoracic Society (Standards for the diagnosis and care of patients with chronic obstructive pulmonary disease. *Am J Respir Crit Care Med.* 1995;152(5 pt 2): S77–121).

CPAP indicates continuous positive airway pressure; ECG, electrocardiogram; BiPAP, bilevel positive airway pressure.

TABLE 14.18

Helpful Rules for Interpreting Arterial Blood Gases in Patients With Acute and Chronic Respiratory Failure

1. Acute Respiratory Acidosis

- For every 10-mmHg acute increase in P_{CO_2}, pH decreases by 0.08
- For every 10-mmHg acute increase in P_{CO_2}, HCO_3 increases by 1 mEq/L
- For ease of calculation, use pH=7.40, P_{CO_2}=40 mmHg, and HCO_3=24 mEq/L as normal values

Example: Well-controlled, young asthmatic patient develops severe respiratory distress and acute respiratory acidosis after pollen exposure.

ABG: pH=7.32, P_{CO_2}=50 mmHg, P_{O_2}=64 mmHg, serum HCO_3=25 mEq/L

Interpretation: Acute respiratory acidosis

One hour later, patient still struggling to breathe.

Repeat ABG: pH=7.24, P_{CO_2}=50 mmHg, P_{O_2}=64 mmHg, serum HCO_3=19 mEq/L

Interpretation: Patient has developed a superimposed metabolic acidosis, in addition to acute respiratory acidosis, most likely secondary to lactic acid from anaerobic metabolism in respiratory muscles.

2. Chronic Respiratory Acidosis

- For every 10-mmHg chronic increase in P_{CO_2} , serum HCO_3 increases by 3.0 mEq/L

Example: 70-year-old asymptomatic male with history of severe COPD presents for routine visits.

Baseline ABG obtained: pH=7.36, P_{CO_2}=50 mmHg, P_{O_2}=65 mmHg, serum HCO_3=27 mEq/L

Interpretation: Patient has chronic respiratory acidosis (patient would be acutely symptomatic, with pH closer to 7.32, in simple, acute respiratory acidosis). There is a superimposed metabolic alkalosis secondary to renal compensation.

TABLE 14.19

Evidence-Based Recommendations for Management of Acute Exacerbations of COPD

1. Admission CXR is useful.
2. Spirometry is *not* helpful in diagnosing or judging severity of exacerbations.
3. Both inhaled anticholinergic bronchodilators (ipratropium) and inhaled short-acting β_2 agonists (albuterol) are beneficial. Use anticholinergic inhalers first, and add second inhaler only after maximal dose of first inhaler reached.
4. Use systemic corticosteroids for up to 2 weeks (may need longer course for patients on chronic steroids).
5. Use oxygen with caution in hypoxemic patients.
6. Consider noninvasive positive-pressure ventilation in severe exacerbations (especially with CO_2 retention).
7. Narrow-spectrum antibiotics (amoxicillin, tetracyclines, trimethoprim-sulfamethoxazole) are reasonable first-choice agents in acute exacerbations.
8. Mucolytic medications, chest physiotherapy, and methylxanthine bronchodilators are *not* beneficial.

Adapted from the American College of Physicians–American Society of Internal Medicine (Snow V, Lascher S, Mottur-Pilson C. Evidence base for the management of acute exacerbations of chronic obstructive pulmonary disease. *Ann Intern Med.* 2001;134:595–599).

COPD indicates chronic obstructive pulmonary disease; CXR, chest X-ray.

TABLE 14.20

Initiating Mechanical Ventilation for Acute Respiratory Failure

1. Whether or not a patient needs mechanical ventilation requires clinical judgment. Most patients with acute respiratory failure present with symptoms and signs of respiratory fatigue, $Pa{O_2} < 60$ mmHg on $Fi{O_2} > 60\%$, $Pa{CO_2} > 50$ mmHg, and $pH < 7.35$.
2. Before initiating mechanical ventilation, consider whether or not patient is a candidate for noninvasive pressure ventilation (BiPAP).
3. If possible, obtain informed consent, particularly in patients with chronic or terminal conditions.
4. Once patient is intubated, place patient on $Fi{O_2}$ 1.0 (100%), tidal volume of 8–10 mL/kg, assist control ventilation with set rate of ~16–20, and PEEP = 5 cm.
5. Set flow rate at ~40–60 L/min and set trigger sensitivity at −2 or −3 cm of inspiratory force.
6. Obtain arterial blood gas 20 minutes later, aiming for a pH ~7.35–7.45 and titrating oxygen down to $Pa{O_2} > 60$ mmHg on <60% oxygen.
7. Consult with pulmonologist regarding the subtleties of managing specific illnesses (ie, asthmatic patients may require higher flow rates and decreased ventilator rates—leading to higher $P{CO_2}$ and lower pH levels—to enhance expiratory flow; lower tidal volumes may be beneficial in ARDS patients).

Adapted from Ahya SH, Flood K, Paranjothi S, Lee H, eds. *The Washington Manual of Medical Therapeutics*. 30th ed. Philadelphia, PA, Lippincott Williams & Wilkins; 2001:201–204.

TABLE 14.21

Brief Guide to Weaning Patients From Ventilators

1. Consult with pulmonary physician if possible.
2. Ensure that patient is alert and aware, has minimal secretions, and has stable cardiovascular status.
3. Ensure that patient's acute and underlying conditions are appropriately treated, including nutritional assessment.
4. Decrease intermittent mandatory ventilation (IMV) rates and/or pressure support ventilation (PSV) pressures rapidly *as long as* respiratory rate of patient remains <30 min, vital signs remain stable, and ABGs remain stable.
5. If the patient is breathing comfortably on PSV 5–8 cm, and the above steps have been followed, then assess patient for withdrawal:

   —Pao_2 >60 mmHg on Fio_2 <50%

   —PEEP ≤5 cm

   —$Paco_2$ and pH normal

   —Vital capacity >10 mL/kg

   —Respiratory rate <30/min

   —Negative inspiratory force >25 cm

   —Spontaneous tidal volume >5 mL/kg

   —Vital signs and ABG stable after 1-hour spontaneous breathing (T-piece) trial

TABLE 14.22

Orotracheal Intubation Technique

1. Gather equipment, including several endotracheal tubes, stylet, lubricant, laryngoscope, tape, 10-cc syringe.
2. Obtain proper head position ("sniff" position).
3. Administer appropriate sedation, "bag" with 100% Fio_2.
4. Suction mouth.
5. After opening patient's mouth with right hand and holding laryngoscope in left hand, insert scope into right side of mouth and sweep tongue away. Apply upward, outward pressure to expose cords.
6. When cords visualized, insert tube's cuff ~2 cm below cords. Have assistant apply cricoid pressure if difficulty visualizing cords.
7. Inflate cuff.
8. Confirm placement by chest auscultation and auscultating epigastrium, and carbon dioxide detector.
9. Secure tube with tape.
10. Check chest x-ray for placement—tube should be 3–5 cm above carina.

TABLE 14.23

Brief Guide to Emergency Chest Tube Insertion

Indications: pneumothorax, empyema, hemothorax
Contraindications (relative): coagulopathy, small, loculated hydrothorax, or pneumothorax

Consult pulmonologist or surgeon if available.

1. Cleanse and drape skin over fourth intercostal space, anterior axillary line.
2. Inject local anesthetic, avoiding nerve bundle immediately below rib.
3. Make 2–4-cm horizontal incision down to muscle.
4. Separate muscle fibers with blunt hemostat and gently puncture parietal pleura.
5. Use finger to enlarge hole, and insert chest tube (12 F for pneumothorax, larger tubes for blood or pus). Direct tube cephalad for pneumothorax, caudad for fluid/pus.
6. Secure tube with suture and attach to pleural drainage system.
7. Check chest x-ray after procedure.

TABLE 14.24

Brief Guide to Thoracentesis

Indications: Evaluation/removal of pleural fluid
Contraindication: Severe coagulopathy

1. Patient should sit down, lean forward, with arms raised and resting on a pillow (see Figure 14.3).
2. Select thoracentesis site several interspaces below percussion level and fluid level on chest x-ray.
3. Apply antiseptic solution to large area at selected site.
4. Anesthetize skin with 1% lidocaine, then inject 1–3 cc *above* rib down to pleura, aspirating as you go.
5. Attach larger needle (20 or 22 gauge) to remove fluid. Vacuum bottles can be used to evacuate large volumes (limit to 1 L).
6. Check postprocedure chest x-ray—rule out pneumothorax.

FIGURE 14.3

Patient in Correct Position for Thoracentesis

He or she should be as comfortable as possible, with arms raised on a pillow.

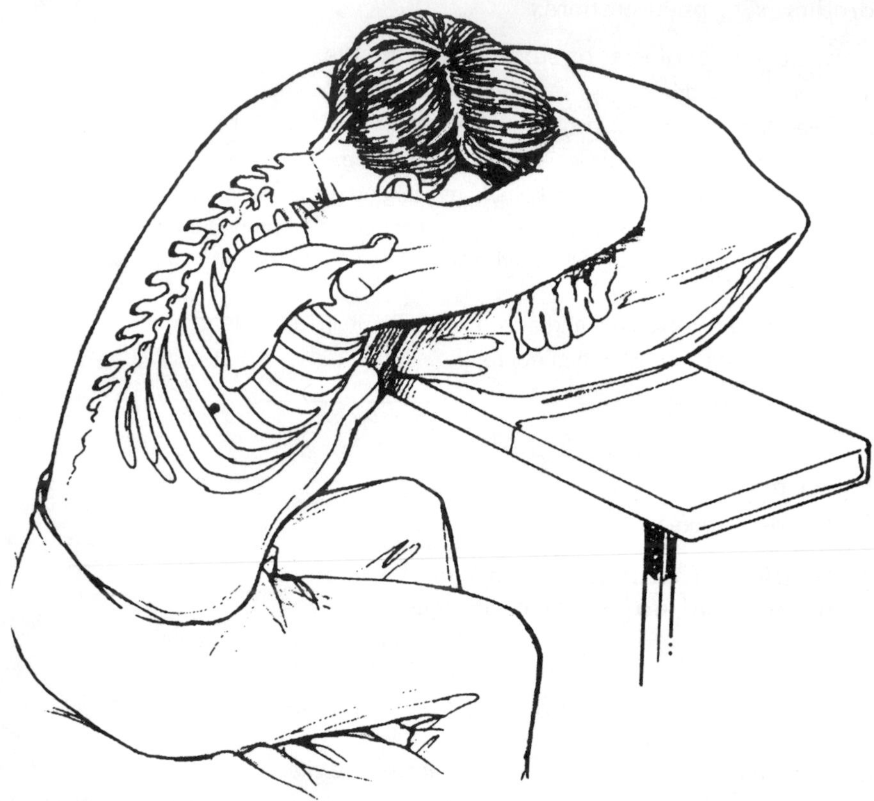

Reproduced with permission from the Practice Management Information Corporation (Driscoll CE, Rakel RE, eds. *Patient Care: Procedures for Your Practice.* 2nd ed. Los Angeles, CA: Practice Management Information Corporation; 1991:68).

chapter 15

The Gastrointestinal System

Robert I. Elliott, MD

IN THIS CHAPTER

- Diagnoses of acute abdomen
- Causes of dysphagia
- Management of gastroesophageal reflux disease
- Evaluation of dyspepsia
- Evaluation of peptic ulcer disease
- Treatment of *Helicobacter pylori*
- Evaluation of abnormal liver function tests
- Viral hepatitis
- Evaluation of ascites
- Management of gallstones
- Acute pancreatitis
- Evaluation of constipation
- Traveler's diarrhea
- Inflammatory bowel disease
- Irritable bowel syndrome
- Evaluation of upper gastrointestinal bleeding
- Evaluation of lower gastrointestinal bleeding
- Anorectal disorders
- Common gastrointestinal procedures

BOOKSHELF RECOMMENDATIONS

- Lipsky MS. *Gastrointestinal Problems*. Philadelphia, PA: Lippincott Williams and Wilkins; 2000.

- Cope Z, Siler W. *Early Diagnosis of the Acute Abdomen*. 20th ed. New York, NY: Oxford University Press; 2000.
- Ahya SN, Flood K, Paranjothi S, et al, eds. *The Washington Manual of Medical Therapeutics*. 30th ed. Philadelphia, PA: Lippincott Williams & Wilkins; 2001.

TABLE 15.1

Evaluation of Patients With GI Complaints

The investigation of patients with symptoms referable to the gastrointestinal tract begins, as in other areas of medicine, with a thoughtful and empathic approach to the patient. This approach is defined by:
■ An ability to listen to the patient
■ Probe for additional pertinent points
■ History should not be limited to the GI system
■ Include associated systems that may contribute to disease in the GI tract
■ Diffuse vascular disease that may suggest intestinal ischemia
■ Medications (NSAIDs) that may predispose to peptic disease
■ Family and social issues that may contribute to conditions
■ Perform a thorough physical exam
■ Additional laboratory and diagnostic options may be needed to supplement findings

GI indicates gastrointestinal; NSAIDs, nonsteroidal anti-inflammatory drugs.

TABLE 15.2

Differential Diagnosis of Acute Abdomen

Gastrointestinal
Appendicitis
Cholecystitis
Crohn disease
Diverticulitis
Duodenal ulcer
Gastroenteritis
Intestinal obstruction
Intussusception
Meckel diverticulitis
Mesenteric lymphadenitis
Necrotizing enterocolitis
Neoplasm (carcinoid, carcinoma, lymphoma)
Omental torsion
Pancreatitis
Perforated viscus
Sigmoid volvulus

Gynecologic
Ectopic pregnancy
Endometriosis
Ovarian torsion
Pelvic inflammatory disease
Ruptured ovarian cyst (follicular, corpus luteum)
Tubo-ovarian abscess

Systemic
Diabetic ketoacidosis
Porphyria
Sickle cell disease
Henoch-Schönlein purpura

Pulmonary
Pleuritis
Pneumonia (basilar)
Pulmonary infarction

Genitourinary
Kidney stone
Prostatitis
Pyelonephritis
Retroperitoneal hemorrhage
Testicular torsion
Urinary tract infection

Vascular
Dissecting abdominal aortic aneurysm
Ischemic bowel

TABLE 15.3

Selected Causes of Dysphagia

Selected Causes of Dysphagia
Neurologic Disorders and Stroke
Cerebrovascular disease
Intracranial hemorrhage
Parkinson disease
Multiple sclerosis
Amyotrophic lateral sclerosis
Poliomyelitis
Myasthenia gravis
Dementias
Structural Lesions
Thyromegaly
Cervical hyperostosis
Congenital web
Zenker diverticulum
Ingestion of caustic material
Neoplasm
Psychiatric Disorder
Psychogenic dysphagia
Connective Tissue Diseases
Polymyositis
Muscular dystrophy
Iatrogenic Causes
Surgical resection
Radiation fibrosis
Medications

TABLE 15.4

Management of Gastroesophageal Reflux Disease

Lifestyle Modifications

- Head of bed elevated 6 inches
- Decreased fat intake
- Smoking cessation
- Weight reduction
- Avoidance of recumbency for 3 hours postprandially
- Avoidance of large meals and certain foods

+

As-Needed Pharmacologic Therapy

- Antacid containing alginic acid
- Over-the-counter histamine H_2–receptor blocker

↓

Scheduled Pharmacologic Therapy

- H_2-receptor blocker or prokinetic agent for 8–12 weeks
- For persistent symptoms, high-dose H_2-receptor blocker or proton pump inhibitor for another 8–12 weeks (or reconsider diagnosis)
- With documented erosive esophagitis use proton pump inhibitor as first-line therapy

↓

Maintenance Therapy

- Appropriate for patient with symptomatic relapse or complicated disease
- Lowest effective dosage of H_2-receptor blocker or proton pump inhibitor

↓

Surgery

- May be appropriate in patient with severe symptoms, erosive esophagitis or disease complications
- Laparoscopic Nissen or Toupet fundoplication procedure

FIGURE 15.1
Evaluation of Dyspepsia

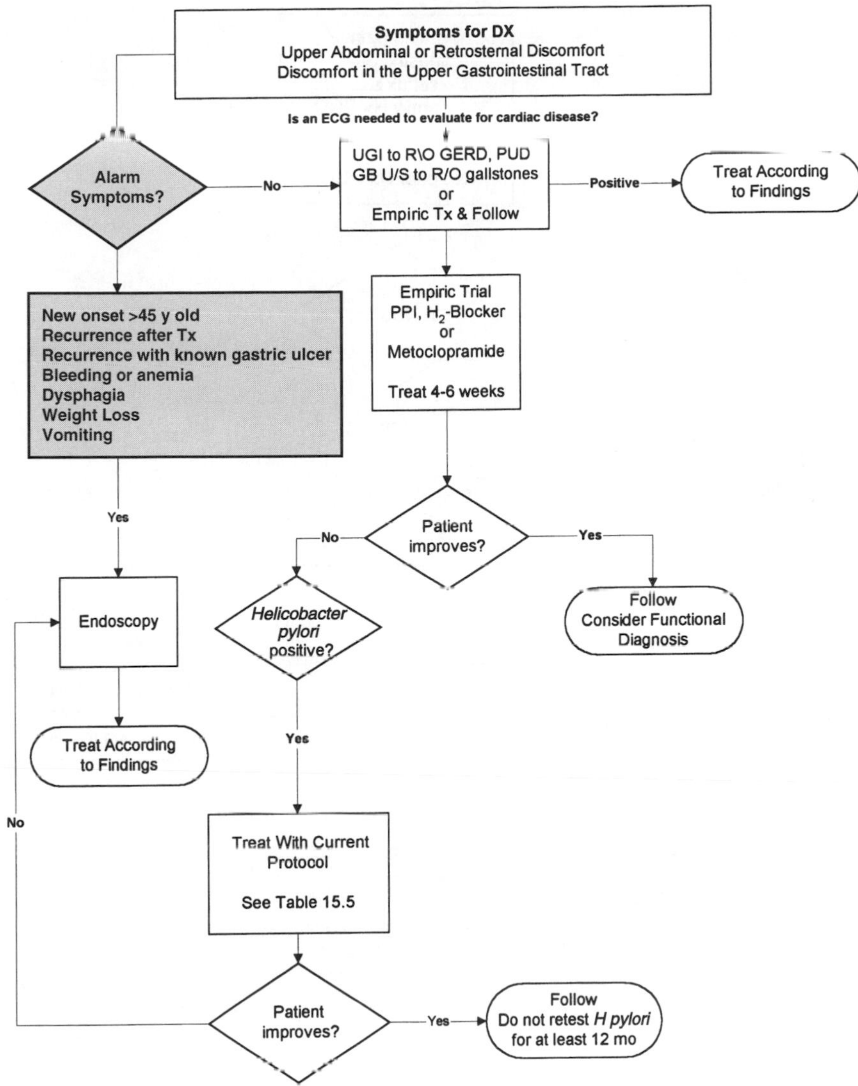

FIGURE 15.2

Evaluation of Peptic Disease

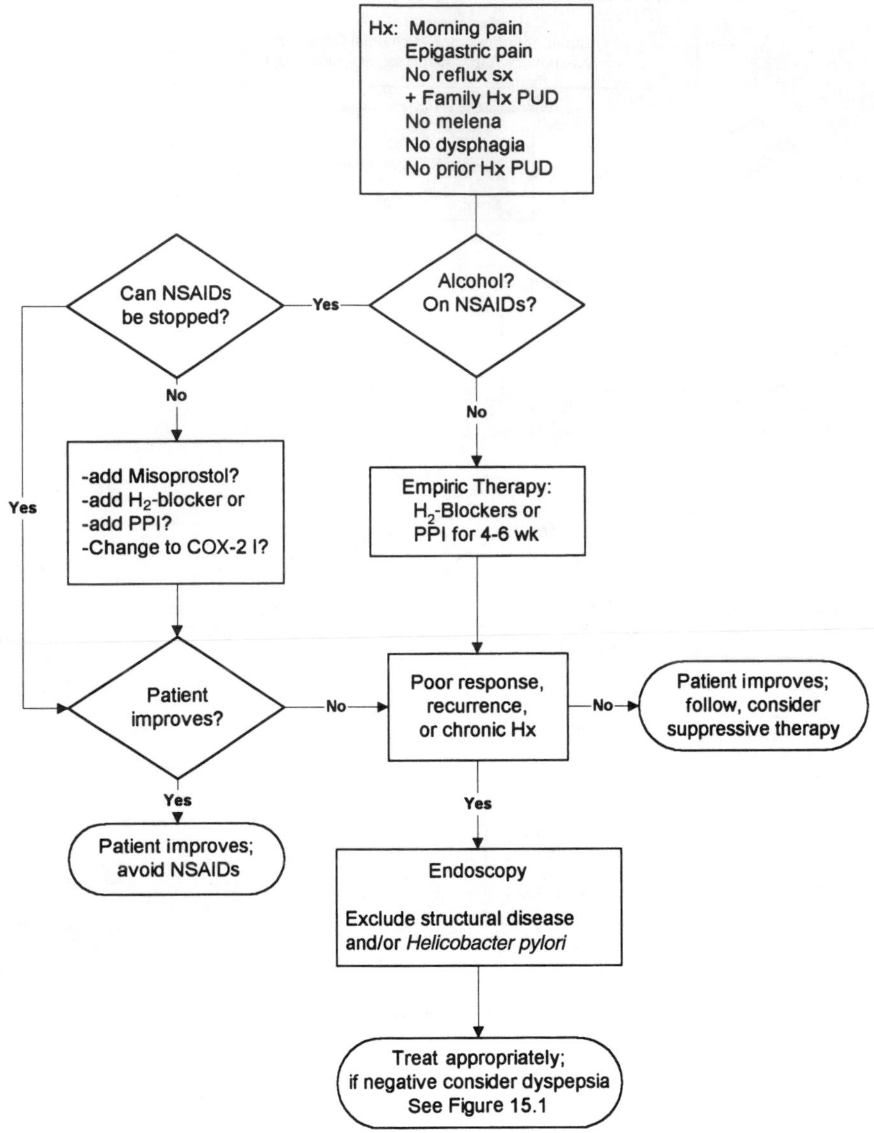

TABLE 15.5
Helicobacter Pylori Eradication Regimen

Therapy	Regimen	Duration	Eradication Rates, %
PPI*-based triple therapy	PPI* dosed bid and amoxicillin 1 g bid and clarithromycin 500 mg bid	2 weeks 1 week	92 86
	OR		
	PPI and metronidazole 1 g bid plus clarithromycin 500 mg bid	2 weeks	88
Ranitidine/bismuth	RBC 400 g bid and clarithromycin	2 weeks	92
Citrate-based triple therapy	500 mg bid and amoxicillin 1 bid		
	OR		
	RBC 400 g bid and metronidazole 250 mg tid plus tetracycline 500 mg tid	2 weeks	80
Bismuth–quadruple therapy	PPI and bismuth subsalicylate 10 mL qid and metronidazole 250 mg qid and tetracycline 100 mg qid	2 weeks	98

*PPI may include omeprazole 20 mg, lansoprazole 30 mg, pantoprazole 40 mg, or rabeprazole 20 mg.

bid indicates twice daily; qid, four times daily; RBC, ranitidine bismuth citrate; tid, three times daily.

FIGURE 15.3

Abnormal ALT/AST (<5 × Normal) in Asymptomatic Patients

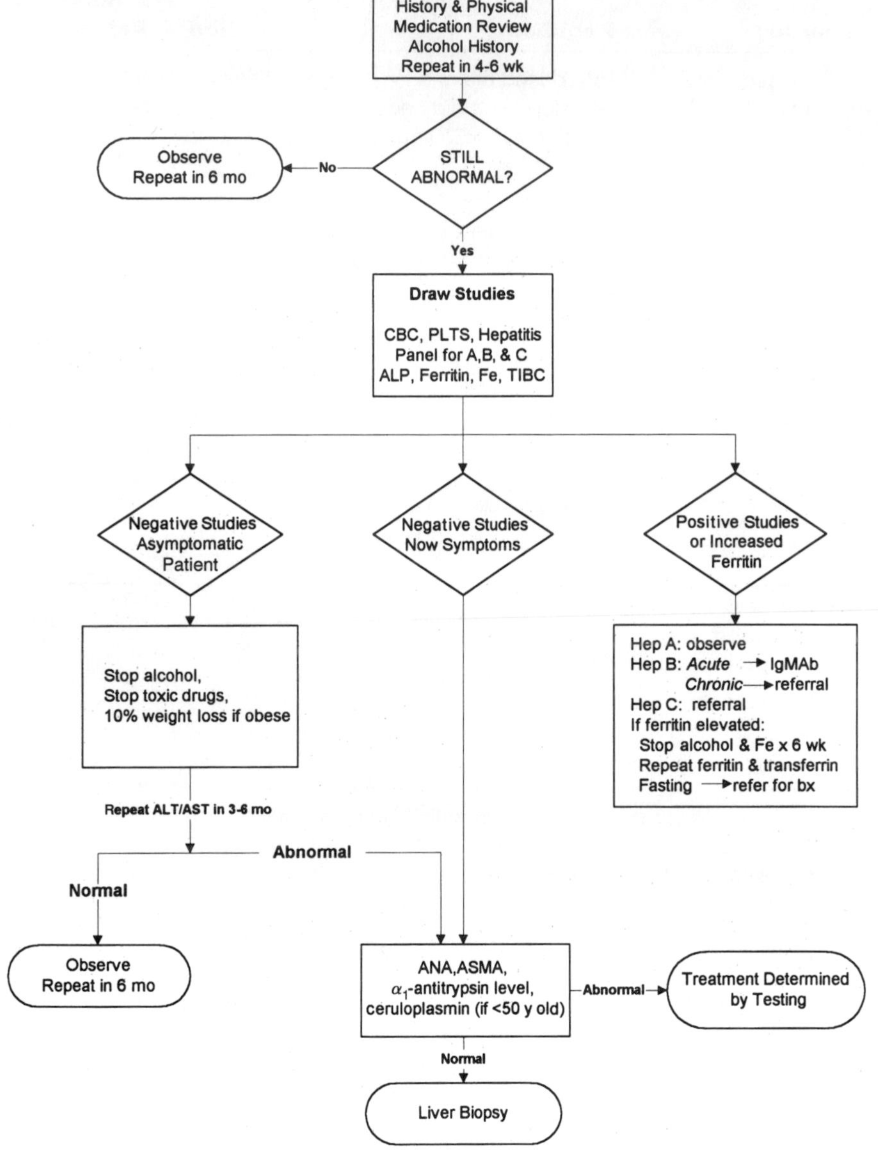

TABLE 15.6

Grading Liver Function Using the Child-Turcotte Class as Modified by Pugh*

	Points		
Feature	**0**	**1**	**2**
Albumin	More than 3.5 g per dL (35 g per L)	2.8 to 3.5 g per dL (28 to 35 g per L)	Less than 2.8 g per dL (28 g per L)
Bilirubin	Less than 2 mg per dL (34 μmol per L)	2 to 3 mg per dL (34 to 51 μmol per L)	More than 3 mg per dL
Prolongation of prothrombin time	Less than 4 seconds	4 to 6 seconds	More than 6 seconds
Ascites	None	Controlled with routine medical therapy	Refractory to medical therapy
Encephalopathy	None	Controlled with routine medical therapy	Refractory to medical therapy

Adapted from Pugh RN, Murray-Lyon IM, Dawson JL, et al. Transection of the oesophagus for bleeding oesophageal varices. *Br J Surg*. 1973;60(8):646–649.

*The Child-Turcotte class, as modified by Pugh, often known simply as the "Child class," is calculated by adding the points as determined by the patient's laboratory results: class A = 0 to 1; class B = 2 to 4; class C = 5 and higher. The classes indicate severity of liver dysfunction: class A is associated with a good prognosis, and class C is associated with limited life expectancy.

TABLE 15.7

Prevention of Hepatitis A Through Active or Passive Immunization: Recommendations of the Advisory Committee on Immunization Practices (ACIP)

Persons at increased risk for hepatitis A virus infection who should be routinely vaccinated:

- Persons traveling to or working in countries that have high or intermediate endemicity of infection
- Men who have sex with men
- Persons who have occupational risk for infection
- Persons who have clotting-factor disorders
- Illegal-drug users
- Patients with chronic liver disease
- Other

TABLE 15.8

Active and Passive Immunization for Hepatitis A

Active

Recommended Dosages of VAQTA*

Vaccine Recipient's Age (yrs)	Dose (U)	Volume (mL)	No. of Doses	Schedule (mos)†
2–17	25	0.5	2	0, 6–18
>17	50	1.0	2	0, 6

*Hepatitis A vaccine, inactivated, Merck Co, Inc.

†0 months represents timing of the initial dose; subsequent numbers represent months after the initial dose.

OR

Vaccine Recipient's Age (y)	Dose (U)†	Volume (mL)	No. of Doses	Schedule (mos)‡
2–18	720	0.5	2	0, 6–12
>18	1440	1.0	2	0, 6–12

*Hepatitis A vaccine, inactivated, SmithKline Beecham Biologicals.

†Enzyme-linked immunosorbent assay (ELISA) units.

‡0 months represents timing of the initial dose; subsequent numbers represent months after the initial dose.

Passive

Setting	Duration of Coverage	IG Dose†
Preexposure	Short-term (1–2 mo)	0.02 mL/kg
	Long-term (3–5 mo)	0.06 mL/kg‡
Postexposure	—	0.02 mL/kg

*Infants and pregnant women should receive a preparation that does not include thimerosal.

†Immune globulin (IG) should be administered by intramuscular injection into either the deltoid or gluteal muscle. For children < 24 months of age IG can be adminstered in the anterolateral thigh muscle.

‡Repeat every 5 months if continued exposure to hepatitis A virus occurs.

FIGURE 15.4

Scheme of Typical Clinical Laboratory Features of Viral Hepatitis Type A

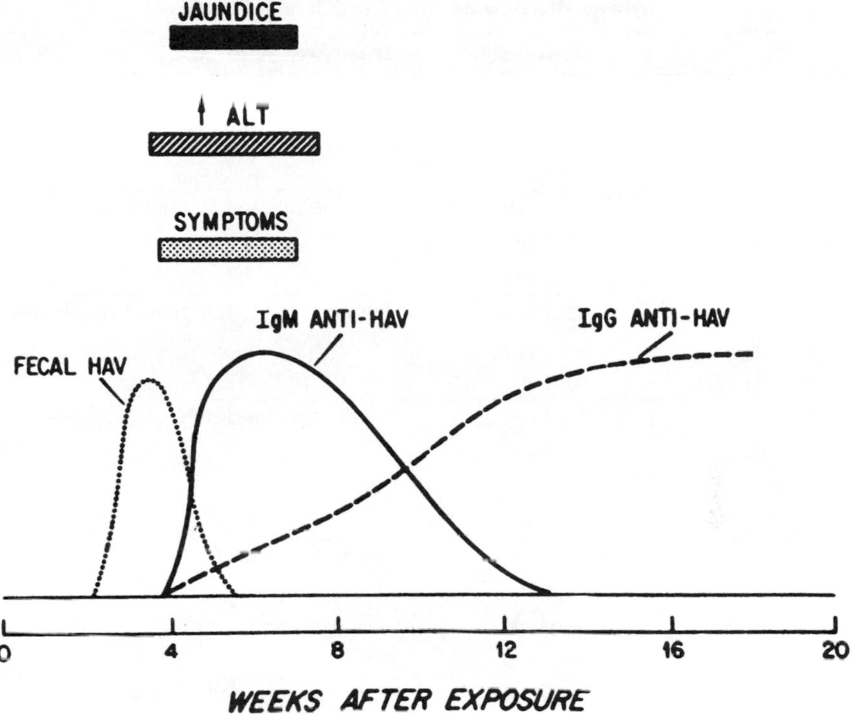

Reproduced with permission from Dienstag JL, Wands JR, Koff RS. Acute hepatitus. In: Petersdorf RG, ed. *Harrison's Principles of Internal Medicine.* 10th ed. New York: McGraw-Hill; 1981.

TABLE 15.9

Viral Hepatitis B

Interpretation of the Hepatitis B Panel		
Tests	**Results**	**Interpretation**
HbsAg	Negative	Susceptible
Anti-HGc	Negative	
Anti-HBs	Negative	
HbsAg	Negative	Immune due to natural infection
Anti-HBc	Positive	
Anti-HBs	Positive	
HbsAg	Negative	Immune due to hepatitis B vaccination
Anti-HBc	Negative	
Anti-HBs	Positive	
HbsAg	Positive	Acutely infected
Anti-HBc	Positive	
IgM anti-HBc	Positive	
Anti-HBs	Negative	
HbsAg	Positive	Chronically infected
Anti-HBc	Positive	
IgM anti-HBc	Negative	
Anti-HBs	Negative	
HbsAg	Negative	Four interpretations possible*
Anti-HBc	Positive	
Anti-HBs	Negative	

Source: National Center for Infectious Disease, Centers for Disease Control, www.cdc.gov/anidod/diseases/hepatitis/b/ Bserology.htm.

*(1) May be recovering from acute hepatitus B virus infection; (2) may be distantly immune and test not sensitive enough to detect very low level of anti-HBs in serum; (3) may be susceptible with a false positive anti-HBc; (4) may be undetectable level of HbsAg present in the serum and the person is actually a carrier.

TABLE 15.10

Recommended Postexposure Prophylaxis for Exposure to Hepatitis B Virus

Vaccination and Antibody Response Status of Exposed Workers[*]	Treatment		
	Source HBsAG[†] Positive	Source HBsAG[†] Negative	Source Unkown or Not Available for Testing
Unvaccinated	HBIG[§] × 1 and initiate HB vaccine series[¶]	Initiate HB vaccine series	Initiate HB vaccine series
Previously vaccinated			
Known Responder**	**No Treatment**	**No Treatment**	**No Treatment**
Known nonresponder	HBIG × 1 and initiate revaccination or HBIG × 2[‖]	No treatment	If known high risk source, treat as if source were HbsAg positive
Antibody response unknown	Test exposed person for anti-HBs[¶¶] 1. If responder,** no treatment is necessary 2. If nonresponder, administer HBIG × 1 and vaccine booster	No treatment	Test exposed person for anti-HBs 1. If responder,** no treatment is necessary 2. If nonresponder,** administer vaccine booster and recheck titer in 1–2 months

*Persons who have previously been infected with HBV are immune to reinfection and do not require postexposure prophylaxis.

†Hepatitis B surface antigen.

§Hepatitis B immune globulin; dose is 0.06 mL/kg intramuscularly.

¶Hepatitis B vaccine.

**A responder is a person with adequate levels of serum antibody to HBsAg (ie, anti-HBs ≥10 mIU/mL). A nonresponder is a person with inadequate response to vaccination (ie, serum anti-HBs <10 mIU/mL).

‖The option of giving one dose of HBIG and reinitiating the vaccine series is preferred for nonresponders who have not completed a second 3-dose vaccine series. For persons who previously completed a second vaccine series but failed to respond, two doses of HBIG are preferred.

¶¶Antibody to HBsAg.

TABLE 15.11

Testing for Hepatitis C Virus

Recommendations for Prevention and Control of Hepatitis C Virus (HCV) Infection and HCV-Related Chronic Disease

Patients who should be tested routinely for HCV infection based on risk for infection:

- Those who ever injected illegal drugs, even if they only injected once or a few times many years ago and do not consider themselves drug users
- Those with selected medical conditions, including the following:
  - Persons who received clotting factor concentrates produced before 1987
  - Persons who were ever on chronic (long-term) hemodialysis
  - Persons with persistently abnormal alanine aminotransferase levels
- Prior recipients of transfusions or organ transplants, including the following:
  - Persons who were notified that they received blood from a donor who later tested positive for HCV infection
  - Persons who received a transfusion of blood or blood components before July 1992

Persons who should be tested routinely for HCV infection based on a recognized exposure:

- Health care, emergency medical, and public safety workers after needle sticks, sharps, or mucosal exposures to HCV-positive blood
- Children born to HCV-positive mothers

FIGURE 15.5

Scheme of Typical Clinical and Laboratory Features of Acute Viral Hepatitis Type B

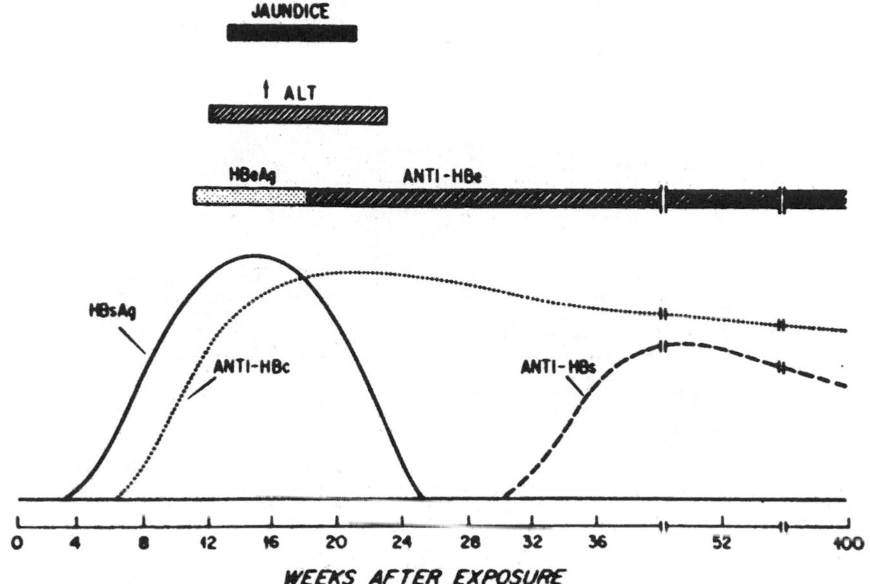

Reproduced with permission from Dienstag JL, Wands JR, Koff RS. Acute hepatitus. In: Petersdorf RG, ed. *Harrison's Principles of Internal Medicine*. 10th ed. New York: McGraw Hill; 1981.

FIGURE 15.6

Hepatitis C Virus Testing for Asymptomatic Persons

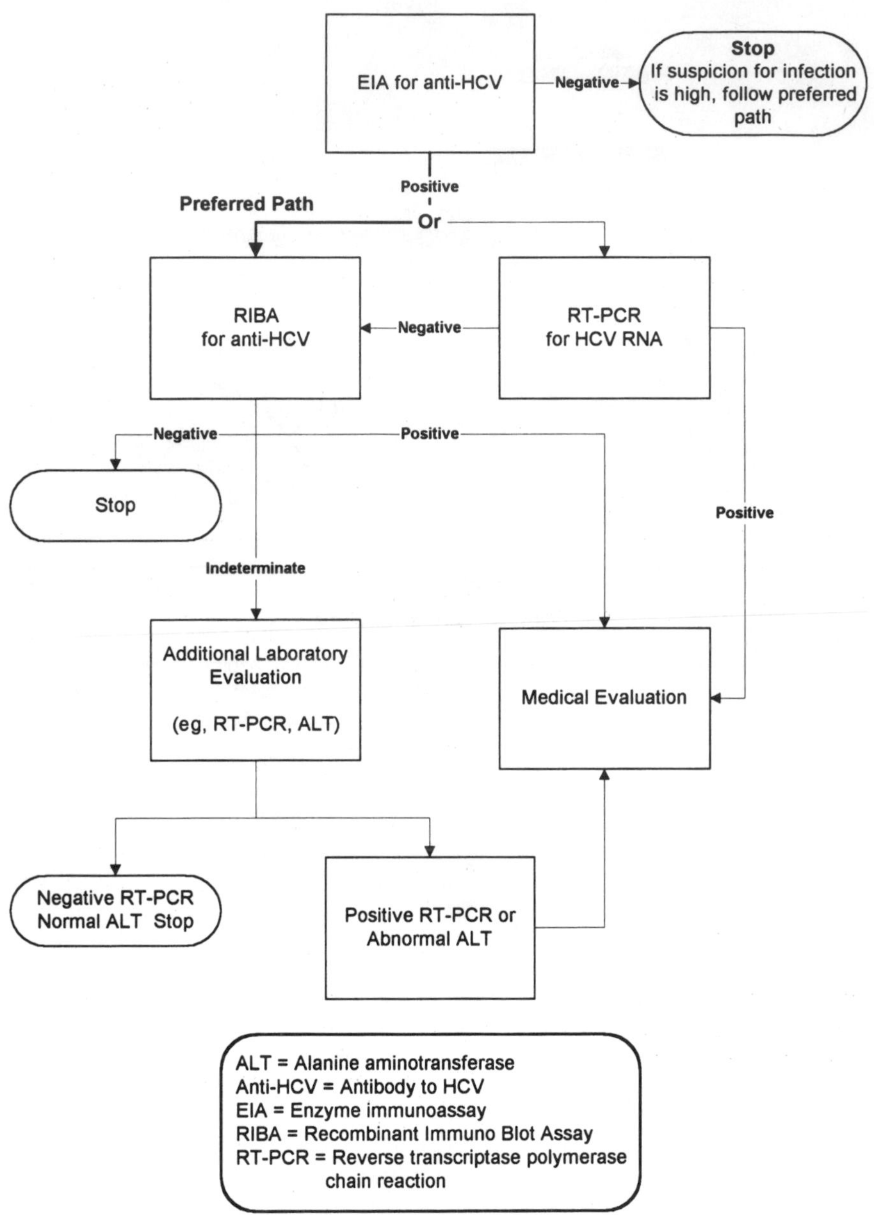

FIGURE 15.7

Evaluation of Ascites

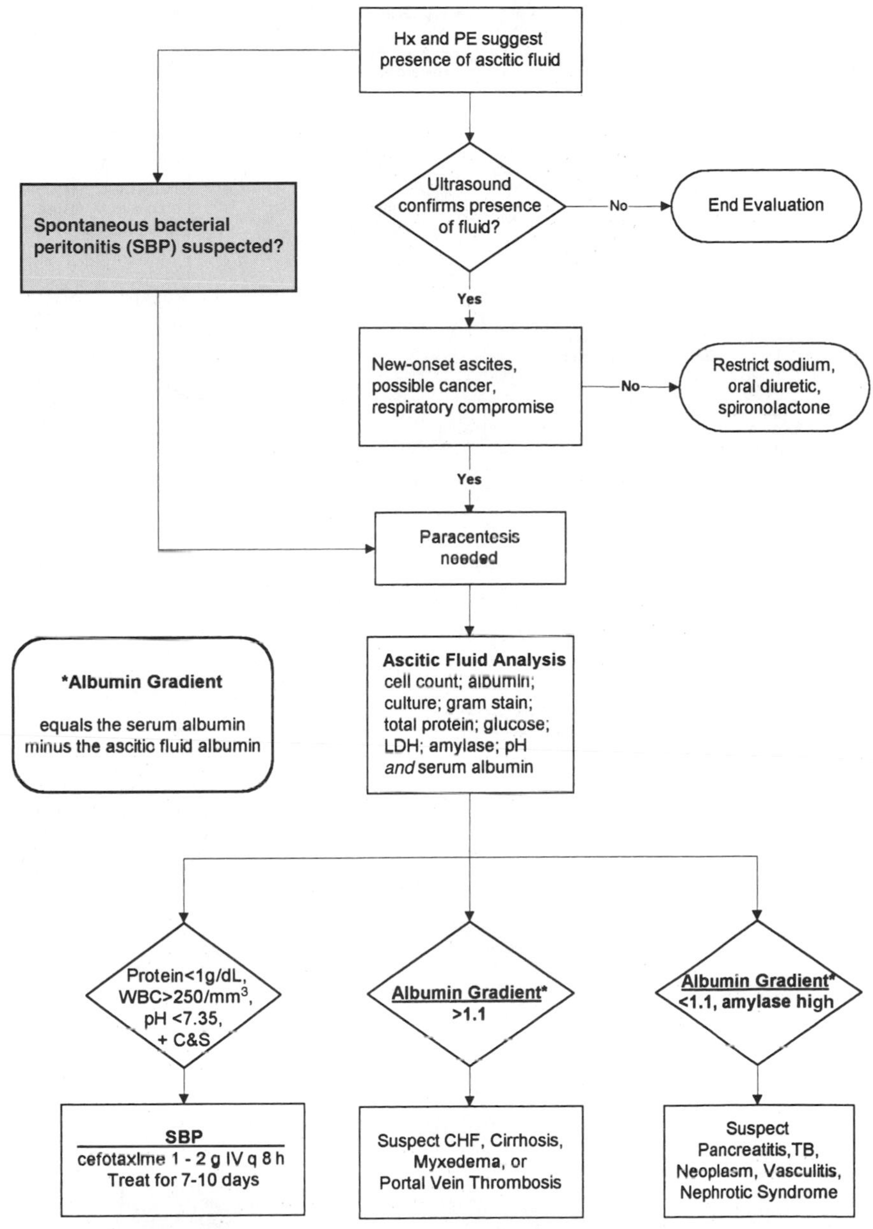

FIGURE 15.8

Decision Tree for Managing Cholelithiasis

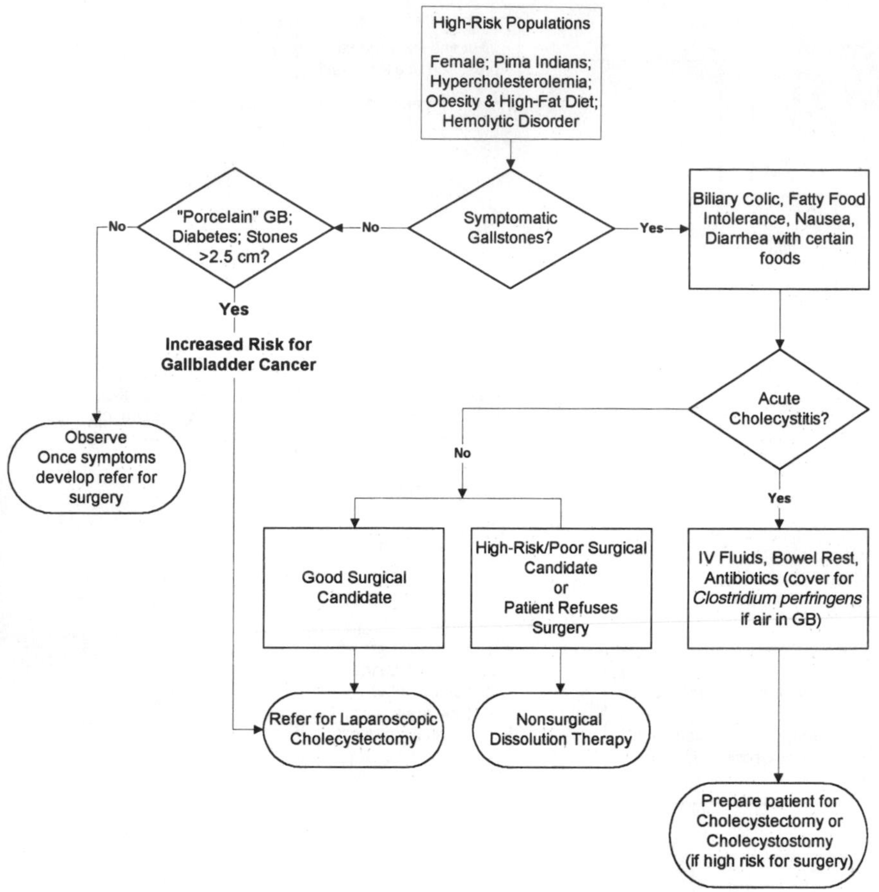

TABLE 15.12

Nonoperative Therapies for Symptomatic Gallstones

Agent	Advantages	Disadvantages
Oral bile acid dissolution: ursodiol (Actigall), at 8 to 10 mg/kg/day	Stone clearance: 30% to 90% with 0% mortality	50% recurrence of stones; dissolves noncalcified cholesterol stones; optimal for stones <5 mm; symptom relief does not start for 3 to 6 weeks; may take 6 to 24 months for results

TABLE 15.13

Potential Causes of Acute Pancreatitis

Obstruction

Cholelithiasis
Ampullary or pancreatic tumor
Parasitic infection (*Ascaris*)
Pancreas divisum with accessory duct obstruction
Hypersensitive Oddi sphincter

Infection

Viral (mumps, hepatitis, Epstein-Barr virus, rubella, human immunodeficiency virus)
Bacterial (*Mycoplasma, Campylobacter*)
Toxins/drugs
Ethanol
Medications

Vascular

Ischemia
Atherosclerotic emboli
Vasculitis (systemic lupus erythematosus, polyarteritis)

Trauma

Accidental
Iatrogenic (endoscopic retrograde cholangiopancreatography, postsurgical)
Metabolic
Hypertriglyceridemia
Hypercalcemia

Miscellaneous

Penetrating peptic ulcer
Cystic fibrosis
Hypothermia

TABLE 15.14

Differential for Elevated Serum Amylase and Lipase Levels

Elevated Amylase
Alcohol intake
Biliary obstruction
Bowel infarction
Chemotherapy
Cirrhosis
Fat emboli
Hepatic failure
Hepatitis
Intestinal obstruction
Mumps
Perforated ulcer
Radiotherapy
Renal failure
Elevated Lipase
Bacterial gastroenteritis
Bile duct obstruction
Bowel obstruction
Diarrhea
Duodenitis
Fallopian tube pathology
Inflammatory bowel disease
Opiate use
Peptic ulcer
Renal failure
Small bower perforation
Viral gastroenteritis

Adapted from Calleja GA, Barkin JS. Acute pancreatitis. *Med Clin North Am.* 1993;77:1037–1056.

TABLE 15.15

Ranson's Early Prognostic Signs of Acute Pancreatitis

At Admission

- Age more than 55 years
- WBC >16,000 cells per mm^3 (16 × 10 per L)
- Blood glucose level >200 mg per dL (11.1 mmol per L)
- Serum lactate dehydrogenase level >350 U per L
- AST level >250 U per L

During Initial 48 Hours

- Hematocrit falls >10 percentage points
- BUN level elevation >5 mg per dL (2.0 mmol per L)
- Serum calcium level falls to <8 mg per dL (2 mmol per L)
- Arterial Po_2 <60 mm Hg
- Base deficit >4 mEq per L
- Estimated fluid sequestration >6 L

Adapted from Ranson JH. Diagnostic standards for acute pancreatitis. *World J Surg.* 1997;21(2):136–142.

AST indicates asparate aminotransferase; BUN, blood urea nitrogen; Po_2, arterial oxygen pressure; WBC, white blood cell count.

≤2 = 1% mortality

3–4 = 15% mortality

≥6 = 100% mortality

FIGURE 15.9

Evaluation of Constipation

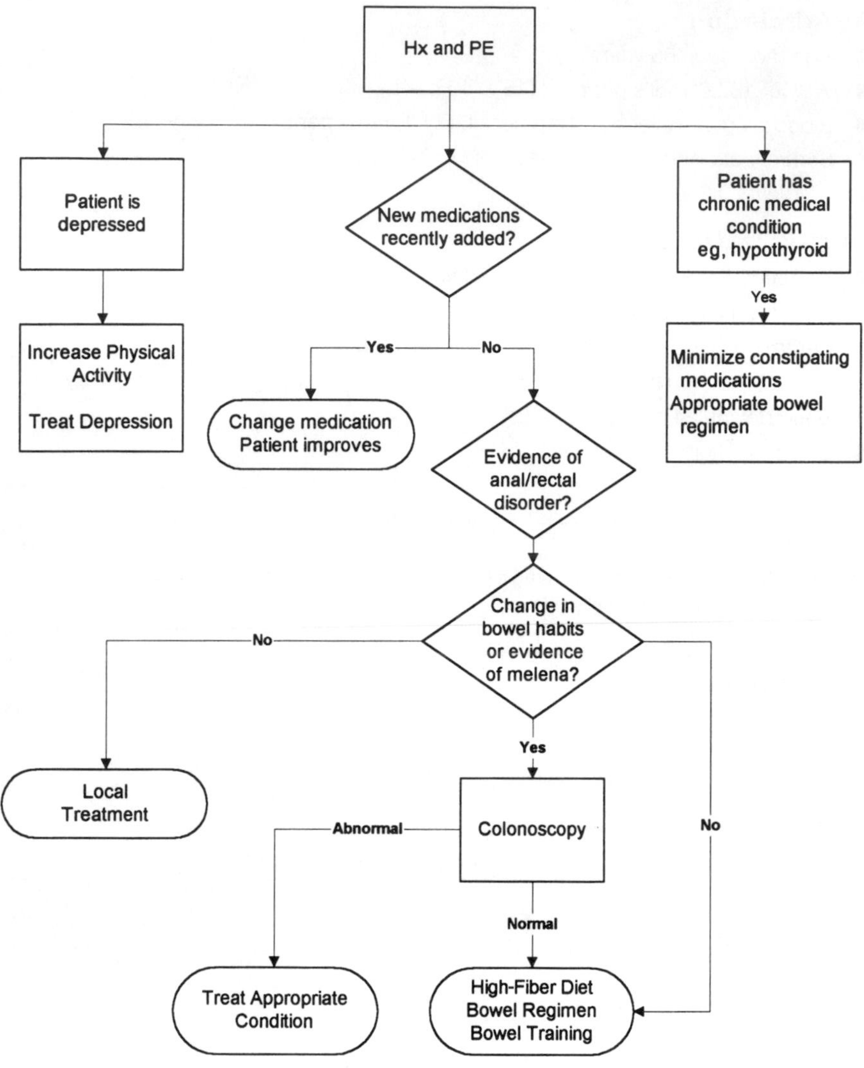

TABLE 15.16
Constipation

Causes	Treatments
Dietary factors (low residue)	■ Increase dietary fiber
Motility disturbances (colonic inertia or spasm such as in irritable bowel syndrome)	■ Increase dietary fiber and give medication based on the underlying disorder (eg, antispasmodic drugs for irritable bowel syndrome)
Sedentary living	■ Increase physical activity level
Structural abnormalities	■ Local treatment
Anorectal disorders (fissures, thrombosed hemorrhoids, rectocele) Strictures Tumor	■ Appropriate evaluation
Endocrine/metabolic disorders Hypercalcemia Hypokalemia Hypothroidism	■ Correct underlying metabolic disorder and give supplements as needed
Neurogenic disorders Cerebrovascular events Parkinson disease Spinal cord tumors Trauma	■ Use enemas for symptomatic treatment, look for underlying metabolic conditions that may contribute to the constipation
Smooth muscle or connective tissue disorders Amyloidosis Scleroderma	■ Increase fiber
Medications Narcotics Nonsteriodal anti-inflammatory drugs Aluminum hydroxide Calcium carbonate Anticholinergic drugs Tricyclic antidepressants Lithium Calcium channel blockers (verapamil) Iron	■ Switch medication class, or stop offending medications(s); check over-the-counter and herbal and other homeopathic preparations as possible causes and stop use if implicated
Psychogenic (especially depression)	■ Treat with counseling and appropriate bowel regimine

TABLE 15.17

Characteristics of Different Laxatives

Type of Laxative	Mechanism of Action	Onset of Action	Potential Adverse Effects
Bulk Laxative Psyllium seed Bran Calcium polycarbophil	Increases fecal bulk as well as the fluid retained in the bowel lumen	12 to 24 hours or more	Increased gas; bloating; bowel obstruction if strictures present, choking if forms are not taken with enough liquid
Emollients and Stool Softeners Dioctyl sodium Calcium sulfosuccinate (docusate sodium)	Lubricates and softens fecal mass	24 to 48 hours	Minor effects such as bitter taste and nausea
Stimulants and irritants Bisacodyl Senna Cascara	Alters intestinal mucosal permeability Stimulates muscle activity and fluid secretions	10 minutes	Dermatitis; electrolyte imbalance; melanosis coli
Osmotic Laxative Lavative Lactulose Magnesium salts Sodium salts Sorbitol	Salts lead to retained fluid in the bowel lumen, with a net increase of fluid secretions in the small intestines	2 to 48 hours	Electrolyte imbalance; excessive gas; hypermagnesemia, hypocalcemia and hyperphosphatemia in patients with renal failure; dehydration
Enema Tap water Saline Sodium phosphate Oil	Causes reflex evacuation	Within 30 minutes	Dehydration; hypocalcemia and hyperphosphatemia in patients with chronic renal failure
Nonabsorbable Solutions Polyethylene glycol	Volume lavage	Within 4 hours	Nausea; abdominal fullness; bloating

TABLE 15.18

Prevention and Management of Traveler's Diarrhea

Risk Factors for Traveler's Diarrhea

Age <30 years

Adventurous travel

Unhygienic primitive environment

Reduced gastric acidity (ie, resulting from histamine H_2-blocker or proton pump inhibitor therapy)

Immunodeficiency disorder

Prior (>6 months previously) residency in an undeveloped country

Causes of Traveler's Diarrhea

Bacteria

Enterotoxigenic *Escherichia coli*

Shigella species

Campylobacter jejuni

Salmonella (nontyphoid) species

Yersinia species

Vibrio (noncholera) species

Aeromonas species

Plesomonas shigelloides

Viruses

Rotavirus

Norwalk virus

Enteroviruses

Protozoa

Entamoeba histolytica

Giardia duodenalis

Cryptosporidium parvum

Cyclospora cayetanensis

Continued

TABLE 15.18

Prevention and Management of Traveler's Diarrhea, cont'd

Dietary Precautions to Prevent Traveler's Diarrhea

Fluids to Avoid

- Tap water, even for brushing teeth
- Bottled water, unless the traveler is the one who breaks the seal
- Ice made from contaminated water
- Unpasteurized milk or dairy products

Fluids That Are Safe to Drink

- Carbonated soft drinks
- Hot drinks, such as tea or coffee, as long as the water was boiled in preparing the drink
- Carbonated or noncarbonated bottled water, as long as the traveler is the one who breaks the seal

Foods to Avoid

- Raw fruits or vegetables, unless they can be peeled and the traveler is the one who peels them
- Lettuce and other leafy vegetables
- Cut-up fruit salad
- Raw or rare meat and fish
- Meat or shellfish that is not hot when it is served
- All food from street vendors

Drug Prophylaxis Against Traveler's Diarrhea in Adults*

Bismuth subsalicylate (Pepto-Bismol), two 262-mg chewable tablets four times daily, taken with meals and once in the evening

Ciprofloxacin (Cipro), 500 mg once daily

Ofloxacin (Floxin), 300 mg once daily

Trimethoprim-sulfamethoxazole (Bactrim DS), 160 mg/800 mg once daily

*Drug prophylaxis against traveler's diarrhea may be taken for up to 3 weeks. Antibiotic prophylaxis is not recommended except in special circumstances, such as in patients who are severely immunocompromised or seriously ill. Prophylactic antibiotic use offers few advantages, because treatment with antibiotics relieves most patients within 24 hours.

TABLE 15.19

Empiric Therapy for Adults and Children With Traveler's Diarrhea

Empiric Therapy for Adults With Traveler's Diarrhea

Fluid and Electrolyte Replacement

Oral rehydration solution, if available; if appropriate solutions are not available, the adult traveler with diarrhea should drink fruit juice, caffeine-free soft drinks, or bottled water and should eat salted crackers

*Antibiotics**

Ciprofloxacin (Cipro), one 500-mg tablet or two 250-mg tablets twice daily for 3 days

OR

Norfloxacin (Noroxin), one 400-mg tablet twice daily for 3 days

OR

Trimethoprim-sulfamethoxazole, double strength (Bactrim DS, Cotrim DS, Septra DS), one tablet twice daily for 3 days

Antimotility Medications

Loperamide (Imodium), two 2-mg tablets after the first loose stool, then one tablet after each loose stool, for a maximum of 16 mg in 24 hours

OR

Diphenoxylate with atropine (Lomotil), two 2.5-mg tablets four times daily for loose stools

Empiric Therapy for Children With Traveler's Diarrhea

Fluid and Electrolyte Replacement[†]

Oral rehydration solution, if available; if appropriate solutions are not available, the child should drink fruit juice, caffeine-free soft drinks, or bottled water and should eat salted crackers

Loperamide (Imodium)[§]

For a child weighing 27.3 to 43.2 kg (60 to 95 lb), the initial dose is 2 tsp, with 1 tsp given after each subsequent loose stool, for a maximum of 6 tsp in 24 hours

For a child weighing 21.8 to 26.8 kg (48 to 59 lb), the initial dose is 2 tsp, with 1 tsp given after each subsequent loose stool, for a maximum of 4 tsp in 24 hours

For a child weighing 10.9 to 21.4 kg (24 to 47 lb), the initial dose is 1 tsp, with 1 tsp given after each subsequent loose stool, for a maximum of 3 tsp in 24 hours

Do not use loperamide in a child weighing less than 10.9 kg (24 lb)

Continued

TABLE 15.19

Empiric Therapy for Adults and Children With Traveler's Diarrhea, cont'd

Antibiotics[‖]
Trimethoprim-sulfamethoxazole (Bactrim, Cotrim, Septra), 4 mg of trimethoprim per kg and 20 mg of sulfamethoxazole per kg twice daily for 3 days

Adapted from Heck JE, Cohen MB. Traveler's diarrhea. *Am Fam Physician.* 1993;48(5):793–800.

*Antibiotics may be used in combination with antimotility medications.

[†]Fluid and electrolyte replacement is critically important in all children with traveler's diarrhea.

[§]Loperamide can be used only if there is no blood in the stools and the child's temperature is less than 38.3°C (101°F).

[‖]Antibiotic therapy may be used if loperamide is not effective or as an alternative to initial therapy.

TABLE 15.20

Diagnosis of Acute Colitis/Proctitis

Diagnosis	Endoscopic Appearance	Barium Enema	Rectal Biopsy
Ulcerative colitis	Diffuse erythema and ulceration (no normal mucosa)	Pseudopolyposis; loss of haustra; involvement from rectum proximally	Goblet cell depletion, pseudopolyps
Crohn disease	Diffuse erythema and ulceration (some normal mucosa)	"Skip" lesions (thickening and luminal narrowing with areas of normal bowel between)	Crypt abscesses, epithelioid granulomas
Salmonella, *Shigella*, or *Campylobacter*	Same as ulcerative colitis	Usually normal	Crypt abscesses
Amebiasis	Diffuse inflammation, ulceration	Usually normal	Trophozoite in ulcer base
Antibiotic-associated colitis	Multiple, discrete yellow plaques	Usually normal	Fibrinous pseudomembrane over inflammation
Gonorrheal proctitis	Erythema and ulceration, limited to rectum	Normal	Intracellular diplococci
Lymphogranuloma venereum	Same as gonorrhea	Normal	Nonspecific inflammation

Adapted from Lewis JH, Clement S, Dobbins WO III. Acute colitis: a logical approach to diagnosis and management. *Postgrad Med.* 198[illegible];70:145–147; 152–164.

TABLE 15.21

Clinical Distinctions Between Crohn Disease and Ulcerative Colitis

Feature	Crohn Disease	Ulcerative Colitis
In the Intestine		
Rectal bleeding	Uncommon	Very common
Sigmoidoscopic findings	Normal or spotty lesions	Diffusely abnormal
Spontaneous fistulas	Common	Never occurs
Perianal disease	Common	Uncommon
Abdominal pain	Very common	Uncommon
Abdominal mass	Common	Only with cancers
Strictures	Common	Rare, suspect cancer
Distribution	Discontinuous, entire gastro-intestinal tract	Continuous, colon and rectum
Shortening from incidence of cancer	Fibrosis increased	Muscle thickening greatly increased
Extraintestinal Manifestations		
Arthritis	Occurs	Occurs
Dermatitis	Occurs	Occurs
Episcleritis and uveitis	Occurs	Occurs
Hydronephrosis	Occurs	Occurs
Liver disease	Occurs	Occurs
Metabolic Manifestations		
Amyloidosis	Incidence increased	Rare
Anemia	Common	Common
Fever	Occurs	Occurs
Gallstones	Incidence increased	Incidence normal
Growth retardation	Occurs	Occurs
Kidney stones	Occurs	Occurs

Adapted from Sessions T. *Viewpoints Dig Dis.* Sept 7, 1975.

TABLE 15.22

Irritable Bowel Syndrome

Diagnostic Criteria: Rome Classification

At least 3 months of continuous or recurrent symptoms of abdominal pain that is:

- Relieved with defecation *and/or*
- Associated with a change in stool frequency *and/or*
- Associated with a change in consistency of stool *plus*

Two or more of the following, at least one fourth the time:

- Altered stool frequency
- Altered stool form
- Altered stool passage
- Passage of mucus
- Bloating

Alarm Symptoms

- Age >50
- Gastrointestinal Bleeding
- Anemia
- Anorexia/weight loss
- Persistent diarrhea
- Prolonged constipation
- FH of gastrointestinal cancers

Differential Diagnosis

- Lactose intolerance
- Enteric infections
- Colon cancer
- Diverticulitis
- Malabsorption
- Endocrine tumors
- Endometriosis
- Intestinal pseudo-obstruction
- Drugs

Mild Symptoms

- Majority of patients
- May only need reassurance
- Dietary changes
- Fiber: the great equalizer (particularly if constipation predominant)

Continued

TABLE 15.22

Irritable Bowel Syndrome, cont'd

Moderate Symptoms
■ Symptom diary
■ Antispasmodics (hyoscyamine [Levsin], Donnatal, dicyclomine [Bentyl])
■ Antidiarrheal agents (loperamide)
■ Bulk laxatives
Severe Symptoms
■ Assess comorbid psychiatric disorders
■ Focus on patient's well-being
■ Set realistic goals
■ Provide therapeutic options
■ Antidepressants (tricyclic better response than SSRI)
■ Schedule brief, regular appointments of fixed duration

TABLE 15.23

Sources of Gastrointestinal (GI) Tract Bleeding

Category	Upper GI Tract	Lower GI Tract
Inflammatory	Peptic ulcer*	Ulcerative colitis*
	Esophagitis*	Crohn disease*
	Gastritis*	Diverticulitis
	Stress ulcer	Enterocolitis; tuberculosis bacterial, toxic, radiation
Mechanical	Hiatal hernia	Diverticulosis*
	Mallory-Weiss syndrome*	Anal fissure*
	Hematobilia	Radiation enteritis
Vascular	Esophageal or gastric varices*	Hemorrhoids*
	Mesenteric vascular occlusion	Mesenteric vascular occlusion
		Aortointestinal fistula
	Aortoduodenal fistula	Aortic aneurysm
	Malformations: hemangioma, Osler-Weber-Rendu disease, blue nevus bleb	Malformations: hemangioma, Osler-Weber-Rendu disease, blue nevus bleb
	Angiodysplasia	Angiodysplasia
Neoplastic	Carcinoma	Carcinoma*
	Polyps; single, multiple, Peutz-Jeghers syndrome	Polyps*; adenomatous and villous, familial polyposis,
		Peutz-Jeghers syndrome
	Leiomyoma	Leiomyoma
	Carcinoid	Carcinoid
	Carcinoid	Leukemia
	Sarcoma	Sarcoma
	Metastatic (eg, melanoma)	Metastatic (eg, melanoma)
Systemic	Blood dyscrasias and clotting abnormalities	Blood dyscrasias and clotting abnormalities
	Collagen diseases	Collagen diseases – Amyloid
	Uremia	Uremia
	Celiac sprue	Celiac sprue
Anomalies	Gastric and duodenal diverticula	Meckel diverticulum

Adapted from Greenberger NH, Norton J. *Gastrointestinal Disorders*. 2nd ed. Chicago: Mosby, Inc; 1981.

*Most common disorders.

FIGURE 15.10

Upper Gastrointestinal Tract Bleeding

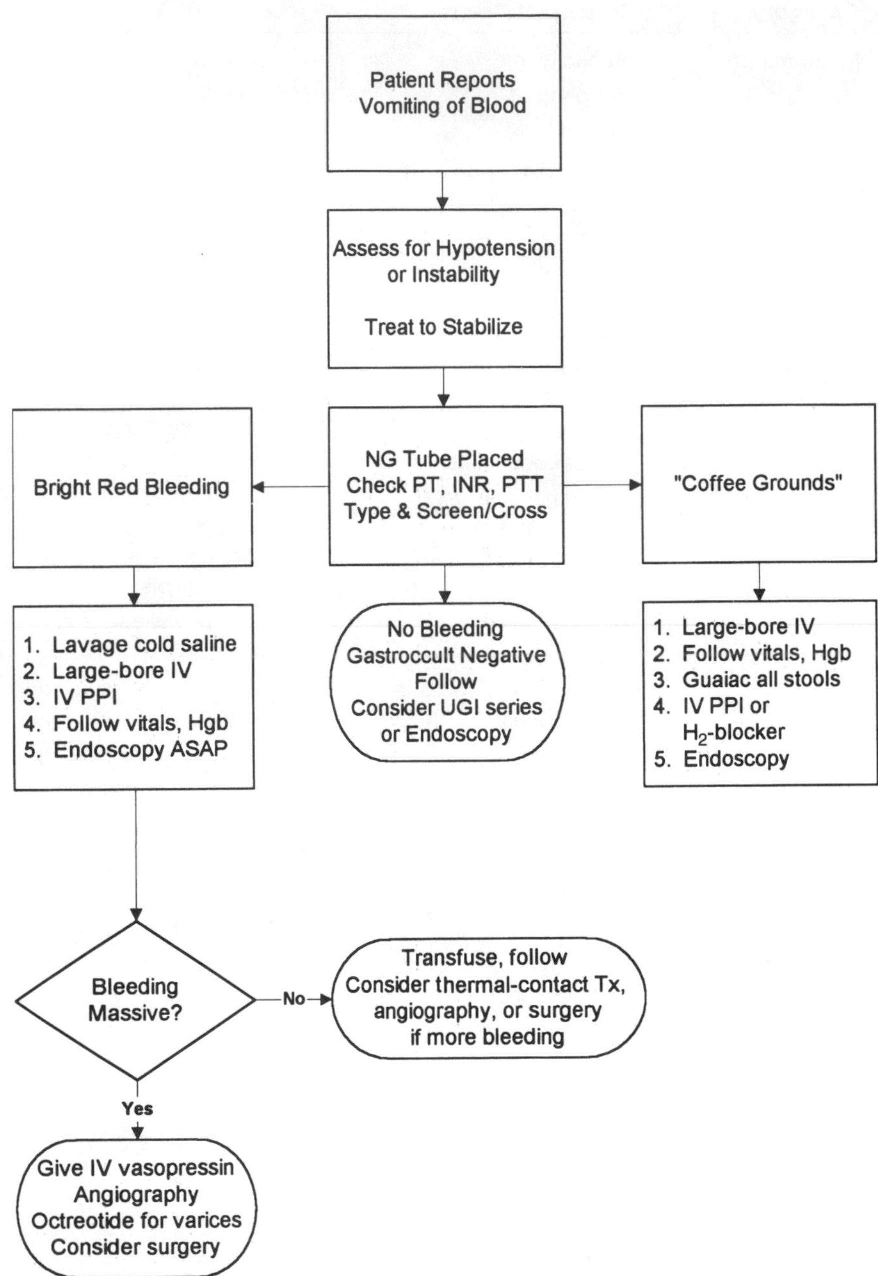

FIGURE 15.11

Lower Gastrointestinal Tract Bleeding

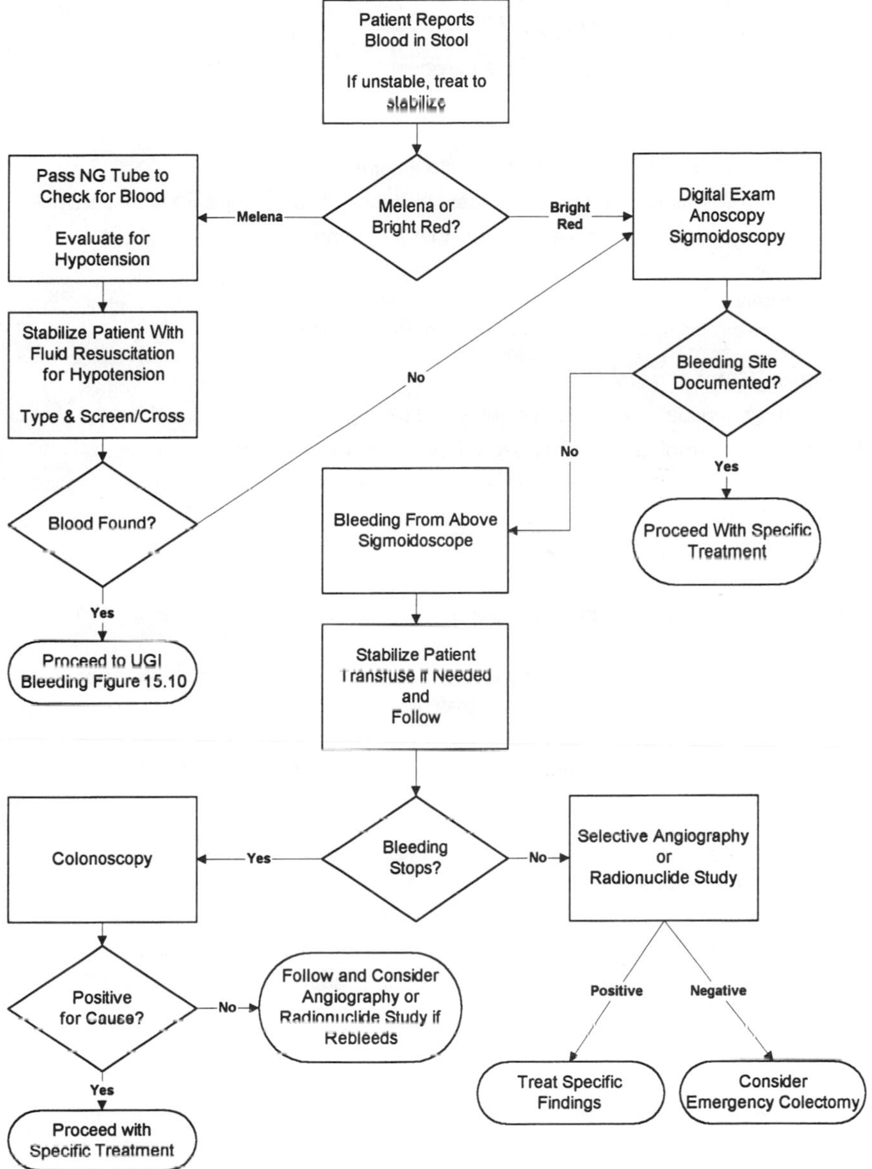

TABLE 15.24

Anorectal Disorders

Hemorrhoids

Thromboses External Hemorrhoids

- Pain is prominent, and bleeding is infrequent
- Examination reveals a bluish perianal mass just below the mucocutaneous junction
- Treatment consists of sitz baths and stool softeners
- Pain usually disappears within 1 week, and the mass disappears within 2 weeks
- Residual skin tags are common and do not indicate chronic hemorrhoidal disease
- If acutely painful, overlying skin may be anesthetized with 1% lidocaine, incised, and the clot removed with resultant immediate pain relief

Internal Hemorrhoids

- Symptoms usually limited to bright red bleeding, almost always painless
- Large hemorrhoids may prolapse out of the rectum at bowel movement
- Digital examination is often negative; diagnosis requires anoscope with a good light source
- Even if hemorrhoids are present on examination, other sources of bleeding such as colon cancer must be excluded
- Small, minimally symptomatic lesions may be treated with observation and a high-fiber diet
- Larger lesions may be treated with sclerotherapy with injection of 5% phenol solution in oil into the submucosal area (care must be exercised not to inject into the vein)
- Very large, prolapsing lesions are best treated by rubber band ligature technique

Anal Fissure

- Characterized by pain associated with a hard bowel movement with minor bleeding on the toilet tissue
- Patients usually mistake them for hemorrhoids
- Mucosal tears are demonstrable, usually at 6 o'clock or 12 o'clock, by everting the buttocks; will often be missed unless specifically sought
- Treat with sitz baths, stool softeners, high-fiber diet, hydrocortisone suppositories, and moist wipes
- Chronic, recalcitrant cases may require sphincterotomy and/or fissurectomy

Pruritus Ani

- Causes are multiple and poorly understood but include poor perianal hygiene, trauma from scratching or excessive cleaning or wiping, excessive moisture, yeast infections, hypersensitivity reactions to local or systemic agents, dietary irritants such as jalapeño peppers, or personality or psychological factors

- Once started, a vicious cycle occurs and is hard to break
- Treatment approaches should include the following:

  1. Correct all predisposing anatomical conditions (eg, hemorrhoids)
  2. Direct attention to meticulous perianal hygiene; use water, not soap. If sitz bath is unavailable, use premoistened towelettes
  3. Avoid scratching; use oral Vistaril, Phenergan, or Benadryl as antipruritic, if necessary
  4. Keep the area dry with loose clothing; consider tucking gauze into the buttocks; cornstarch or other drying powder may help
  5. Medications should be minimized; topical steroids are contraindicated except for a short, initial course; avoid local anesthetic such as benzocaine, which is highly sensitizing. Yeast infections are often secondary and should be treated with nystatin or miconazole cream
  6. Efforts should be directed toward complete normalization of stool patterns. Overly soft stool may be as irritating as constipated stool
  7. Consider the importance of psychological factors

TABLE 15.25

Procedures in the Gastrointestinal Tract

Flexible Sigmoidoscopy

1. The patient should administer two Fleets enemas on the morning of the procedure. If patient had chronic constipation, preparation of the bowel requires three bisacodyl (Dulcolax) tablets the afternoon before the test in addition to the enemas on the morning of the procedure.
2. Place patient in left lateral decubitus position.
3. Perform digital examination and anoscopy first.
4. Hold shaft of instrument in right hand and control head of endoscope with left hand.
5. Apply water-soluble lubricant to endoscope shaft.
6. Guide scope into rectum with finger.
7. Advance scope, always with lumen in view.
8. Insufflate air periodically to distend collapsed bowel.
9. Aspirate liquid with suction control as needed.
10. Extra care is required to negotiate the angle at the rectosigmoid junction.
11. If colonic spasm occurs, pull back 3–4 cm and reinsert.
12. Examine mucosa on withdrawal of scope.
13. Biopsy suspicious lesions on withdrawal.

Diagnostic Paracentesis

1. Turn patient on left side for 5 minutes.
2. After the bladder has been emptied, insert a 19-gauge, short, beveled spinal needle halfway between the umbilicus and pubis at the left lateral edge of the rectus sheath.
3. If you do *not* use local anesthesia, pain signals entering peritoneum.
4. Apply gentle suction with 15- to 20-mL syringe.
5. If no fluid is obtained, repeat on the right side.

Alternate Method

1. Use intracath.
2. Insert in lower abdominal midline, 1 inch below umbilicus.
3. Pass catheter and withdraw needle; apply gentle suction.
4. If no fluid is obtained, infuse 500 mL of sterile saline over 10–15 minutes.
5. Aspirate and check fluid for pH, bile, amylase, white blood cells, red blood cells, cytology, and cultures, as indicated.

Insertion of Nasogastric Tube

1. Measure from the xiphoid to either ear lobe. This is the distance the tube should be passed.
2. The tube should be placed in ice or refrigerated before insertion to facilitate passage through the pharynx.
3. Insert gently through the nose to the posterior pharynx.

4. Ask the patient to swallow, or have patient drink sips of water. Tube should be passed synchronous with swallowing.
5. Aspiration of gastric contents and/or auscultation of borborygmi with air insertion confirms proper placement in the stomach.
6. Tube should be carefully taped to the nose, avoiding excessive pressure of the tube on the nares.

chapter 16

Infections

Dawn Mattern, MD
Edward T. Bope, MD

IN THIS CHAPTER

- Otitis media
- Chronic or recurrent otitis media
- Community-acquired pneumonia
- Urinary tract infection
- Pyelonephritis
- Prostatitis
- Sexually transmitted diseases
- Pelvic inflammatory disease
- Skin and soft tissue infections
- Diarrhea-stool studies
- Traveler's diarrhea
- Cerebrospinal fluid findings in meningitis
- Subacute bacterial endocarditis prophylaxis
- Human immunodeficiency virus initial evaluation
- Anthrax

BOOKSHELF RECOMMENDATIONS

- Gorbach SL, Bartlett JG, Blacklow NR, eds. *Infectious Diseases*. 2nd ed. Philadelphia, PA: WB Saunders Company; 1998.
- Gilbert DN, Moellering RC Jr, Sande MA, eds. *The Sanford Guide to Antimicrobial Therapy*. 32nd ed. Hyde Park, VT: Antimicrobial Therapy, Inc; 2002.
- Pickering LK, ed. *2000 Red Book: Report of the Committee on Infectious Diseases*. 25th ed. Elk Grove Village, IL: American Academy of Pediatrics; 2000.

FIGURE 16.1

Acute Otitis Media

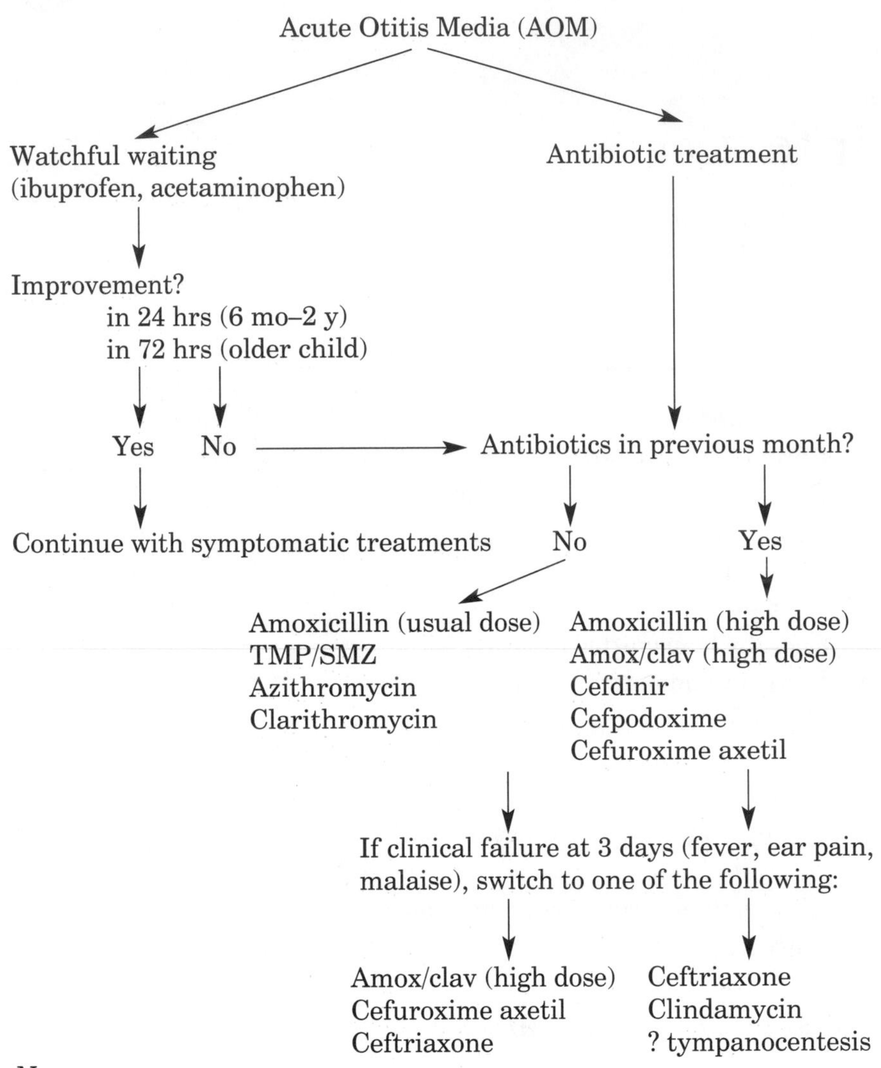

Notes

1. 81% of untreated AOM undergoes spontaneous resolution
   95% of treated AOM undergoes resolution
2. Otitis media with effusion: 70% at 2 weeks
   50% at 1 month
   10% at 3 months

Consider hearing evaluation if bilateral fluid after 3 months, definitely if it persists after 6 months

TABLE 16.1

Pediatric Dosages for Otitis Media Antibiotics

Amoxicillin (usual dose)	40–45 mg/kg/d ÷ q 12 h or q 8 h
Amoxicillin (high dose)	80–90 mg/kg/d ÷ q 12 h or q 8 h
Amoxicillin clavulanate (high dose)	80–90 mg/kg/d of amoxicillin (use either 875/125 q 12 h or 500/125 + regular amoxicillin q 8 h)
TMP/SMZ	8 mg/kg TMP & 40 mg/kg SMZ per day ÷ q 12 h
Azithromycin	10 mg/kg on day 1, 5 mg/kg on days 2–5
Clarithromycin	15 mg/kg/d ÷ q 12 h
Cefdinir	7 mg/kg q 12 h or 14 mg/kg q 24 h
Cefpodoxime	10 mg/kg/d (single dose) (max 400 mg/d)
Cefuroxime axetil	30 mg/kg/d ÷ q 12 h (max 1000 mg/d)
Cefriaxone	50 mg/kg IM × 3 days
Clindamycin	20–30 mg/kg/d ÷ QID

TABLE 16.2

Chronic or Recurrent Otitis Media

1. Treat acute exacerbations
2. Secondary prevention (3 or more episodes in 6 months, 4 or more episodes in 12 months)

Options for Secondary Prevention

- Prophylaxis
  —Amoxicillin 20 mg/kg/d
  —Sulfisoxazole 75 mg/kg/d
- Pneumococcal vaccine
- Tympanostomy tubes
- ± adenoidectomy

FIGURE 16.2

Community-Acquired Pneumonia Risk Factor Assessment

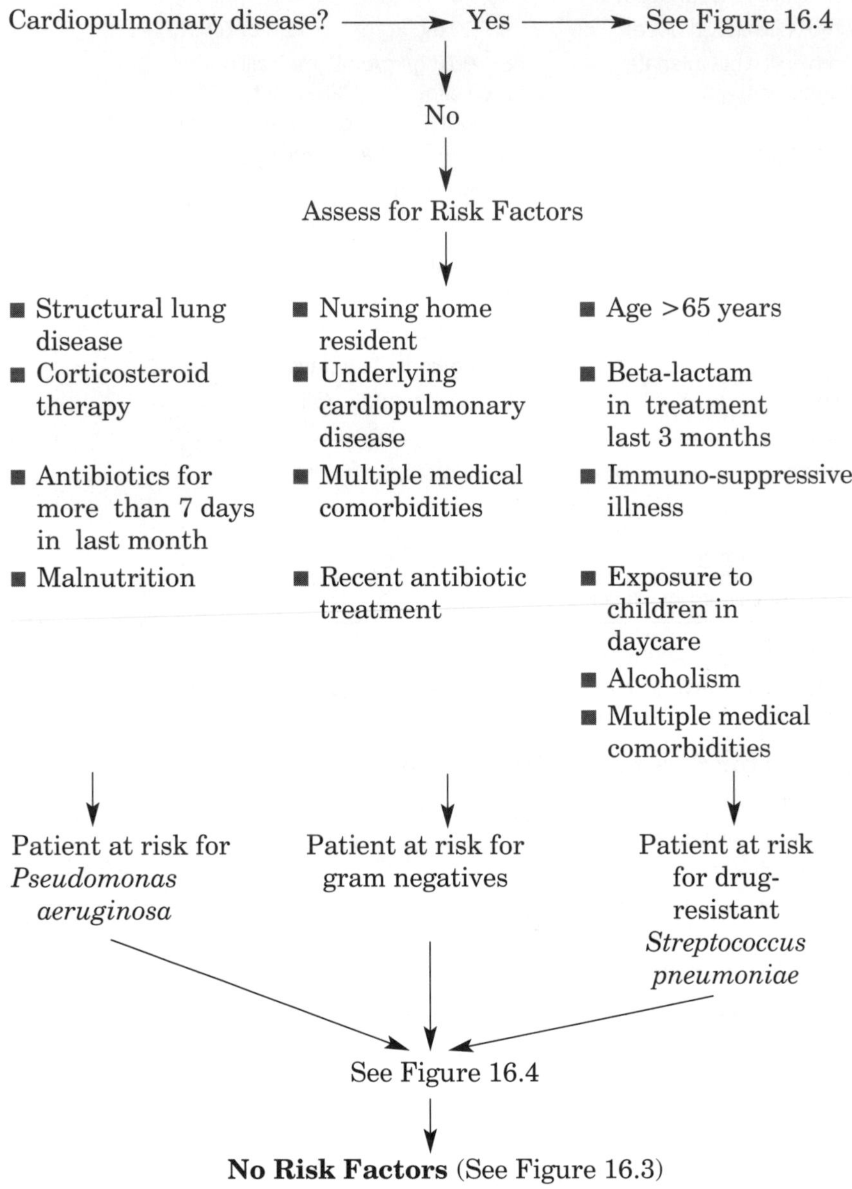

FIGURE 16.3

Treatment of Community-Acquired Pneumonia

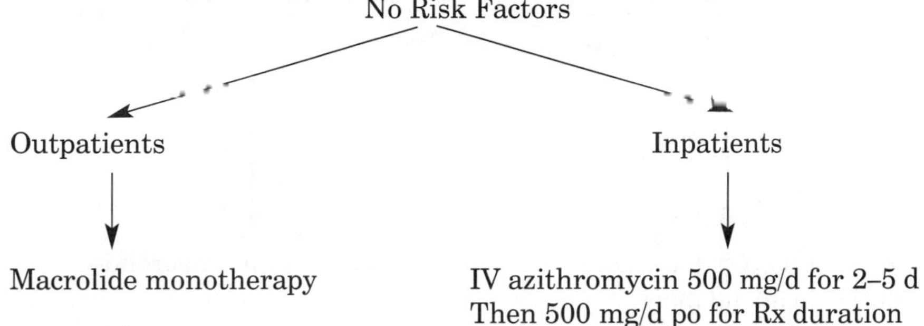

(Azithromycin 500 mg/d po × 1
then 250 mg/d clarithromycin
500 mg po bid)

Options

Doxycycline 100 mg po bid

Rx duration varies, usually treat until afebrile for 3–5 days

Total duration of antibiotic therapy is 7–14 days

FIGURE 16.4

Treatment of Community-Acquired Pneumonia

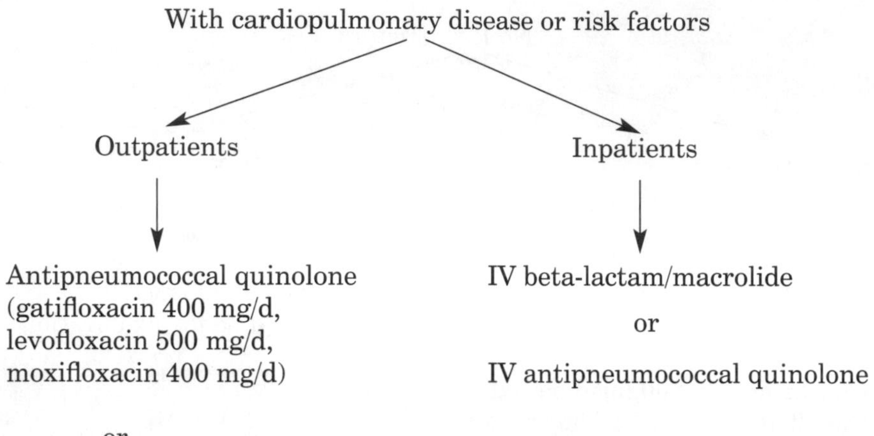

or

selected beta-lactams plus a macrolide

- The Centers for Disease Control recommends using fluoroquinolones only when patient fails other regimens or has documented high-level DRSP
- Outpatient beta-lactams—cefuroxime 250–500 mg po q 12 h, amoxicillin/clavulanate 875/125 mg po bid, cefpodoxime 300 mg po q 12 h
- Inpatient beta-lactams—cefuroxime 1.5 g IV q 8 h, ceftriaxone 2 g/d IV, cefotaxime 2 g IV q 4–8 h, ampicillin/sulbactam 1.5-3 g IV q 6 h, cefepime 2 g IV q 12 h

FIGURE 16.5

Urinary Tract Infections

Symptomatic patient
or
Patient with functionally, metabolically, or anatomically abnormal urinary tract (stones, obstruction, DM, sickle cell disease, polycystic kidneys)
or
Hx of UTI pathogens resistant to antibiotics

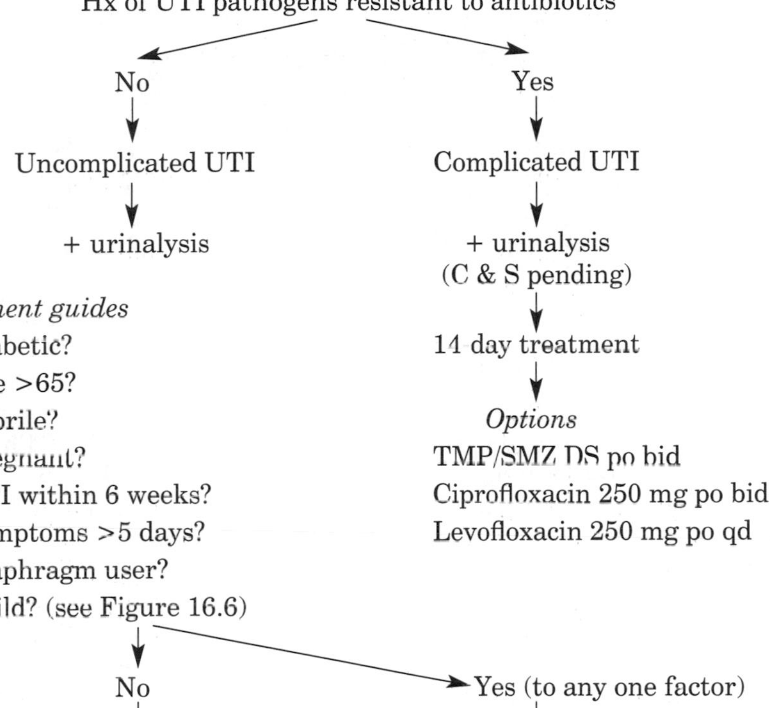

Treatment Options
TMP/SMZ DS po bid (8 mg/kg/d TMP in 2 divided doses for pediatrics)
Trimethoprim 100 mg po bid
Ciprofloxacin 250 mg po bid
Levofloxacin 250 mg/d po
Oral cephalosporins
Doxycycline 100 mg po bid

In Pregnancy
Nitrofurantoin 100 mg po bid
Amoxicillin 500 mg po tid

FIGURE 16.6

Urinary Tract Infection

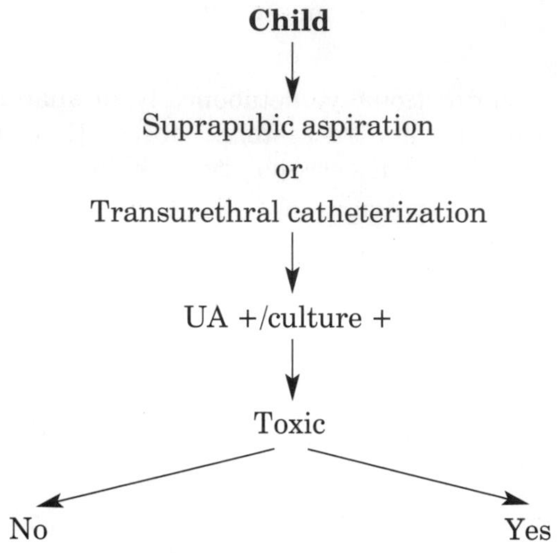

Oral antibiotics	IV antibiotics
TMP/SMZ 4 mg TMP/kg bid	Ampicillin 50–100 mg/kg/24 h ÷q 6 h
Amoxicillin 10 mg/kg tid	and
Nitrofurantoin 2.5 mg/kg tid	Gentamicin 6–7.5 mg/kg/24 h ÷q 8 h
	3rd-generation cephalosporins

Treat for 10 days total. May switch from IV to po when clinically stable.

FIGURE 16.7

Pyelonephritis

Nausea/vomiting

Ill appearing/dehydrated

Age >65

Pregnancy

Immunosuppression

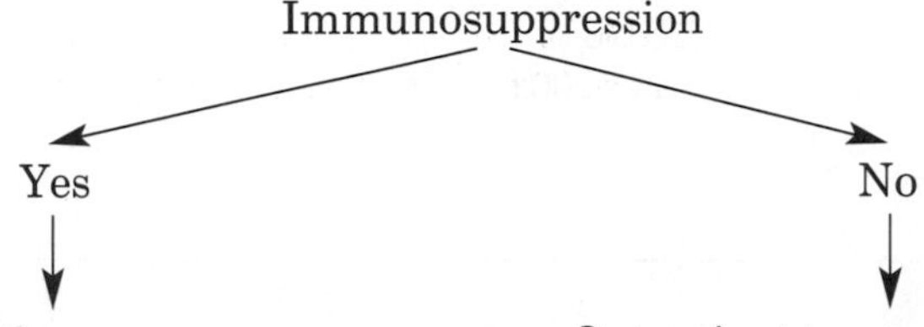

Yes	No
Hospitalization	Outpatient treatment
Treat for 14 d (total po & IV)	Treat for 10–14 days
Ciprofloxacin 400 mg IV bid Levofloxacin 500 mg/d IV Ampicillin and gentamicin Cefotaxime 1 g q 12 h–2 g q 4 h IV Ceftriaxone 1–2 g/d IV (use 2 g age <40) Piperacillin 3 g IV q 6 h	Ciprofloxacin 500 mg po bid Levofloxacin 250 mg/d po TMP/SMZ DS po bid

Note: May change to po from IV when tolerating diet.

TABLE 16.3

Prostatitis

	Acute	**Chronic**
Presenting Symptom	Fever, malaise	Mild low back pain, perineal discomfort
Voiding	Frequency, dysuria, and obstruction	Minimal symptoms unless urine is infected
Prostate	Swollen and tender	Normal exam
Treatment	TMP/SMZ DS bid or quinolones 400–500 mg bid	Quinolones 400–500 mg bid or doxycycline 100 mg bid
Length of Treatment	3–4 weeks	3–4 months

TABLE 16.4

Sexually Transmitted Diseases*

Urethritis/Cervicitis	
Gonorrhea (one-time dose)	Ceftriaxone 125 mg IM Cefixime 400 mg po Ciprofloxacin 500 mg po Ofloxacin 400 mg po *Options:* Spectinomycin 2 g IM Ceftizoxime 500 mg IM Cefotaxime 500 mg IM Cefotetan 1 g IM Cefoxitin 2 g IM with probenicid 1 g po Enoxacin 400 mg po Lomefloxacin 400 mg po Gatifloxacin 400 mg po
Chlamydia	Doxycycline 100 mg po bid × 7 days Azithromycin 1 g po × 1 *Options:* Erythromycin base 500 mg qid × 7 days Ofloxacin 300 mg q12 h po × 7 days

*Treat for both infections and treat partners.

TABLE 16.5

Pelvic Inflammatory Disease

Outpatient Regimens		
Ofloxacin 400 mg po bid × 14 d	*plus*	metronidazole 500 mg po bid × 14 d
Ceftiaxone 250 mg IM Or Cefoxitin 2 g IM/probenecid 1 g Or Parenteral 3rd-generation cephalosporin	*plus*	doxycycline 100 mg po bid × 14 d
Parenteral (Inpatient)		
Cefotetan 2 g IV q 12 h Or Cefoxitin 2 g IV q 6 h	*plus*	doxycycline 100 mg IV/po q 12 h
Clindamycin 900 mg IV q 8 h	*plus*	gentamicin IV/IM (2 g/kg load & 1.5 g/kg q 8 h or single daily dosing)
Options		
Ofloxacin 400 mg IV q 12 h *plus* Metronidazole 500 mg IV q 8 h		
Ampicillin/sulbactam 3 g IV q 6 h *plus* Doxycycline 100 mg IV/po q 12 h		
Ciprofloxacin 200 mg IV q 12 h *plus* Doxycycline 100 mg IV/po q 12 h *plus* Metronidazole 500 mg IV q 8 h		

TABLE 16.6

Skin and Soft Tissue Infections

Type of Infection	Organisms	Treatments
Impetigo, ecythyma, erysipelas, folliculitis	*Staphylococcus aureus, Streptococcus pyogenes*	■ Cephalexin 250 mg po qid ■ Cloxacillin, dicloxacillin 250 mg po qid ■ Clindamycin 250 mg po qid ■ TMP/SMZ DS po bid ■ Erythromycin 500 mg po qid
Infected wounds (not bites or postsurgical)	Polymicrobic	■ Amoxicillin/clavulanate 875/125 mg po bid or 500/125 mg tid ■ Cephalexin 250/500 mg po qid ■ Cefadroxil 500 mg po bid ■ Erythromycin 500 mg po qid ■ Azithromycin 500 mg × 1, then 250 mg × 4 ■ Clarithromycin 500 mg po bid ■ Clindamycin 250 mg po qid ■ Levofloxacin 500 mg/d po

TABLE 16.7

Diarrhea (Stool Studies)

Stain for Fecal Leukocytes

Positive: invasive bacterium, idiopathic inflammatory disease

Negative: preformed toxin, viral/parasite/toxigenic bacterium, small bowel process

Ova and Parasites

Giardia lamblia, *Entamoeba hystolytica*, *Cryptosporidium*

Stool Culture

Salmonella, *Shigella*, *Campylobacter*, *Yersinia*

Cholera (*Vibrio parahaemolyticus*, *Vibrio cholerae*) should be plated on special media

Virus Culture

Rotavirus, Norwalk, enteric adenovirus

TABLE 16.8

Traveler's Diarrhea*

Causes	Treatment
Toxigenic *Escherichia coli*, *Shigella*, *Salmonella*, *Campylobacter*, amebiasis, *Cyclospora*, *Cryptosporidia*	Ciprofloxacin 750 mg × 1 or azithromycin 500 mg × 1, then 250 mg/d × 4 d (children, 5–10 mg/kg/d) If severe, Ciprofloxacin 500 mg bid × 3 d Levofloxacin 500 mg bid × 3 d Ofloxacin 300 mg × 3 d

*If afebrile and no blood in the stool, can use loperamide for loose stools.

TABLE 16.9

CSF Findings in Meningitis

	Bacterial	Viral
Cells	500–100,000	50–1000
Cell Types	PMNs	Monocytes
Protein	High–very high	Slightly elevated
Glucose	Low–very low	Normal
Pressure	Usually elevated	Normal–slightly elevated

CSF indicates cerebrospinal fluid; PMNs, Polymorphonuclear leukocytes.

TABLE 16.10

Empiric Meningitis Treatment

Age	Primary	Alternative
Preterm-1 month	Ampicillin and cefotaxime	Ampicillin and gentamicin
1 month-50 years	Cefotaxime or ceftriaxone, dexamethasone and vancomycin	Meropenem, dexamethasone, and vancomycin
>50 yrs/alcoholism/ debilitated illnesses	Ampicillin, vancomycin, dexamethasone, and ceftriaxone or cefotaxime	Meropenem, vancomycin, and dexamethasone

Dosages

Ampicillin	150 mg/kg/d IV ÷ q 12 h for infants < 1 week 200 mg/kg/d IV ÷ q 6 h for infants 1–4 weeks 2 g IV q 4 h for adults
Cefotaxime	100 mg/kg/d IV ÷ q 12 h for infants < 1 week 150–200 mg/kg/d IV ÷ q 8 h for infants 1–4 weeks 200 mg/kg/d IV ÷ q 6–8 h for children 2 g IV q 4–6 h for adults
Gentamicin	5 mg/kg/d IV ÷ q 12 h for infants < 1 week 7.5 mg/kg/d IV ÷ q 8 h for infants 1–4 weeks
Ceftriaxone	100 mg/kg/d IV ÷ q 12 h for children 2 g IV q 12 h for adults
Dexamethasone	0.4 mg/kg q 12 h IV × 2 d (give before or with first dose of antibiotic)
Vancomycin	15 mg/kg q 6 h IV for children 500–750 mg q 6 h IV for adults
Meropenem	40 mg/kg IV q 8 h for children 1 g IV q 8 h for adults

TABLE 16.11

Prophylaxis for Subacute Bacterial Endocarditis

Conditions Requiring Prophylaxis

- Prosthetic cardiac valves
- History of previous bacterial endocarditis
- Cyanotic congenital heart disease
- Surgically constructed systemic-pulmonary shunts
- Acquired valvular dysfunction
- Hypertrophic cardiomyopathy
- Mitral valve prolapse *with* regurgitation

TABLE 16.12

Procedures Requiring Prophylaxis for Subacute Bacterial Endocarditis

Dental

- Extractions
- Periodontal procedures
- Dental implant placement
- Reimplantation of avulsed teeth
- Endodontic procedures (root canal)
- Prophylactic cleaning (bleeding is anticipated)
- Initial placement of orthodontic bands (not brackets)

Respiratory Tract

- Tonsillectomy and/or adenoidectomy
- Surgical procedures that involve respiratory mucosa
- Bronchoscopy with a rigid bronchoscope

Gastrointestinal Tract

- Sclerotherapy for esophageal varices
- Esophageal stricture dilation
- Endoscopic retrograde cholangiopancreatography with biliary obstruction
- Biliary tract surgery
- Surgical procedures that involve intestinal mucosa

Genitourinary Tract

- Prostatic surgery
- Cystoscopy
- Urethral dilation

TABLE 16.13

Subacute Bacterial Endocarditis Prophylaxis

Prophylactic Regimens

Route	Drug	Dosage	Timing
PO	Amoxicillin	2 g (adults) 50 mg/kg (children)	1 h before procedure
IV/IM	Ampicillin	2 g (adults) 50 mg/kg (children)	Within 30 minutes of procedure
Allergic to penicillin			
PO	Clindamycin	600 mg (adults) 20 mg/kg (children) or	1 h before procedure
	Cefadroxil or cephalexin	2 g (adults) 50 mg/kg (children) or	1 h before procedure
	Azithromycin or clarithromycin	500 mg (adults) 15 mg/kg (children)	1 h before procedure
IV/IM	Clindamycin (IV)	600 mg (adults) 20 mg/kg (children) or	Within 30 minutes of procedure
	Cefazolin (IM/IV)	1 g (adults) 25 mg/kg (children)	

IM indicates intramuscularly; IV, intravenously; PO, orally.

TABLE 16.14

Human Immunodeficiency Virus (HIV) Initial Evaluation

HIV serology (confirmatory)	Chest x-ray
CD4 cell count and %	PPD
Viral load	Pap smear
CBC	Vaccinations
Chemistry panel	Pneumovax
Liver function tests	Hepatitis A vaccine
Hepatitis serology	Hepatitis B vaccine
Toxoplasma titer (IgG)	Influenza vaccine
CMV IgG	Varicella vaccine for household members without history of chickenpox
VDRL/RPR	
G6PD level (if indicated)	

CBC indicates complete blood cell count; CMV, cytomegalovirus; PPD, purified protein derivative; RPR, rapid plasma reagin.

FIGURE 16.8
Anthrax

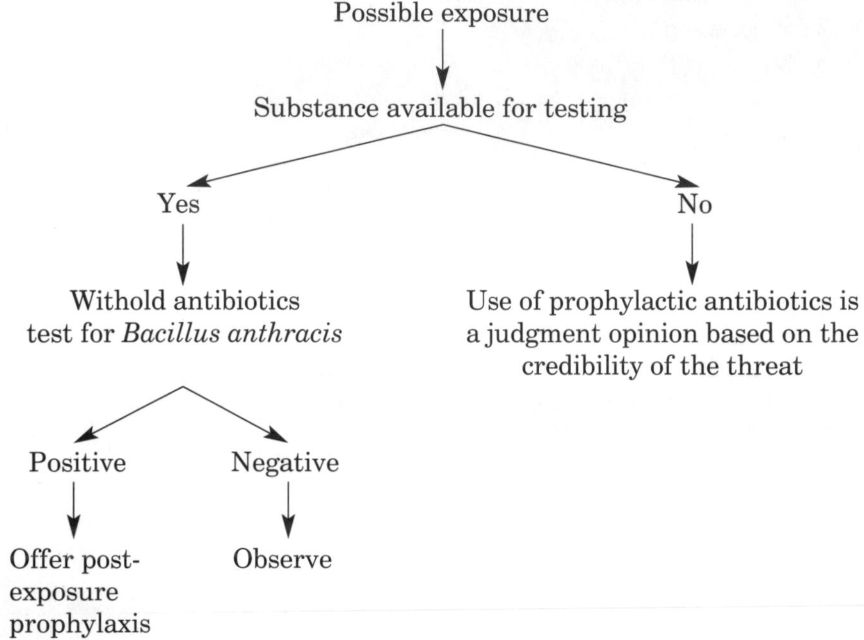

Ciprofloxacin 500 mg po bid × 60 days
or
doxycycline 100 mg po bid × 60 days

chapter 17

Musculoskeletal Conditions

George C. Wortley, MD

IN THIS CHAPTER

- Neck pain: evaluation
- Neck pain: treatment
- Low back pain: differential diagnosis
- Low back pain: evaluation
- Low back pain: treatment
- Shoulder pain
- Shoulder physical exam
- The elbow
- The wrist
- The hand
- The hip
- The knee
- Knee effusions (causes)
- Joint fluid analysis
- Knee examination
- Pittsburgh rules for acute knee injuries
- Ankle sprains
- Ottawa ankle rules
- The foot
- Osteoarthritis
- Rheumatoid arthritis: diagnosis
- Conditions with a positive rheumatoid factor
- Rheumatoid arthritis: treatment
- Ankylosing spondylitis
- Polymyalgia rheumatica
- Juvenile rheumatoid arthritis
- Fibromyalgia
- Osteoporosis
- Developmental dysplasia of the hip
- Transient synovitis of the hip

- Legg-Calve-Perthes disease
- Slipped capital femoral epiphysis
- Scoliosis
- Sports injuries
- Medications
- Physical therapy
- Arthrocentesis
- Intra-articular injection
- Casting techniques

BOOKSHELF RECOMMENDATIONS

- Anderson BC. *Office Orthopedics for Primary Care: Diagnosis and Treatment*. Philadelphia, PA: WB Saunders; 1998.
- Hoppenfeld S, Hutton R. *Physical Examination of the Spine and Extremities*. Norwalk, CT: Appleton & Lange; 1976.
- Mellon M, Walsh WM, Putukian M, Madden C. *Team Physician's Handbook*. 3rd ed. Philadelphia, PA: Hanley & Belfus; 2001.

TABLE 17.1A

Neck Pain: Evaluation

Two thirds of people will experience neck pain at some time in their lives. Common causes include:

- Cervical muscle strain (including whiplash-type injuries)
- Cervical arthritis
- Emotional stress
- Cervical disk disease

Physical exam (with specific attention to):

- Limited range of motion
- Spasm of cervical and upper back muscles
- Tender trigger points
- Neurologic defects

TABLE 17.1B

Cervical Spine Neurology

Root	Disk	Reflex	Sensation	Muscles
C5	C4–C5	Biceps	Lateral upper arm	Deltoid/biceps
C6	C5–C6	Brachioradialis	Lateral forearm	Biceps/wrist extension
C7	C6–C7	Triceps	Middle finger	Wrist flexors
C8	C7–T1	None	Medial forearm	Finger flexors/hand intrinsics
T1	T1–T2	None	Medial elbow	Hand intrinsics

TABLE 17.1C

Specific Tests

Spurling test	To test for narrowing of the neural foramen or painful facet joint *Technique*: Press down upon the top of the patient's head. A positive test will increase pain in the neck or pain radiating down the extremity.
Adson Test	To test for compression of subclavian artery (thoracic outlet syndrome) *Technique*: Palpate the patient's radial pulse. As you continue to feel the pulse, abduct, extend, and externally rotate the arm. Then have the patient take a deep breath and turn his head toward the arm being tested. A positive test will have an absent or markedly diminished pulse.

Imaging

- Plain films of cervical spine used to exclude bony pathology
- May show loss of normal lordotic curve due to muscle spasm
- If neurologic findings present, magnetic resonance imaging is the preferred test to evaluate spinal cord and nerve roots

TABLE 17.2

Neck Pain: Treatment

Treatment

Cervical strain *without* radiculopathy:

- Gentle stretch exercises
- Heat and massage
- Mild analgesics
- Nighttime muscle relaxants

If no response:

- Gentle cervical reaction (5 lbs for 5–10 minutes twice daily)
- Trigger point injection
- Tricyclic antidepressant

Cervical strain *with* radiculopathy:

- Proper nighttime sleeping position with cervical pillow
- Analgesics
- Nighttime muscle relaxant
- Soft collar
- Cervical traction
- Neurosurgical referral

TABLE 17.3

Low Back Pain: Differential Diagnosis

Ninety percent of adults will experience back pain at some time in their life. It is the second most common symptomatic reason for a physician visit, behind upper respiratory tract symptoms. It results in a yearly estimated direct and indirect cost of $50 billion in the US. Low back pain has a self-limited course in 90% of patients, with most improving with conservative management.

Differential Diagnosis of Low Back Pain (LBP)

Mechanical LBP	Nonmechanical Spine Pathology	Referred Pain
Lumbar strain	Inflammation:	Abdominal aortic aneurysm
Degenerative disease	Rheumatoid arthritis	Renal disease:
Spondylolysis	Ankylosing spondylosis	Pyelonephritis
Spondylolisthesis	Reiter syndrome	Nephrolithiasis
Herniated disk	Polymyalgia rheumatica	Gastrointestinal disease:
Compression fracture	Infection:	Pancreatitis
Spinal stenosis	Osteomyelitis	Cholecystitis
Congenital kyphoscoliosis	Septic diskitis	Perforated bowel
	Paraspinal abscess	Inflammatory
	Epidural abscess	bowel disease

Neoplasm	Pelvic Disease
Metastatic disease	Prostatitis
Multiple myeloma	Endometriosis
Lymphomas	Pelvic inflammatory disease
Spinal cord tumors	
Retroperitoneal tumors	

TABLE 17.4

Low Back Pain: Evaluation

Physical Exam

Inspection	Undress the patient to expose back. Look for curves or asymmetry. Bend forward to screen for scoliosis and evaluate range of movement. Observe gait.
Palpation	Examine for trigger points, muscle spasm, spondylolisthesis and spodylolithesis step off. Examine abdomen for tenderness or masses including prostate. Feel peripheral pulse.

LS Neurologic Exam

Root	Disk	Reflex	Sensation	Muscle
L4	L3-L4	Patellar	Medial foot and ankle	Anterior tibialis-dorsiflex foot
L5	L4-L5	None	Dorsum of foot	Extensor hallucis-toe raise
S1	L5-S1	Achilles	Lateral foot	Peroneus longus-toe walking

Specific Tests

Straight leg raising test	Test to reproduce pain in the back and leg caused by nerve root irritation. With patient supine lift leg upward by supporting the foot around the heel. Keep the knee straight. Note extent to which the leg can be raised without discomfort. Normal range is 60° to 90°. Hamstring tightness will cause posterior thigh pain. Sciatic pain can extend all the way down the leg. Positive test is associated with herniated disk, spinal stenosis, or any other external pressure upon nerve.

Continued

TABLE 17.4

Low Back Pain: Evaluation, cont'd

Imaging

Plain films are rarely useful in initial evaluation of acute low back pain except in patients who meet certain criteria (see below). Computed tomographic scan provides better imaging of bone, whereas magnetic resonance imaging provides better images of soft tissues (cord, disk). All abnormal findings must correlate with symptoms and exam to be considered significant.

Indications for Radiological Imaging in Acute Low Back Pain

- Significant trauma
- Neurologic symptoms
- Unexplained fever
- Unexplained weight loss
- History of cancer
- History of chronic corticosteroid use
- History of intravenous drug use or alcohol abuse
- Suspected ankylosing spondylitis

True Surgical Emergency Suspected (cauda equina syndrome, cord tumor, massive midline disk herniation)

- Severe or progressive neurologic defect in lower extremity
- Recent onset of bladder dysfunction
- Saddle anesthesia

TABLE 17.5

Low Back Pain: Treatment

Treatment

- Maintain activity except in severe cases
- Modify activities such as avoiding prolonged sitting, standing, or heavy lifting
- Analgesics (acetaminophen, NSAIDs, short-term use of narcotics)
- Muscle relaxants
- Physical therapy modalities (heat, cold, massage)
- Spinal manipulation
- Patient education

Evidence-Based Recommendations

Acute low back pain

- Beneficial
  1. NSAIDs
  2. Advise to stay active
- Likely to be beneficial
  1. Analgesics
  2. Spinal manipulation
- Tradeoff between benefits and harms
  1. Muscle relaxants
- Likely to be ineffective or harmful
  1. Bed rest
  2. Traction

Chronic low back pain

- Beneficial
  1. Back exercises
  2. Multidisciplinary treatment programs
- Likely to be beneficial
  1. Analgesics
  2. NSAIDs
  3. Trigger point and ligamentous injections
  4. Back school
  5. Spinal manipulation
  6. Behavioral therapy
- Unlikely to be beneficial
  1. Bed rest
  2. EMG biofeedback
- Likely to be ineffective or harmful
  1. Facet joint injections
  2. Traction

Adapted from Vantulder M, Koes B. Low back pain and sciatica. In: Barton S, ed. *Clinical Evidence*, June 2001.

EMG indicates electromyogram; NSAIDs, nonsteroidal anti-inflammatory drugs.

TABLE 17.6

Shoulder Pain

Diagnosis	Character of Pain	Physical Findings	X-ray Findings	Treatment
Glenohumeral osteroarthritis	Dull, aching, not severe	Crepitus, decreased ROM	Degenerative changes	Conservative
Bicipital tendinitis	Pain in anterior shoulder; radiates to biceps and forearm	Tender to palpation in bicipital groove; pain with resisted elbow flexion	Usually normal	Conservative plus steroid injection over bicipital groove
Rotator cuff injury	Chronic pain with overhead movement	Painful arc of movement, positive "drop arm" sign	MRI and arthrogram	Rehabilitation surgery
Frozen shoulder	Pain following prior shoulder condition	Restricted active and passive ROM	Usually normal	Active and passive ROM, steroid injection
Subacromial bursitis	Sudden, severe, diffuse pain; radiates to deltoid; cannot sleep on side	Positive Neer and Hawkins tests	Occ. fluffy calcium deposit	Conservative, steroid injection

Diagnosis	Character of Pain	Physical Findings	X-ray Findings	Treatment
Glenoid labrial tear	Throwing athlete with painful click or pop with throwing	Clunk test with overhead movement	Abnormal MRI	Rehabilitation, possible arthroscopic repair
Acromioclavicular sprain	Pain upon palpation of AC joint and movement of shoulder	Tender AC joint crossover test	Weighted stress films may show laxity	Conservative, possible surgery

AC indicates acromioclavicular; MRI, magnetic resonance imaging; ROM, range of motion.

TABLE 17.7

Shoulder Physical Exam

Painful arc of movement	Ask patient to actively abduct arm from side to overhead. Pain between 60° and 120° degrees suggests subacromial impingement or rotator cuff pathology
Drop arm test	Ask patient to abduct arm to 90°. Them ask him to slowly lower the arm to his side. This is done with and without manual pressure from the examiner. If the patient is not able to smoothly lower his arm, this suggests a torn rotator cuff.
Neer test	The examiner fixes the scapula with one hand while elevating the patient's arm in the frontal plane. Pain in shoulder is a positive test. Note the degrees of elevation at which the pain appeared. A positive test is often caused by subacromial impingement.
Hawkins test	Arm forward, elevated to 90°, then internally rotated. Pain in shoulder suggests subacromial impingement or rotator cuff tendinitis.
Crossover test	Arm raised to 90° then actively crossed over the chest. Pain in the acromioclavicular joint suggests a problem in that joint.
Apprehension test	Place shoulder in 90° abduction, externally rotate shoulder while applying slight anterior pressure to the humerus. Pain or the appearance of apprehension by the patient to the maneuver suggests anterior glenohumeral instability.

TABLE 17.8

The Elbow

Lateral Epicondylitis ("tennis elbow")

Symptoms	Pain over lateral side of elbow during and after activity
Cause	Degenerative changes in wrist extensor tendons
Signs	Point tenderness over lateral epicondyle Pain increased with resisted wrist extension "Coffee cup" test (pain increased with picking up a full cup of coffee)
Imaging	X-rays usually not needed
Treatment	Ice, NSAIDs, wrist splint, tennis elbow strap Steroid injection, surgery for refractory cases

Medial Epicondylitis ("golfer's elbow")

Symptoms	Pain over medial epicondyle
Cause	Degenerative changes in tendon insertion on medial epicondyle
Signs	Point tenderness over medial epicondyle Pain increased with resisted wrist flexion
Imaging	X-rays usually not needed
Treatment	Ice, NSAIDs, rest, wrist splint, steroid injection

Olecranon Bursitis

Symptoms	Swelling over posterior aspect of elbow
Cause	Repetitive trauma to olecranon bursa 5% gout, 5% infection (usually staphylococcal)
Signs	Swollen, fluctuant bursa
Imaging	Usually not needed unless foreign body or fracture suspected
Treatment	Aspirate bursa. Send fluid for culture/crystal analysis if suspected Compression dressing after aspiration Steroid injection if no infection present Surgical excision if chronic/recurrent

NSAIDs indicates nonsteroidal anti-inflammatory drugs.

TABLE 17.9

The Wrist

DeQuerevain Tenosynovitis	
Symptoms	Pain in radial side of wrist with grip
Cause	Stenosing tenosynovitis of first dorsal compartment of the wrist Usually caused by repetitive use of thumb
Signs	Tenderness to palpation at the tip of radial styloid. Pain aggravated by thumb abduction and extension. Finkelstein test is diagnostic. Tuck thumb in palm and ulnarly deviate the wrist. A positive test will be painful
Imaging	Usually not needed
Treatment	Splint thumb, nonsteroidal anti-inflammatory drugs, ice Steroid injection if not responding Surgical release if conservative measures fail
Carpal Tunnel Syndrome	
Symptoms	Numbness or pain in median nerve distribution Worse at night Pain may travel retrograde up the arm
Cause	Entrapment of median nerve in carpal tunnel of wrist often associated with repetitive hand motions
Signs	Loss of sensation in median nerve distribution Tinel sign: paresthesias in median nerve distribution by percussion over flexor side of wrist Phalen sign: reproduction of tingling sensation by maximally flexing wrist for up to 60 seconds Atrophy of thenar muscles with weak thumb opposition Abnormal nerve conduction velocity test
Imaging	Not needed
Treatment	Night splinting, reduce repetitive wrist movements Treat underlying problems (rheumatoid arthritis, hypothyroidism) Steroid injection in carpal tunnel Surgical decompression

TABLE 17.10
The Hand

Dupuytren Contracture	
Symptoms	Finger stiffness and loss of motion of affected fingers
Cause	Fibrosis of the palmer fascia typically involving the fourth and fifth fingers
Signs	Fixed flexion contracture of the fourth and fifth fingers
	Painless palmar nodules
Imaging	Not needed
Treatment	Tendon stretching
	Surgical release
	Educate patient about the recurrent and progressive nature
Trigger Finger	
Symptoms	Locking or catching of the finger in flexion Occasionally painful
Cause	Inflammation of the flexor tendons of the finger as they cross the metacarpophalangeal (MCP) head in the palm at the A1 pulley
Signs	Mechanical locking of the finger in flexion
	Local tenderness at the MCP head
Imaging	Not needed
Treatment	Ice over MCP head, splint, limit gripping
	Steroid injection over metacarpal head
	Gentle stretch exercises for fingers
	Surgical release if not better with conservative measures

TABLE 17.11

The Hip

Osteoarthritis of Hip

Symptoms	Hip, groin, or thigh pain
Cause	Degenerative changes in articular cartilage of the hip
Signs	Pain upon weight bearing Loss of internal and external rotation
Imaging	Plain films often abnormal May show loss of joint space, sclerotic changes in acetabulum, and osteophyte formation
Treatment	Analgesics, continue daily activity as able but restrict high-impact activity Weight loss and range of motion exercise may be helpful If pain becomes intractable or activity severely limited consider joint replacement

Trochanteric Bursitis

Symptoms	Pain over the outer thigh, often worse with activity
Cause	Inflammation of the bursa overlying the trochanter Often there is an underlying back, sacroiliac, or leg problem
Signs	Localized tenderness over the greater trochanter Normal range of motion of the hip
Imaging	X-rays may be needed to exclude underlying pathology such as degenerative joint disease or stress fractures
Treatment	Nonsteroidal anti-inflammatory drugs Correct any underlying biomechanical abnormality If symptoms persist consider steroid injection

TABLE 17.12
The Knee

Osteoarthritis of the Knee

Symptoms	Knee pain, usually better in the morning and worse in the evening Osteoarthritis is the most frequent cause of knee pain
Cause	Degenerative changes in the articular cartilage often caused by prior injury, obesity, genu valgum, or other biomechanical abnormality
Signs	Crepitus over joint line, effusion, and bony deformity due to osteophytes
Imaging	X-ray recommended to confirm diagnosis Will show joint space narrowing (less than 6 mm) Osteophytes seen in advanced disease
Treatment	Analgesics Weight loss if overweight Limit squatting and kneeling Encourage low impact or non-weight-bearing activity If symptoms persist consider steroid injection (limit to three injections per year) If pain is intractable or significant disability consider joint replacement

Patellofemoral Pain Syndrome

Symptoms	Anterior knee pain often worse descending stairs or slopes
Causes	Abnormal tracking of the patella in the femoral grove
Signs	Painful patellar crepitation, abnormal Q angle (greater than 20°)
Imaging	X-rays of knee including "sunrise view" are helpful but may be normal in early disease
Treatment	Avoid squatting or kneeling Ice after activity NSAIDs Quadriceps strengthening exercises to improve patellar tracking

Prepatellar Bursitis

Symptoms	Pain and swelling anterior to the patella
Causes	Repetitive trauma to the bursa is the most common cause Other causes include gout (5%) or staphylococcal infection (5%)
Signs	Swelling and inflammation directly over the patella Aspiration of the bursa may be needed to exclude infectious causes

Continued

TABLE 17.12

The Knee, cont'd

Imaging	Not necessary
Treatment	Protect from further trauma Ice NSAIDs Aspirate Compressive dressing Consider steroid injection if infection has been excluded Recurrent cases may need bursectomy

Baker Cyst

Symptoms	Swelling behind the knee
Causes	Collection of synovial fluid in the popliteal fossa
Signs	Cystic mass in the popliteal fossa with limited knee flexion
Imaging	X-ray unrevealing Ultrasound will show cystic mass
Treatment	Treat underlying knee pathology (osteoarthritis or rheumatoid arthritis) Aspirate cyst If cyst reaccumulates inject with steroid Consider surgical removal if cyst interferes with function

TABLE 17.13

Knee Effusions: Causes

Osteoarthritis Trauma

- Fractures
- Ligamentous injury
- Meniscus injury

Inflammatory Diseases

- Rheumatoid arthritis
- Juvenile rheumatoid arthritis
- Reiter disease
- Systemic lupus erythematosus
- Rheumatic fever

Crystals

- Gout (urate crystals)
- Pseudogout (calcium pyrophosphate crystals)

Tumors

- Benign
  —Osteochondroma
  —Osteoid osteoma
  —Pigmented villonodular synovitis
  —Fibrous dysplasia
- Malignant
  —Chondroblastoma
  —Giant cell tumor
  —Ewing sarcoma
  —Osteosarcoma
  —Synovial sarcoma
  —Eosinophilic granuloma
  —Lymphoma

Infection

- Blood-borne seeding
- Lyme disease
- Gonorrhea
- Tuberculosis

TABLE 17.14

Joint Fluid Analysis

Diagnosis	Color	Viscosity	WBC Count/mL	% PMNs	Protein (g/dL)	Glucose
Normal	Clear/straw	High	<200	<20	1.0–4.0	Same as serum
Trauma	Bloody or xanthochrome	High	<2000	<30	1.3–5.0	Same as serum
Osteoarthritis	Clear/straw	High	<2000	<25	2.9–5.5	Same as serum
Gout	Turbid/white	Low	>100,000	50–95	1.5–3.5	Same as serum
Pseudo-gout	Clear/turbid	Fair/Low	50,000–75,000	30–90	1.5–3.5	Same as serum
Rheumatoid arthritis	Turbid/green-yellow	Low	3000–50,000	60–95	3.0–6.0	75%–100% of serum
Infection	Turbid/yellow	Low	50,000–300,000	>90	2.8–3.8	<50% of serum

PMNs indicates polymorphonuclear leukocytes; WBC, white blood cell.

TABLE 17.15

Knee Examination

Medial Collateral Stress	With the patient supine and thigh muscle relaxed, the examiner places one hand on the lateral side of the knee and the other hand around the ankle. Force is applied to the lateral knee in an attempt to open up the knee on the medial side. Watch and feel for medial joint opening. Determine if there is a "firm" or "soft" endpoint. This test is done with the knee straight and in 30° of flexion. Laxity at 30° indicates instability of the medial collateral ligament. Laxity when straight suggests associated posterior cruciate instability. Perform the test on the uninjured knee to establish a "normal" for the patient.
Lateral Collateral Stress	With the patient supine and the thigh muscle relaxed, the examiner places one hand on the medial side of the knee and the other hand around the ankle. Force is applied to the medial side of the knee in an attempt to open up the lateral side of the knee. Watch and feel for lateral joint opening. Determine if there is a "firm" or "soft" endpoint. This test is done with the knee straight and in 30° of flexion. Laxity at 30° indicates instability of the lateral collateral ligament. Because other ligaments contribute to lateral stability, even a complete isolated tear of the lateral collateral ligament may appear stable. Laxity at 0° of flexion suggests an associated posterior cruciate instability. Compare findings with the uninjured knee to determine what is normal.
Anterior Drawer Test	Position patient supine with hip flexed 45° and the knee flexed 90°. Externally rotate the foot 30° and sit on the foot to stabilize it. Grasp the proximal tibia with your thumbs on the medial and lateral joint line and pull forward. A positive test will have the tibia sliding forward. This suggests a tear of the anterior cruciate ligament. If the anterior drawer test is done with the foot in the neutral or internally rotated position, ligaments other than the anterior cruciate contribute to stability.
Posterior Drawer Test	Position the patient the same as for anterior drawer test but with the foot in the neutral position. Posterior force is applied to the proximal tibia. A positive test will have the tibia sliding posterior to the femur and suggest a tear of the posterior cruciate ligament.

Continued

TABLE 17.15

Knee Examination, cont'd

Lachman Test	Position the patient supine with the thigh muscles relaxed. Grasp the distal femur with one hand while grasping the proximal tibia with the other hand. This may be difficult with a large patient or an examiner with small hands. With the knee flexed 15°, the tibia is pulled forward. A positive test will show anterior translation of the tibia forward and lack a firm endpoint. This suggests a tear of the anterior cruciate ligament. Compare with the uninjured knee.
McMurray Test	Position the patient supine with the leg relaxed. Flex the knee maximally. Rotate the tibia externally. Extend the knee while palpating the medial joint line. A palpable or audible click suggests a tear of the medial meniscus. Repeat the test with the tibia internally rotated while palpating the lateral joint line. A click would indicate a tear of the lateral meniscus.
Apley Compression Test	Position the patient prone with the knee flexed 90° and the muscles relaxed. Push down on the heel to compress the medial and lateral menisci between the tibia and femur. Rotate the tibia medially and laterally. Pain in the medial side of the knee suggests medial meniscus damage. Pain on the lateral side suggests lateral meniscus damage.
Apprehension Test	Position the patient supine with the leg straight and the thigh relaxed. With both thumbs, the examiner attempts to push the patella laterally. Pain or extreme apprehension by the patient indicates subluxation or instability of the patella.

TABLE 17.16

Pittsburgh Rules for Acute Knee Injuries

Which patients presenting with an acute knee injury require x-rays to exclude a fracture? Only 6% of patients with knee trauma have a fracture. The Pittsburgh Knee Rules were developed to guide clinicians in the appropriate use of x-rays in acute knee injuries. In clinical practice these rules have been shown to have a sensitivity of 99% and a specificity of 60%. When applied, they have reduced x-ray use by up to 50%.

X-rays of the knee **should be obtained** when blunt trauma or a fall is the mechanism of injury *and* either

1. The patient is younger than 12 years or older than 50 years of age

or

2. The injury causes an inability to walk four weight-bearing steps

The Pittsburgh Rules are *not* applicable in knee injuries:

- Sustained more than 6 days before presentation.
- With a history of previous surgery or fracture.
- Being reassessed for the same injury.
- With lacerations or abrasions on the knee.

Adapted from Bauer SJ, Hollander JE, Fuchs SH, Thode HC Jr. A clinical decision rule in the evaluation of acute knee injuries. *J Emerg Med.* 1995;13:661–665.

TABLE 17.17

Ankle Sprains

Ankle Sprain

Each day 30,000 Americans seek medical care for an ankle sprain. A sprain is a ligamentous injury. Ninety percent of ankle sprains involve the lateral ligament. The usual mechanism of injury is an inversion of the ankle.

Examine the ankle and foot, noting swelling, ecchymosis, tenderness, and neurovascular status. Test for ligamentous laxity with the anterior drawer test and the inversion stress test. Test the patient's ability to bear weight. Based upon these findings, the extent of the sprain can be graded. Accurate grading can provide useful information for treatment and prognosis.

West Point Ankle Sprain Grading System

Criteria	Grade I	Grade II	Grade III
Edema, ecchymosis	Slight, local	Moderate, local	Significant, diffuse
Weight bearing	Full or partial	Difficult	Impossible without pain
Ligament damage	Stretched	Partial tear	Complete tear
Instability	None	None or slight	Definite

Grades I and II can be treated conservatively. Grade III may require referral and consideration for surgical repair.

Treatment

- Emphasis is on early treatment
- Ice for 20 minutes every 4 hours for initial 48 hours
- Compression
- Elevation
- Protected weight bearing (aircast or stirrup brace)
- Crutches if unable to bear weight
- Analgesics if needed
- Adequate rehabilitation (range of motion, strength, proprioception) is vital

Prognosis by West Point Grading System (Return to Sporting Activity)

- Grade I: Average 11 days
- Grade II: 2 to 6 weeks
- Grade III: 4 to 26 weeks

Chronic Pain in a Sprained Ankle May Be Due to

- Chronic instability
- Degenerative joint disease
- Loose body
- Occult fracture
- Peroneal tendon injury
- Intra-articular meniscoid injury

TABLE 17.18

Ottawa Ankle Rules

The Ottawa Ankle Rules were developed to determine which patients need x-rays of the ankle and/or foot in the setting of an acute injury. If none of the clinical criteria are present, the sensitivity for excluding a fracture approaches 100%. These rules are only valid in adults not under the influence of drugs or alcohol.

An ankle x-ray series is only necessary if there is pain near the malleoli and either of these findings:

- Inability to bear weight (four steps) immediately and in the emergency department

or

- Bone tenderness at the posterior edge or tip of either malleolus

A foot x-ray series is only necessary if there is pain in the midfoot and either of these findings:

- Inability to bear weight (four steps) immediately and in the emergency department

or

- Bone tenderness at the navicular or base of fifth metatarsal

Adapted from Stiell IG, Greenberg GH, McKnight RD, Nair RC, McDowell I, Worthington JR. A study to develop clinical decision rules for the use of radiography in acute ankle injuries. *Ann Emerg Med.* 1992;21:384–390.

TABLE 17.19

The Foot

Plantar Fasciitis

Symptoms	Pain and point tenderness at the origin of the plantar fascia (medial heel and arch)
	The pain is typically worse with initial weight bearing upon arising in the morning
Cause	Microtears and inflammation at the origin of the plantar fascia
	This is typically associated with tight heel cords
Differential diagnosis	Entrapment of the medial calcaneal branch of the tibial nerve
	Tarsal tunnel syndrome
	Calcaneal stress fracture
	Fat pad syndrome (atrophy of heel pad)
	Plantar facia tear
Imaging	Usually not necessary
	May show "heel spur," which is usually not the cause of pain
Treatment	Shock-absorbing heel pad or heel cup
	Well-fitting shoe with good arch support
	Heel cord stretching
	NSAIDs
	Steroid injection if conservative measures fail

Achilles Tendinitis

Symptoms	Tenderness in heel cord or insertion on calcaneus
Causes	Usually associated with tight heel cords, overpronation, or change in shoes or running routine
Signs	Tenderness and thickening at the insertion site or along the tendon
	Occasionally crepitation is noted along the tendon
Imaging	Plain x-rays usually unrevealing
	MRI or ultrasound may show degeneration or partial tear
Treatment	Ice
	NSAIDs
	Stretching program
	Heel lift for several weeks
	Correct pronation with orthotics if present
	Correct training errors
	Never inject with steroid (may lead to rupture of tendon)

Continued

TABLE 17.19

The Foot, cont'd

Morton Neuroma	
Symptoms	Burning pain in the middle toes, usually worse with weight bearing
Causes	Entrapment of interdigital nerve between metatarsal heads
	Typically between the third and fourth but can occur between the second and third metatarsals
Signs	Manual compression of the metatarsal heads will reproduce the pain
	May be point tender at site of impingment
Imaging	Not necessary
Treatment	Metatarsal pads to spread the metatarsal heads
	Avoid tight shoes
	NSAIDs
	Steroid injection
	Surgical resection of nerve

MRI indicates magnetic resonance imaging; NSAIDs, nonsteroidal anti-inflammatory drugs.

TABLE 17.20

Osteoarthritis

Osteoarthritis (OA) is the most common joint disorder. While x-ray findings of osteoarthritis can be found in most people over the age of 60 years, clinically significant disease affects 10% to 20% of the population. The disease process involves damage to the articular cartilage with associated remodeling of the underlying bone and mild synovitis. The most commonly involved joint are the hands, knees, hip, and spine.

Risk factors for the development of osteoarthritis include obesity (strongly related to knee OA), prior joint injury, and age-related impairments of joint-protective neural, mechanical, and muscular functions.

Treatment

- There is no proven disease-modifying agent for OA; the goal of treatment is symptomatic relief and preservation of function

Analgesics

- Acetaminophen is the first choice based upon safety and effectivness
- NSAIDs (may require concurrent use of misoprostol or proton pump inhibitor for gastric protection; the elderly, patients with prior peptic ulcer disease and renal disease are at high risk for significant side effects)
- Topical analgesics (capsaicin)
- Glucosamine/chondroitin may be of benefit

Lifestyle Modification

- Activity (maintain regular physical activity, avoiding high-impact activity and any activity that is stressful to a particularly painful joint)
- Strengthening and aerobic activity
- Weight loss for knee OA

Intra-articular Medications

- Steroids reduce pain (maximum usage 3 times a year)
- Hyaluronic acid (weekly for 3 to 5 weeks)

Surgery

- Joint replacement for severe OA

Evidence-Based Recommendations

Based upon currently available systematic reviews and randomized clinical trials the following recommendations can be supported as being beneficial in the management of osteoarthritis.

Continued

TABLE 17.20
Osteoarthritis, cont'd

Beneficial

- Systemic analgesics (short-term pain relief and improved function)
- Systemic NSAIDs (short-term pain relief)
- Topical agents (short-term pain relief)
- Hip replacement

Likely to Be Beneficial

- Exercise (pain relief and improved function)
- Education, dietary advice and support (improved knowledge of disease and pain relief)
- Physical aids
- Knee replacement in older patients

Trade-off Between Benefits and Harms

- Hip replacement in younger patients
- Hip replacement in obese patients
- Knee replacement in younger patients

Unknown Effectiveness

- Knee replacement in obese patients

Unlikely to Be Beneficial

- Intra-articular injection of the knee

Likely to be Ineffective or Harmful

- Systemic analgesics in patients with existing liver damage
- Systemic NSAIDs in older patients and patients at risk for renal disease or peptic ulceration

Adapted from Dieppe P, Chard J. Osteoarthritis. In: Barton S, ed. *Clinical Evidence*, June 2001.
NSAIDs indicates nonsteroidal anti-inflammatory drugs.

TABLE 17.21

Rheumatoid Arthritis: Diagnosis

Rheumatoid arthritis (RA) is a chronic, systemic, polyarticular, inflammatory arthritis. Females outnumber males 3 to 1. Peak onset is in the fourth to sixth decade. RA initially affects the small joints of the wrist, MCP, PIP, ankle, and MTP. The DIP is usual spared, in contrast to osteoarthritis (OA). The clinical course is usually that of a gradually progressive, symmetrical polyarthritis. The diagnosis is clinical and may be difficult because there are no pathognomonic findings.

American College of Rheumatology Classification Criteria for Diagnosis of RA

- Patient must have at least four of the following present with items 1–4 present for at least 6 weeks:
  1. Morning stiffness
  2. Arthritis of three or more joints
  3. Arthritis of hand joints
  4. Symmetrical arthritis
  5. Rheumatoid nodules
  6. Serum rheumatoid factor
  7. Radiological changes

Differential Diagnosis

- Post-viral infection symptoms (hepatitis C, rubella, parvovirus)
- Spondyloarthopathy
- Systemic lupus erythematosus
- Adult-onset Still disease
- OA (most frequent cause of arthritis)

RA vs OA (How to Differentiate)

- DIP (usually spared in RA; frequently involved in OA)
- Joint fluid analysis

  RA: WBC 3000 to 50,000/mL, 60% to 95% PMNs, low viscosity

  OA: WBC <2000/mL, <25% PMNs, high viscosity

Radiologic Findings in RA

- Periarticular soft-tissue swelling
- Osteopenia
- Progressive marginal erosions
- Synovial cyst formation
- Joint space narrowing in the classic joint distribution

Continued

TABLE 17.21

Rheumatoid Arthritis: Diagnosis, cont'd

Laboratory Findings

- Rheumatoid factor positive in 75% of RA patients
- Elevated sedimentation rate
- Elevated C-reactive protein
- Thrombocytosis
- Normocytic, normochromic anemia

TABLE 17.22

Conditions Associated With a Positive Rheumatoid Factor

Rheumatologic Diseases

- RA
- SLE
- JRA
- Sjogren syndrome
- Ankylosing spondylitis
- Enteropathic arthritis

Viral Disease

- Rubella
- CMV
- Influenza
- Hepatitis B and C

Chronic Bacterial Infections

- Subacute bacterial endocarditis
- Leprosy
- TB
- Syphilis

Parasitic Disease

Mixed Cryoglobulinemia

Dermatomyositis

Psoriatic Arthritis

Chronic Inflammatory Diseases

- Sarcoid
- Periodontal disease
- Pulmonary interstitial disease
- Liver disease

TABLE 17.23

Rheumatoid Arthritis: Treatment

The ultimate goal of treatment is disease remission with resolution of morning stiffness, fatigue, joint pain and swelling, and normalization of lab values. Treatment for RA is multifaceted and includes:

- Analgesics and NSAIDs for pain control
- Disease-modifying Antirheumatic drugs (DMARDs): begin early! (DMARDs are the only way to achieve remission)
- Systemic and local corticosteroids as bridge therapy and for disease flares

NSAIDs

- Decrease pain and swelling but do not modify the disease

Corticosteroids

- Decrease erosions and improve systemic symptoms but there is risk of significant side effects. Doses >10 mg/d of prednisone rarely indicated

DMARDs

- Methotrexate (most frequently used DMARD)
  Dosage: 7.5 to 20 mg once weekly along with folic acid
  Toxicity: Hypersensitivity pneumonitis, elevated LFTs, infections
  Monitoring: CBC, liver, renal, chest x-ray
- Hydroxychloroquine (second most commonly used DMARD)
  Dosage: 6.5 mg/kg/day in divided doses
  Toxicity: Retinal
  Monitoring: Regular eye exams recommended
- Sulfasalazine
  Dosage: 1 to 3 g/d in divided doses
  Monitoring: CBC, liver, renal
- Gold (intramuscular) (slow onset of action, 3 to 6 months; oral gold not as effective)
  Dosage: 10 to 50 mg IM weekly; after 1 g reached, dose 50 mg q 3 wk
  Toxicity: Hematologic, renal
  Monitoring: CBC, U/A regularly checked

Other Agents

- Penicillamine
- Azathioprine
- Cyclophosamide
- Leflunomide
- Minocycline
- Tumor necrosis factor antagonists

Evidence-Based Recommendations

Based upon currently available systematic reviews and randomized clinical trials the following recommendations can be supported as being beneficial in the management of rheumatoid arthritis.

Beneficial

- Early intervention with DMARDs
- Methotrexate
- Antimalarials
- Sulfasalazine
- Parenteral gold
- Short-term low-dose oral corticosteroids

Likely to Be Beneficial

- Oral gold
- Minocycline
- Leflunomide (long term safety unclear)
- Tumor necrosis factor antagonists (long-term safety unclear)

Trade-off Between Benefits and Harms

- Penicillamine
- Azathioprine
- Cyclophosphamide
- Cyclosporine
- Longer-term low-dose oral corticosteroids

Adapted from Suarez-Almazor ME, Foster W. Rheumatoid arthritis. In: Barton, S, ed. *Clinical Evidence*, June 2001.

TABLE 17.24
Ankylosing Spondylitis

Ankylosing spondylitis is the most common inflammatory disorder of the axial skeleton. The onset is often insidious with low back pain and stiffness. The classic finding of sacroilitis may take years to develop. The hip joints may also be involved. Extra-articular involvement can include the eye (uveitis), heart (aortitis, aortic insufficiency, pericarditis, and conduction defects) and lung (pulmonary fibrosis). Symptoms begin in the second or third decade. Onset after the age of 40 years is rare. Males outnumber females 4:1.

X-ray Findings
Include sacroilitis and the classic "bamboo spine"

Laboratory Findings
Include elevated sedimentation rate, elevated C-reactive protein, and anemia of chronic disease. HLA-B27 may be present in up to 50% but is not necessary to make the diagnosis.

Treatment
Current treatments cannot cure the disease. All patients should be counseled regarding exercise to maintain mobility, diet, rest, and vocational choices.

Medications
- NSAIDs (except salicylates)
- Sulfasalazinie
- Methotrexate
- Intra-articular steroid injection

NSAIDs indicates nonsteroidal anti-inflammatory drugs.

TABLE 17.25

Polymyalgia Rheumatica*

Clinical	Physical	Laboratory	Treatment
Age >50 y; Proxmial muscle pain in hips, spine, and shoulders	Usually negative	ESR >50 mm/h; often >100 mm/h	Rapid response to steroids confirms diagnosis
May have fatigue and stiffness		Anemia of chronic disease	Prednisone 10 to 20 mg/d until response; then maintain at 1 to 2.5 mg/d for 6 to 12 months

ESR indicates erythrocyte sedimentation rate.

*Polymyalgia rheumatica can be associated with giant cell arteritis. Symptoms include new onset of severe headache, visual loss, jaw claudication, and stroke. Examination may show tenderness or loss of pulsation in the temporal artery. Treatment should begin immediately if giant cell arteritis is suspected with high-dose Prednisone (1 mg/kg/day). Biopsy of the temporal artery should be obtained within 1 week of starting steroids to confirm the diagnosis.

TABLE 17.26

Juvenile Rheumatoid Arthritis

Juvenile Rheumatoid Arthritis is the most common rheumatic disease of childhood. There are three subsets, each with its characteristic presentation, treatment, and prognosis.

Syndrome	Signs and Symptoms	Prognosis	Treatment
Systemic-onset disease (Still Disease)			
■ Male = Female Median age at onset 5 years	■ Fever, rash, arthritis, myalgias. ■ Extra-articular manifestations include lymphadenopathy, hepatosplenomegaly, pericarditis, pleuritis. ■ ANA and RF negative	■ One third become disabled ■ Chronic, progressive	■ Indomethacin ■ Pulse steroid
Polyarticular Disease			
■ Seronegative: F > M 3:1 Median age at onset, 2 years	■ Insidious onset, initially involves small joints of hand and feet ■ RF negative in 90% ■ ANA positive in 40%	■ One sixth become disabled	■ NSAIDs ■ DMARD
■ Seropositive: F > M Median age at onset, 12 years	■ Insidious onset, initially involves hands and feet ■ Tendonitis, nodules ■ RF positive ■ ANA negative ■ HLA-B27 in 75%	■ Rapidly progressive	■ NSAIDs ■ DMARD
Pauciarticular Disease			
■ F > M 4:1 Mean age at onset 2–4 years	■ Involves <5 joints ■ Usually knees and ankles ■ 20% with iritis ■ RF negative ■ ANA positive in 70%	■ Good prognosis ■ Mild disability	■ Intra-articular steroid ■ If no response then give DMARD

TABLE 17.27

Fibromyalgia

Symptoms

- Gradual onset of chronic, diffuse, poorly localized musculoskeletal pain, typically accompanied by fatigue and sleep disorder

Cause

- Unknown
- Most likely produced by a central nervous system mechanism
- Patients with fibromyalgia have a high rate of major depression, migraine, irritable bowel, and panic disorder

Diagnostic Criteria

- American College of Rheumatology Criteria:
    1. History of chronic, widespread pain (above and below the waist on both sides of the body) of greater than 3 months' duration
    2. Pain in 11 of 18 trigger points on digital palpation. The trigger points are located at the occiput, low cervical, trapesius, supraspinous, second rib, lateral epicondyle, gluteus, greater trochanter, and knee

Differential Diagnosis

- Polymyalgia rheumatica
- Hypothyroidism
- Polymyositis
- Systemic lupus erythematosus
- Rheumatoid arthritis

Treatment

- Reassurance, education
- Low-level aerobic exercise
- Amitriptyline (low dose), SSRI may also be helpful
- Cyclobenzaprine at night
- NSAIDs have not been shown to be helpful

NSAIDs indicates nonsteroidal anti-inflammatory drugs; SSRI, selective serotonin reuptake inhibitor.

TABLE 17.28

Osteoporosis

Risk Factors for Osteoporosis

- Female
- Low body weight
- White or Asian ancestry
- Sedentary lifestyle
- Nulliparity
- Increasing age
- High caffeine intake
- Renal disease
- Smoking
- Alcoholism
- Postmenopausal
- Lifelong low calcium intake

Bone Mineral Density Testing Recommended in:

- All women older than 65 years.
- Postmenopausal women younger than 65 years with risk factors other than being postmenopausal
- Radiographic evidence of bone loss
- Patients on long-term glucocorticoid therapy (more than 3 months at a dosage of 7.5 mg of prednisone per day or higher)
- Hyperparathroidism
- Monitor for therapeutic response in women undergoing treatment for osteoporosis if the result would affect clinical decisions

Medicare Reimbursement for Bone Mass Density Testing

- Medicare will reimburse for testing every 2 years if one of the following qualifications is met:
    1. An estrogen-deficient woman at clinical risk for osteoporosis
    2. An individual with vertebral abnormalities
    3. An individual receiving long-term glucocorticoid therapy
    4. An individual with primary hyperparathyroidism
    5. An individual being monitored to assess the response to or efficacy of an FDA-approved osteoporosis drug therapy

Osteoporosis Treatment

- Adequate calcium intake (1500 mg/d)
- Estrogen (while this has been a time-honored treatment, the FDA has removed this treatment benefit from the label)
- Selective-estrogen receptor modulators (Raloxifen 60 mg/d)
- Calcitonin (200 IU/d intranasally)
- Bisphosphonates (alendronate [Fosamax] 10 mg/d or 70 mg/wk; risedronate [Actonel] 5 mg/d)
- Fall prevention (home safety checks; increase muscular strength; eyesight correction; restricting use of drugs that alter the CNS)

Source: National Osteoporosis Foundation. Available online at www.nof.org.

TABLE 17.29

Developmental Dysplasia of the Hip

Formerly known as congenital dislocation of the hip	
Incidence	1 to 2 per 1000 children
Risk Factors	Positive family history Breech presentation Foot deformity Oligohydramnios Female gender
Physical Exam	Hip exam should be done at all regular well-child visits until child is walking
Ortolani Maneuver	Opposite hip is stabilized The hip is abducted and gently pulled anteriorly A positive test will have the sensation of instability with a palpable and some times audible "clunk" High-pitched "clicks" without sensation of instability have no pathologic significance
Barlow Maneuver	Adduct the hip and push the thigh posteriorly A positive test will have the hip going out of the socket The Ortolani maneuver will relocate the hip
Other Signs	Irreducible dislocation is suspected by limited abduction of the thigh Look for apparent shortening of the femur Look for asymmetrical skin folds in thigh
Imaging	X-rays are not useful in children less than 3 months of age until the femoral nucleus of ossification has appeared Ultrasound evaluation can be useful if interpreted by an experienced clinician Best done at 4 to 6 weeks of age
Treatment	If irreducible or positive Ortolani sign refer to pediatric orthopedist If dislocatable (positive Barlow sign) referral may be delayed 2 to 4 weeks Many hips will stabilize within that time Use abduction pillow for the first 2 to 4 weeks

TABLE 17.30

Transient Synovitis of the Hip

Transient synovitis of the hip is the most common cause of limping and hip pain in children. Usual age range is 3 to 10 years. It is more common in boys. It is an acute inflammatory reaction in the hip joint, usually following an upper respiratory infection.

Symptoms	Painful hip with limp without fever
Lab	Normal CBC; ESR can be elevated Joint aspiration is sterile
Imaging	X-ray may show joint effusion
Differential diagnosis	Septic hip joint Legg-Calve-Perthes disease
Treatment	Bed rest for comfort Usually self-limited to a few days Analgesics may be needed for comfort Follow-up x-ray to look for Legg-Calve-Perthes disease

CBC indicates complete blood cell count; ESR, erythrocyte sedimentation rate.

TABLE 17.31

Legg-Calve-Perthes Disease

Legg-Calve-Perthes disease is an avascular necrosis of the femoral head. Usual age range is 5 to 9 years, but children 2 to 11 years of age can be affected. Male > female 5:1.

Symptoms	Insidious onset of hip pain with limp
Lab	CBC and ESR are normal
	Joint aspirates are also typically normal
Imaging	If done early, the x-ray may be normal
	Joint effusion may be seen
	A radioisotope bone scan may show decreased uptake in the femoral head
	Decreased bone density in and around the joint can be seen after several weeks
	Later on as new bone is added to the femoral head, there will be increased bone density with deformity of the femoral head
Differential diagnosis	Septic joint Transient synovitis
Treatment	Orthopedic referral
	The hip is maintained in abduction and internal rotation by a brace

CBC indicates complete blood cell count; ESR, erythrocyte sedimentation rate.

TABLE 17.32

Slipped Capital Femoral Epiphysis

A slipped capital femoral epiphysis most frequently occurs in the 11- to 14-year age range. Obese boys are the typical victims. The onset of pain can be gradual or sudden. These can be bilateral in up to 30% of patients.

Symptoms	Pain in the hip with limp
	The pain can be referred to the thigh or medial side of the knee
	It is important to examine the hip joint in any child complaining of knee pain
	There will be limited internal rotation and abduction of the hip
Imaging	X-rays will show the slipped epiphysis
Treatment	Urgent orthopedic referral
	Usually requires surgical stabilization

FIGURE 17.1

Scoliosis

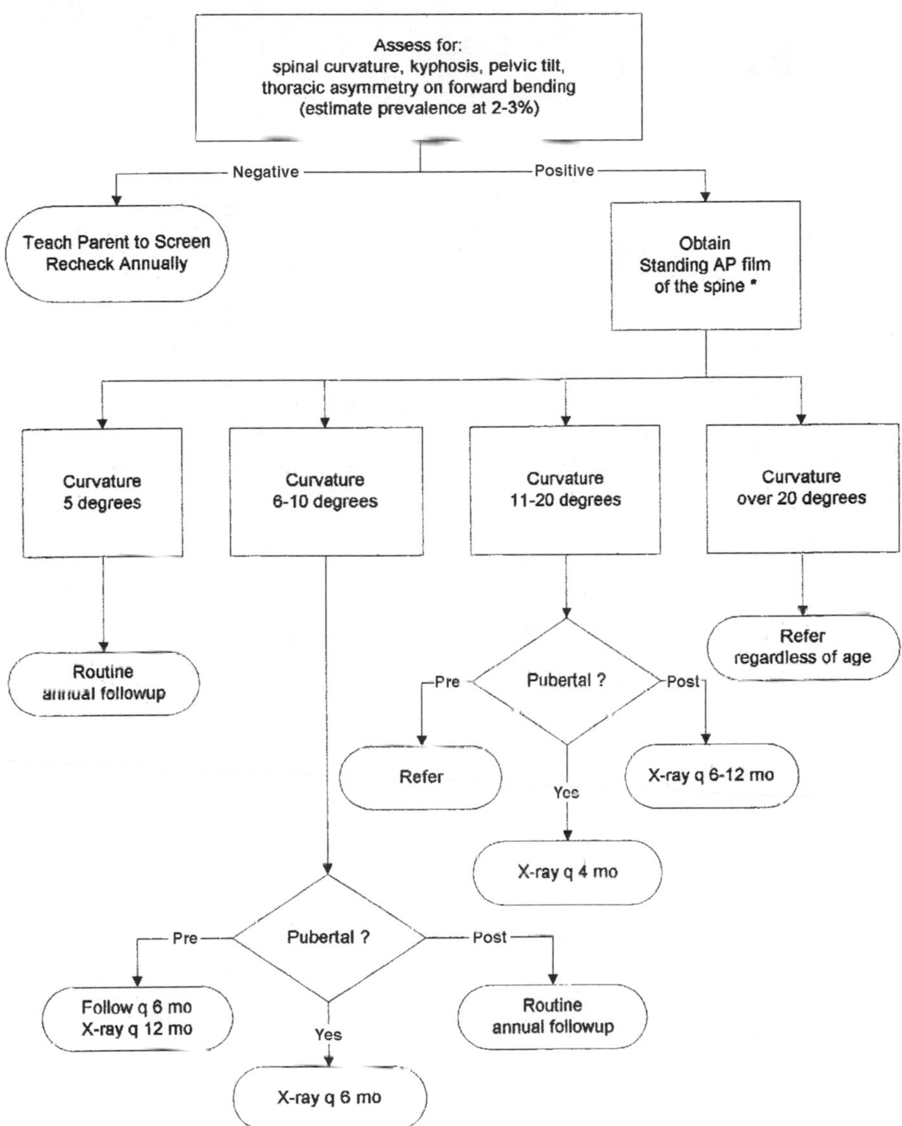

*Cobb method of angle measurement:

1. Find the lowest vertebra whose bottom tilts toward concavity of curve.
2. Erect a perpendicular line from extension of bottom surface.
3. Find highest vertebra as in Step 1 and erect perpendicular from extension of top surface.
4. Measure intersecting angle = ° of scoliosis.

AP indicates anteroposterior; q 6 mo, every 6 months.

TABLE 17.33

Sports Injuries

Injury/Condition	History	Special Testing/History	Treatment	Resumption of Sports
Ligamentous injuries of the knee:	Twisting, deceleration, or contact injuries with pain and swelling	Testing is specific for ligament injured	Treatment is dependent on grade of injury	
Medial collateral	Lateral force	Valgus stress test	Grade I (pain, swelling, stable): RICE, rehab; grade II (pain, swelling, moderately unstable): RICE, protected weight bearing with crutches; grade III (marked instability): usually surgical but may improve with immobilization	When knee is minimally painful, stable, range of motion is good, and patient can run in place, hop on affected leg, run figure-of-8 in both directions, start and stop quickly
Lateral collateral	Medial force	Varus stress test		
Anterior cruciate	"Pop" or "snap" heard in 50%	Anterior drawer sign		
Posterior cruciate		Posterior drawer sign		
Meniscus tear	Twisting injury followed by swelling, locking, pain, and negative ligament stress test	Joint line tenderness; McMurphy's and Apley's tests	NSAIDs for pain/swelling; protected ROM, rehab of quads/hamstrings; surgical intervention if significant mechanical symptoms despite conservative therapy	Minimal pain, good range of motion and strength; completion of functional rehab, including sport-specific drills
Patella subluxation	Generally bilateral knee pain, squatting, climbing stairs	Clicking on squatting and pain on climbing stairs	Quadriceps strengthening; patellar cut-out brace	When comfortable

Injury/Condition	History	Special Testing/History	Treatment	Resumption of Sports
Corns, calluses, blisters	Painful hypertrophic skin changes	May need x-ray examination to see if there is underlying structural deformity	Padding, reduction of source of friction	When comfortable
Subungual hematoma	Traumatic hematoma with pain	Trauma	Evacuation of hematoma with perforation of nail by hot paper clip or needle	When comfortable
Stress fractures	Repetitive stress like running; sudden onset of pain and swelling	Plain x-ray may not show fracture for several weeks; bone scan or MRI may show defect sooner	Relative rest until pain subsides; look for underlying causes; femoral neck and mid fibia with "dreaded backine" will require more aggressive treatment	Gradually when asymptomatic
Achilles tendinitis	Repeated stress to the achilles tendon, pain and swelling		Limit running while acute; anti-inflammatory drug	When asymptomatic with agressive achilles tendon stretch program
Shin splints	Aching pain in posteromedial aspect of lower leg after running	May require x-ray to exclude tibial stress fracture	Ice and rest; tendon stretching	When asymptomatic, tendon stretch program; avoid hard surfaces

Continued

TABLE 17.33

Sports Injuries, cont'd

Injury/Condition	History	Special Testing/History	Treatment	Resumption of Sports
Hamstring pull	Pain in back of thigh or at hamstring origin in pelvis	X-ray examination may show avulsion injury	Ice, rest, stretch program	When asymptomatic, good warm-up needed to avoid reinjury
Brachial plexus injury	Hyperextension of neck with counter-traction of arm	Numbness in arm and fingers lasting ≤5 minutes	Protect shoulder	If lasting <5 min, may resume
Mallet finger	Ball hits tip of extended finger. Unable to extend DIP joint	X-ray may show avulsion fracture	Splint DIP joint in full extension for 6 to 8 weeks	May play if splinted

DIP indicates distal interphalangeal.

TABLE 17.34

Medications Useful to Treat Musculoskeletal Conditions

Medication	Dosage	Cost*	Adverse Reactions
Analgesics			
Acetaminophen (Tylenol)	650 to 1000 mg q 6 h	$8.99 generic (500) $12.99 brand (250)	Hepatotoxicity, nephrotoxicity
Tramadol (Ultram)	50 mg qid	$21.73 brand (30)	Seizures, anaphylaxis
Acetaminophen with codeine 30 mg	1 to 2 q 6 h	$6.35 generic (30)	Hepatotoxicity, respiratory depression
Propoxyphene/ Acetaminophen 100/650 (Darvocet N-100)	1 q 6 h	$7.31 generic (30) $24.37 brand (30)	Dependency, abuse, hepatotoxicity
Hydrocodone/ ibuprofen (Vicoprofen)	7.5/200 1 q 6 h	$30.12 brand (28)	Pancytopenia, respiratory depression
Nonsteroidal Anti-inflammatory Drugs (NSAIDs)			
Ibuprofen (Motrin)	200 to 800 mg qid	$5.49 generic (30) $12.78 brand (30)	Anaphylaxis, gastrointestinal bleed, renal failure, bronchospasm
Naproxen (Naprosyn)	375 to 500 mg bid	$13.66 generic (60) $78.98 brand (60)	Same as above
Sulindac (Clinoril)	150 to 200 mg bid	$21.22 generic (60) $84.86 brand (60)	Same as above
Diclofenac (Cataflam/Voltaren)	50 mg tid	$ 32.58 generic (60) $110.00 brand (Cataflam) (60) $72.41 brand (Voltaren) (60)	Same as above
Diclofenac/ misoprostol (Arthrotec)	bid	$82.34 brand (60)	Same as above
Indomethacin (Indocin)	25 mg tid	$5.49 generic (30) $19.29 brand (30)	Same as above
Salsalate (Disalcid)	1000 mg tid	$15.55 generic 500 mg (100) $62.19 brand 500 mg (100)	Same as above

Continued

TABLE 17.34

Medications Useful to Treat Musculoskeletal Conditions, cont'd

Medication	Dosage	Cost*	Adverse Reactions
Celecoxib (Celebrex)	200 mg/d	$65.33 brand (30)	Same as above
Rofecoxib (Vioxx)	25 mg/d	$70.76 brand (30)	Same as above
Disease-Modifying Antirheumatic Drugs (DMARDs)			
Methotrexate (Rheumatrex)	7.5 to 15 mg weekly	$13.29 generic 2.5 mg (12) $53.10 brand 2.5 mg (12)	Neurotoxicity, seizures, renal failure, bone marrow suppression, hepatotoxicity, pulmonary fibrosis
Hydroxy-chlorquine (Plaquenil)	200 mg/d	$39.00 generic (60) $86.64 brand (60)	Bone marrow suppression, seizure, visual changes, exfoliative dermatitis
Steroids			
Prednisone	2.5 to 20 mg/d	$5.49 generic 5 mg (30) $5.49 generic 20 mg (30)	Adrenal insufficiency, steroid psychosis, peptic ulcer
Muscle Relaxants			
Cyclobenzaprine (Flexeril)	10 mg tid	$7.50 generic (30) $35.84 brand (30)	Arrhythmias, seizures
Methocarbinol (Robaxin)	500 mg 2 qid	$5.49 generic 500 mg (30) $20.88 brand 500 mg (30)	Seizures, anaphylaxis
Metaxalone (Skelaxin)	400 mg 2 tid	$22.55 brand 400 mg (30)	Hemolytic anemia, leukopenia, hepatotoxicity

*All prices are the posted prices at a nationwide discount pharmacy as of August 1, 2001. Prices may vary between regions and individual stores.

TABLE 17.35

Physical Therapy

Modality	Action	Indications	Contraindications	How to Order
Moist Heat				
Hot packs	Circulation Muscle relaxation	Muscle spasm Joint contraction	Sensory loss Malignant tumor Open lesion	20 minutes
Whirlpools	Cleansing Muscle relaxation	Open lesions Muscle spasm	Poor heat tolerance Cortisone withdrawal	20 minutes
Therapeutic pools	Decrease gravity to aid in exercise	To aid exercise and ambulation training	Cardiovascular disease	Temperature 9[illegible]°–96°; progress from shallow to deep water; continue exercise after leaving water
Dry Heat				
Diathermy	Circulation Muscle relaxation	Muscle spasm Chronic pain Adhesive capsulitis	Metallic implants Coagulation defects Sensory loss Open lesions Malignancy	20 minutes, 3 times/week, for 1–2 weeks
Infrared		Muscle spasm Relief of pain Promotes healing of open lesions	Sensory loss Excessive scar tissue	Buy infrared bulb, keep 20 inches from skin; direct it perpendicular to skin for 30 minutes; may repeat after cooling skin 1 hour

Continued

TABLE 17.35

Physical Therapy, cont'd

Modality	Action	Indications	Contraindications	How to Order
Deep Heat Ultrasound	Muscle relaxation	Joint pain Contractures	Application to eyes Pregnancy, malignancy Caution after laminectomy	10–15 minutes
Cold packs, ice massage	Reduce pain and swelling	Acute trauma	Raynaud phenomenon Cryoglobulinemia	Freeze water in paper cups; peel away paper at open end; massage affected area with circular motion
Intermittent traction	Spine distraction	Cervical DJD Lumbar DJD Herniated disk	Unstable vertebrae Malignancy Pregnancy	50–60 lb (maximum of 10 for neck) intermittently; need PT instruction
Paraffin baths	Minimizes pain Heat joint Capsule	Arthritis	Sensory loss that could lead to burns	5–10 minutes per treatment; home units and MITS are available with PT instruction

TABLE 17.36

Arthrocentesis

Indications

- Analysis of joint fluid
- Relief of pain by drainage of an effusion
- Instillation of medication (Table 17.37)
- Drainage of hemarthrosis

Contraindications

- Infection in skin or soft tissue
- Coagulation disorder

General Technique

- Identify landmarks and mark site with indelible ink or skin indentation
- Use antiseptic technique
- Inject local anesthesia in the overlying skin and subcutaneous tissues
- Choose syringe appropriate for effusion size: 3–50 mL
- Advance needle with negative pressure
- Remove effusion
- Apply sterile bandage

Technique (Site Approach)

Shoulder (Anterior Approach)

- Seat patient with hand in lap
- Palpate the glenohumeral joint (between the coracoid process and humeral head)
- Internally rotate shoulder and feel joint groove lateral to the coracoid
- Direct needle (20–22 gauge) dorsally and medially into the joint space; a slight superior direction will avoid the neurovascular bundle

Shoulder (Posterior Approach)

- Rotate the patient's arm internally by having the patient place the hand on the opposite shoulder
- Palpate the acromion process
- Insert needle 1 cm below the posterior tip of the acromion
- Direct it anteriorly and medially to the humeral head

Continued

TABLE 17.36

Arthrocentesis, cont'd

Wrist (Dorsal Approach)

- Patient should be sitting with pronated palm flexed slightly over a rolled towel
- Mark the bony process of the distal radius and ulna
- Direct the needle into the groove between the two bony processes just lateral to the extensor pollicis longus tendon

Elbow

- Place patient's relaxed arm on pillow in lap 45° from full extension
- Turn palm toward abdomen or pillow
- Palpate the lateral epicondyle
- The shallow depression distal to it represents the joint
- Enter perpendicular to the joint with a 22-gauge needle

Ankle (Medial Approach)

- Place foot at 45° plantar flexion with heel on table
- Palpate medial malleolus
- Insert needle 1.2 cm proximal and volar to the distal end of medial malleolus
- Direct the needle 45° posteriorly, slightly upward and medial

Knee (Medial Approach)

- Patient should be supine with a relaxed knee (patella freely movable)
- Mark the inferior plane of the patella (the underside)
- Direct the needle (18 gauge) parallel to the inferior plane of the patella
- Compression of the suprapatellar pouch may help aspiration

TABLE 17.37

Intra-articular Injection

Mix 1% lidocane or 0.25% bupivacaine and steroid; lidocaine provides rapid but short-duration pain relief. Bupivacaine has a slower onset of action but provides a longer duration of pain relief:

- For elbow or ankle, 10–40 mg of methypredisolone acetate in 0.5 mL of anesthetic
- For knee or shoulder, 40–80 mg of methypredisolone acetate in 1 mL of anesthetic

Use the approaches listed in Table 17.36 to enter the joint.
Aspirate to be sure you are not in a vessel.
Inject and apply a sterile bandage.
Advise a patient that there may be an initial irritation from the steroid lasting less than 24 hours.
This may need to be repeated for severe inflammation.
Bursae overlie these joints and can be injected with the same preparation.

Volume of Steroid for Injection*

Area	Volume (mL)
Large joints	0.5–2.0
Small joints	0.2–1.0
Bursae	0.5–1.5
Tendon sheaths	0.1–0.5
Ganglia	0.2–1.0

*Volume is steroid only. Most often the volume is doubled by adding local anesthetic as vehicle.

TABLE 17.38

Casting Techniques

General Principles

Fiberglass

1. Lightweight and can endure moisture
2. Wear gloves. Use specially designed nylon stockinette and padding, which is designed to dry quickly if it gets wet
3. Use small width such as 4-inch for leg, 2-inch for hand, and 3-inch for wrist; wrap around forearm, so that "tucks" are not needed as with plaster
4. Wet the roll; there will be a thermal reaction during the curing, which is not a hazard
5. Apply fiberglass spirally with a little more tension than plaster
6. Trimming is difficult but can be done with Bohler scissors before the fiberglass sets
7. Be sure to evert the edges
8. The cast can be trimmed or cut after it has set with cast removal saw

Plaster

1. The hotter the water, the faster the plaster will set
2. Stockinette should be the first layer applied
3. Next, line the extremity with padding (eg, Webril)
4. Extra padding or felt should be applied to bony prominences
5. Wear gloves (protection and smoothing of plaster)
6. Soak plaster until bubbling stops, squeeze gently, then apply
7. Start plaster at either end
8. Advance plaster about one-third to one-half width of roll per turn
9. Six or seven layers are the usual thickness needed
10. Turn stockinette onto plaster and incorporate into cast to form smooth soft edge
11. Sculpt plaster with both hands while applying
12. Do not pull plaster tight as you roll it
13. Check capillary filling and for parenthesias every 1–2 hours for the first 24 hours while awake; office follow-up in 24–48 hours

Short Arm Cast

1. For nondisplaced fractures of the forearm and wrist
2. Have an assistant hold the patient's arm in 90° flexion with arm partially extended while applying cast
3. Extend cast to, not beyond, metacorpophalangeal joints
4. Include thumb, if for navicular fracture
5. Hold wrist in 15–20° extension
6. If thumb spica, hold thumb in "neutral" position
7. Use 3-inch plaster (2-inch may be used for hand and thumb)

Short Leg Cast

1. For nondisplaced fractures of the lower leg and ankle
2. Apply with patient on end of table, knee at 90° flexion
3. Keep ankle in neutral position avoiding plantar flexion
4. Use 6-inch plaster (4-inch may be used around ankle)
5. After applying one or two layers, fold four 4-inch splints longitudinally and place one on each side and front and back of ankle
6. Apply one additional layer and trim as needed
7. If walking cast is desired, fill arch of foot with splints to make a flat surface; apply rubber "walker" and secure with a plaster bandage

chapter 18

The Skin

Dana Nottingham, MD

IN THIS CHAPTER

- Preventive measures
- Describing skin lesions
- Diagnosis
- Seasonal skin diseases
- Common problems and treatments
- Compresses
- Steroid usage
- Drugs that commonly cause dermatological reactions
- Procedures

BOOKSHELF RECOMMENDATIONS

- Habif TP. *Clinical Dermatology: A Color Guide to Diagnosis and Therapy*. 3rd ed. St Louis, MO: Mosby, Inc; 1996.
- Hall JC. *Sauer's Manual of Skin Diseases*. 8th ed. Philadelphia, PA: Lippincott Williams & Williams; 1999.
- Pfenninger JL, Fowler, GC. *Procedures for Primary Care Physicians*. St Louis, MO: Mosby, Inc; 1994.
- Rakel RE, ed. *Textbook of Family Practice*. 6th ed. Philadelphia, PA: WB Saunders Company; 2001.
- Weinstock MB, Neides DM, Schumick D. *The Resident's Guide to Ambulatory Care*. 4th ed. Columbus, OH: Anadem Publishing; 2000.

FIGURE 18.1

Dermatologic Silhouettes

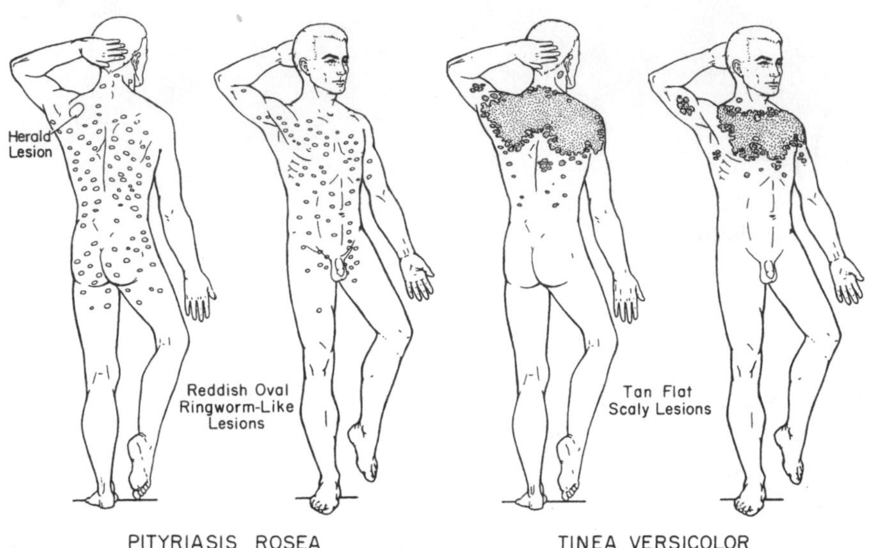

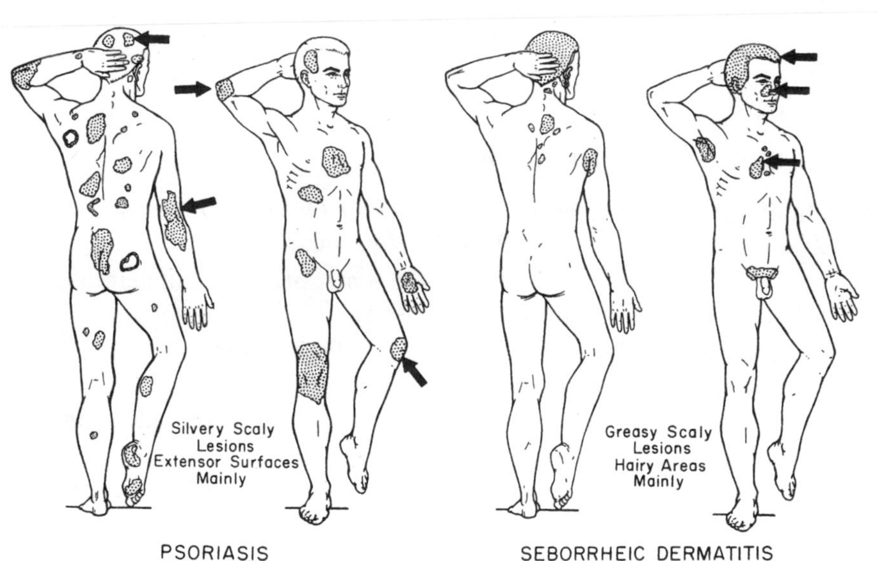

FIGURE 18.2

Dermatologic Silhouettes

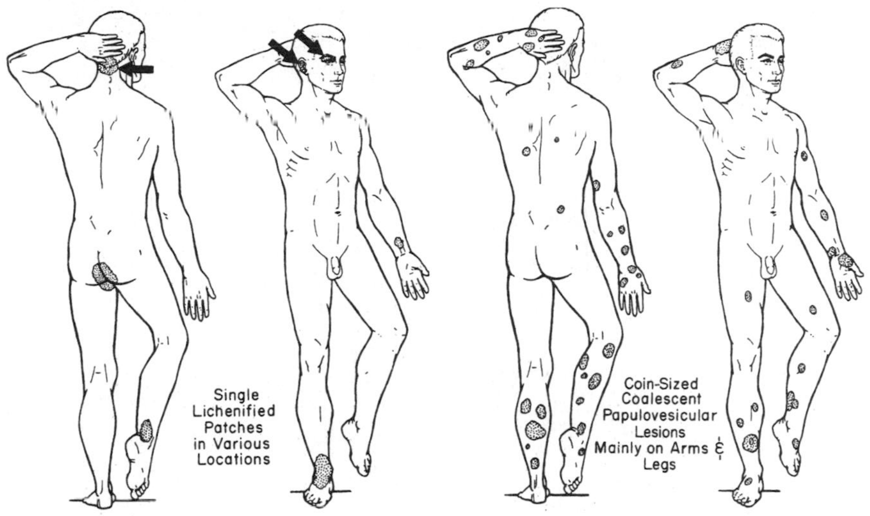

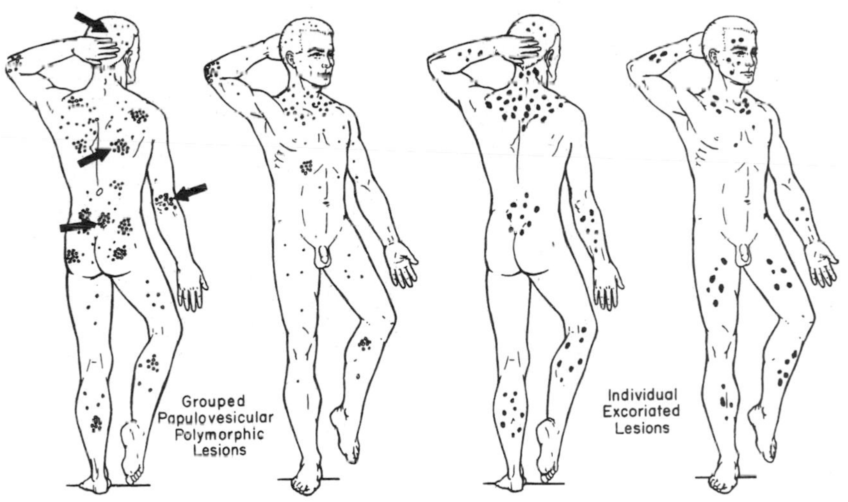

FIGURE 18.3

Dermatologic Silhouettes

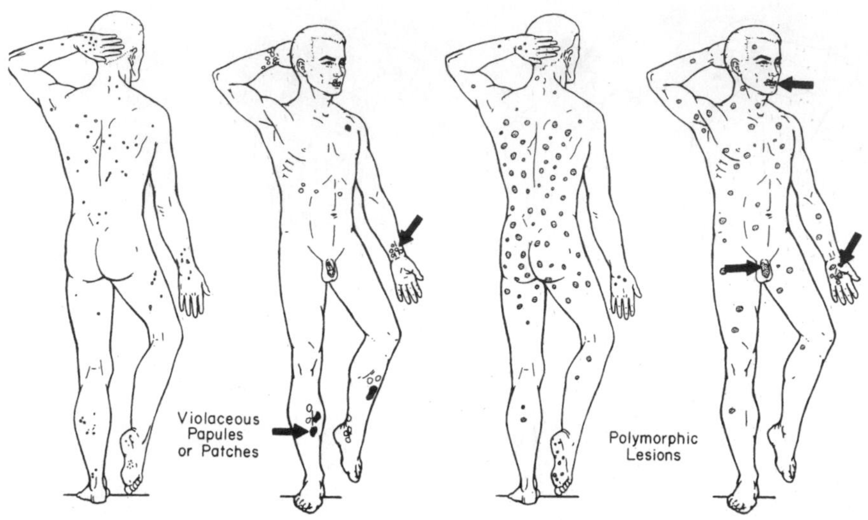

Diaper Area Usually Clear

Mainly on Flexor Surfaces

INFANTILE FORM of ATOPIC ECZEMA

ADULT FORM of ATOPIC ECZEMA

FIGURE 18.4

Dermatologic Silhouettes

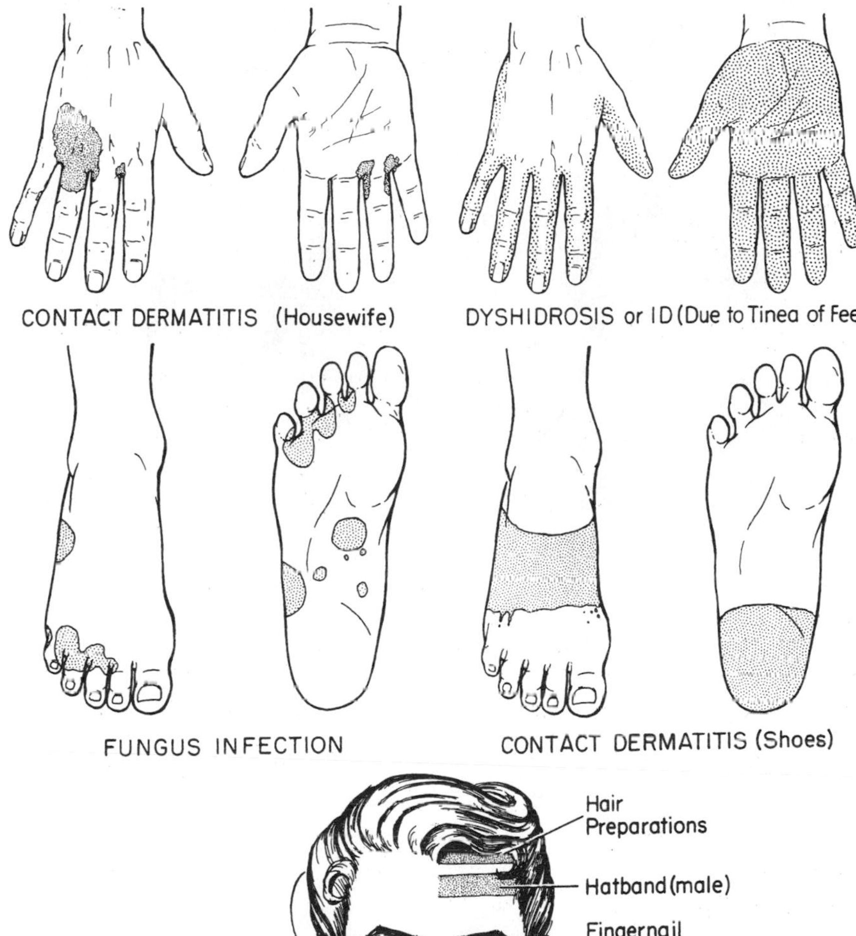

FIGURE 18.5

Dermagrams for Comparison of Tinea of Crural Area and Candidiasis of Crural Area

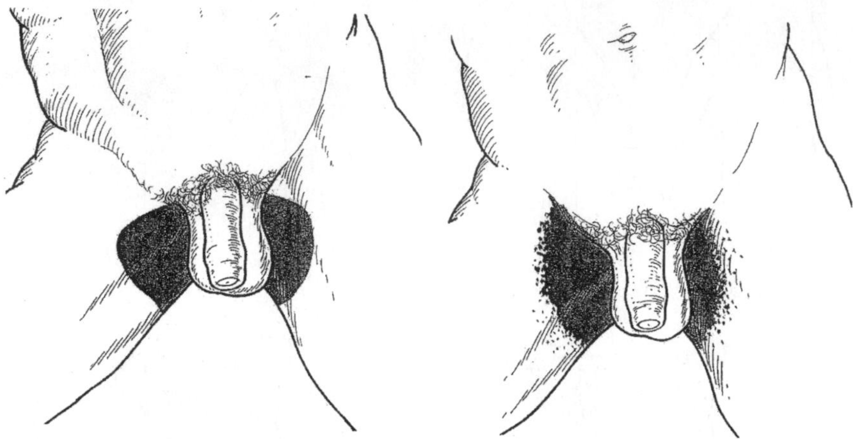

Tinea of crural area (left). Note sharp border of lesions. Candidiasis of crural area (right). Note indefinite border with satellite pustule-like lesions at edge. Candidiasis can also involve the scrotum.

PREVENTIVE MEASURES

Although such measures are perhaps prudent, the US Preventive Services Task Force did not find enough evidence to recommend for or against either periodic skin exams or regular use of sunscreen. The task force did, however, recommend counseling patients at increased risk for skin cancer to avoid excess sun exposure.

TABLE 18.1

Describing Skin Lesions: Definitions

Lesion	Definition
Macule	1 cm or smaller, flat, circumscribed
Patch	Greater than 1 cm, flat, circumscribed
Papule	1 cm or smaller, raised, solid, circumscribed
Plaque	Greater than 1 cm, raised, solid, circumscribed
Nodule	1 cm or smaller, solid with depth
Tumor	Greater than 1 cm, solid with depth
Vesicle	1 cm or smaller, raised, circumscribed, fluid-containing
Bulla	Greater than 1 cm, raised, circumscribed, fluid-containing
Pustule	Variably sized, raised, circumscribed, pus-containing
Furuncle	Large infected hair follicle or boil
Carbuncle	Collection of boils
Petechiae	Circumscribed blood deposits, 1 cm or smaller
Purpura	Circumscribed blood deposits, greater than 1 cm
Erosion	Localized loss of epidermis
Ulcer	Localized loss of epidermis and dermis
Comedone	Sebaceous/keratinous plug lodged in the opening of a hair follicle; open (blackhead) vs closed (whitehead)

DIAGNOSIS

TABLE 18.2

Diagnosis by Distribution and Type of Lesion

Distribution	Description	Likely Condition
Scalp	White nits	Pediculosis
Face	Vesicles/golden crusts	Impetigo
	Vesicles/painful ulcer(s)	Herpes simplex
	Pustules/blackheads/ whiteheads	Acne
	Nodule	Skin cancer
Trunk	Scale with depigmentation	Tinea/pityriasis versicolor
	Dermatomal/vesicles	Herpes zoster
	Dermatomal/macules	Pityriasis rosea
	With fever and erythematous rash	Viral exanthem
Limbs	Pruritic papules/vesicles	Insect bites
	Chronic lesion	Warts
Flexures	Pruritic patch (red, moist)	Candida
	Circinate spreading lesion with clear center	Tinea
Nails	With discoloration of distal nail bed	Tinea
	With ridged nail	*Candida*
Penis/ Vulvovaginal	Pruritic nodules with erythematous base	Scabies
	Erythematous itchy white patches	*Candida*
	Recurrent erosions or pigmented plaques	Fixed drug eruption 2° to deodorants/ cosmetics
Perianal	Intense pruritus with excoriation, worst in arm	Pinworms
Widespread	Silvery scales	Psoriasis
	Raised itchy wheal	Urticaria
	With family history of atopy	Atopic dermatitis
	On medication	Drug eruption

Adapted from Jamison JR. *Differential Diagnosis for Primary Practice.* Philadelphia, PA: Churchill Livingstone; 1999:230.

TABLE 18.3

Diagnosis of Scaly Skin Rash

Lesion Type	Description	Likely Condition
Flaking skin	Finely fissured, superficial, itchy	Winter itch
	Limited to scalp	Dandruff
	Generalized but spares face and scalp	Ichthyosis (congenital)
	Freely exfoliating, laminated	Exfoliative dermatitis
Fissured orange-red patches	Dry or greasy	Seborrheic dermatitis
Reddish macules	Clear center with advancing edge	Tinea
	Clear center, symmetrical	Pityriasis rosea
	Weeping patches	Contact dermatitis
	Silvery foam cells	Psoriasis
Red Plaques	Cornified, dry, adherent scales	Discoid lupus

Adapted from Jamison JR. *Differential Diagnosis for Primary Practice*. Philadelphia, PA: Churchill Livingstone; 1999:229.

TABLE 18.4

Diagnosis of Generalized Pruritus

Character of Lesion	Additional Signs/Symptoms	Likely Condition
Tickling/crawling pruritus	Alcohol withdrawal	Psychoses
	Worst when stressed/anxious	Psychogenic
	Associated with eating	Allergic dermatitis (food)
	Wheals or papules	Insect bites (fleas, mosquitoes)
	Worst at night, associated with nodules with a red base	Scabies
	Intense itch with marked excoriation	Lice
No visible lesion	Precipitated by hot shower or alcohol and associated with:	
	Pallor	Leukemia
	Rubor	Polycythemia rubra vera
	Night sweats	Lymphoma
	Steatorrhea	Cholestatic jaundice
	Restless legs, lethargy	Renal failure
	Glucosuria	Diabetes
	Episodes of severe pruritus in elderly patient	Senile pruritus
	Amenorrhea	Pregnancy
	Pallor	Iron deficiency anemia
	Generalized itch	Occult cancer or psychogenic
Dry, fine scales	Associated with cold, windy climate	Winter itch
	Constipation, cold intolerance	Hypothyroidism
Vesicles	Associated with humid environment	Prickly heat
	Weeping lesions	Allergic dermatitis (plant)
Concurrent vesicles, papules, scabs	Centripetal distribution	Chickenpox

Adapted from Jamison JR. *Differential Diagnosis for Primary Practice*. Philadelphia, PA: Churchill Livingstone; 1999:181.

TABLE 18.5

Characteristics of Malignant and Benign Pigmented Skin Lesions

Feature	Melanoma	Benign Skin Lesion
Size	Over 1 cm, increasing in size	Less than 1 cm, stable size
Color	Varied, resembling an autumn maple leaf, "flag sign"*	Brown, often becomes pale with increasing age
Surface	Hard, elevated area; scaling; oozing; bleeding	Macule progresses to soft papule with increasing age
Surrounding skin	Fingers of pigment penetrate, erythematous	Unremarkable or white, halo
Patient-reported sensations	Itchiness, tenderness	None
Location	Back most common	Over entire body but more common on sun-exposed surfaces
Precursors	Family history, dysplastic nevi, congenital nevi, giant hairy nevus, excess sun exposure, type I/II (easily burned) skin	Excess sun exposure in youth; family history of similar lesions at same or mirror-image site
Skin marking†	Absent	Often present

Adapted from Lovo R. *Principles of oncology*. Monograph ed 125, Home study self-assessment program. Kansas City, MO: American Academy of Family Physicians; October 1989.

*The "flag sign" is the appearance of red, white and blue colors in a pigmented lesion.

†With a magnifying glass, normal skin has crisscrosses of grooves. These normal lines are obliterated by the disordered malignant growth of melanomas.

TABLE 18.6

Seasonal Skin Diseases

Winter	Spring
Contact dermatitis (hands)	Acne (flares)
Eczema (atopic, nummular)	Erythema multiforme
Ichthyosis	Pityriasis rosea
Psoriasis	
Seborrheic dermatitis	
Winter itch and dry skin (xerosis)	
Summer	**Fall**
Candidal intertrigo	Acne (flares)
Contact dermatitis (poison ivy)	Atopic eczema
Impetigo and other pyodermas	Contact dermatitis (ragweed)
Insect bites	Pityriasis rosea
Miliaria or prickly heat	Senile pruritus
Polymorphous light eruption	Tinea of scalp (schoolchildren)
Tinea (feet and groin)	Winter itch
Tinea versicolor	

Adapted from Hall JC. *Sauer's Manual of Skin Diseases*. 8th ed. Philadelphia, PA: Lippincott Williams & Williams; 1999:22.

COMMON PROBLEMS AND TREATMENTS

Diaper Rash

A good history and examination may reveal whether the rash is due to an irritant or a yeast infection. Yeast generally affects the skin creases more than irritants do.

If irritant, remove irritant. If urine, leave the baby undiapered several times per day. Use very mild topical steroid such as 1% hydrocortisone cream. If yeast (*Candida albicans* or other species), use an antifungal, such as nystatin or clotrimazole, or antifungal-steroid compound.

Corns and Calluses

These are areas of thickened skin over areas where repeated, prolonged friction or pressure occurs. These areas are very painful, but pain is eradicated on the removal of thickened skin.

Surgical Debridement
Use a No. 15 blade and 1% Xylocaine for anesthesia, if needed.

Intermittent Debridement
Use 50% salicylic acid plaster, applied with tape, for 1–7 days and then remove. Soak foot and debride dead tissue. Repeat as needed to keep the lesion flat.

Warts (nongenital)

There will be spontaneous regression in two thirds of children within 2 years.

Warts that are treated by one or more of the treatments below should have a 60%–70% cure rate but may require repeated treatments from several weeks to months. Some of the modalities also can be used for genital warts.

Chemical Agents
Acids: trichloroacetic, salicylic
Chemotherapeutics: podophyllin, fluorouracil, interferons
Immunotherapy

Physical Agents
Cryotherapy
Electrodesiccation
CO_2 laser
Surgical excision

Topical Preparations for Home Therapy
10% salicylic acid, 10% lactic acid in flexible collodion or 40% salicylic acid plaster

TABLE 18.7

Acne Therapy Guide

Lesion/Stage	Therapy
Comedones	Retinoic acid cream/gel (see Table 18.8)
Mild inflammation; comedones and papules present	Topical antibiotic or benzoyl peroxide lotion or gel bid; (consider retinoic acid)
Moderate to severe inflammation; papules and pustules, some cysts present	Benzoyl peroxide and oral or topical antibiotic (see Table 18.9); consider retinoic acid; referral of treatment failures
Abscesses and severe scarring	Referral to dermatologist

bid indicates twice daily.

TABLE 18.8

Topical Acne Products*

Drug	Concentrations and Strengths	Acne Severity	Comments
Benzoyl peroxide liquid lotion, cream, gel, soap (generic)	2.5%, 5%, 10%	Mild to moderate	Wash face before applying. Begin with 2.5% once daily for several days, then bid. Slowly increase strength if needed. Most are nonprescription.
Sulfur, salicylic acid, resorcinol combinations	Various strengths and combinations	Mild to moderate	Some products have alcohol, phenol, or zinc oxide. Most are nonprescription.
Erythromycin solution (generic, ETS-2%)	1.5%, 2%	Moderate	Wash face and apply bid. All products require a prescription.
Clindamycin gel, solution (Cleocin T)	10 mg/mL	Moderate	Apply bid. Diarrhea and pseudomembranous colitis have occurred with topical and systemic clindamycin. Prescription only.

Continued

TABLE 18.8

Topical Acne Products, cont'd

Drug	Concentrations and Strengths	Acne Severity	Comments
Metronidazole gel (MetroGel)	0.75%	Moderate	Apply bid. Prescription only
Tetracycline solution (Topicycline)	2.2 mg/mL	Moderate	Apply bid. Safety in pregnancy not established
Tretinoin (Retin-A)	Cream: 0.025%, 0.05%, 0.1% Gel: 0.025%, 0.01% Liquid: 0.05%	Moderate to severe	Apply at bedtime. Not contraindicated in pregnancy, but it should be avoided. Prescription only

*Cream is better for dry skin; gel for oily skin.

bid indicates twice daily.

TABLE 18.9

Oral Therapy for Acne

Drug	Concentration Strengths	Acne Severity	Comments
Erythromycin capsules and tablets (generic)	250 mg, 500 mg	Moderate to severe	Dose of 250 mg qid
Tetracycline capsules (generic)	250 mg, 500 mg	Moderate to severe	Contraindicated in pregnancy. Initial dose is 250 mg qid followed by 125–500 mg daily. Do not take with dairy products, iron, or antacids
Minocycline	50 mg, 100 mg	Moderate to severe	Dose of 50 mg bid or 100 mg/d
Isotretinoin capsules (Accutane)	10 mg, 20 mg, 40 mg	Severe recalcitrant cystic acne	Absolutely contraindicated in pregnancy. Dose is 0.5–2.0 mg/kg/d divided into two doses over 15–20 weeks. Numerous adverse reactions may occur

bid indicates twice daily; qid, four times daily.

TABLE 18.10

Disorders of the Hair and Scalp

Disease	Description	Etiology	Treatment
Alopecia areata	Well-defined single or multiple patches of balding	Probably autoimmune	Reassurance, intralesional steroids
Dandruff	Noninflammatory scaling occurring on scalp	Physiological desquamation	Selenium sulfide 2.5%
Seborrheic dermatitis	Inflammatory scaling in sebaceous areas: scalp, face, trunk	*Pityrosporum ovale*	Selenium sulfide 2.5%, corticosteroid cream, ketoconazole shampoo
Psoriasis	Chronic proliferative epidermal disease	Unclear	Tar shampoo, intralesional steroids
Fungal infection	Superficial epidermis infections	Dermatophytes	Antifungal agents topically and rarely orally
Hair loss	Loss of hair in front or crown	Male pattern baldness	Minoxidil topically for crown balding; Propecia 1 mg/d orally
Folliculitis	Infection around hair follicles	*Staphylococcus*	Antibiotics

TABLE 18.11

Compresses

Mix any of the following with one quart of cool to warm water:

1. Bath oil: 1 capful
2. Baking soda: 2 tablespoons
3. Epsom salts: 2 tablespoons
4. Vinegar: 2 tablespoons
5. Domeboro: 1 tablet
6. Saline: 2 teaspoons
7. Balnetar: 1 part Balnetar to 5 parts cool or warm water

Technique

1. Dip towel in one of the above solutions, wring out slightly, and wrap soaked towel around affected area for 15–20 minutes two to four times daily.
2. Dry area gently and apply prescribed cream, ointment, or lotion.

TABLE 18.12

Steroid Usage

Topical

The most potent topical steroids are fluorinated and should be used only for a short time. In general, ointment and gel vehicles are superior to cream or lotion vehicles.

Intralesional

Provides high local concentration with minimal systemic side effects and a prolonged depot effect. Use a 1:4 dilution of one of the following with saline or lidocaine:

- Betamethasone acetate suspension
- Triamcinolone acetonide
- Triamcinolone diacetate
- Triamcinolone hexacetonide
- Methylprednisolone

Indications: acne cysts, psoriatic plaques, circumscribed neurodermatitis, keloids

Oral

Indications: severe contact dermatitis, sunburn, acne
A taper lasting 2–3 weeks is often required.

Sample Rx: Prednisone 10 mg #40 day 1, 2, 3 take five at once, day 4, 5, 6 take 4, day 7, 8, 9 take 3, day 10, 11, 12 take 2 then 1 each day until gone.

TABLE 18.13

Prescribing Guidelines for Creams and Ointments

Amount Needed for One Application to:			
2 g	**3 g**	**4 g**	**30–60 g**
Hands Head Face Anogenital area	One arm Anterior trunk Posterior trunk	One leg	Entire body

TABLE 18.14

Topical Steroid Potency

Drug	Brand Name	Dosage Form	Strength
Very High Potency			
Augmented betamethasone dipropionate	Diprolene Embeline/Cormax	Ointment Cream, ointment Cream, ointment	0.05% 0.05%
Clobetasol propionate	Temovate	Ointment	0.05%
Diflorasone diacetate	Florone, Maxiflor, Psorcon		
Halobetasol propionate	Ultravate	Cream, ointment	0.05%
High Potency			
Amcinonide	Cyclocort	Cream, lotion, ointment	0.1%
Augmented betamethasone dipropionate	Diprolene AF	Cream	0.05%
Betamethasone dipropionate	Generic, Diprosone, Maxivate, others	Cream, ointment	0.05%
Betamethasone valerate	Generic, Betatrex, Beta-Val, Valisone	Ointment	0.1%
Desoximetasone	Generic, Topicort	Cream, ointment, gel	0.25% 0.05%
Diflorasone diacetate	Florone, Maxiflor, Psorcon	Cream, ointment (emollient)	0.05% 0.05%
Fluocinolone acetonide	Synalar-HP, Flurosyn	Cream	0.2%
Fluocinonide	Generic, Fluonex, Lidex, Lidex-E	Cream, ointment, gel	0.05%
Halcinonide	Halog, Halog-E	Cream, ointment	0.1%
Triamcinolone acetonide	Generic, Kenalog	Ointment, cream	0.5%
Medium Potency			
Betamethasone benzoate	Uticort	Cream, gel, lotion	0.025%
Betamethasone dipropionate	Generic, Diprosone, Maxivate	Lotion	0.05%
Betamethasone valerate	Generic, Betatrex, Beta-Val, Valisone	Cream	0.1%
Clocortolone pivalate	Cloderm	Cream	0.1%
Desoximetasone	Generic, Topicort LP	Cream	0.05%
Fluocinolone acetonide	Generic, Flurosyn, Synalar, Synemol	Cream, ointment	0.025%

Drug	Brand Name	Dosage Form	Strength
Flurandrenolide	Generic, Cordran	Cream, ointment	0.025%
	Cordran SP	Cream, ointment, lotion	0.05%
	Cordran	Tape	4 μg/cm^2
Fluticasone propionate	Cutivate	Cream	0.05%
		Ointment	0.005%
Hydrocortisone butyrate	Locoid	Ointment, solution	0.1%
Hydrocortisone valerate	Westcort	Cream, ointment	0.2%
Mometasone furoate	Elocon	Cream, ointment, lotion	0.1%
Triamcinolone acetonide	Generic, Kenalog	Cream, ointment, lotion	0.025%
	Aristocort	Cream, ointment, lotion	0.1%
Low Potency			
Aclometasone dipropionate	Aclovate	Cream, ointment	0.05%
Desonide	Desonide, DesOwen, Tridesilon	Cream	0.05%
Dexamethasone	Aeroseb-Dex	Aerosol	0.01%
	Decaspray	Aerosol	0.04%
Dexamethasone sodium phosphate	Decadron Phosphate	Cream	0.1%
Fluocinolone acetonide	Generic, Flurosyn, Synalar, Synemol, Fluonid	Cream, solution	0.01%
Hydrocortisone	Cetacort	Lotion	0.25%
	Generic	Cream, ointment, lotion, aerosol	0.5%
	Generic	Cream, ointment, lotion, solution	1%
	Generic	Cream, ointment, lotion	2.5%
Hydrocortisone acetate	Cortaid	Cream, ointment	0.5%
	Lanacort, others	Cream, ointment	1%

TABLE 18.15
Drugs That Commonly Cause Dermatological Reactions

Drug	Most Common Reactions
Allopurinol	Epidermal necrolysis, maculopapular
Ampicillin	Urticaria, maculopapular
Angiotension-converting enzyme inhibitors	Pemphigus, exfoliative erythroderma, lichen planus-like reaction, pityriasis rosea-like reaction, angioedema
Antimetabolites	Alopecia, maculopapular
Barbiturates	Epidermal necrolysis, exfoliative dermatitis, Stevens-Johnson syndrome, bullous, erythema multiforme
Carbamazepine	Erythematous purpuric rashes
Cephalosporins	Maculopapular, urticaria, eczematous
Chlordiazepoxide	Maculopapular
Codeine	Urticaria, erythema nodosum
Corticosteroids	Acneiform
Estrogens	Photosensitive
Griseofulvin	Photosensitive, erythema multiforme, maculopapular, urticaria
Gold	Purpura, maculopapular, exfoliative dermatitis, urticaria, photosensitive, bullous, erythema multiforme
Hydralazine	Lupus erythematosus-like syndrome
Iodides	Acneiform, bullous, erythema nodosum, urticaria
Isoniazid	Acneiform, maculopapular, exfoliative dermatitis
Latex	Urticaria, severe rhinitis, respiratory problems, anaphylactic reaction
Lithium	Acneiform, maculopapular, urticaria, alopecia
Macrolides	Urticaria
Nitrofurantoin	Urticaria, maculopapular, exfoliative dermatitis
Nonsteroidal anti-inflammatory drugs	Urticaria, maculopapular, bullous
Opioids	Pruritus, urticaria, erythematous rash
Oral contraceptives	Photosensitive, acneiform, erythema nodosum, urticaria, alopecia
Penicillins	Urticaria, maculopapular, epidermal necrolysis, erythema nodosum, erythema multiforme, exfoliative dermatitis, Stevens-Johnson syndrome
Phenothiazines	Photosensitive, erythema multiforme, urticaria, epidermal necrolysis, exfoliative dermatitis

Drug	Most Common Reactions
Phenytoin	Epidermal necrolysis, exfoliative dermatitis, Stevens-Johnson syndrome, erythema multiforme, urticaria, acneiform
Procainamide	Lupus erythematosus-like syndrome
Quinidine	Purpura, maculopapular, photosensitive
Salicylates	Maculopapular, erythema nodosum, urticaria, purpura
Sulfonamides	Epidermal necrolysis, urticaria, photosensitive, maculopapular, bullous, erythema nodosum, erythema multiforme, Stevens-Johnson syndrome, purpura
Sulfonylureas	Epidermal necrolysis, urticaria, photosensitive, maculopapular, bullous, erythema nodosum, erythema multiforme, Stevens-Johnson syndrome, purpura
Tetracycline	Epidermal necrolysis, urticaria, photosensitive, maculopapular, erythema multiforme
Thiazides	Photosensitive, erythema multiforme, urticaria, purpura, maculopapular
Valproic acid	Rashes, stomatitis

Adapted from Young LY, et al. *Handbook of Applied Therapeutics*. Vancouver: Applied Therapeutics, Inc; 1989.56.

PROCEDURES

Potassium Hydroxide (KOH) Examination

KOH causes a destruction of the stratum corneum cells and thus a cleaning of debris so that exogenous materials like hyphae, spores, and fiberglass fibers can be seen.

FIGURE 18.6

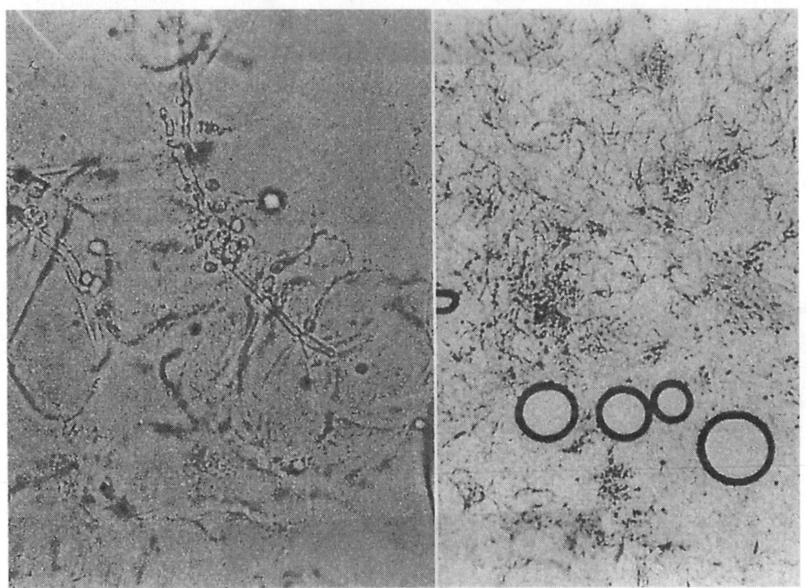

(A) Spores, budding spores, and hyphae of *Candida* (x400). *Candida* hyphae cross the epidermal cell walls, as do dermatophyte hyphae. (B) Hyphae and spores of tinea versicolor (x100). The findings are often called "spaghetti and meatballs." Short and long hyphae and clusters of spores are seen. In this field, long hyphae predominate. Large circles are oil droplets.

Reproduced with permission from Elsevier Science. (Eaglstein WH, Pariser DM. *Office Techniques for Diagnosing Skin Disease*. St Louis: Mosby; 1978.)

Indications

- Scaling disorders
- Blisters of the hands and feet
- Patches of missing or broken hair
- Disorders of the nails
- Excoriated papules in skin creases
- Warty nodules containing tiny black dots (chromomycosis)

Technique

1. Remove all powders or creams with acetone or alcohol.
2. Collect scale on a clean slide by scraping the advancing edge of the lesion with a round-bellied blade.
3. Place a drop of 10% KOH solution on the material and apply the coverslip.
4. Gently warm but do not boil the slide over an alcohol burner.
5. Examine microscopically.

SCABIES DETECTION

Preparing a Scabies Slide

1. Select an unexcoriated papule or tract.
2. Place a drop of immersion oil over the lesion. Scrape off the epidermis over the tract or tease the tract open with a scalpel blade. The mite will grasp the scalpel blade and can be transferred to a slide.

FIGURE 18.7

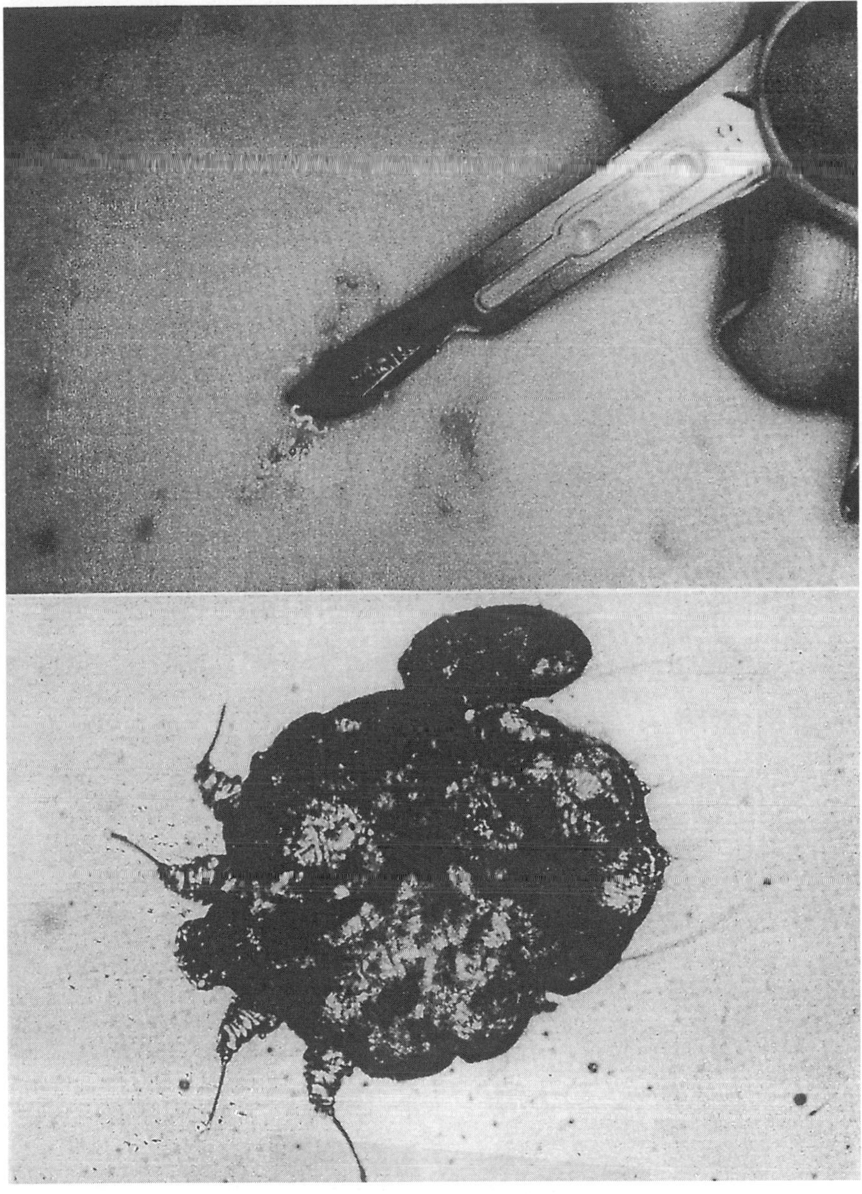

(A) With immersion oil over the lesion, use scalpel blade to scrape off epidermis. (B) Female mite with four of eight legs in focus. An egg is adjacent to the mite at the top of the picture. Reproduced with permission from Elsevier Science. (Eaglstein WH, Pariser DM. *Office Techniques for Diagnosing Skin Disease.* St Louis: Mosby; 1978.)

WOOD'S LIGHT EXAMINATION

A Wood's light produces an invisible long-wave ultraviolet radiation that will induce visible fluorescence that can aid in differential diagnosis. It is very safe.

Technique

1. A Wood's lamp must be on for several minutes to get to optimum intensity.
2. Seat the patient securely so that she or he does not fall in the dark.
3. Turn off room lights and allow the patient's eyes to adjust.
4. Hold Wood's lamp 4 to 5 inches from area being inspected.

TABLE 18.16

Wood's Light Examination Diagnostic Table

	Findings
Condition	**Fluorescent Color**
Tinea Capitis	
Microsporum audouinii	Brilliant green
Microsporum canis	Brilliant green
Trichophyton schoenleinii	Pale green
Erythrasma	Coral-red or pink*
Pigmentary Alterations	
Depigmentation	Cold bright white
Hypopigmentation	Blue-white
Hyperpigmentation	Purple-brown
Vitiligo	Cold bright white and blue-white
Albinism	Cold bright white
Leprosy	Blue-white
Ash-leaf spot of tuberous sclerosis	Blue-white
Pseudomonas aeruginosa infections	Aqua-green or white-green (rarely yellow-green)
Porphyria cutanea tarda (urine)	Pink to pink-orange
Tinea versicolor	Yellow

Adapted from Eaglstein WH, Pariser DM. *Office Techniques for Diagnosing Skin Disease.* St Louis: Mosby; 1978.

*Patients who bathe shortly before Wood's light examination may show little or no fluorescence.

TICK REMOVAL

1. Disinfect area with antibacterial cleanser.
2. Using blunt forceps, tweezers, or gloved fingers, grasp tick as close to skin surface as possible and pull straight upward with steady, even pressure.
3. Do not twist or jerk the tick, as this may break off mouthparts. Do not squeeze, crush, or puncture the body of the tick because its fluids may contain infectious agents.
4. Tick may be placed in container of alcohol and frozen in case subsequent identification is needed.
5. Again disinfect site with antibacterial cleanser and thoroughly wash hands.

In cases of especially difficult removal or retained mouthparts:

1. Disinfect site with antibacterial cleanser. Infiltrate area beneath bite with lidocaine.
2. Apply punch biopsy instrument so it encompasses tick. Stretch skin on each side of lesion. Perform "punch biopsy" of tick attached to skin.
3. Remove punch and specimen. Tissue may be submitted for histological study.
4. Disinfect area again and apply pressure with gauze. If further hemostasis is required, cauterize with silver nitrate stick or aluminum chloride solution or close with suture. Apply bandage.

SKIN BIOPSY TECHNIQUES

Punch Biopsy

Indications: for diagnosis of most inflammatory diseases and tumors.
Technique:

1. Clean the lesion with 70% alcohol.
2. Use infiltration with 0.5% to 1.0% lidocaine for anesthesia.
3. Use a 3- to 4-mm punch. Simultaneously twist and press the cutting edge into the tissue.
4. Incise as deeply as possible.
5. Elevate the specimen, handling the edges only, and cut the base with scissors or a scalpel. Put the specimen in a specimen container.

FIGURE 18.8

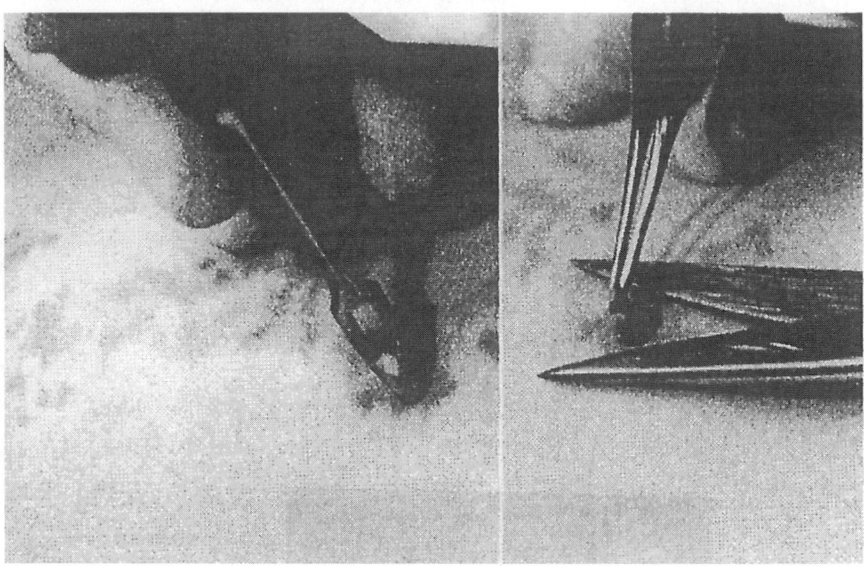

Punch biopsy technique.

Shave Biopsy

Indications: For removing superficial benign lesions and biopsy of basal cell and squamous cell carcinomas. This procedure is contraindicated in patients with melanoma.

Technique:

1. Clean the biopsy site with 70% alcohol.
2. Inject 0.5% to 1.0% lidocaine beneath or directly into the lesion.
3. With scalpel parallel to the skin, shave the lesion from the skin. Pinching the skin may facilitate this step.
4. Complete the incision and place the thin disk of tissue in a specimen bottle.
5. Achieve hemostasis with pressure, silver nitrate, or ferric subsulfate solution.

FIGURE 18.9

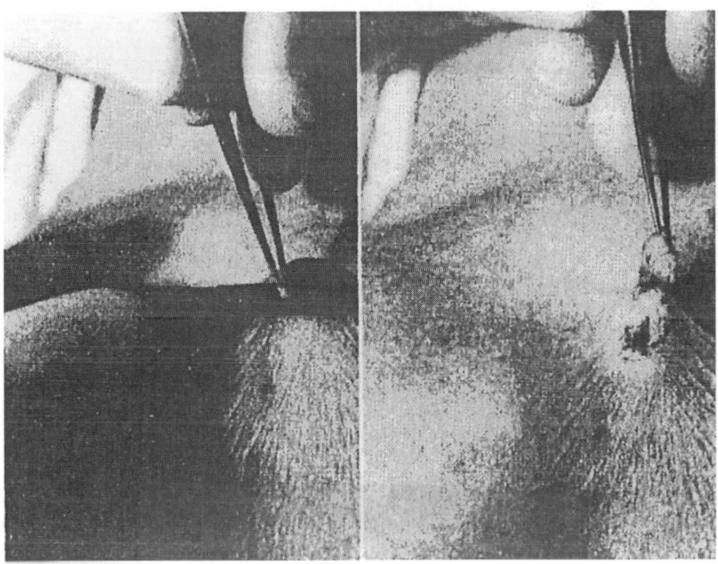

Shave biopsy techniques.

CRYOSURGERY

Useful for treatment of warts, actinic keratoses, hypertrophic scars, and other minor skin lesions. There are several methods of application, including cryogun, Verruca Freeze, Histofreezer, liquid nitrogen, and a nitrous oxide unit.

General Technique

Freeze lesion until ice ball extends 2–3 mm beyond edge of involved tissue (about 1 min for most skin lesions; vascular lesions require longer). It works best to perform a cycle of rapid freeze-thaw-refreeze. It is not necessary to apply a bandage unless the lesion remains irritated or begins to weep.

chapter 19

The Ears, Nose, and Throat

Curtis L. Gingrich, MD
Edward T. Bope, MD

IN THIS CHAPTER

- Normal middle ear anatomy
- Audiometry and tympanometry
- Assessment of hearing loss
- Infections of ear, nose, and throat
- Otitis externa
- Otitis media with effusion
- Rhinosinusitis
- Pharyngitis
- Rhinitis
- Epistaxis
- Tinnitus
- Dizziness/vertigo
- Indirect mirror laryngoscopy
- Emergency airway

BOOKSHELF RECOMMENDATIONS

- Ballenger JJ. *Diseases of the Nose, Throat, and Ear*. 14th ed. Philadelphia, PA: Lea and Febiger; 1991.
- DeWeese EE, et al. *Otolaryngology-Head and Neck Surgery*. 8th ed. St Louis, MO: Mosby, Inc; 1994.

FIGURE 19.1

Normal Middle Ear Anatomy

Otoscopic view of normal tympanic membrane and middle ear structures.

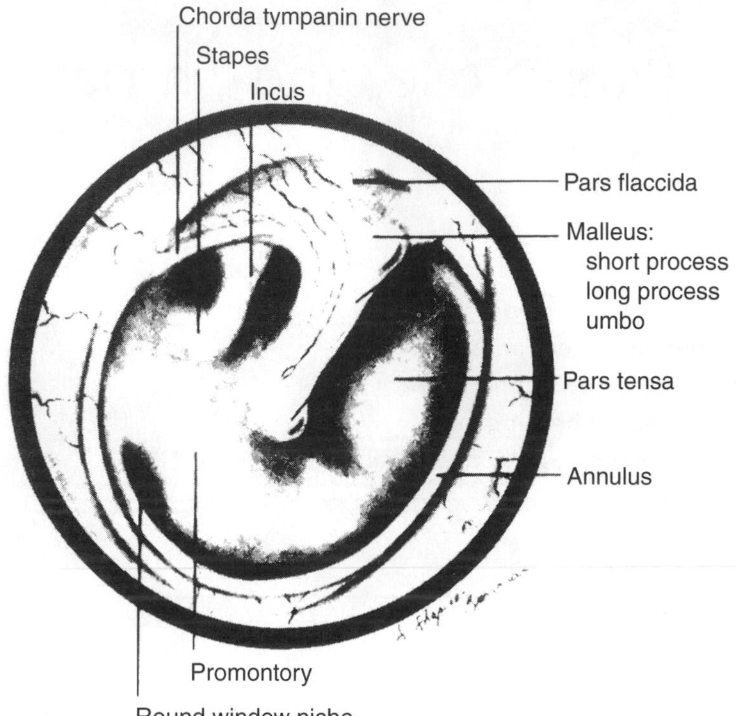

There are many quick and effective office hearing tests, which can be used to screen patients for both conductive and neurosensory loss. Table 19.1 lists the more common tests with their interpretations.

TABLE 19.1

Office Hearing Tests

Test	Method	Interpretation
Weber's test	512-Hz tuning fork placed in midline on top of head; patient is asked which ear tone is heard.	*Normal*: sound heard in midline. *Conductive loss*: sound heard on affected side. *Neurosensory loss*: sound heard on unaffected side.
Rinne's test	512-Hz tuning fork held against mastoid; when sound is no longer heard fork is transferred to $\frac{1}{2}$inch from ear; air conduction should be twice as long as bone and louder.	*Air > bone*: normal (+) test *Bone > air:* conductive loss (−) test.
Whispered voice	Occlude opposite ear and whisper softly, from 2 feet away; do not use a "yes"/"no" question.	Correlates with at least a 20-dB hearing loss if not perceived.
Watch tick	Hold watch 2 inches from ear.	Indicates high frequency loss if not perceived. If heard, 98% chance of hearing all lower frequencies normally.

Audiometric testing and tympanometry can be used when a more detailed evaluation is required. Common types of audiometric tests used by the primary care physician as well as their indications and interpretation are provided in Table 19.2. Examples of audiogram and tympanometry findings are shown in Figure 19.2 and Figure 19.3, respectively.

TABLE 19.2

Audiometric Testing

Test	Indication	Interpretation
Pure tone audiometry	Persistent abnormality on office hearing screening tests	Conductive, sensorineural, or combined deficit identified
Speech audiometry	Learning disability; poor school performance; evaluation of need for speech therapy	Shows altered speech reception threshold of diminished speech discrimination
Bekesy audiogram	Sensorineural hearing loss	Helps differentiate between cochlear and eighth nerve hearing loss
Short increment sensitivity index	Sensorineural hearing loss	Positive in early cochlear disease
Threshold tone decay	Sensorineural hearing loss	Positive in cochlear disease

FIGURE 19.2

Sample Audiograms

Examples of a normal audiogram (A) and each of the three major hearing loss types: conductive (B), sensorineural (C), and mixed (D). Results are shown for right ear only.

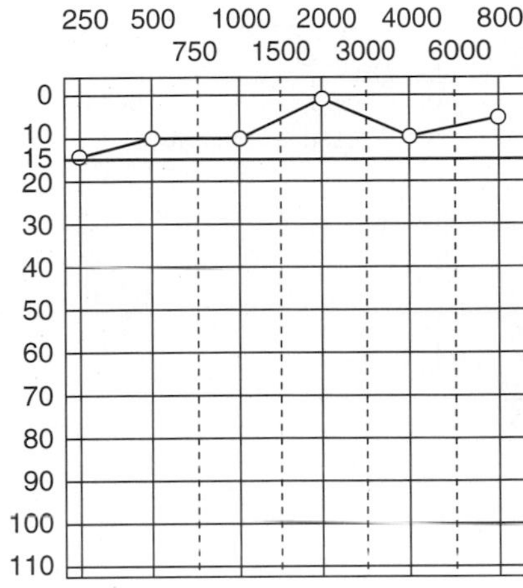

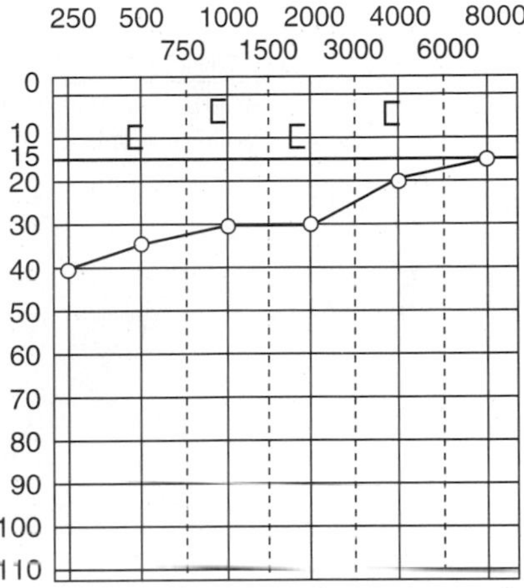

○ Air conduction
< Bone conduction
[Masked bone conduction

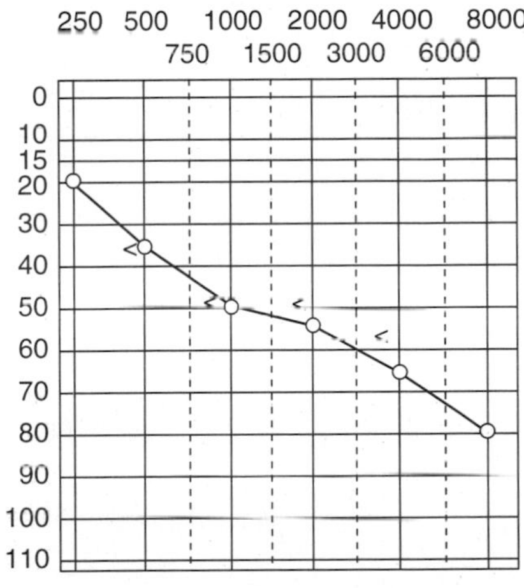

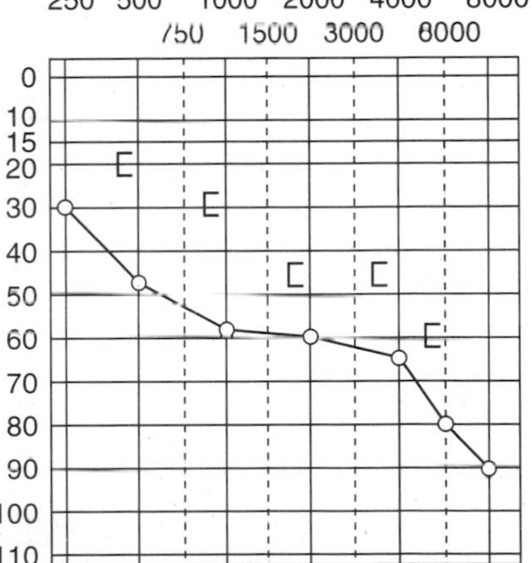

FIGURE 19.3

Tympanometry

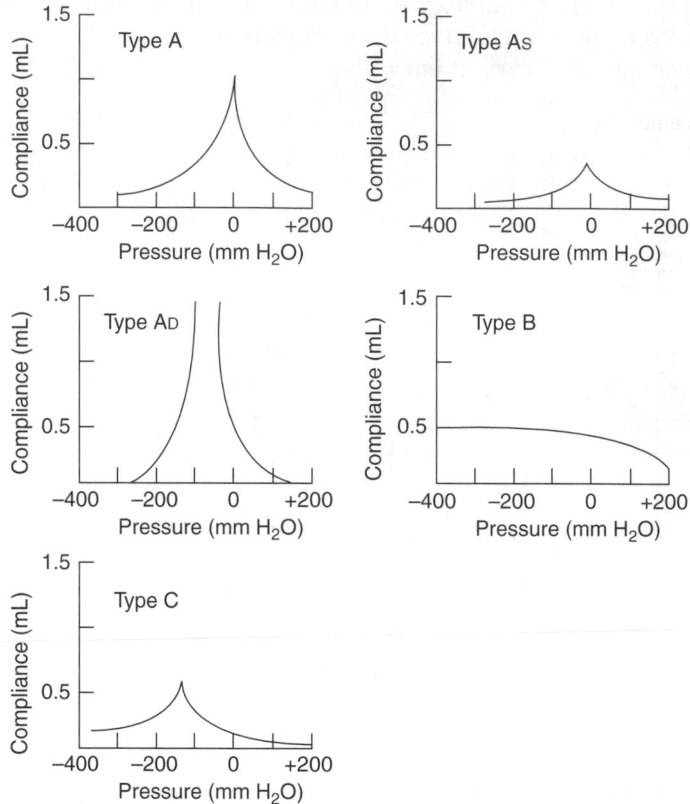

Tympanogram Pattern	Interpretation
Type A	Normal
Type As	Stiff ossicles (tympanosclerosis)
Type AD	High tympanic membrane (TM) compliance (monomeric TM)
Type B	Middle ear fluid, thickened drum, impacted cerumen
Type C	Retracted TM, eustachian tube dysfunction

FIGURE 19.4

Diagnosis and Treatment of Hearing Loss

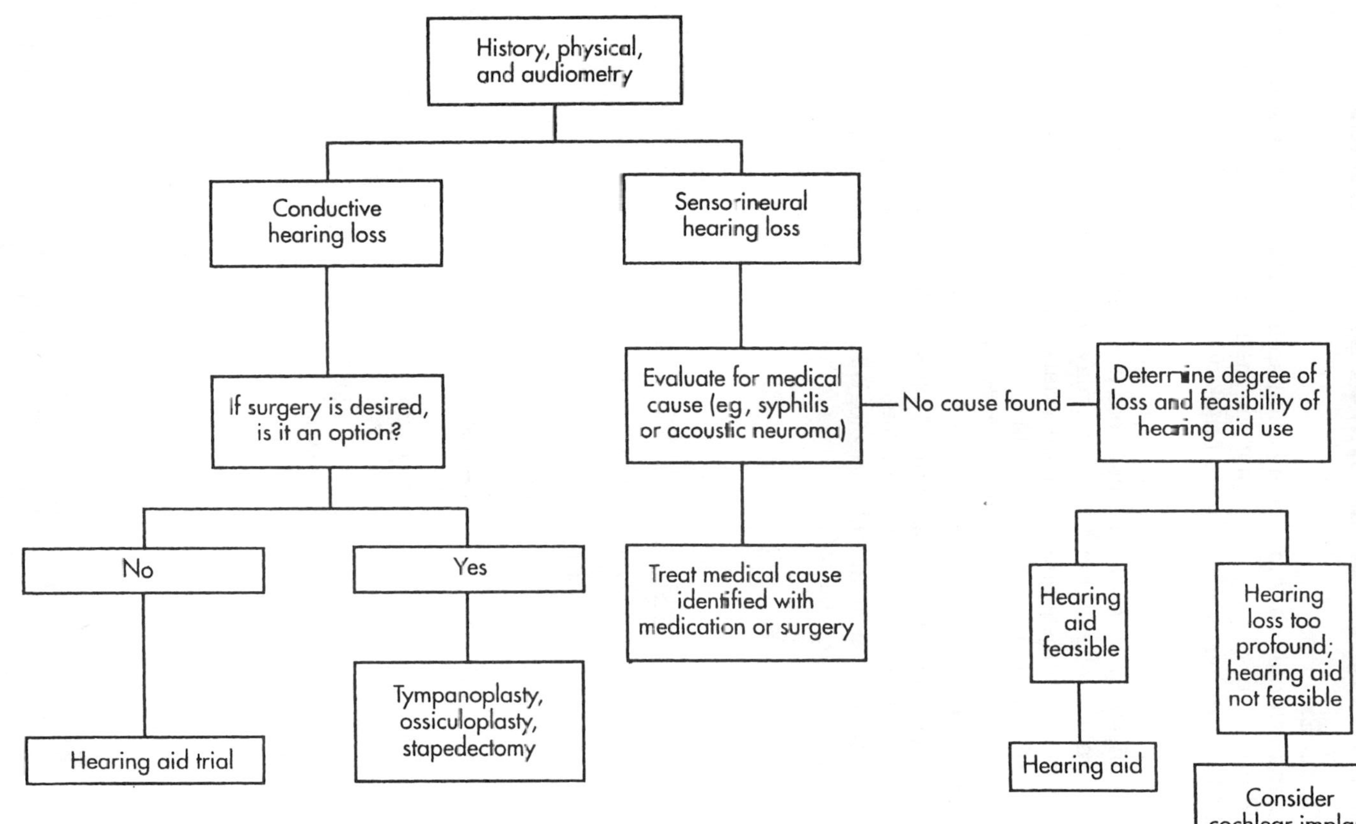

INFECTIONS OF EAR, NOSE, AND THROAT

Otitis Externa

Otitis externa is a common infection seen in children and sometimes in adults. Predisposing factors include instrumentation of the ear canal and swimming, which serve to break down the normal defense mechanisms to infection. *Pseudomonas aeruginosa*, *Staphylococcus aureus*, *Proteus mirabilis*, and *Peptostreptococcus* species are the most common organisms involved. A rare but potentially life-threatening condition known as malignant otitis externa may occur in poorly controlled diabetic or immunosuppressed individuals. This condition is caused by *P aeruginosa* and involves spread of the infection from the external auditory canal to the underlying soft tissues, bone, and potentially the skull base. The diagnosis is made on the basis of progression of the infection with signs of granulation tissue in the ear canal. Treatment requires topical medications and long-term broad-spectrum antibiotics. Prompt referral to an otolaryngologist is also recommended. Table 19.3 summarizes basic treatments for otitis externa.

TABLE 19.3

Treatment of Otitis Externa

Preparation Name	Active Agents	Dosage
Corticosporin otic solution and suspension	Polymyxin B Neomycin Hydrocortisone	3–4 drops 3–4 times a day
Otic Domeboro	Acetic acid in aluminum acetate	4–6 drops every 2–3 hrs
VoSol otic solution	Acetic acid in propylene glycol	5 drops 3–4 times a day
VoSol HC otic solution	Acetic acid Hydrocortisone in propylene glycol	5 drops 3–4 times a day
Cipro HC otic suspension	Ciprofloxacin Hydrocortisone in benzyl alcohol	3 drops 2 times a day

TABLE 19.4

Predisposing Factors for Acute Otitis Media

Age (6 months–18 months most common)	Secondhand smoke
Preceding upper respiratory infection	Pacifier use
Children in group care settings	History of chronic otitis media
Bottle feeding in bed	Ethnicity (Polynesians, Native Americans, American and Canadian Eskimos)

TABLE 19.5

Diagnosis of Acute Otitis Media

Must have the presence of fluid under pressure plus one of the following	Earache	Vomiting
	Fever	Anorexia
	Cough	Lethargy
	Otorrhea	Headache
	Hearing Loss	Irritability

Adapted from Semchenko A. Management of acute sinusitis and acute otitis media. *Am Fam Physician*. Monograph No.1, 2001.

TABLE 19.6

Usual Bacterial Organisms in Otitis Media

Organism	Percent of cases
Streptococcus pneumoniae	35
Haemophilus influenzae, nontypeable	23
Moraxella catarrhalis	14
Sterile aspirate	16
Other bacterial organisms	12

TABLE 19.7

Antibiotic Treatment of Acute Otitis Media and Acute Bacterial Rhinosinusitis

Drug	Pediatric Dosage	Adult Dosage
Amoxicillin	20–40 mg/kg per day divided every 8 hours for uncomplicated otitis media	500 mg every 8 hours
Amoxicillin-clavulanate (Augmentin)	45 mg/kg per day every 12 hours	500-mg tablet every 12 hours
Cefuroxime axetil (Ceftin)	30 mg/kg per day twice daily	125 mg to 500 mg twice daily
Cefpodoxime (Vantin)	10 mg/kg per day twice daily	100–400 mg twice daily
Cefdinir (Omnicef)	7 mg/kg every 12 hours or 14 mg/kg every 24 hours	300 mg every 12 hours or 600 mg every 24 hours
Cefprozil (Cefzil)	30 mg/kg per day every 12 hours	250 mg to 500 mg twice daily
Ceftriaxone (Rocephin)	50 mg/kg IM as one-time dose	1 to 2 gm one or two times daily
TMP/SMX (Bactrim, Septra, Cotrim)	10 mg/kg TMP daily every 12 hours	160 mg TMP/800 mg SMX two times daily
Gatifloxacin (Tequin)	**Do not use in children**	400 mg every 24 hours
Levofloxacin (Levaquin)	**Do not use in children**	500 mg every 24 hours
Moxifloxicin (Avelox)	**Do not use in children**	400 mg every 24 hours
Azithromycin (Zithromax)	10 mg/kg day 1; 5 mg/kg days 2 through 5	500 mg day 1; 250 mg days 2 through 5
Clarithromycin (Biaxin)	15 mg/kg per day every 12 hours	500 mg every 12 hours

IM indicates intramuscularly.

FIGURE 19.5

Management of Otitis Media With Effusion (OME)*

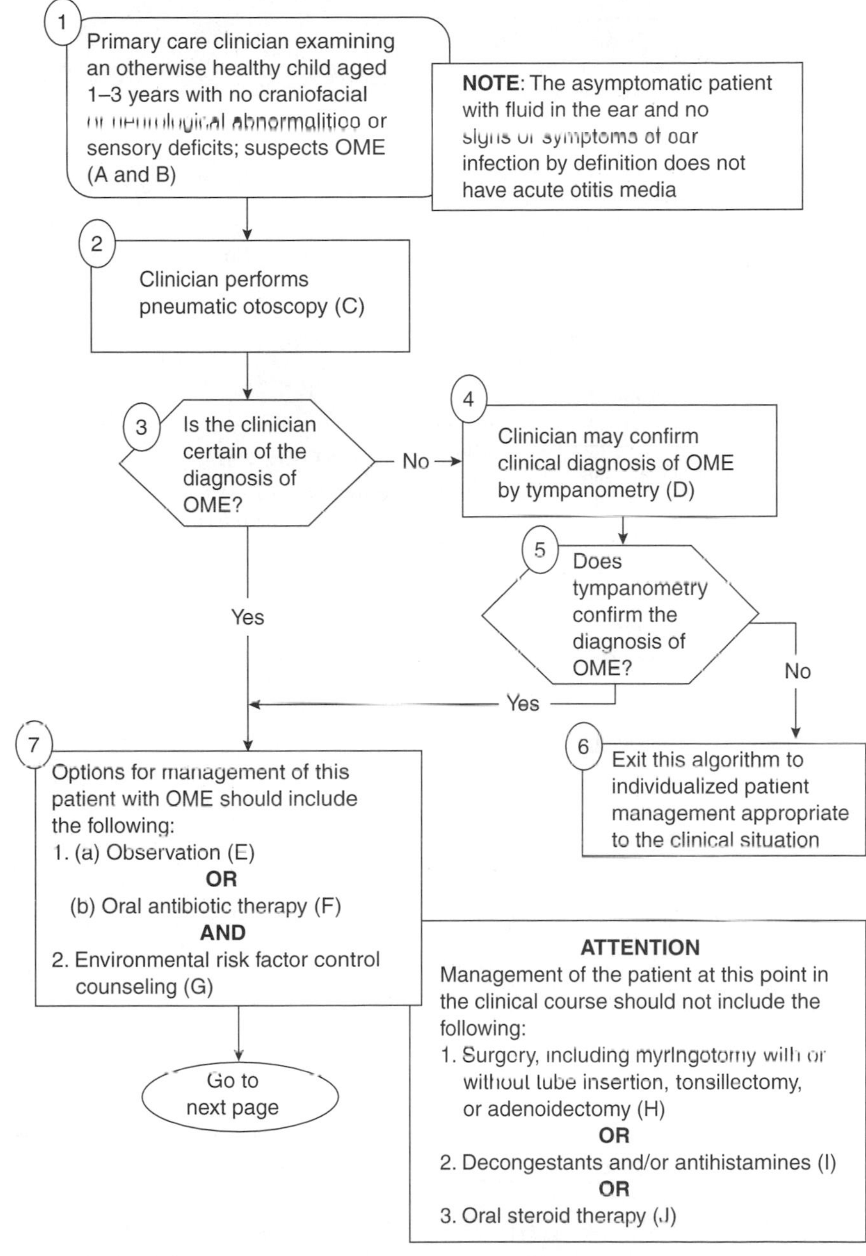

Continued

FIGURE 19.5

Management of Otitis Media With Effusion, cont'd

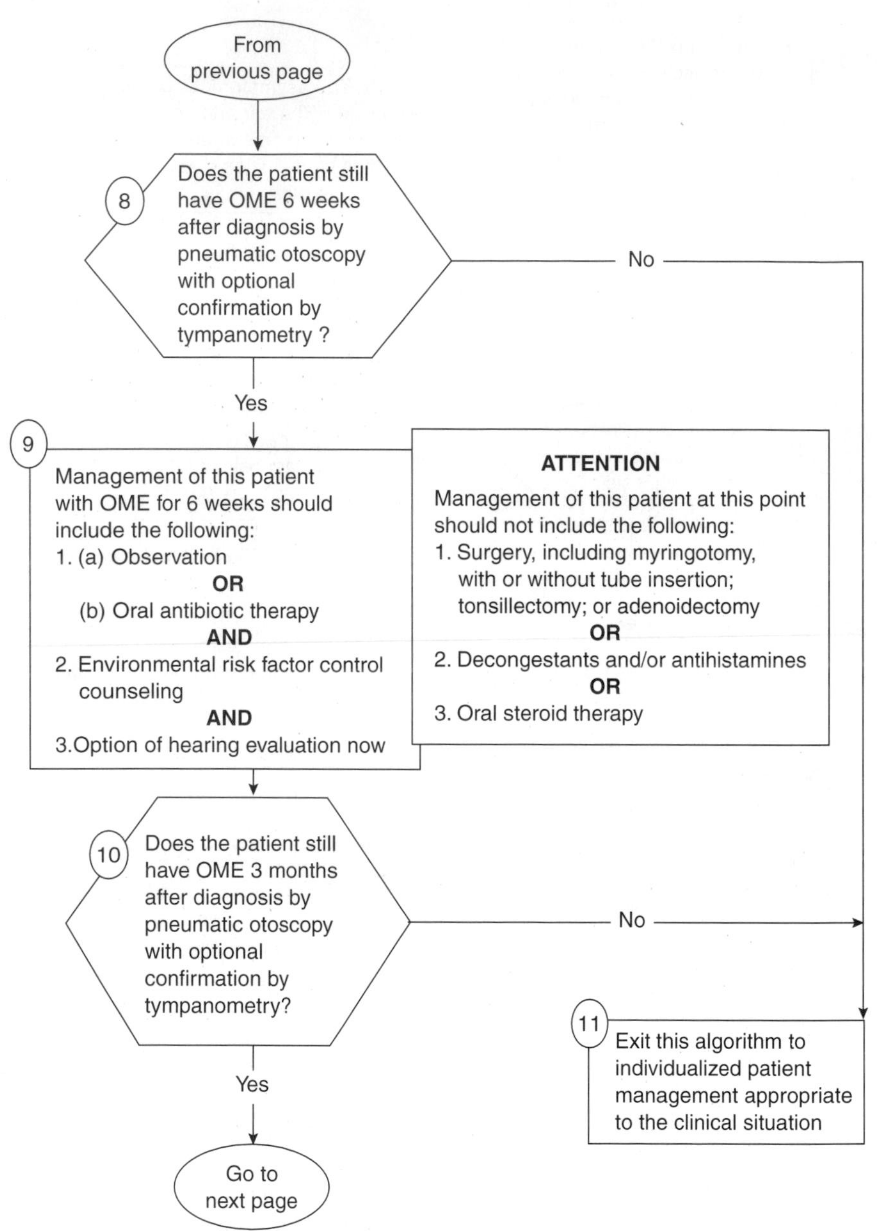

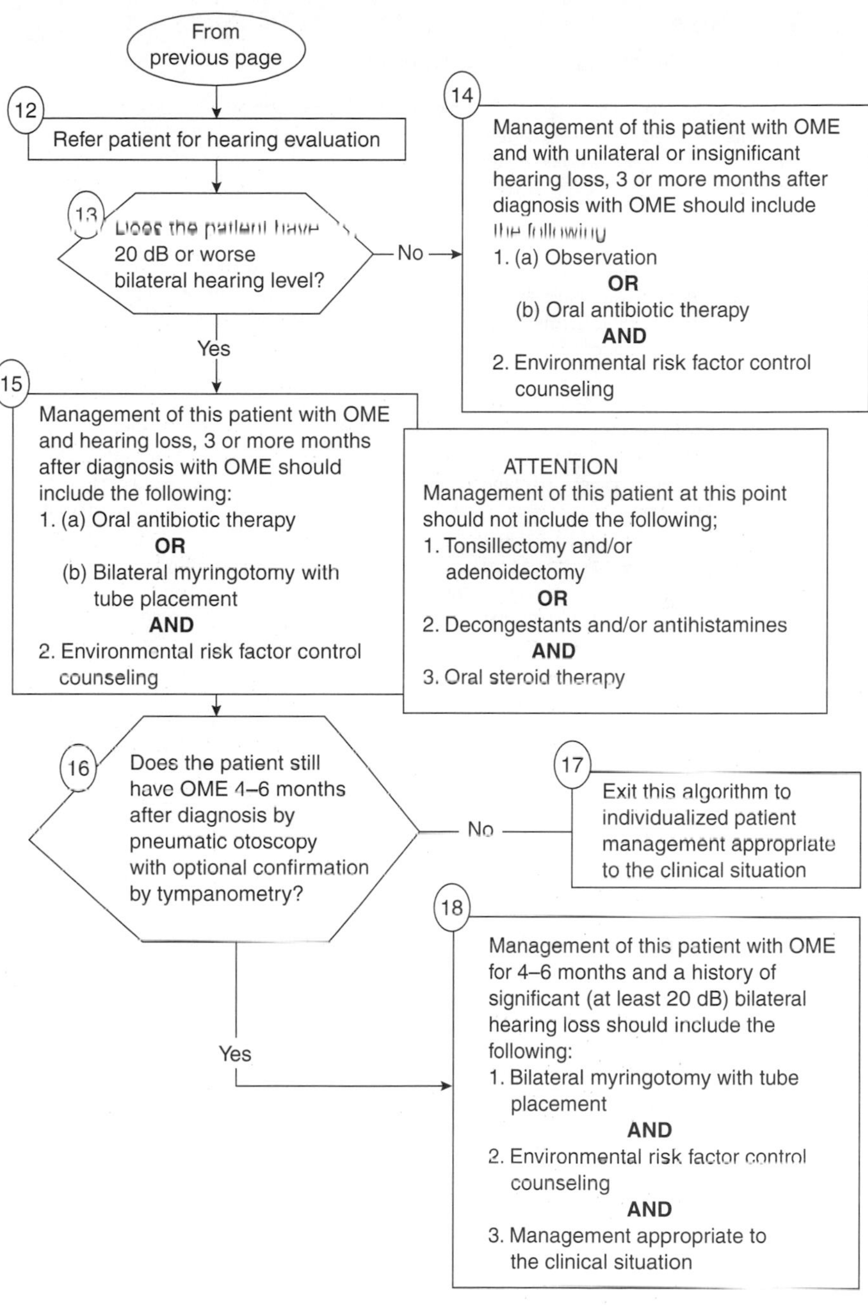
From previous page
12
Refer patient for hearing evaluation
13
Does the patient have 20 dB or worse bilateral hearing level?
No
Yes
14
Management of this patient with OME and with unilateral or insignificant hearing loss, 3 or more months after diagnosis with OME should include the following
1. (a) Observation
OR
(b) Oral antibiotic therapy
AND
2. Environmental risk factor control counseling
15
Management of this patient with OME and hearing loss, 3 or more months after diagnosis with OME should include the following:
1. (a) Oral antibiotic therapy
OR
(b) Bilateral myringotomy with tube placement
AND
2. Environmental risk factor control counseling
ATTENTION
Management of this patient at this point should not include the following;
1. Tonsillectomy and/or adenoidectomy
OR
2. Decongestants and/or antihistamines
AND
3. Oral steroid therapy
16
Does the patient still have OME 4–6 months after diagnosis by pneumatic otoscopy with optional confirmation by tympanometry?
No
17
Exit this algorithm to individualized patient management appropriate to the clinical situation
Yes
18
Management of this patient with OME for 4–6 months and a history of significant (at least 20 dB) bilateral hearing loss should include the following:
1. Bilateral myringotomy with tube placement
AND
2. Environmental risk factor control counseling
AND
3. Management appropriate to the clinical situation

Continued

FIGURE 19.5

Management of Otitis Media With Effusion, cont'd

*Algorithm for managing otitis media with effusion in an otherwise healthy child age 1 to 3 years. (A) Otitis media with effusion (OME) is defined as *fluid in the middle ear without signs or symptoms of infection*. OME is not to be confused with acute otitis media (inflammation of the middle ear with signs of infection). The guideline and this algorithm apply only to the child with otitis media with effusion. This algorithm assumes follow-up intervals of 6 weeks. (B) The algorithm applies only to a child aged 1 to 3 years with no craniofacial or neurological abnormalities or sensory deficits (except as noted) who is healthy except for otitis media with effusion. The guideline recommendations and algorithm do not apply if the child has any craniofacial or neurological abnormality (eg, cleft palate or mental retardation) or sensory deficit (eg, decreased visual acuity or preexisting hearing deficit). (C) There is found some evidence that pneumatic otoscopy is more accurate than otoscopy performed without the pneumatic test of eardrum mobility. (D) Tympanometry may be used as confirmation of pneumatic otoscopy in the diagnosis of OME. Hearing evaluation is recommended for the otherwise healthy child who has had bilateral OME for 3 months; before 3 months, hearing evaluation is a clinical option. (E) In most cases, OME resolves spontaneously within 3 months. (F) The antibiotic drugs studied for treatment of OME were amoxicillin, amoxicillin-clavulanate potassium, cefaclor, erythromycin, erythromycin-sulfisoxazole, sulfisoxazole, and trimethoprim-sulfamethoxazole. (G) Exposure to cigarette smoke (passive smoking) has been shown to increase the risk of OME. For bottle-feeding vs breastfeeding and for child-care facility placement, associations were found with OME, but evidence did not show decreased incidence of OME with breastfeeding or removal from child-care facilities. (H) The recommendation against tonsillectomy is based on the lack of added benefit from tonsillectomy when combined with adenoidectomy to treat OME in older children. Tonsillectomy and adenoidectomy may be appropriate for reasons other than OME. (I) The panel found evidence that decongestants and/or antihistamines are ineffective treatments for OME. (J) Meta-analysis failed to show a significant benefit for steroid medications without antibiotic medications in treating OME in children.

RHINOSINUSITIS

Rhinosinusitis represents a common problem confronting primary clinicians. It may be divided into three major categories: acute rhinosinusitis, subacute rhinosinusitis, and chronic rhinosinusitis. Acute rhinosinusitis is defined as symptoms lasting less than 4 weeks. It may be treated with antibiotics listed in Table 19.7. Ten to 14 days of treatment usually suffices. The duration of symptoms for subacute rhinosinusitis is 4–12 weeks and may require treatment for up to 6 weeks. Chronic rhinosinusitis represents a more indolent course of infection with symptoms lasting greater than 12 weeks. Treatment for this condition should continue for at least 3–6 weeks. Consideration must be given to the fact that these patients may harbor more resistant organisms secondary to prolonged and repeated antibiotic exposure. They also are more likely to be infected with gram-negative organisms and anaerobes. Therefore, broad-spectrum antibiotics such as amoxicillin/clavulanate (Augmentin), second- or third-generation cephalosporins, or quinolones should be strongly considered.

TABLE 19.8

Predisposing Factors for Acute Rhinosinusitis

Allergic rhinitis	Hormone factors
Anatomic variations (deviated septum, nasal polyps)	Immunodeficiency disease
Barotrauma	Inhalation of irritants
Dental infections and procedures	Mechanical ventilation
Preceding upper respiratory infection	Nasal dryness
	Nasotracheal and nasogastric tubes

TABLE 19.9

Signs and Symptoms Commonly Associated With Acute Bacterial Rhinosinusitis*

Malaise/fatigue	Cough
Maxillary pain**/pressure/fullness	Halitosis
Nasal obstruction/blockage	Mouth breathing
Fever	Snoring
Nasal or postnasal discharge/purulent discharge** (by history or physical exam)	Hyponasal speech "Double-sickening"[†] history

Adapted from Semchenko A. Management of acute sinusitis and acute otitis media. *Am Fam Physician*. Monograph No.1, 2001.

*None of these signs and symptoms is specific for acute bacterial rhinosinusitis

**In the absence of sinus aspiration and culture, these symptoms increase diagnostic certainty of bacterial infection.

[†]"Double-sickening" implies an initial upper respiratory infection that starts to improve and then worsens.

ACUTE PHARYNGITIS

The majority of cases of acute pharyngitis are viral. It has been estimated that group A beta-hemolytic streptococci (GABHS) account for 15% of the adult and 40% of the pediatric cases of pharyngitis. Determination of the etiology is important, however, when one considers the complications of untreated group A beta-hemolytic streptococcal pharyngitis. These complications include rheumatic fever, scarlet fever, tonsillar abscess, and rapid spread of the disease to household, daycare, and classroom contacts. Figure 19.6 provides one approach to determining if GABHS is present. Table 19.10 provides common treatments for GABHS.

FIGURE 19.6

Algorithm for Determining Probability of Group A Streptococcal Pharyngitis*

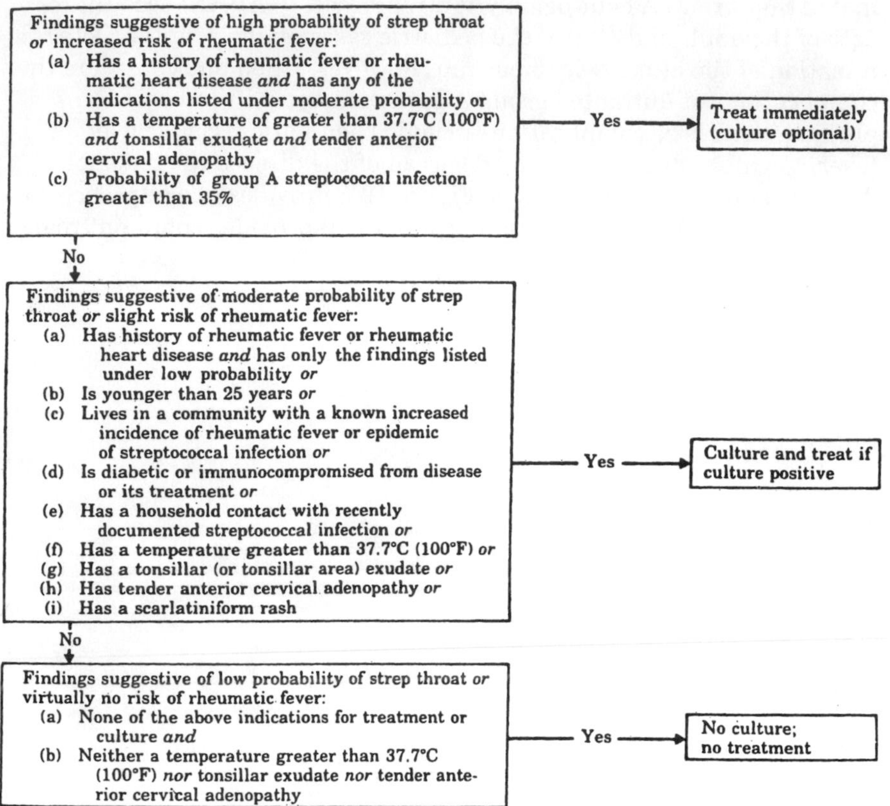

Reproduced with permission from Komaroff AL. Coryza, pharyngitis, and related infections in adults. In: Branch WT, ed. *Office Practice of Medicine*. 2nd ed. Philadelphia, PA: WB Saunders; 1987.

*Algorithm describing an evaluation of the probability of group A streptococcal pharyngitis and the risk of developing acute rheumatic fever. Note: Rapid (10-minute) strep test may be substituted for culture. Immediate treatment is preferred for those individuals whose throat culture results will not be complete for 9 days into the illness (as treatment after that time has not been shown to be protective against rheumatic fever).

TABLE 19.10

Antibiotic Treatment of Group A Beta-Hemolytic Streptococcal Pharyngitis

Antibiotic	Adult Dose	Pediatric Dose
Penicillin V (Pen-Vee K)	1000 mg bid × 10 days	25 mg/kg bid for 10 days
Benzathine penicillin (Bicillin)	1.2 million units × 1 dose	2500 units/kg × 1 dose up to 40 kg
Amoxcillin	500 mg tid × 10 days	40 mg/kg/d tid × 10 days
Cephalexin (Keflex)	500 mg bid × 10 days	25 mg/kg bid × 10 days
Amoxicillin-clavulanate (Augmentin)	500 mg bid × 10 days	40 mg/kg bid × 10 days
Azithromycin (Zithromax)	500 mg day 1 then 250 mg daily days 2–5	10 mg/kg day 1 then 5 mg/kg days 2–5
Clarithromycin (Biaxin)	500 mg bid × 10 days	7.5 mg/kg bid × 10 days

bid indicates twice daily.

RHINITIS

TABLE 19.11

Causes of Rhinitis*

Allergic	Nonallergic
Seasonal	Infectious (acute and chronic)
Perennial	NARES syndrome (nonallergic rhinitis with eosinophilia syndrome)
Episodic	Vasomotor rhinitis
Occupational	Ciliary dyskinesia syndrome
	Atrophic rhinitis
	Hormonally induced
	Exercise induced
	Drug induced (nasal sprays, OCPs, aspirin, NSAIDs)
	Reflex induced (gustatory rhinitis, chemicals, posture reflexes, nasal cycle, emotional factors)

*Rhinitis may be defined as an inflammatory process of the nasal mucous membranes causing the classic symptoms of rhinorrhea, congestion, sneezing, and postnasal drip.

TREATMENT OF RHINITIS

Nonpharmacological treatments include avoidance of inciting factors and the consideration for allergy skin testing if determination of the inciting factor is not possible by history alone. The Joint Task Force on Practice Parameters in Allergy, Asthma, and Immunology lists the second-generation antihistamines as first-line therapy for the treatment of allergic rhinitis (Table 19.12). They are effective in reducing symptoms of itching, sneezing, and rhinorrhea but have little documented effect on nasal congestion. Nasally inhaled corticosteroid sprays have been shown to be more efficacious than nasal cromolyn sodium or oral antihistamines in controlling all four allergic rhinitis symptoms. This includes nasal congestion. The effectiveness of these preparations may be limited by patient compliance and tolerability. One study by Juniper et al found that at least 50% of patients need to take both nasal corticosteroids and oral antihistamines to adequately control symptoms of seasonal allergic rhinitis. Nasal spray preparations are summarized in Table 19.13.

TABLE 19.12

Second-Generation Oral Antihistamines

Agent	Usual Adult Dose	Available With Decongestant	Reduce Dose With Liver Disease?	Reduce Dose With Renal Impairment?	Pregnancy Category
Cetirizine (Zyrtec)	5–10 mg/d	Yes	5 mg/d	5 mg/d	B
Fexofenadine (Allegra)	60 mg bid 180 mg/d	Yes No	60 mg/d	No change	C
Loratadine (Claritin)	10 mg/d	Yes	Start at 10 mg QOD	Start at 10 mg QOD	B

TABLE 19.13

Prescription Nasal Sprays for Rhinitis

Agent	Trade Name(s)	Dose per Inhalation	Usual Adult Dose
Intranasal Corticosteroids			
Beclomethasone dipropionate	Beconase Beconase AQ Vancenase Pockethaler	42 μg	1–2 sprays per nostril 2 times a day
	Vancenase AQ Double Strength	84 μg	1–2 sprays per nostril 1 times a day
Budesonide	Rhinocort Rhinocort AQ	84 μg	2 sprays per nostril 2 times a day or 4 sprays per nostril 1 time a day
Flunisolide	Nasarel Nasalide	25 μg	2 sprays per nostril 2 times a day
Fluticasone propionate	Flonase	50 μg	2 sprays per nostril 1 time a day or 1 spray per nostril 2 times a day
Mometasone	Nasonex AQ	50 μg	2 sprays per nostril 1 time a day
Triamcinolone acetonide	Nasacort Nasacort AQ	55 μg	2 sprays per nostril 1 time a day
Dexamethasone sodium phosphate	Dexacort	84 μg	2 sprays per nostril 2–3 times a day
Intranasal Cromolyn			
Cromolyn sodium	Nasalcrom	5.2 mg	1 spray per nostril every 4 hours
Intranasal Anticholinergics			
Ipatropium bromide	Atrovent Nasal Spray 0.03%	21 μg	2 sprays per nostril 2–3 times a day
	Atrovent Nasal Spray 0.06%	42 μg	2 sprays per nostril 3–4 times a day
Intranasal Antihistamines			
Azelastine hydrochloride	Astelin Nasal Spray	136 μg	2 sprays per nostril 2 times a day

EPISTAXIS

Epistaxis is a common medical problem. The majority of nosebleeds originate anteriorly in the region of Kiesselbach plexus. Predisposing factors include infections, allergic rhinitis, trauma, atrophic rhinitis, local irritants (nasal sprays, illegal drug use), hypertension, and hereditary bleeding disorders.

The majority of nosebleeds can be controlled with firm pressure applied to the elastic areas of both nostrils for 10 minutes. The pressure should be constant and timed with a clock. If the bleeding is not controlled at this point, vasoconstrictive agents may be used. Once the bleeding has been controlled, identification of the source and then cautery using silver nitrate is appropriate. Table 19.14 lists the commonly used vasoconstrictive agents.

TABLE 19.14

Vasoconstricitve Agents Used in Epistaxis

Epinephrine 0.25 mL of 1:1000 concentration mixed with 20 mL of 4% lidocaine
Oxymetazoline (Afrin) 0.05% concentration mixed with 4% lidocaine
Phenylephrine (Neo-Synephrine) 0.5%–1.0% concentration mixed with 4% lidocaine

If the bleeding is determined to be anterior but cannot be controlled with the above measures, anterior packing should be considered. If the bleeding originates from the posterior region, an ear, nose, and throat consultation should be strongly considered. The technique for posterior packing of the nose is given in Table 19.15.

TABLE 19.15

Technique for Posterior Nasal Packing

1. Insert small rubber catheter through nose, clasp, and then pull from nasopharynx through oropharynx with Kelly clamp.
2. Roll a 4 × 4-inch pad and tie two 8-inch and one 3-inch lengths of 3-0 silk suture to the middle of the roll. Apply Vaseline to gauze pad.
3. Attach two of the ties to the catheter.
4. Pull the catheter and the pad back through the nose, placing the pad, if necessary, with the index finger.
5. Fix by tying two sutures around another 4 × 4-inch pad placed across the nares.
6. The third, shorter string hangs from the nasopharynx for removal of the pack in 48 hours.
7. Anterior pack may then be placed if bleeding continues.

Materials for epistaxis management and nasal packing (see Figure 19.7):

- Head mirror
- Nasal speculum
- Suction equipment
- Tongue blades
- Cotton balls
- Lidocaine with epinephrine (1:1000)
- Bayonet forceps
- Silver nitrate sticks
- Scissors
- Vaseline gauze (1/2 inch)
- Cotton-tipped applicators
- Kelly clamp
- Posterior packs or Epistat catheter (Xomed, Inc)
- Gauze pads (4 × 4 inches)
- Long, 25-gauge needle
- 5-cc syringe
- Cetacaine spray

FIGURE 19.7

Algorithm of Epistaxis Management

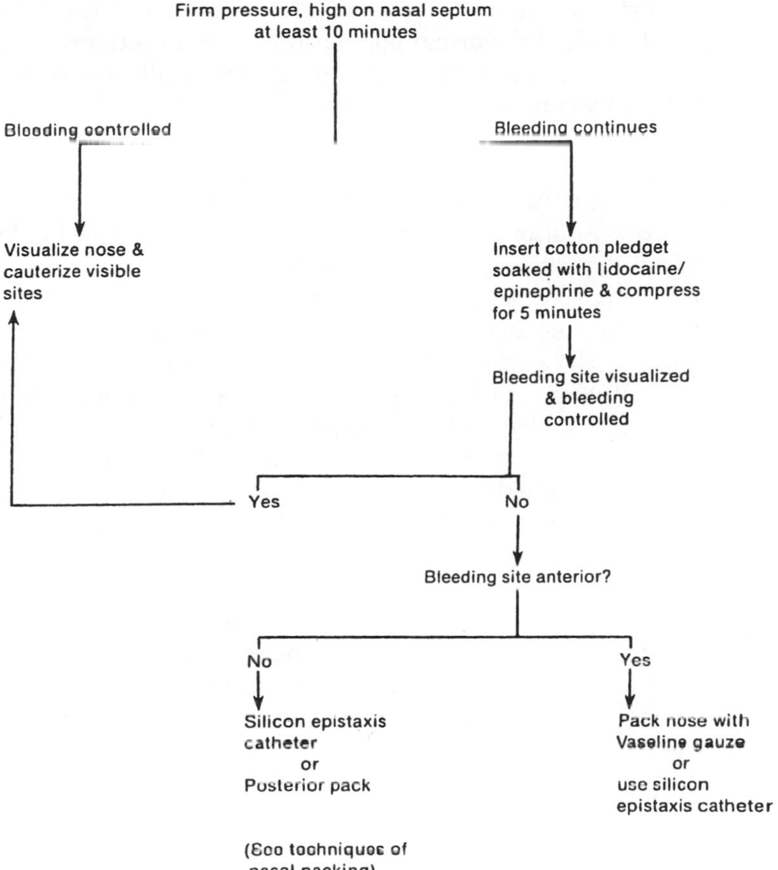

TINNITUS

Tinnitus can be defined as the sensation of noise heard in the head or ears without external stimuli. It is relatively common, and it has been estimated that 95% of the normal population would experience tinnitus if placed in a quiet environment.* Tinnitus is usually associated with hearing loss and most frequently noticed at bedtime. Patients with progressive unilateral tinnitus associated with hearing loss should be evaluated for acoustic neuroma.

The source for tinnitus may be divided into auditory and extra-auditory sources. Auditory sources include sensorineural hearing loss, Meniere disease, infections, external auditory canal obstruction, conductive hearing loss, and ototoxic medications. (See Table 19.16.) Extra-auditory sources include vascular etiologies such as cerebrovascular disease, arteriovenous malformations, and glomus tumors. Other extra-auditory etiologies include a patulous eustachian tube, temporomandibular joint disorder, and cervical arthritis.

The mainstay of management of tinnitus is to identify and treat the underlying cause if possible. This may require removal of potentially offending medications, surgical evaluation in the case of an arteriovenous malformation, glomus tumor, or acoustic neuroma, and treatment with assistive hearing devices if the main cause appears to be sensorineural hearing loss. Many alternative medicine options are available including magnet therapy, acupuncture, and herbal therapy but as of yet have not been proven effective in controlled trials.

Source: Marion MS, Cevette MJ. *Tinnitus.* Mayo Clinic Proceedings. 1991;66:614–620.

TABLE 19.16

Ototoxic Agents

- Salicylates
- Nonsteroidals
- Loop diuretics
  - Ethacrynic acid
  - Furosemide
  - Bumetadine
- Quinine
- Antibiotics
  - Aminoglycosides
  - Erythromycin
  - Vancomycin
- Chemotherapeutic agents
  - Cisplatin
  - Carboplatin
  - Vinblastine
  - Vincristine

Topical Agents

- Solvents
  - Propylene glycol
- Antiseptics
  - Ethanol
- Antibiotics
  - Polymyxin B
  - Neomycin

DIZZINESS/VERTIGO

Dizziness is a common complaint seen in the primary care office. The first step in the evaluation is to differentiate dizziness from vertigo. Dizziness may be defined as a feeling of imbalance or unsteadiness while vertigo describes the sensation of motion of the patient's environment. When evaluating the dizzy patient, the physician must rule out many potential causes including central and peripheral neurological disease, cardiac disease, cerebrovascular disease, and psychogenic causes. In one study looking at the etiology of dizziness, peripheral vestibular causes accounted for 44% of the cases and psychiatric sources were found to be the major cause in 16% of patients. Serious treatable causes including cerebrovascular disease, cardiac arrhythmia, and brain tumor accounted for less than 9% of the patients affected.

Vertigo may be classified as peripheral or central in origin. Peripheral vertigo tends to be more acute in onset, episodic, and more severe than central vertigo. Recovery from peripheral vertigo also tends to occur faster.

TABLE 19.17

Comparison of Symptoms of Peripheral vs Central Vertigo

Symptom	Peripheral Vertigo	Central Vertigo
Vertigo	Strong	Weak
Nausea and vomiting	Strong	Weak
Suppression with fixation	Yes	None
Hearing loss	Common	Rare
Facial weakness	Occasional	Common
Ataxia	Rare	Common
Oscillopsia	Rare	Common
Other CNS symptoms	Rare	Common

Adapted from Rakel RE, Bope ET, eds. *Conn's Current Therapy*. Philadelphia: WB Saunders; 2001.

CNS indicates central nervous system.

TABLE 19.18

Common Causes of Vertigo

Central Vertigo

- Central nervous system infection
- Vertebrobasilar insufficiency
- Cerebrovascular accidents involving cerebellum, brainstem, or vestibular tracts
- Migraine headache
- Central nervous system tumor
- Multiple sclerosis
- Trauma

Peripheral Vertigo

- Labrynthitis
- Vestibular neuronitis
- Meniere disease
- Benign paroxysmal positional vertigo
- Otitis media or serous otitis media
- Cholesteatoma
- Perilymphatic fistula
- Cerebellopontine angle tumor
- Temporal bone fracture

TABLE 19.19

Evaluation of Vertigo

1. History to include onset, precipitating events, duration, exacerbating causes, and associated symptoms
2. Physical exam to include complete neurologic exam of cranial nerves, assessment of cerebellar function, Romberg test, and gait testing as well as otologic exam to rule out infection, middle ear fluid, and canal obstruction.
3. Positional testing to include observing for nystagmus after placing the patient in the upright, recumbent with left ear down, recumbent with right ear down, and with head hanging, pointing at the floor.
4. Other testing such as audiometry, electronystagmography, and radiographic assessment as indicated.

BENIGN PAROXYSMAL POSITIONAL VERTIGO

One of the more common forms of peripheral vertigo is benign paroxysmal positional vertigo (BPPV). BPPV has certain characteristics that distinguish it from other causes of vertigo. First, there is a delay of onset of the vertigo after the provocative movement. Second, there tends to be a limited duration and fatigue of the symptoms with repetition of the provocative movement. A Hallpike maneuver can be performed in which the patient is placed in an upright position with the head turned 30° to one side. The patient is then moved to a supine position with the head hanging in a dependent position. The ear being tested is the one in the downward position. A rotatory nystagmus should be elicited for the test to be considered positive.

The treatment for BPPV is the canolith repositioning procedure more commonly known as the Eply maneuver. This procedure attempts to remove debris floating in the posterior semicircular canal and allow it to drop into the vestibule. This maneuver is described in Figure 19.8.

FIGURE 19.8

The Canolith Repositioning Procedure

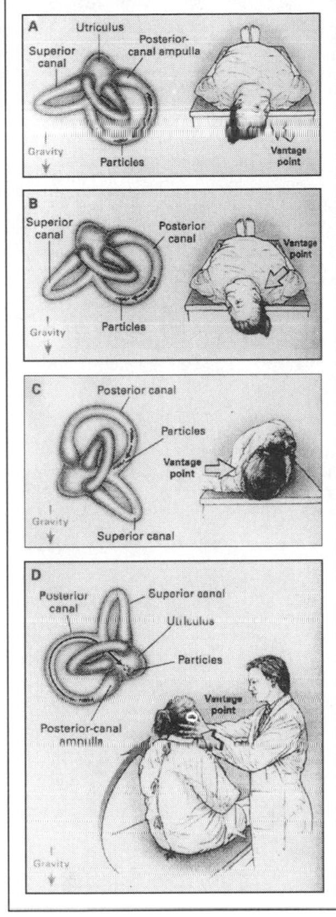

Bedside maneuver for the treatment of a patient with benign paroxysmal positional vertigo affecting the right ear. The presumed position of the debris within the labyrinth during the maneuver is shown in each panel. The maneuver is a three-step procedure. First, a Dix-Hallpike test is performed with the patient's head rotated 45° toward the right ear and the neck slightly extended with the chin pointed slightly upward. This position results in the patient's head hanging to the right (panel A). Once the vertigo and nystagmus provoked by the Dix-Hallpike test cease, the patient's head is rotated about the rostral-caudal body axis until the left ear is down (panel C). The vertex of the head is kept tilted downward throughout the rotation. The maneuver usually provokes brief vertigo. The patient should be kept in the final, face-down position for about 10 to 15 seconds. With the head kept turned toward the left shoulder, the patient is brought into the seated position (panel D). Once the patient is upright, the head is tilted so that the chin is pointed slightly downward.

TABLE 19.20

Common Medications Used to Treat Vertigo

Medication	Class	Dosage (mg)	Side Effects
Oral Medications			
Meclizine (Antivert)	Antihistamine	25 q 6 h	Drowsiness, dry mouth
Promethazine (Phenergan)	Antihistamine	12.5–25 q 4 h	Drowsiness, xerostomia, extrapyramidal effect
Dimenhydrinate (Dramamine)	Antihistamine	50 q 4 h	Drowsiness, xerostomia, extrapyramidal effect
Prochlorperazine (Compazine)	Phenothiazine	5–10 q 6 h	Drowsiness, dizziness, amenorrhea, xerostomia
Chlorpromazine (Thorazine)	Phenothiazine	25 q 6 h	Strong sedative, jaundice, xerostomia
Diazepam* (Valium)	Benzodiazepine	2–10 q 8 h	Strong sedative, fatigue, ataxia
Ondansetron* (Zofran)	$5\text{-}HT_3$-receptor antagonist	4 q 6 h	Diarrhea, headache, fever, akathisia, acute dystonic reaction
Intramuscular Medications			
Promethazine	Antihistamine	12.5–25 q 4 h	Drowsiness, xerostomia, extrapyramidal effect
Dimenhydrinate	Antihistamine	50 q 4 h	Drowsiness, xerostomia, extrapyramidal effect
Prochlorperazine	Phenothiazine	5–10 q 6 h	Drowsiness, dizziness, amenorrhea, xerostomia
Chlorpromazine	Phenothiazine	25 q 6 h	Strong sedative, jaundice, xerostomia

Medication	Class	Dosage (mg)	Side Effects
Diazepam*	Benzodiazepine	2–10 q 8 h	Strong sedative, fatigue, ataxia
Ondansetron*	$5\text{-}HT_3$-receptor antagonist	4 q 6 h	Diarrhea, headache, fever, akathisia, acute dystonic reaction
Intravenous Medications			
Promethazine	Antihistamine	12.5–25 q 4 h	Drowsiness, xerostomia, extrapyramidal effect
Ondansetron*	$5\text{-}HT_3$-receptor antagonist	4 q 4 h	Diarrhea, headache, fever, akathisia, acute dystonic reaction
Transdermal Medications			
Scopolamine (Transderm Scop)	Anticholinergic	1 q 3 d	Drowsiness, xerostomia, extrapyramidal effect
Suppository Medications			
Promethazine	Antihistamine	12.5–25 q 4 h	Drowsiness, xerostomia, extrapyramidal effect
Dimenhydrinate	Antihistamine	100 q 8 h	Drowsiness, extrapyramidal effect
Prochlorperazine	Phenothiazine	25 q 12 h	Drowsiness, extrapyramidal effect

Adapted with permission from Rakel RE, Bope ET, eds. *Conn's Current Therapy*. Philadelphia, PA: WB Saunders; 2001.

$5\text{-}HT_3$ indicates 5-hydroxytryptamine 3, q 6 h, every 6 hours.

*Not approved by the Food and Drug Administration for this indication.

Vestibular rehabilitation is also an option when medical treatment alone does not suffice. These exercises allow for progressive stimulation of the semicircular canals in an attempt to compensate for the peripheral vestibular deficit. An example of these exercises can be found in Table 19.21.

TABLE 19.21

Cawthorne Head Exercises

Exercises to be carried out for 15 minutes twice a day, increasing to 30 minutes:

Eye Exercises

1. Look up, then down—at first slowly then quickly; 20 times.
2. Look from one side to other—at first slowly, then quickly; 20 times.
3. Focus on finger at arm's length, moving finger 1 foot closer and back again; 20 times.

Head Exercises

1. Bend head forward then backward with eyes open—slowly, later quickly; 20 times.
2. Turn head from one side to other side—slowly then quickly; 20 times.
3. As dizziness decreases, these exercises should be done with eyes closed.

Sitting

1. While sitting, shrug shoulders; 20 times.
2. Turn shoulders right, then left; 20 times.
3. Bend forward and pick up objects from ground and sit up; 20 times.

Standing

1. Change from sitting to standing and back again; 20 times with eyes open.
2. Repeat with eyes closed.
3. Throw a small rubber ball from hand to hand above eye level; 10 times.
4. Throw a ball from hand to hand under one knee.

Moving About

1. Walk across room with eyes open, then closed; 10 times.
2. Walk up and down a slope with eyes open, then closed; 10 times.
3. Walk up and down steps with eyes open, then closed; 10 times.
4. Any game involving stooping or turning is good.

Adapted from Cawthorne T. Surgical treatment of the endolymphatic hydrops. In: Chambaugh GE Jr, Glasscock ME III, eds. *Surgery of the Ear*. 3rd ed. Philadelphia, PA: WB Saunders; 1980:589.

SELECTED PROCEDURES IN EAR, NOSE, AND THROAT

TABLE 19.22

Technique of Indirect Mirror Laryngoscopy

1. Patient should sit upright and lean slightly forward.
2. Spray posterior pharynx with anesthetic (2% to 4% lidocaine or 14% benzocaine) spray.
3. Warm mirror over alcohol lamp or in warm water to prevent fogging. Test temperature on back of own hand prior to inserting.
4. Cover protruded tongue with gauze and grasp firmly with thumb and middle finger.
5. Have patient breathe in and out through mouth or "pant like a dog."
6. Place back side of mirror against uvula and lift out of the way. Avoid touching posterior pharynx, as this will cause the gag reflex.
7. Ask patient to say "EEE" to observe approximation of the vocal cords.

TABLE 19.23

Emergency Airway

1. Place patient supine with support under shoulders and neck hyperextended.
2. Palpate space between thyroid and cricoid cartilage.
3. Make horizontal incision about 1 inch wide over this space (cricothyroid membrane).
4. Bluntly dissect tissues down to membrane.
5. Make 1-cm incision through cricothyroid membrane.
6. Insert flat instrument (eg, scalpel handle) through incision and rotate 90° to hold incision open.
7. If available, insert a small tube through incision.
8. As soon as possible, convert cricothyrotomy to standard tracheostomy.

chapter 20

The Eye

Edward T. Bope, MD

IN THIS CHAPTER

- Vision evaluation
- Pediatric eye and vision screening guidelines
- Strabismus, pseudostrabismus, and amblyopia
- Lacrimal duct obstruction
- Geriatric eye moisture problems
- Differential diagnosis of red eye
- Glaucoma
- Conjunctival abnormalities
- Herpes infections of the eye
- Retinal examination
- Painless loss of vision
- Extraocular muscles
- Common eye symptoms
- Common eye signs
- Ocular manifestations of systemic disease
- Refractive surgery
- Eye trauma
- Treatment for chemical burn
- Blunt injury to the eye
- Ophthalmic antimicrobials
- Treatment of allergic conjunctivitis
- Ocular manifestations of common drugs
- Alternative medicine for ocular conditions

BOOKSHELF RECOMMENDATIONS

- Goldberg S. *Ophthalmology Made Ridiculously Simple*. 2nd ed. Miami, FL: Medmaster; 2001.
- Krachmer JH, Palay DA, eds. *Ophthalmology for the Primary Care Physician*. St Louis, MO: Mosby, Inc; 1997.
- Trobe JD. *Physician Guide to Eye Care*. 2nd ed. San Francisco, CA: American Academy of Ophthalmology; 2000.
- Yanoff M, Duker JS. *Ophthalmology*. St Louis, MO: Mosby, Inc; 1999.

VISION EVALUATION

TABLE 20.1

Percentage of Visual Loss (American Medical Association Method)*

Use best-correcting glasses and measure both distance vision by the Snellen chart and near vision by the Jaeger test. In this method, near and distant vision are weighted equally.

Snellen Chart for *Distance Visual Acuity*	*% Loss*
20/20	0
20/25	5
20/40	15
20/50	25
20/80	40
20/100	50
20/160	70
20/200	80
20/400	90
Jaeger Test for *Near Visual Acuity*	*% Loss*
1	0
2	0
3	10
6	50
7	60
11	85
14	95

*Percent vision acuity = 100 − [(% near loss + % distance loss) ÷ 2].

FIGURE 20.1

Jaeger Test for Near Visual Acuity

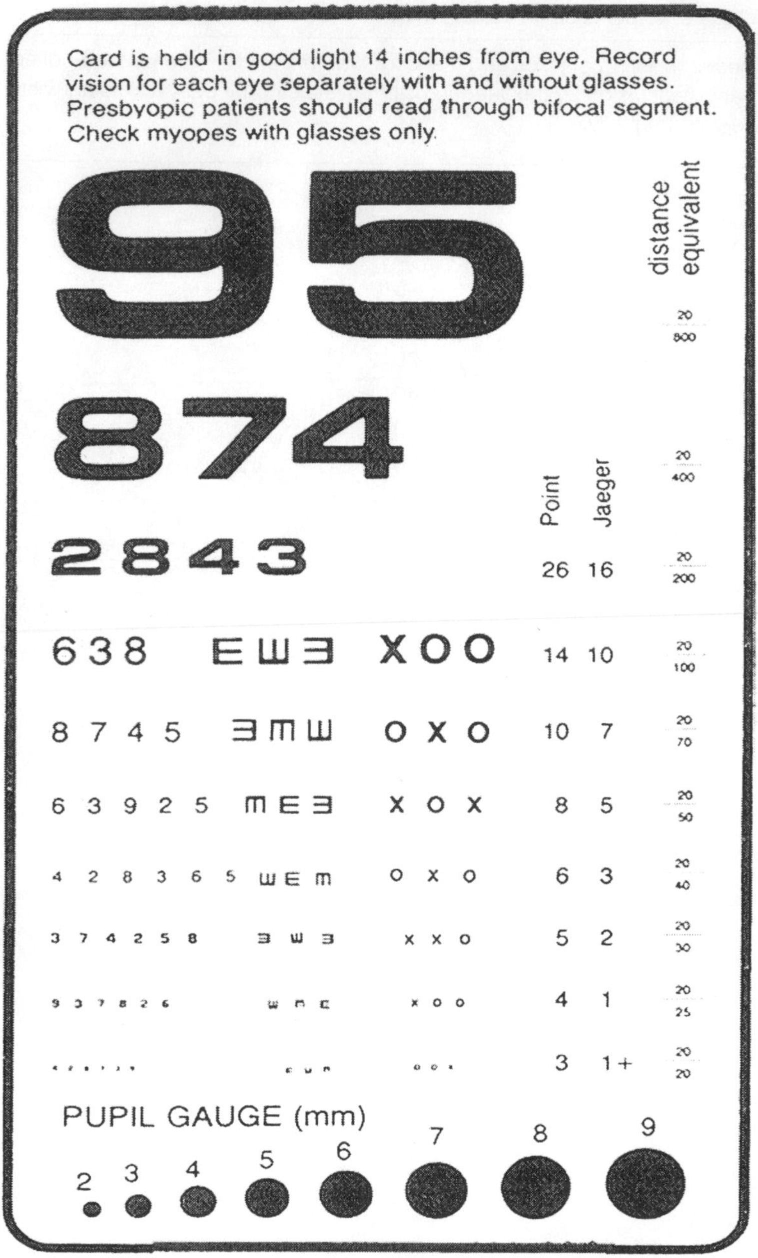

Card is held in good light 14 inches from eye. Record vision for each eye separately with and without glasses. Presbyopic patients should read through bifocal segment. Check myopes with glasses only.

	Point	Jaeger	distance equivalent
95			20/800
874			20/400
2843	26	16	20/200
638 EШƎ XOO	14	10	20/100
8745 ƎmШ OXO	10	7	20/70
63925 mEƎ XOX	8	5	20/50
428365 ШEm OXO	6	3	20/40
374258 ƎШƎ XXO	5	2	20/30
937826	4	1	20/25
	3	1+	20/20

PUPIL GAUGE (mm)

2 3 4 5 6 7 8 9

CHILDHOOD EYE CARE

TABLE 20.2

Pediatric Eye and Vision Screening Guidelines

Test	0–3 Months	6–12 Months	3½ Years	5 Years
Red reflex	X	X	X	X
Symmetric corneal reflex	X	X	X	X
Inspection	X	X	X	X
Differential occlusion (resisting one eye being covered more than the other)		X		
Ability to fix and follow		X		
Cover/uncover (see Table 20.3)		X	X	X
Visual acuity testing			X	X

Reproduced courtesy Gerald R. Page, OD, Columbus, OH.

TABLE 20.3

Strabismus, Pseudostrabismus, and Amblyopia

Amblyopia

Loss of vision in one eye caused by (1) physical occlusion (eg, cataract, ptosis), (2) refractive error (unilateral), or (3) strabismus

Mechanism:

The brain receives a confusing image from the affected eye and selectively suppresses the image

Strabismus

Deviation of the eye in an inward direction (esotropia, crosseyed), outward direction (exotropia, walleyed), or vertical direction (hypertropia)

Mechanism:

Paralytic: Caused by damage to cranial nerves III, IV, or VI or by a lesion in the extraocular muscle itself. May be caused by brain tumor, encephalitis, intracranial aneurysm, vascular accident, thyrotropic exophthalmos, myasthenia gravis, or orbital cellulitis

Nonparalytic: The most common form, resulting in suppression amblyopia

Detection:

Corneal light reflex: Normal eye position will show a penlight reflected in the exact center of each pupil. Displacement of corneal light reflex in one eye suggests strabismus

Cover/uncover test: To diagnose strabismus, cover the disconjugate eye and then remove the cover. The eye remains deviated. Cover the other eye; the deviated eye straightens and the covered eye turns inward (under the cover)

Treatment:

If not corrected by age 6 months, seek consultation. The ophthalmologist will probably follow this outline:

1. *Nonparalytic*:

Refractive error: Correct it. Remember that if eye is farsighted it will converge to accommodate, producing esotropia

No refractive error: Alternately patch the eyes to exercise the extraocular muscles and stimulate vision in both eyes. Consider surgical intervention if this fails

2. *Paralytic*: Specific to neurological diseases

Pseudostrabismus

An optical illusion, usually secondary to broad epicanthal folds. Corneal light reflex is normal

TABLE 20.4

Common Causes of Impaired Tear Drainage in Children

Diagnosis	Features	Treatment
Dacryostenosis	Excessive tearing beyond 2 weeks of age; no global irritation; no distress due to tearing and discharge	Nasolacrimal massage twice a day; cleanse lids with warm water four times daily antibiotics if mucopurulent discharge on eyes and eyelids **96% resolve spontaneously before 1 year of age** If it does not resolve after 1 year old: nasolacrimal probing If it does not resolve after 1 year old *and* nonresponsive to probing: advanced surgical procedures
Dacryocystitis (with or without pericystitis)	Sac area swollen, red, and tender; possible fever and irritation due to infection	Hot compress to affected area four times daily Antibiotics: erythromycin 30–50 mg/kg/d or dicloxacillin 12.5–25 mg/kg/d May be indication for surgical intervention
Mucocele (proximal and distal obstruction)	Firm, bluish subcutaneous mass below medial canthus of eyelid	Initial warm compress, massage as for dacryostenosis; probing at first sign of inflammation

TABLE 20.5

Geriatric Eye Moisture Problems

Cause	Signs and Symptoms	Mechanism	Treatment	Differential Diagnosis
Dry eye syndrome	Ocular burning, foreign body sensation, photophobia, blurred vision	Decrease in tear production by lacrimal gland with increasing age. Exacerbated by orbicular muscle weakness and incomplete lid closure	Artificial tears, lubricants, ointments; punctal occlusion in severe cases	Seasonal allergic conjunctivitis, drug-induced conjunctivitis, superior limbic conjunctivitis, trichiasis, Sjogren syndrome
Excessive tearing	Watery eyes, tears rolling down face, condition worsens in cold weather	Hypersecretion of tears or impaired lacrimal drainage	Wipe tears as necessary, no intervention indicated unless there is a punctal occlusion or a large ectropion	Keratitis, blepharitis, conjunctivitis, atopy, sinusitis, facial palsy, reflex tearing of red eye, dacrocystitis, punctal obstruction, ectropion, obstruction of lacrimal sac, Sjogren syndrome

COMMON OPHTHALMIC CONDITIONS

TABLE 20.6

Differential Diagnosis for Common Causes of Red Eye

Aspect	Acute Conjunctivitis	Acute Iritis (Uveitis)	Angle-Closure Glaucoma	Corneal Ulcer or Trauma
Redness	Diffuse; more toward fornices	Circumcorneal	Diffuse; mainly circumcorneal	Diffuse; mainly circumcorneal
Vision	Normal	Slightly blurred	Markedly blurred	Blurred
Discharge	Large	None	None	Watery or purulent
Pain	None	Moderate	Severe	Moderate to severe
Cornea	Clear	Anterior chamber may be cloudy	Cloudy	Opacity, fluorescein positive
Pupil size	Normal	Small, irregular	Moderately dilated	Normal or small if secondary iritis
Pupil light response	Normal	Poor	Unreactive to light	Normal
Intraocular pressure	Normal	Normal	Increased	Normal
Smear/culture	Causative organism	No organisms	No organisms	Organisms found only in corneal ulcers due to infection
Therapy	Antibiotics	Ophthalmology referral	Ophthalmology referral	Antibiotics
Prognosis	3–5 days	Definitive treatment needed to avoid serious complications		

TABLE 20.7

Glaucoma

Diagnosis	Symptoms	Treatment
Primary open-angle glaucoma	The anterior chamber angle anatomy appears normal, but aqueous outflow is reduced. Progressive visual field loss begins in the periphery and occurs so insidiously that affected individuals may be unaware until late in the disease course	1. Request consultation for confirmation and management 2. Topical medications (may be additive in their effects): ■ Topical beta-adrenergic antagonists ■ Alpha-2 selective adrenergic agonists ■ Nonselective adrenergic agonists ■ Carbonic anhydrase inhibitors ■ Prostaglandin analogs ■ Cholinergic agonists 3. Laser trabeculoplasty (if glaucoma not controlled by medication) 4. Glaucoma surgery (trabeculectomy) (if medical therapy and laser trabeculoplasty do not lower intraocular pressure to acceptable level)
Angle-closure glaucoma	Red, painful eye Nausea and vomiting are common The pupil is usually fixed in a mid-dilated position and nonreactive to light, and the cornea appears cloudy due to pressure-driven edema	*Requires immediate treatment to decrease intraocular pressure and urgent referral to ophthalmologist.* 1. Topical antiglaucomatous medications: ■ Beta-adrenergic antagonists ■ Alpha-adrenergic agonists ■ Carbonic anhydrase inhibitors ■ Osmotic diuretics

Diagnosis	Symptoms	Treatment
	The iris is bowed forward by posterior accumulation of aqueous humor, thereby sealing off the anterior chamber angle	2. Topical pilocarpine (2%) (to facilitate breaking pupillary block) 3. Acetazolamide (500 mg) **Strong miotics and mydriatic-cycloplegic agents exacerbate condition and should be avoided** The contralateral eye is treated prophylactically on an elective basis
Secondary glaucomas	Inflammatory debris may clog trabecular meshwork in uveitis Angle recession glaucoma may follow blunt trauma up to several years after inciting event Congenital glaucoma may result from malformation (eg, aniridia) causing mechanical dysfunction of trabecular meshwork Retinal ischemia from diabetic retinopathy or vascular occlusion may cause neovascularization of the anterior chamber angle leading to neovascular glaucoma	Treatment requires panretinal laser photocoagulation

TABLE 20.8

Conjunctival Abnormalities

	Subconjunctival Hemorrhage	Pinguecula	Pterygium
Physical findings	Focal, bright red lesion that obscures underlying sclera No pain or vision loss	Conjunctival thickening that is elevated, white to yellow in color, and horizontally oriented May become red with surface keratinization	Focal conjunctival thickening in the palpebral fissure area Inflammation may cause redness and irritation
Distinguishing characteristics	Lacks any vascular injection in or around the lesion	Less transparent than normal conjunctiva, often have a fatty appearance, are usually bilateral, and more often nasally than temporally; avoids the cornea	More often nasally than temporally, although both occur *Invasion of the cornea distinguishes a pterygium from a pinguecula*
Etiology	Blunt trauma, severe coughing or retching, or long-term anticoagulation therapy	Causes unknown Likely associated with increasing age and ultraviolet light exposure Seen in most eyes by 70 years of age, and in almost all by 80 years of age	Associated with ultraviolet light exposure
Prognosis	Benign, although may enlarge due to dispersion of blood	Rarely associated with any symptoms other than a minimal cosmetic defect When inflamed, the diagnosis of pingueculitis may be given	Good prognosis with treatment, although incidence of recurrence is high
Treatment	Cold compress first 12 hours, then warm compress next 48 hours Complete resolution takes 5–10 days Nonresolving condition requires referral to rule out rare pathological conditions (eg, Kaposi sarcoma, lymphoma)	Pingueculitis responds to a brief course of topical corticosteroids. Chronically inflamed or cosmetically unsatisfactory pingueculae rarely warrant simple excision	Treatment indicated when it encroaches upon the visual axis, induces significant regular or irregular astigmatism, or becomes cosmetically bothersome. Simple excision of the pterygium on the cornea and sclera. For larger and recurrent pterygia the goal of treatment has been prevention of recurrence

TABLE 20.9

Herpes Infections of the Eye

Simplex: Ulcers on the eyelid may be inoculated into the eye, and this forms a dendritic corneal ulcer (a zigzag surface lesion). These are difficult to treat and may cause corneal scarring. Most often they are referred for care. Oral acyclovir can be used. (Note: Topical corticosteroids should not be used because they will encourage corneal spread of the virus.)

Zoster: When involving the eye, it is in the typical unilateral trigeminal distribution. The conjunctiva is red, and the cornea shows discrete white subepithelial opacities. Fine dendritic ulcers may occur. Cycloplegics, antivirals, topical corticosteroids, and pain medications should be used. Consultation is suggested.

RETINAL EXAMINATION

FIGURE 20.2

Normal Retina

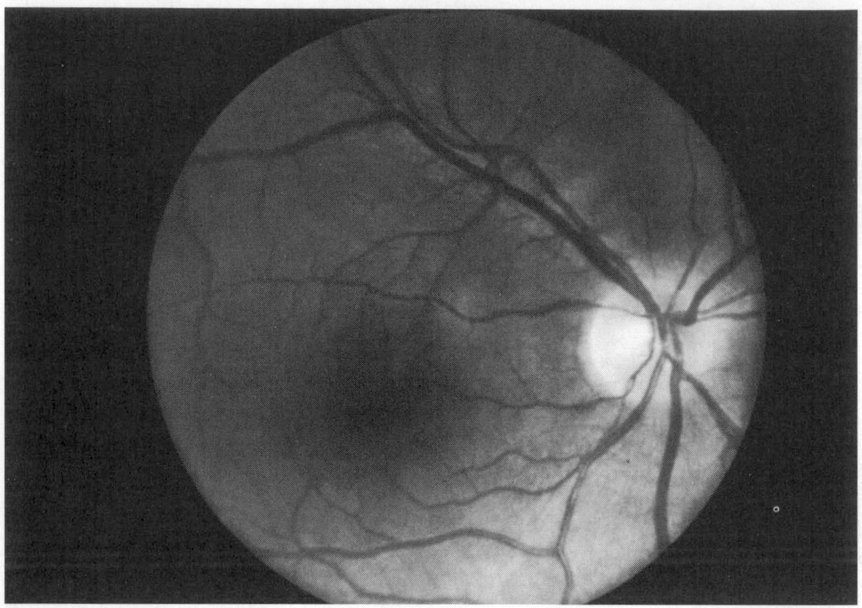

FIGURE 20.3

Glaucoma

Cupping due to glaucoma extends to edge of the optic disc.

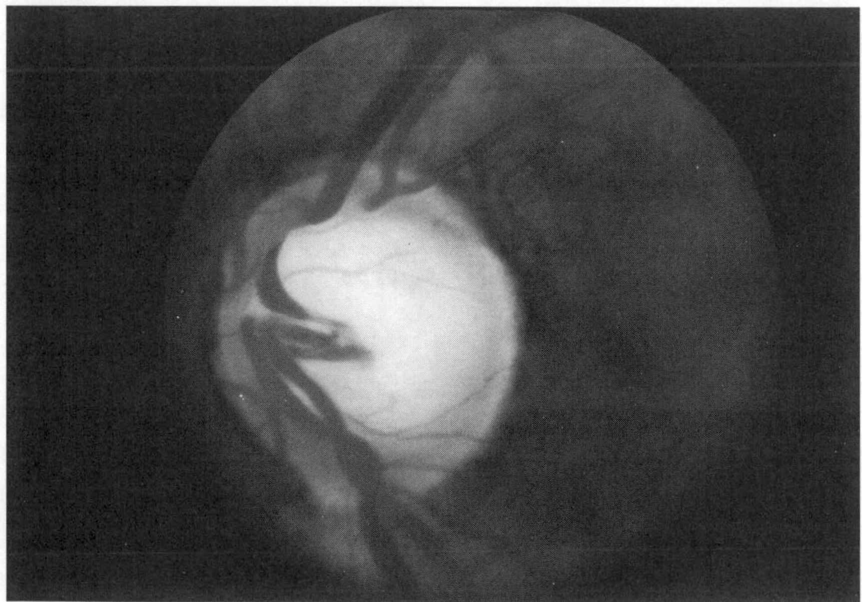

FIGURE 20.4

Senile Macular Degeneration

Note scattered exudates in the macular area and absent foveal light reflex. There may be scattered hemorrhages.

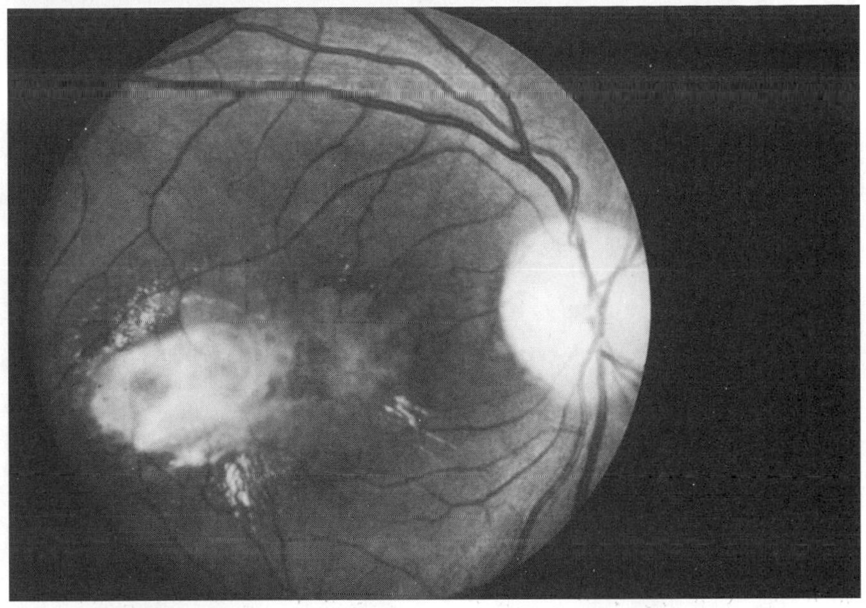

FIGURE 20.5

Diabetic Retinopathy

Note small hemorrhages and scattered exudates.

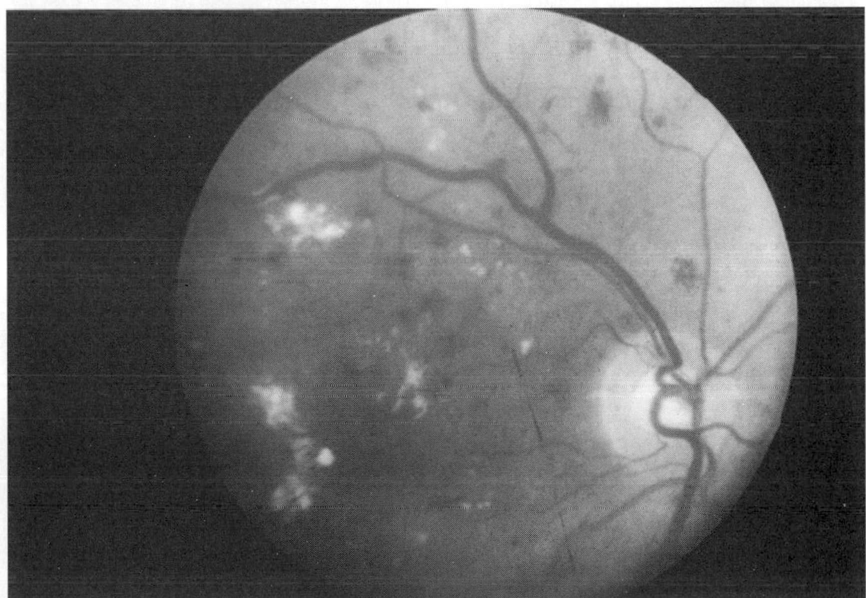

FIGURE 20.6

Diabetic Retinitis Proliferans

Note sheets of connective tissue and new blood vessels near the optic disc.

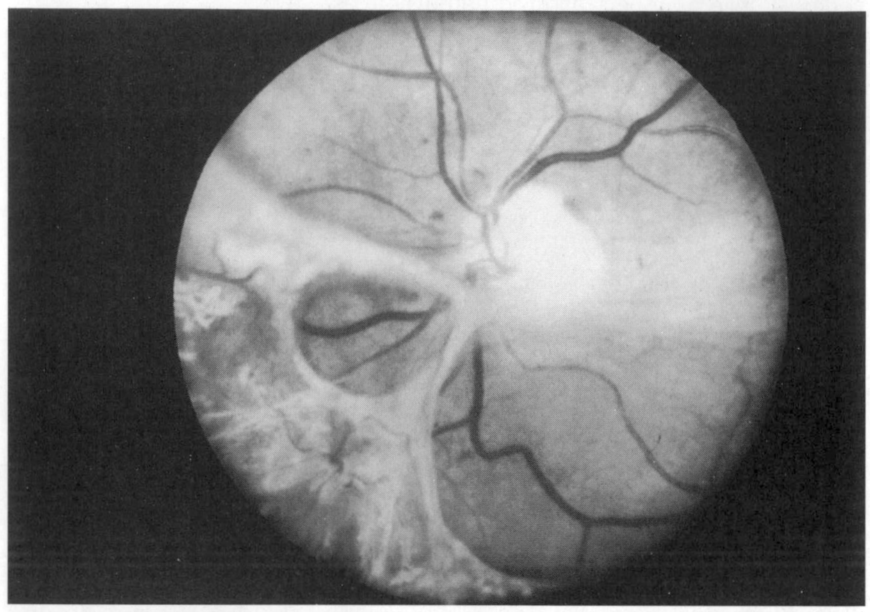

FIGURE 20.7

Hypertensive Retinopathy

Note arteriovenous nicking and hard exudates.

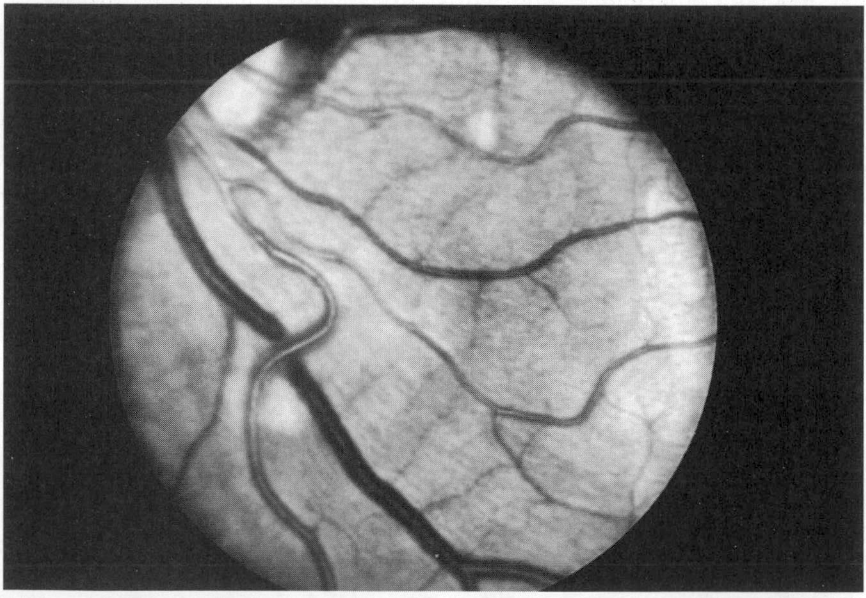

TABLE 20.10

Painless Loss of Vision

Disorder	Onset	Pupil Response	Retinal Examination
Cataract	Slow	Normal	Clouded due to lens opacities
Chronic glaucoma	Slow	Normal	Optic disc cupping
Central retinal artery occlusion	Fast	Absent	Cherry-red macula, pale fundus with thin branching fundus
Central retinal vein occlusion	Fast	Normal	Tortuous vessels, congestion, hemorrhages
Diabetic retinopathy	Slow	Normal	Dot hemorrhages, cotton wool exudates
Macular degeneration	Slow	Normal	Mottling and pigment changes in macular area
Optic atrophy	Slow	Absent	Optic disc pallor
Optic neuritis	Fast	Absent	Optic disc normal, swollen, possibly pale
Retinal detachment	Fast	Normal	Ballooning of retina
Vitreous hemorrhage	Fast	Variable	Exam obscured by blood, red reflex variable

EXTRAOCULAR MUSCLES

TABLE 20.11

Extraocular Muscle Innervation

Nerve	Cranial No.	Muscle	Function	Results of Deficit
Oculomotor	III	Medial rectus	Moves eye toward nose	Eye looks downward because of unopposed action of lateral rectus and superior oblique
		Superior rectus	Upward gaze	Weakness of upward gaze
		Inferior rectus	Downward gaze	Weakness of downward gaze
		Inferior oblique	Moves eye up when looking nasally Rotates eye when looking temporally	Vertical diplopia; head remains tilted to compensate
		Levator of upper eyelid (levator palpebrae superioris)	Moves eye up and out when in forward gaze	Severe ptosis
Trochlear	IV	Superior oblique	Moves eye down when looking nasally Rotates eye when looking temporally Moves eye down and out when in forward gaze	Vertical diplopia; head remains tilted to compensate
Abducens	VI	Lateral rectus	Moves eye temporally	Inability to look temporally
Cervical sympathetics		Müller	Elevates upper lid	Mild ptosis

TABLE 20.12

Common Eye Symptoms

Eye Symptoms	Most Common Diagnoses
Acute spontaneous loss of vision in one eye, transient	Transient ischemic attack involving blood circulation to retina; lasting deficit may indicate central retinal artery occlusion or arteriolar or venous hemorrhage
	Migraine
Acute spontaneous loss of vision in both eyes, transient	Transient ischemic attack involving blood circulation to visual areas of the brain
	Migraine
Floaters; no other visual difficulties	Vitreous opacities, usually insignificant
Lightning flashes	Migraine (often also manifest as "wavy" appearance of environment)
	May accompany traction on retina or retinal detachment
Curtain drawn over an eye	Retinal detachment or hemorrhage
Blurred vision—far only	Myopia
Blurred vision—near only	Hyperopia; use of cycloplegic drops; presbyopia
Double vision	Nerve or muscle damage; if monocular, may reflect lens dislocation or cataract
Vertigo (sensation of spinning, either the patient or the environment)	Dysfunction of vestibular apparatus or its connection in the brainstem

TABLE 20.13

Common Eye Signs

Sign	Diagnosis	Treatment
Tender pimple on lid margin	Hordeolum (stye)	Warm compresses qid Topical antibiotic Referral or I&D if persistent
Tender nodule in lid away from margin	Chalazion	Warm compress Antibiotics of little value Referral for excision if persistent
Ulcerated lesion with pearly border (lower lid)	Basal cell carcinoma	Excision or referral for excision
Soft, yellow, raised lid lesions	Xanthelasma	Can be cosmetically removed Check for diabetes and hyperlipidemia
Lower conjunctiva exposed and red	Ectropion	Plastic repair
Foreign body sensation; lid margin not seen	Entropion	Plastic repair
Ecchymosis of lid	Black eye	Examine eye for diplopia Ice for 24 hours
Red hemorrhagic sclera	Subconjunctival hemorrhage	No treatment
Warm, tender swelling in superolateral aspect of upper lid	Lacrimal gland inflammation	Treat infection Rule out tumor
Warm, tender swelling of nasal aspect of lower lid	Lacrimal sac inflammation	Antistaphylococcal topical antibiotics Warm compresses Massage lacrimal sac
Crusty, sore eyelids with scaling	Blepharitis	Topical antibiotics Dandruff control
Ocular pain—eye injected temporally	Episcleritis	Consultation Steroids
Ocular pain—halos around lights	Glaucoma	Measure pressure Consultation
Soft yellow patches on sclera at 3 o'clock and 9 o'clock	Pinguecula	No treatment

Sign	Diagnosis	Treatment
Scleral vascularization extending to nasal cornea	Pterygium	Can be cosmetically removed
Mild ptosis, small pupil and same-sided decreased facial sweating	Horner syndrome	Consultation, chest x-ray film A large differential, including tumor

TABLE 20.14

Ocular Manifestation of Systemic Disease

AIDS: Retinopathy with "cotton wool" spots on retina; Kaposi sarcoma of eyelids and conjunctiva; keratitis; herpes zoster; uveitis; *Candida* chorioretinitis; molluscum contagiosum of eyelids; cytomegalovirus (CMV) retinitis.

Albinism: Light fundus background (choroidal vessels seen easily with ophthalmoscope as pigment epithelium is unpigmented); nystagmus; poor vision (high refractive errors and poor macular development); pink-blue iris (iris transilluminates).

Alkaptonuria: Melanin deposits in sclera (at 9 o'clock and 3 o'clock positions around the cornea).

Amyloidosis: Weakness of extraocular muscles; vitreous opacities; pupillary abnormalities; amyloid nodules in lids and conjunctiva.

Anemia: Conjunctiva appears pale; retinal hemorrhages and exudates present.

Ankylosing spondylitis: Uveitis; scleritis; scleromalacia perforans (thinning of the sclera with exposure of the uveal tissue).

Atopic dermatitis: Cataracts; keratoconus.

Behçet syndrome: Uveitis.

Crohn disease: Uveitis.

Cystic fibrosis: Papilledema; retinal hemorrhages.

Cystinosis: Deposits of cystine crystals in cornea and conjunctiva.

Cytomegalic inclusion disease (congenital): Chorioretinitis, cataracts.

Dermatomyositis: Extraocular muscle palsies; lid edema; scleritis; uveitis; retinal exudates.

Diabetes mellitus: Extraocular muscle palsies; xanthelasmas; retinal microaneurysms; hemorrhages, exudates, and neovascularization of the retina; cataracts; rubeosis iridis (neovascularization of the iris); glaucoma.

Down syndrome: Up-and-out obliquity to the lids; Brushfield spots (white speckling of iris); cataracts; myopia; strabismus.

Ehlers-Danlos syndrome: Blue sclera; strabismus; epicanthal folds.

Friedreich ataxia: Nystagmus; strabismus; retinitis pigmentosa.

Galactosemia: Cataracts.

Glomerulonephritis: Periorbital edema; hypertensive retinopathy.

Gout: Episcleritis, uveitis; deposition of uric acid crystals in cornea.

Hereditary hemorrhagic telangiectasia (Osler-Weber-Rendu disease): Telangiectasis of conjunctiva and retina.

Herpes zoster: Dermatitis along ophthalmic branch of cranial nerve V; uveitis; keratitis.

Histoplasmosis: Chorioretinal scars, retinal hemorrhage.

Homocystinuria: Dislocated lens.

Hyperlipidemia: Xanthelasma, arcus juvenilis, lipemia retinalis (milky retinal vessels secondary to excessive lipids in the blood).

Hyperparathyroidism: Band keratopathy (gray-white band containing calcium deposits, extending horizontally across the cornea); optic atrophy.

Hyperthyroidism: Proptosis, lid retraction; infrequent blinking (staring); lid lag on downward gaze, weakness of upward gaze; poor convergence; diplopia, corneal erosion (from poor lid closure); papilledema; papillitis.

Hypoparathyroidism: Cataracts; papilledema; optic neuritis.

Hypothyroidism (congenital cretinism): Strabismus; farsightedness; cataracts; swollen lids with narrow slits between lids; wide-set eyes; retrobulbar neuritis; optic atrophy; loss of outer half of eyebrows.

Impending stroke: Amaurosis fugax (transient blindness from intermittent vascular compromise in arteriosclerotic disease); Hollenhorst plaques (glistening emboli seen at branch points of retinal arterioles).

Kernicterus (erythroblastosis fetalis): Strabismus; nystagmus; retinal hemorrhage.

Lead poisoning: Papilledema; optic atrophy.

Lupus erythematosus: Retinal hemorrhages; cotton wool exudates; papilledema; lid lesions similar to lesions elsewhere; episcleritis; keratitis; uveitis; nystagmus; extraocular muscle palsies; cataracts.

Macroglobulinemia: Venous occlusion (engorged retinal veins with hemorrhages and exudates); papilledema.

Marchesani syndrome: Dislocated lens.

Marfan syndrome: Dislocated lens.

Migraine: Throbbing eye pain: transient visual compromise (eg, flashing lights, waves, hemianopia); miotic (small) pupil (sympathetic axon compromise with carotid artery wall edema).

Mucopolysaccharidoses: Corneal clouding.

Multiple sclerosis: Retrobulbar neuritis; optic atrophy; internuclear ophthalmoplegia; strabismus.

Continued

TABLE 20.14

Ocular Manifestation of Systemic Disease, cont'd

Myasthenia gravis: Ptosis; extraocular muscle paresis.

Myotonia: Cataracts.

Neurofibromatosis: Lid and orbital tumors; optic gliomas.

Osteogenesis imperfecta: Blue sclera (choroid shows through thin sclera).

Polyarteritis nodosa: Episcleritis; corneal ulcers, uveitis; retinal hemorrhages and exudates; papilledema; hypertensive retinopathy; arteriolar occlusion.

Polycythemia: Markedly dilated retinal veins; papilledema.

Pseudoxanthoma elasticum: Angioid streaks (reddish bands radiating from disc region, resembling blood vessels, probably representing defects in the choroidal membrane [Bruch membrane] just outside the pigment epithelium. Also found in Paget diseases of the bone and sickle cell disease).

Radiation exposure: Cataracts; retinopathy.

Reiter syndrome: Triad of arthritis, urethritis, and uveitis.

Rheumatoid arthritis: Uveitis; band keratopathy; scleromalacia perforans (degeneration and thinning of anterior sclera with bulging out of underlying bluish choroid).

Riley-Day syndrome (familial dysautonomia): Decreased tear production; decreased corneal sensation with subsequent exposure keratitis.

Rosacea: Blepharitis; conjunctivitis; keratitis; episcleritis.

Rubella (congenital): Cataracts; microphthalmia; cloudy corneas; uveitis; pigmentary retinopathy.

Sarcoid: Uveitis; whitish perivenous infiltrates in retina; band keratopathy.

Sickle cell anemia: Retinal hemorrhages, exudates, microaneurysms, neovascularization (vascular and hemorrhagic changes are worse in sickle cell-hemoglobin C disease than in sickle cell-hemoglobin S disease); papilledema; angioid streaks.

Sjogren syndrome: Dry eyes; corneal erosions.

Stevens-Johnson syndrome: Purulent conjunctivitis with scarring of conjunctiva and cornea.

Subacute bacterial endocarditis: Conjunctival and retinal hemorrhages; Roth spots (retinal hemorrhages with white centers).

Sturge-Weber syndrome: Congenital glaucoma on side of facial nevus.

Syphilis: Interstitial keratitis (inflammation, edema, and vascular infiltration of cornea, particularly the corneal periphery); uveitis; optic neuritis; cataracts; chorioretinitis; lens dislocation; Argyll-Robertson pupil.

Tay-Sachs disease: Cherry red spot (cloudiness of retina, except in fovea region).

Temporal arteritis: Transient or permanent loss of vision from vasculitis affecting the optic nerve.

Toxemia: Hypertensive retinopathy.

Toxoplasmosis: Chorioretinitis.

Trichinosis: Inflammation of extraocular muscles.

Tuberculosis: Uveitis; chorioretinitis.

Tuberous sclerosis: Retinal tumor.

Ulcerative colitis: Uveitis (also found in Crohn disease).

Vitamin deficiencies:

Vitamin A deficiency: Night blindness; xerophthalmia (drying of cornea and conjunctiva).

Thiamine deficiency (beriberi): Optic neuritis; extraocular muscle weakness.

Niacin deficiency (pellagra): Optic neuritis.

Riboflavin deficiency: Photophobia; inflammation of conjunctiva and cornea.

Vitamin C deficiency (scurvy): Hemorrhages within and outside the eye.

Vitamin D deficiency: Cataracts; papilledema (as in hypoparathyroidism).

Von Hippel-Lindau disease: Retinal hemangiomas.

Wilms tumor: Aniridia (absence of iris).

Wilson disease: Copper deposits in Descemet membrane in the peripheral cornea (Kayser-Fleischer ring) and in the lens (copper cataracts).

Adapted from Goldberg S. *Ophthalmology Made Ridiculously Simple*. 2nd ed. Miami: MedMaster; 2001.

AIDs indicates acquired immunodeficiency syndrome.

TABLE 20.15
Refractive Surgery

	LASIK	Photorefractive Keratectomy (PRK)	Radial Keratotomy (RK)	Intrastromal Corneal Ring Segments
Definition	A corneal flap is raised and a laser is used to change the shape of the cornea beneath	No corneal flap A laser is used to change the corneal shape	A scalpel is used to make radial cuts to flatten the cornea	Small transparent ring segments implanted into the periphery of the cornea
Indication	To correct distance vision. Best procedure for keloid formers and high refractive error	To correct distance vision Best for low to moderate refractive error	To correct distance vision	To correct distance vision Only used for low refractive error and over age 21 with stable vision
Limitation	Cannot correct presbyopia and is not reversible	Cannot correct presbyopia and is not reversible Contraindicated in rheumatoid arthritis, lupus, immuno-compromised patients, systemic illness, and keloid formers	Cannot correct presbyopia Glare at night Unpredictable vision correction Vulnerable to rupture Not reversible	Reversible
Healing	Fast vision recovery, steroids and antibiotics for 4 days	More painful, slower healing time Steroids and antibiotics for 1–4 months	Fast recovery	Fast recovery

Reproduced courtesy Gerald R. Page, OD, Columbus, OH.

LASIK indicates laser in situ keratomiteusis.

EYE TRAUMA

TABLE 20.16

Treatment for Chemical Burn

1. Identify the chemical, if possible
2. Rule out globe perforations from explosion pieces
3. Use topical anesthetics
4. Irrigate eye with water or saline for at least 20 minutes
5. Test pH in the inferior cul-de-sac
6. Repeat irrigation at 20- to 30-minute intervals until pH is nearly neutral (pH = 7)
7. Examine cornea:

   A. *Clear cornea*: Stain with fluorescein to estimate damage

   Mild to moderate epithelial damage:

   - Topical antibiotic
   - Patch
   - Examine daily until healed (2–3 days)

   Marked epithelial damage:

   - Consult ophthalmologist

   Pupillary constriction (indicates intraocular irritation):

   - Consult ophthalmologist
   - Consider emergency use of cycloplegic drop on recommendation of ophthalmologist

   B. *Cloudy cornea*: Irreversible damage; consult ophthalmologist

FIGURE 20.8

Blunt Injury to the Eye

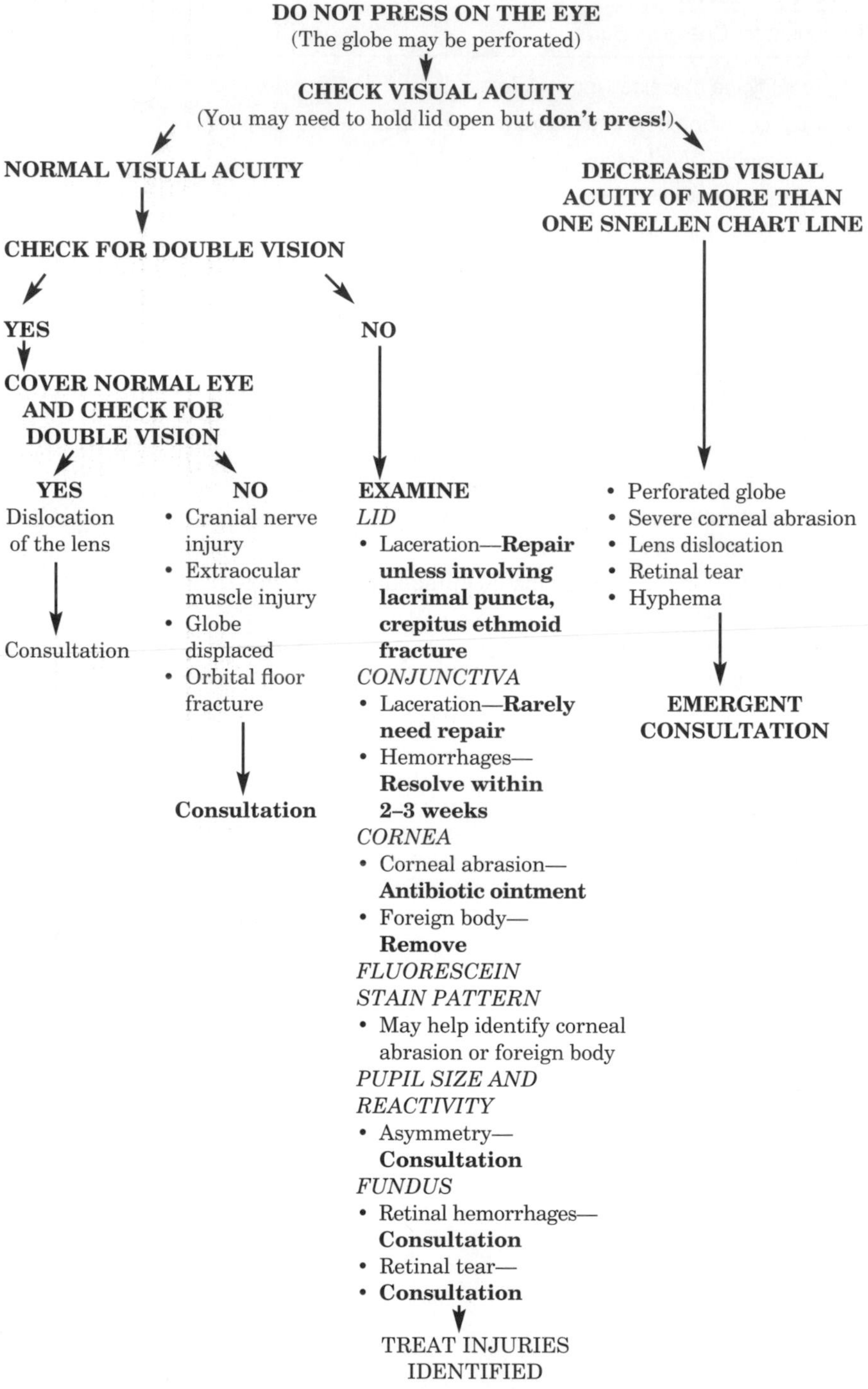

DO NOT PRESS ON THE EYE
(The globe may be perforated)
↓
CHECK VISUAL ACUITY
(You may need to hold lid open but **don't press!**)

↙ **NORMAL VISUAL ACUITY**
↓
CHECK FOR DOUBLE VISION

↙ **YES**
↓
COVER NORMAL EYE AND CHECK FOR DOUBLE VISION

↙ **YES**
Dislocation of the lens
↓
Consultation

↘ **NO**
- Cranial nerve injury
- Extraocular muscle injury
- Globe displaced
- Orbital floor fracture

↓
Consultation

↘ **NO**
↓
EXAMINE

LID
- Laceration—**Repair unless involving lacrimal puncta, crepitus ethmoid fracture**

CONJUNCTIVA
- Laceration—**Rarely need repair**
- Hemorrhages—**Resolve within 2–3 weeks**

CORNEA
- Corneal abrasion—**Antibiotic ointment**
- Foreign body—**Remove**

FLUORESCEIN STAIN PATTERN
- May help identify corneal abrasion or foreign body

PUPIL SIZE AND REACTIVITY
- Asymmetry—**Consultation**

FUNDUS
- Retinal hemorrhages—**Consultation**
- Retinal tear—
- **Consultation**

↓
TREAT INJURIES IDENTIFIED

↘ **DECREASED VISUAL ACUITY OF MORE THAN ONE SNELLEN CHART LINE**
↓
- Perforated globe
- Severe corneal abrasion
- Lens dislocation
- Retinal tear
- Hyphema

↓
EMERGENT CONSULTATION

OCULAR THERAPY

TABLE 20.17

Ophthalmic Antimicrobials

Drug	Dosage Form/Strength
Bacitracin	Ointment (500 U/g)
Chloramphenicol	Ointment (1%); solution (0.16%, 0.5%)
Ciprofloxacin	Solution (0.3%)
Erythromycin	Ointment (5%)
Gentamicin	Ointment or solution (0.3%)
Levofloxacin	Solution (0.5%)
Norfloxacin	Solution (0.3%)
Ofloxacin	Solution (0.3%)
Sulfacetamide	Solution (1%, 10%, 15%, 30%); ointment (10%)
Tobramycin	Solution or ointment (0.3%)
Combination Antibiotic Products	
Neomycin 0.35%; polymyxin B 10,000 U/g, bacitracin 400 U/g in ointment	
Polymyxin B 10,000 U/g; bacitracin 500 U/g in ointment	
Polymyxin B 10,000 U/g or mL; neomycin 0.175%; gramicidin 0.0025% in solution	
Oxytetracycline 0.5% and polymyxin B 10,000 U/g in ointment	
Trimethoprim 0.1% and polymyxin B 10,000 U/g in solution	

Reproduced courtesy Miriam Chan, PharmD, and Matt D. Roth, Columbus, OH.

TABLE 20.18

Some Agents for Allergic Conjunctivitis

Drug (Active Ingredient)	Dosage	Comments
Oral Antihistamine Therapy		
Chlorpheniramine	4–12 mg once or twice daily	Reserve for patients with systemic allergic symptoms Other oral antihistamines are acceptable but much more expensive
Antihistamine Ophthalmic Solution		
Livostin (levocabastine 0.05%)	One drop in affected eye(s) four times daily	H_2-receptor antagonist; preservative—benzalkonium Cl 0.15 mg
Optivar (azelastine HCl 0.05%)	One drop in affected eye(s) two times daily	H_1-receptor antagonist; preservative—benzalkonium Cl 0.125 mg
Patanol (olopatadine HCl 0.1%)	One or two drops in affected eye(s) two times daily	H_1-receptor antagonist and antihistamine; preservative—benzalkonium Cl 0.01%
Zaditor (ketotifen 0.025%)	One drop in affected eye(s) every 8 to 12 hours	H_1-receptor antagonist; preservative—benzalkonium Cl 0.01%
Decongestant Ophthalmic Solution		
Naphcon (naphazoline 0.012%, 0.02%, 0.03%, 0.1%)	One or two drops in affected eye(s) every 3 to 4 hours	Preservative—benzalkonium Cl
Visine LR (oxymetazoline HCl 0.025%)	One or two drops in affected eye(s) every 6 hours	Over-the-counter; preservative—benzalkonium Cl 0.01%, EDTA 0.1%
Visine Original (tetrahydrozoline HCl 0.05%)	One or two drops in affected eye(s) four times daily	Over-the-counter; Preservative-Benzalkonium Cl 0.01%, EDTA 0.1%
Antihistamine/Decongestant Combination Ophthalmic Solution		
Naphcon A (pheniramine maleate 0.3%; naphazoline HCl 0.025%)	One or two drops in affected eye(s) four times daily	Over-the-counter; preservative—Benzalkonium Cl 0.01%
Vasocon A (antazoline 0.5%; naphazoline 0.05%)	One or two drops in affected eye(s) four times daily	Preservative—benzalkonium Cl 0.01%

Drug (Active Ingredient)	Dosage	Comments
Mast Cell Stabilizer Ophthalmic Solution		
Alamast (pemirolast K 0.1%)	One or two drops in affected eye(s) four times daily	Preservative—lauralkonium Cl 0.005%
Alocril (nedocromil Na 2%)	One or two drops in *each eye* two times daily	Preservative—benzalkonium Cl 0.01%
Opticrom (cromolyn Na 4%)	One or two drops in affected eye(s) four to six times daily *for up to 6 weeks*	Preservative—benzalkonium Cl 0.01%
Nonsteroidal Anti-inflammatory Ophthalmic Solution		
Acular (ketorolac tromethamine 0.5%)	One drop in affected eye(s) four times daily	Preservative—benzalkonium Cl 0.01%

Reproduced courtesy Miriam Chan, PharmD, and Matt D. Roth, Columbus, OH.

Cl indicates chloride; EDTA, edetic acid; HCl, hydrochloride; K, potassium; Na, sodium.

TABLE 20.19

Ocular Manifestations of Common Drugs

Allopurinol: Cataracts.

Amantadine: Visual hallucination (reversible) more common in the elderly.

Amiodarone: Corneal deposits.

Antianxiety agents: Diplopia.

Antihistamines: Blurred vision, mydriasis, decreased lacrimal secretions.

Antimalarials: Corneal deposits and edema, ptosis, decreased accommodation.

Antituberculosis drugs: Optic neuritis and optic atrophy.

Contraceptives: Corneal edema (may interfere with contact lens wearing), papilledema, migraine.

Corticosteroids: Cataracts, increased intraocular pressure, retinal edema, papilledema.

Digitalis: Yellow hue to vision (xanthopsia), conjunctivitis, decreased vision.

Diuretics: Retinal edema, retinal hemorrhages, myopia.

Gold: Corneal, conjunctival, and lens gold deposits, ptosis.

Haloperidol: Oculogyric crisis.

Ibuprofen: Reduced vision and change in color vision.

Indomethacin: Reduced vision and change in color vision.

Metoclopramide: Oculogyric crisis.

Pentazocine (Talwin): Constriction of pupils and visual hallucinations.

Phenothiazines: Posterior corneal deposits, Horner syndrome, oculogyric crisis.

Phenytoin: Frequent nystagmus, ophthalmoplegia and resulting diplopia, cataracts.

Sildenafil citrate (Viagra): Temporary vision loss, reduced vision, causes blue tint to color perception.

Tamoxifen: Corneal opacities, reduced vision, retinopathy.

Tetracycline: Blurring of vision, diplopia, papilledema (reversible).

Thioridazine (Mellaril): Pigment deposits on retina.

Tricyclic antidepressants: Mydriasis, angle-closure glaucoma, cycloplegia.

Vitamin A: Papilledema, nystagmus, diplopia, color vision disturbance.

Vitamin D: Band keratopathy.

TABLE 20.20

Alternative Treatments Used for Ocular Conditions

	Other Names/Forms	Used for	Proposed Mechanism of Action	Effectiveness	Safety
Areca (*Areca catechu*)	Betel nut, *Areca* nut	Glaucoma	Cholinergic effect	Insufficient information	Likely unsafe when used orally because of carcinogenic potential
Eyebright	Euphrasia, clary sage, clear eye	Conjunctivitis, blepharitis, eye fatigue, inflamed eyelids and conjunctiva	Components of flower have antibacterial and astringent properties	Likely not effective. Originally used because flower resembles an open eye	Safe if ingested in moderate amounts Potentially unsafe as ophthalmic agent because of hygienic concerns
Glutathione	GSH, glutamyl-cysteinylglycine	Glaucoma and cataracts	Naturally synthesized in liver, serves as antioxidant; natural deficiency leads to macular degeneration	Likely ineffective when ingested because not absorbed	Likely safe when used orally

	Other Names/Forms	Used for	Proposed Mechanism of Action	Effectiveness	Safety
Jaborandi (*Pilocarpus microphyllus*)	Arruda bravam, Jamguarandi	Glaucoma	Cholinergic effect	Effective and FDA approved when used in small amounts (lethal dose = 60 mg)	**Potentially fatal** Unsafe when leaves ingested because contain large amount of pilocarpine (lethal dose is 5–10 g of leaves). Used industrially for manufacture of pilocarpine
Lutein	Xanthophyll, zeaxanthin (isomer)	Cataracts and macular degeneration	Antioxidant and blue light filter protection from photodamage	Possibly effective, not known if supplementation is effective	Likely safe Naturally found in high amounts in broccoli, spinach, and kale
Marijuana	Tetrahydro-cannabinol, THC, cannabis, pot	Glaucoma	Decrease intraocular pressure	Possibly effective	Possibly unsafe when inhaled

Continued

TABLE 20.20

Alternative Treatments Used for Ocular Conditions, cont'd

	Other Names/Forms	Used for	Proposed Mechanism of Action	Effectiveness	Safety
Nux vomica (*Strychnos nux-vomica*)	Poison nut, Quaker buttons, strychni semen	Diseases of eye	Centrally acting neurotoxins	Likely ineffective	**Potentially fatal** Unsafe, contains strychnine; 30–50 mg of nux vomica has 5 mg of strychnine, which has severe side effects; 1–2 g has lethal dose of strychnine
Vitamin A	Retinoids, retinol, retinal, beta carotene	Glaucoma, cataracts, and promote good vision	Fat-soluble, essential vitamin involved in number of mechanisms including growth and cellular differentiation, immune function, and transduction of light into neural signals for production of vision	Effective in treating ocular problems associated with vitamin A deficiency (night blindness, xeropthalmia). Possibly effective for other ocular disorders (not known if supplementation is effective)	Safe in adults in doses <10,000 U/d, potentially unsafe in larger doses. Naturally found in large amounts in various precursors in eggs, milk, butter, meat, green and leafy vegetables, and carrots

Reproduced courtesy Matt D. Roth, Columbus, OH.

chapter 21

The Kidney and Urinary System

Charles E. Driscoll, MD
Anitha Lokesh, MD

IN THIS CHAPTER

- Examination of the urine
- Renal function
- Urine collection from infants
- Urinary tract infection in children
- Urinary tract imaging in children
- Urinary tract infection in adults
- Management of the urinary system in paralyzed persons
- Prevention of catheter-related infections
- Obstructive uropathy
- Urolithiasis
- Prostate specific antigen interpretation
- Prostatic diseases
- Benign prostatic hypertrophy
- Urinary incontinence
- Prevention of renal insufficiency
- Hematuria
- Hematospermia
- Interstitial cystitis

- Acute and chronic renal failure
- Scrotal problems
- Urological emergencies
- Incidental adrenal masses
- Nephrotic syndrome
- Urologic management of the stroke patient

BOOKSHELF RECOMMENDATIONS

Lipshultz LI, Kleinman I. *Urology and the Primary Care Practitioner*. Baltimore, MD: Gower Medical Publishing; 1996.

Nseyo UO, Weinman E, Lamm DL, eds. *Urology for Primary Care Physicians*. Philadelphia, PA: WB Saunders; 1999.

TABLE 21.1

Substances in Urine That May Change Urine Color

Substance	Colors Produced in Urine
Acetanilid	Yellow to red
Acetophenetidin (metabolite)	Yellow (dark brown to wine color)
Alcohol	Lightens color
Aloin	Red-brown to yellow-pink (alkaline urine), yellow-brown (acid urine)
Aminopyrine	Red-brown
Aminosalicylic acid (para-aminosalicylic acid)	Discoloration (no distinctive color)
Amitriptyline	Blue-green
Anisindione	Orange (alkaline urine), pink to red-brown
Anthraquinone laxatives	Reddish (alkaline urine)
Antipyrine	Yellow to red-brown
Azuresin	Blue or green
Beets	Red
Benzene	Red-brown
Biliverdin	Yellow-green
Carbon tetrachloride	Red-brown
Carrots	Yellow
Cascara	Yellow brown (acid urine), yellow-pink (alkaline urine), darkens to brown to black on standing
Chloroquine	Rust-yellow to brown
Chlorzoxazone	Orange to purple-red
Cinchophen	Red-brown
Creosote	Dark green
Cresol	Dark color on standing
Danthron	Pink to red
Deferoxamine mesylate	Reddish
Dihydroxyanthraquinone	Pink to orange (alkaline urine)
Dinitrophenol	Red-brown
Diphenylhydantoin	Pink to red to reddish brown
Dithiazanine hydrochloride	Blue
Doan's kidney pills	Greenish-blue
Doxorubicin	Red-brown
Emodin (in cascara)	Pink to red-brown (alkaline urine)
Ethoxazene	Orange to red
Ferrous salts	Black
Fluorescein (intravenous)	Yellow-orange
Furazolidone (metabolite)	Brownish to rust-yellow

Continued

TABLE 21.1

Substances in Urine That May Change Urine Color, cont'd

Substance	Colors Produced in Urine
Ibuprofen	Red or pink
Indanediones	Orange (alkaline urine)
Indomethacin	Green (biliverdinemia)
Iron sorbitex	Dark to black on standing
Lead	Red-brown
Levodopa	Dark red-brown
Melanin	Black-brown
Mercury	Red-brown
Methocarbamol	Dark brown, black or green on standing
Methyldopa	Dark (red or black) on standing
Methylene blue	Greenish yellow to blue
Metronidazole	Dark brown in acidic urine
Naphthol	Dark color on standing
Nitrobenzene	Dark color on standing
Nitrofurantoin and derivatives	Brown or rust-yellow
Oxamniquine	Red-orange
Pamaquine naphthoate	Rust-yellow or brown
Phenacetin	Yellow (dark brown to wine color)
Phenazopyridine	Orange-red to red-brown (HNO_3 turns orange to pink)
Phenindione	Reddish brown to pink, orange in alkaline urine
Phenolphthalein	Pink to red to magenta (alkaline urine), yellow-brown (acid urine)
Phenolsulfonphthalein	Red (alkaline urine)
Phenols	Dark green to brownish black (darkens on standing)
Phenothiazines	Pink to red-brown
Phensuximide	Pink to red to red-brown
Phenyl salicylate	Dark green
Phenytoin	Pink to red to reddish brown
Picric acid	Yellow to red-brown
Porphyrins	Burgundy red, darkens on standing
Primaquine phosphate	Rust-yellow to brown
Pyocyanin	Blue-green
Pyrogallol	Brown to black (darkens on standing)
Quinacrine hydrochloride	Yellow (deep yellow on acidification)
Quinine and derivatives	Brown to black

Substance	Colors Produced in Urine
Resorcinol	Dark green to green-blue, darkens on standing
Rhubarb	Yellow-brown (acid urine), yellow-pink (alkaline urine), darkens to brown to black on standing
Riboflavin	Yellow
Rifampin	Red to orange
Salicylazosulfapyridine	Orange-yellow (alkaline urine)
Salol	Dark color on standing
Santonin	Bright yellow (NaOH changes to pink or scarlet)
Senna	Yellow-brown (acid urine), yellow-pink (alkaline urine), darkens on standing
Sulfonamides	Rust-yellow or brown
Sulfonethylmethane	Red
Sulfonmethane	Red-brown
Tetralin (tetrahydronaphthalene)	Greenish blue
Thiazosulfone	Pink to red
Thymol	Greenish blue
TNT (trinitrotoluene)	Red-brown
Tolonium (Blutene)	Blue-green
Triamterene	Bluish color (pale blue fluorescence)
Warfarin sodium	Orange

Adapted from Martin EW. *Hazards of Medication.* Philadelphia, PA: JB Lippincott; 1978 and Raymond JR, Yarger WE. Abnormal urine color: differential diagnosis. *South Med J.* 1988;81:837–841.

FIGURE 21.1

Microscopic Appearance of Urine Sediment

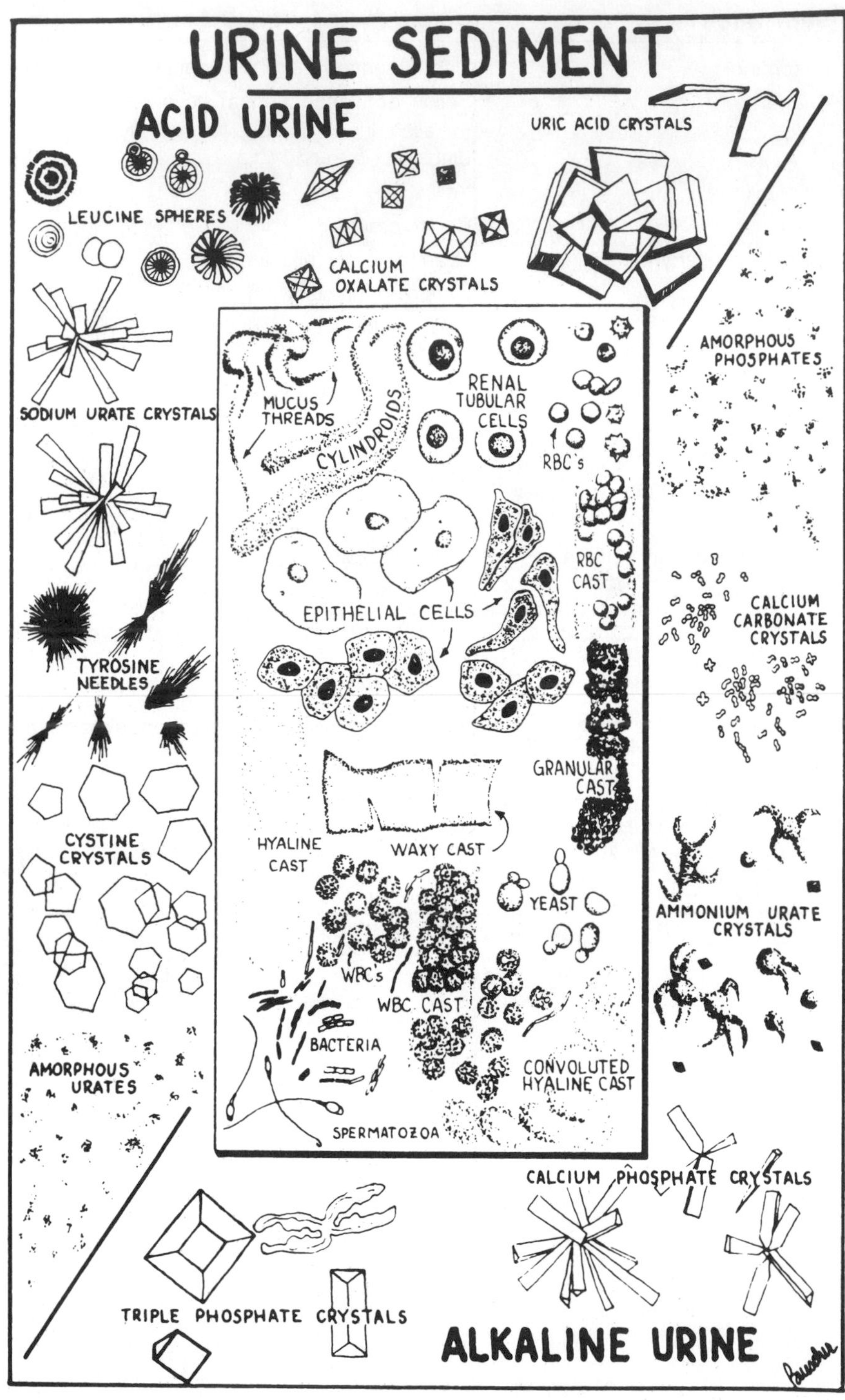

TABLE 21.2

Twenty-four-Hour Urine Collections

Collection Technique	
As soon as awakening from sleep, void into toilet and discard. Collect all urinations for the next 24 hours, including first urine after awakening next day. Check with laboratory to see if preservatives are needed in collection container.	
Normal Values	
Calcium	<150 mg/24 h on low-calcium diet
Chloride	140–250 mEq/L
Citrate	2.4–5.1 mmol/24 h
Creatinine	
Males	19–26 mg/kg of body weight/24 h
Females	14–21 mg/kg of body weight/24 h
Cystine	0
Osmolality	500–1200 mOsm/L
Oxalate	
Males	≤55 mg/24 h
Females	≤50 mg/24 h
pH	5.6–7.0 (>9 indicates old specimen)
Phosphorus	1 g/24 hrs
Protein	0–100 mg/24 h
Sodium	<200 mEq/L
Uric acid	≤750 mg/24 h
Normal Volumes	
Adults	600–2500 mL/24 h (average 1200)
Children	0.3–2.0 mL/kg/h

FIGURE 21.2

Estimating Relative Urinary Function*

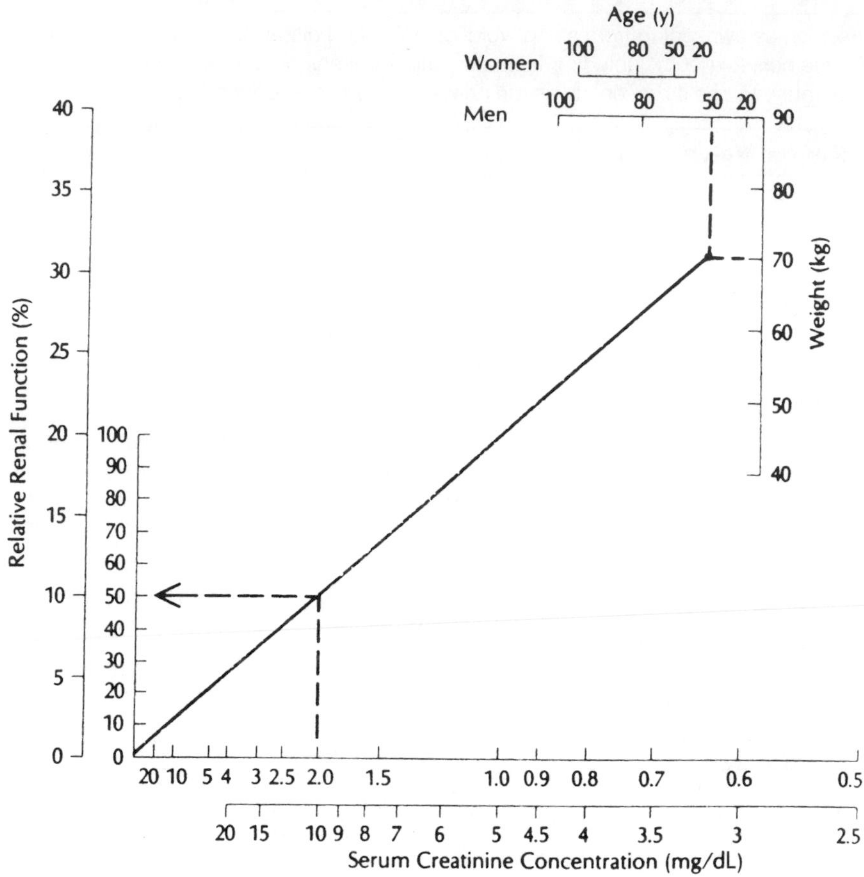

Adapted from Anderson RF. Drug prescribing for patients in renal failure. *Hosp Pract.* 1983;18:155.

*Estimating relative renal function. Nomogram graphically depicts patient's relative renal function from the serum creatinine concentration. To prepare, a line is drawn from the point of intersection of individual's sex, age, and weight to the origin; the percent of renal function remaining for a given serum creatinine value is read on the ordinate, using the outer scales for serum creatinine values above 2.5 mg/dL. For example, renal function is 50% of normal in a 50-year-old man weighing 70 kg with a serum creatinine of 2 mg/dL.

TABLE 21.3

Estimating Creatinine Clearance

Cockcroft-Gault Equation*:

$$\text{CrCl} = \frac{(140 - \text{age}) \times \text{weight (kg)}}{72 \times S_{cr}}$$

Multiply by 0.85 for females

Weight: Lean weight in kg
CrCl: Creatinine clearance
S_{cr}: Serum creatinine

Note: A 75-year-old woman (60 kg/lean) who has a "normal" serum creatinine value of 1.0 may not have "normal" renal function:

$$\frac{(140 - 75) \times 60 \text{ kg}}{72(1.0)} \times 0.85 = 46 \text{ mL/min}$$

The following equation may be used for drugs that are primarily excreted by the kidney. The change in dosing interval is estimated by using the estimated creatinine clearance and the usual dosing interval in the following equation:

$$\frac{100 \text{ kg}}{\text{Estimated creatinine clearance}} \times \text{Usual interval in hours}$$

Adapted from Cockcroft DW, Gault MN. Production of creatinine clearance from serum creatinine. *Nephron*. 1976;16:31–41.

*In young, healthy persons with stable renal function. May be less accurate in the elderly.

TABLE 21.4

Collection of Urine From Infants and Children

Noninvasive

- Stimulation of the Perez reflex (see Figure 21.3)
- Useful if male and circumcised; not useful in females
- Hold infant as shown near collection container
- Stroke the midline from sacrum to cephalad
- As infant perceives the stimulus, back will arch
- Position over collection container and obtain urine

Catheterization

- Use when Perez reflex fails or in females
- Cleanse around urethral orifice with antiseptic solution
- Insert lubricated, sterile 5 or 8 French polyethylene pediatric feeding tube until it enters bladder

Bladder Aspiration

- Wait until at least 1 hour since last void to make sure urine is present
- Administer liquids to ensure a full bladder; can check with ultrasound
- Gently restrain child in frog-leg, supine position
- Cleanse suprapubic area with antiseptic solution and drape
- With sterile gloved index finger, palpate symphysis which should be at or just above the fat crease of the lower abdomen
- Use 10-mL syringe with $1\frac{1}{2}$ inch 23 gauge needle and insert in midline just above the palpating finger
- Aim at the coccyx and apply negative pressure as needle advances
- Do *not* move needle from side to side, but rather straight in until urine is aspirated
- If no urine is aspirated after needle advanced to its hub, withdraw completely before redirecting
- Prevent urination by having an assistant apply gentle pressure to urethra during the aspiration
- After aspiration, apply sterile dressing over needle insertion site

FIGURE 21.3

Perez Reflex

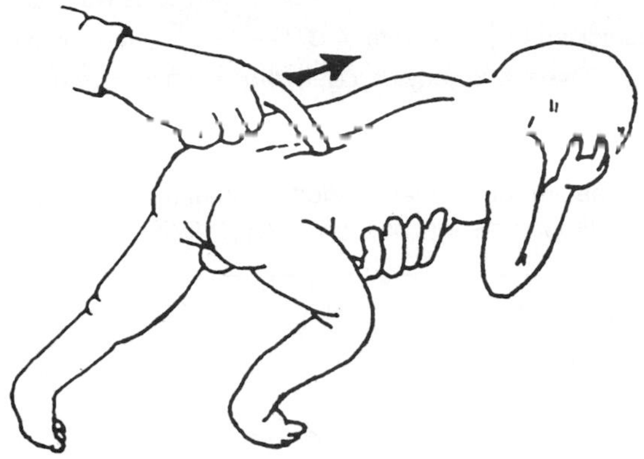

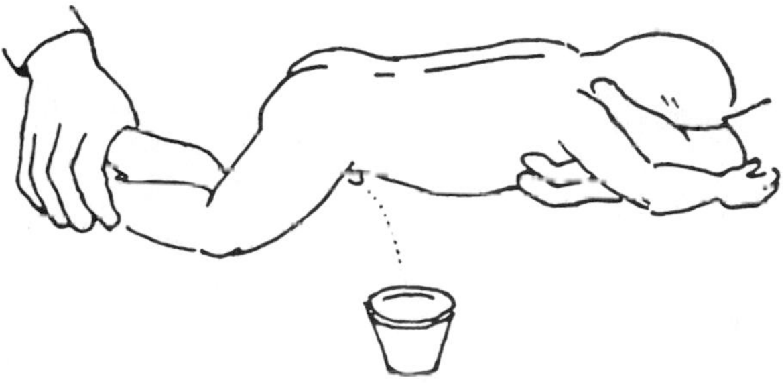

Collection of urine from children may be done noninvasively in the male by stimulating the Perez reflex. Holding the infant in ventral suspension, stroke along the midline cephalad. As the infant's back is arched, position the infant over a sterile collection cup.

Reproduced with permission from Kuhlberg A. *Top Emerg Med.* 1983;5:50.

TABLE 21.5

Management of Initial UTIs in Children

- Stronger concern for the presence of UTI in febrile children is warranted.
- In girls and uncircumcised boys, the rate of UTIs in febrile infants is 8%.
- In infants 2 months to 2 years, toxicity and dehydration should be assessed.
- If a febrile infant is ill enough to merit consideration for antibiotics in the absence of an obvious diagnosis, a sterile collection of urine should be done first.
- Figure 21.4 outlines the approach to evaluation and management. Table 21.6 gives evidence-based recommendations for imaging studies.

UTIs indicates urinary tract infections.

FIGURE 21.4

Evaluation and Management of Urinary Tract Infections in Young Children*

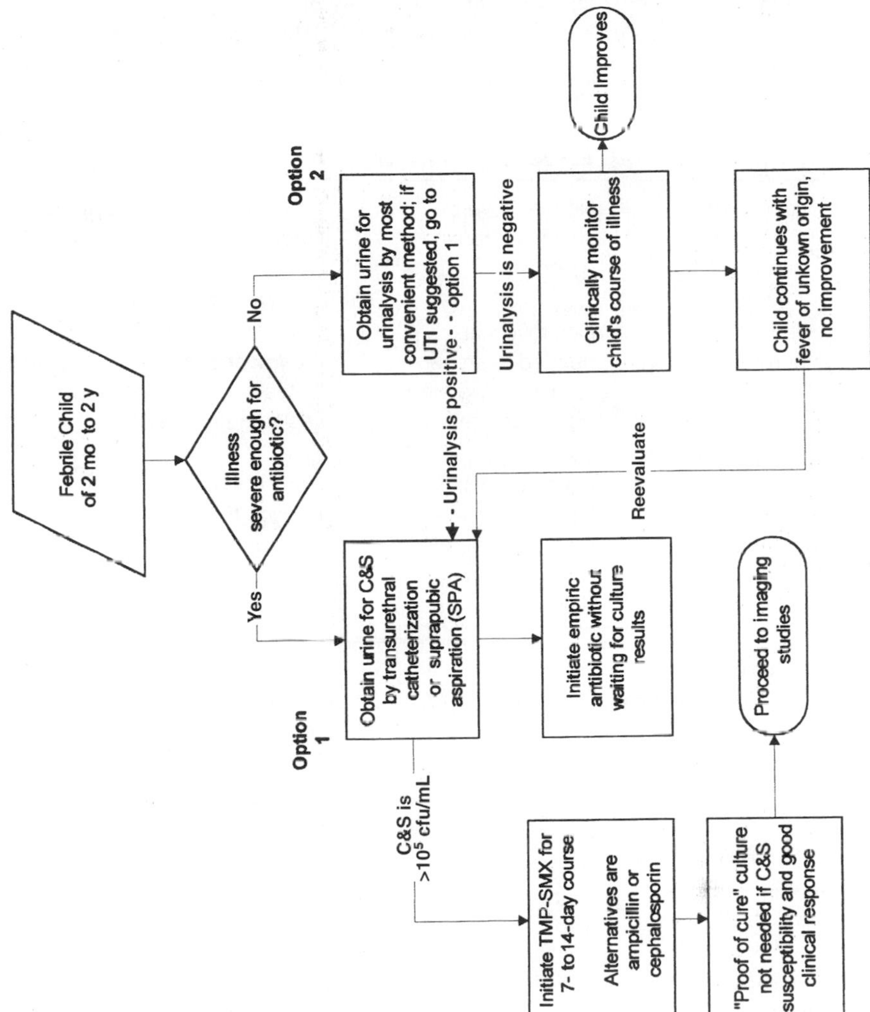

*Information is based on material included in the American Academy of Pediatrics Practice Parameter on the Diagnosis, Treatment, and Evaluation of the Initial Urinary Tract Infection in Febrile Infants and Young Children. Available online at www.aap.org/policy/ac9830.htm.

TABLE 21.6

Imaging of the Urinary Tract in Children*

- UTI in young children may be a marker for structural abnormality.
- Every febrile child 2 months to 2 years with a first UTI should have an imaging study.
- No distinction is made on the basis of gender.

Imaging Study	Evidence Strength	Utility of Test
Ultrasonography	Noncontroversial; should be routine (good)	Detects dilatation of ***upper tract*** due to distal obstruction. Detects renal cysts. May miss vesicoureteral reflux.
VCUG (cystourethrography)	Controversial; needed to prevent renal scarring of high-grade reflux (fair)	Necessary to image the ***lower tract***. Detects and grades vesicoureteral reflux
RNC (radionuclide cystography)	Controversial; needed to prevent renal scarring of high-grade reflux (fair)	Does not require catheter. Images ***lower tract*** like VCUG

UTI indicates urinary tract infection.

*Information is based on material included in the American Academy of Pediatrics Practice Parameter on the Diagnosis, Treatment, and Evaluation of the Initial Urinary Tract Infection in Febrile Infants and Young Children. Available online at www.aap.org/policy/ac9830.htm.

FIGURE 21.5

Evidence-Based Management of Urinary Tract Infection

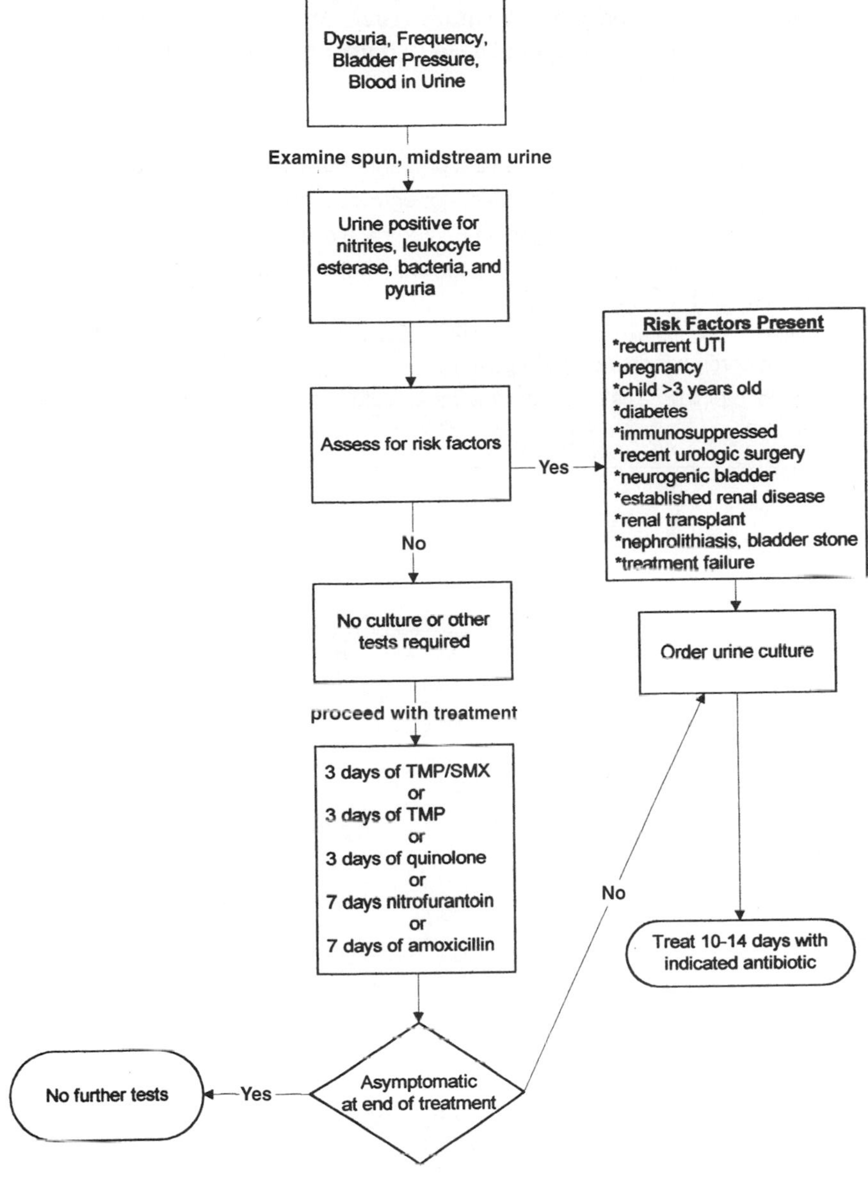

TABLE 21.7

Management of the Urinary Tract in Paralyzed Persons

The populations most affected are MS (multiple sclerosis) and SCI (spinal cord injury) patients. Urinary tract infection is the most frequent medical complication of these two groups and responsible for one third of hospitalizations.

Evidence-based findings in the published literature are:

- Bacteriuria is common and, when accompanied by pyuria, may indicate infection
- Fever as a symptom should suggest upper tract infection
- Multiple organisms or urea-splitting bacteria are associated with calculi formation
- Indwelling catheterization is associated with more infections than is intermittent catheterization
- Antibiotic prophylaxis reduces infection rates in acute SCI patients; the benefit is lost for chronic (nonacute) SCI patients
- Antibiotic prophylaxis is responsible for a twofold increase in antibiotic-resistant bacteria

TABLE 21.8

Prevention of Catheter-Related Infections

Using 18 randomized controlled trials, the following **evidence-based recommendations** have been developed:

- Use of surgical sterile technique for catheter insertion was not significantly different in infection rates vs use of clean catheterization technique
- There is a slight reduction of bacteriuria with "In-out" intermittent catheterization vs indwelling catheters
- Always use sealed drainage system for urine collection when using indwelling catheters
- Use good personal hygiene with soap and water around the meatal area on a daily basis
- Silver-impregnated catheters may slightly reduce the incidence of chronic bacteriuria in some subsets of patients, but a specific group was not identified for this intervention
- Keep drainage bags below bladder level

There was **no evidence** or **negative evidence** for the following:

- Use of antibacterial or antiseptic ointments for meatal care does not reduce bacteriuria
- No significant difference in infection rates noted between silicon and latex catheters
- No significant reduction in bacteriuria when disinfectant added to drainage bags or irrigation performed
- No significant difference in infection rates when postoperative catheters were left in place for 1 day vs 3 days

TABLE 21.9A

Obstructive Uropathy

Significance

- Common cause of acute and chronic renal failure
- Diagnosis requires a high index of suspicion—symptoms are usually mild
- Obstruction at any level leads to increased intraluminal ureteral pressure and it is eventually transmitted directly to the nephron
- As pressures rise, GFR falls and renal blood flow decreases

Prevalence

- Men over 60, 20%–35% prevalence
- Adults, 3%–4%
- Children, 2%

High-Risk Scenarios

- Uremia occurs without hypertension, diabetes, or prior renal disease
- Gross or microscopic hematuria (stone, papillary necrosis, tumor)
- Recurrent UTIs
- Sudden worsening of previously controlled hypertension
- Polycythemia
- History of gynecological or abdominal surgery
- Symptoms of prostatism
- Palpable mass in flank or abdominal
- Phimosis or meatal stenosis

Laboratory and Imaging Studies

- Urinalysis
- Serum electrolytes, BUN, creatinine, calcium, and uric acid
- Complete blood cell count
- Postvoid residual test (should be >100 mL)
- Ultrasonography
- Spiral CT
- Intravenous pyelography

BUN indicates serum urea nitrogen; CT, computed tomography; GFR, glomerular filtration rate; UTIs, urinary tract infections.

TABLE 21.9B

Causes of Obstructive Uropathy

- Treatment is specific to the cause.
- The goal is to alleviate obstruction and restore blood flow to the nephron.

Age Group	Urethral and Bladder Outlet Obstruction	Ureteral Obstruction
Infants and children	Urethral atresia Phimosis, meatal stenosis Urethral valves (males) Calculus Blood clot Meningomyelocele Ureterocele	Vesicoureteral reflux (females) Ureterovesical junction narrowing Ureterocele Retrocaval ureter Retroperitoneal tumor Prune belly syndrome Blood clot Ureteropelvic junction narrowing
Adults	Phimosis Stricture (males) STDs, particularly HSV in females Trauma Blood clot Calculi Benign prostatic hypertrophy Cancer (prostate, colon, cervix, bladder) Neurogenic bladder (diabetes, MS, drugs, Parkinson disease)	Vesicoureteral reflux (females) Calculi, uric acid crystals Blood clot Trauma Papillary necrosis (sickle cell, diabetes, pyelonephritis) Inflammatory bowel disease Pregnancy Aortic aneurysm Cancer (ureter, uterus, prostate, bladder, colon, rectum, multiple myeloma) Retroperitoneal fibrosis Tuberculosis Sarcoidosis Chronic UTI Uterine leiomyomata Stricture (radiation, NSAIDs, tuberculosis, schistosomiasis) Accidental surgical ligation

HSV indicates herpes simplex virus; MS, multiple sclerosis; NSAID, nonsteroidal anti-inflammatory drug; STD, sexually transmitted disease; UTI, urinary tract infection.

FIGURE 21.6

Acute Renal Colic With Ureteral Stone

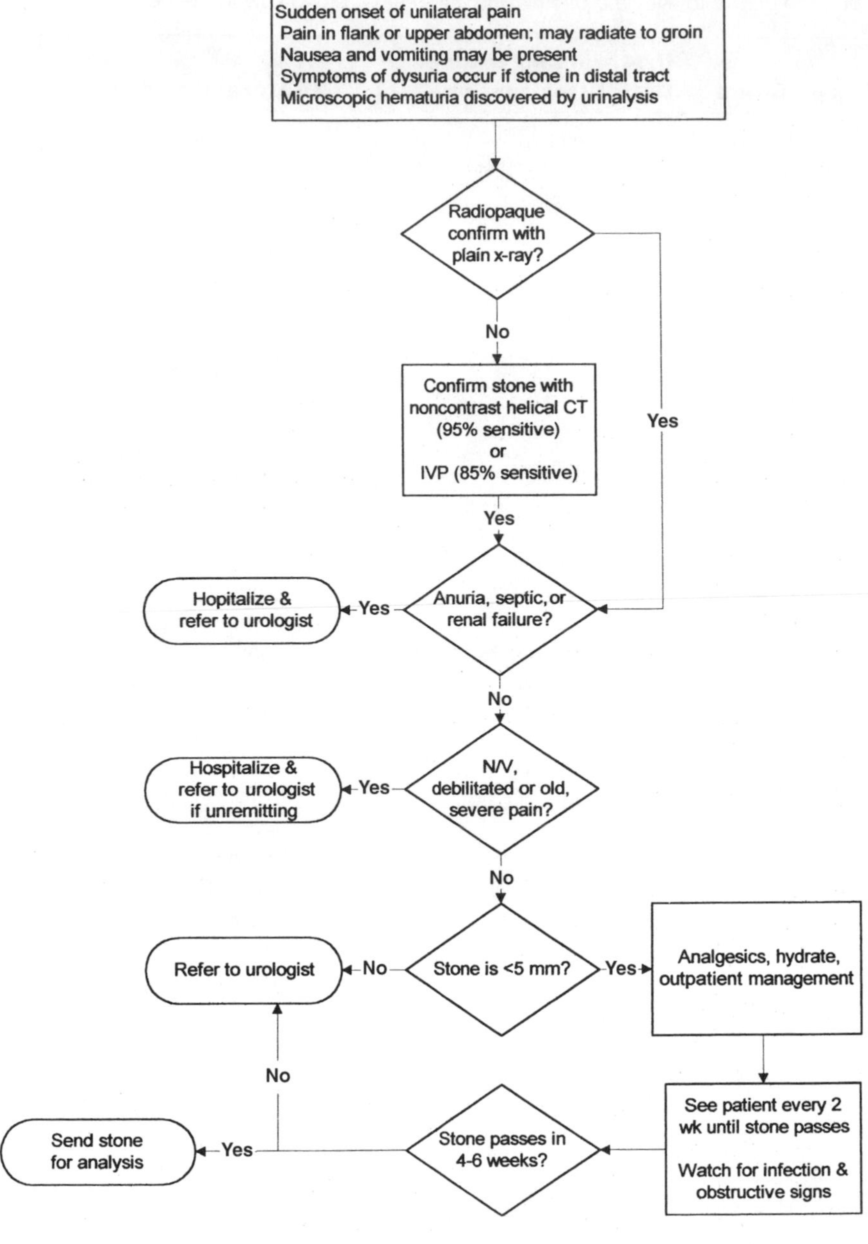

TABLE 21.10

Urolithiasis

Significance: occurs in 15% of white males, 6% of women, <1% of black males	
Acute Illness	**Chronic Illness**
Severe pain, nausea and vomiting, hypotension and acute obstruction	Slow painless process of obstruction leads to parenchymal damage or infection

High-Risk Scenarios

- Dehydration and reduced renal output
- Increased protein intake
- Heavy physical exertion
- Drugs promoting urolithiasis

Drugs Promoting Stone Formation

Calcium Stones
antacids, glucocorticoids, acetazolamide, loop diuretics, theophylline, vitamins D & C

Uric Acid Stones
thiazides, salicylates, probenecid, allopurinol

Drug Nidus Stones
triamterine, acyclovir, indinavir

Differential Diagnoses	
Hypercalciuria/Calcium Stones	**Hyperuricosuria/Uric Acid Stones**
Primary hyperparathyroidism	Diet high in purines
Malignancy	Gout
Sarcoid	Myeloproliferative disorders
Thyrotoxicosis	Tumor lysis syndrome
Immobilization	Salicylism
Familial hypercalciuria	Thiazide diuretics
Hyperoxaluria (increased intake of rhubarb, tea, nuts, beans, coffee, spinach, chocolates)	Lesch-Nyhan syndrome
Hypocitraturia (renal failure, potassium depletion, tubular acidosis, chronic diarrhea)	

Continued

TABLE 21.10
Urolithiasis, cont'd

Struvite or Triple Phosphate Stones	Cystine Stones
Bacteriuria Alkaline urine	Hypercystinuria

Diagnosis
Stone analysis, urinalysis, and a 24-hour urine for volume, Ca^{++}, Na^{+}, urate, creatinine, phosphate, citrate, and oxalate (see Table 21.2 for normal values)

General Management of Stone Disease	
Acute Stones	**Chronic Stones**
■ Narcotic analgesics and ■ IV nonsteroidal anti-inflammatory drug (eg, ketorolac 30–60 mg IV) ■ Increase diuresis with fluids	■ Sensible diet ■ Increase water intake to 2 L/d ■ Low-protein diet of 1 g/kg/d ■ Limit dietary calcium and sodium ■ See below for specific therapies

Specific Therapies for Patients With Metabolically Active Stone Disease
Calcium stones with hypercalciuria: Thiazide diuretic at 25–50 mg/d; potassium citrate to maintain potassium and improve citrate excretion in the renal tubules
Calcium stones with hyperoxaluria: Increase fluid intake and reduce oxalate in the diet; increase dietary calcium with calcium carbonate 1000 mg tid; potassium citrate 450 mg tid and magnesium gluconate 1 g/d
Calcium stones with hypocitraturia: Potassium citrate 450 mg tid to maintain urinary citrate concentration above 2.5–5.1 mmol/d
Calcium stones with renal tubular acidosis: High doses of potassium to prevent stone formation
Uric acid stones: Low-purine diet and urinary alkalinization with potassium citrate to get pH to 6.5 or above.
Struvite stones: Early urological intervention to rid the patient of the stone nidus; continue antibiotics for 3 months after removal. Oral phosphate binders reduce stone phosphate content
Cystine stones: Increase urinary solubility by increase in fluids to more than 4 L/d and alkalinize the urine with potassium citrate to >7.4 pH. Restrict dietary sodium

Recommended reference: Bihl G, Meyers A. Recurrent renal stone disease: advances in pathogenesis and clinical management. *Lancet*. 2001;358:651–655.

TABLE 21.11

Reference Ranges for the Prostate Specific Antigen (PSA) Test by Age and Race

Reference Range Based on 5th Percentile of Distribution of PSA Levels		
Age (y)	**Blacks**	**Whites**
	PSA, ng/mL	
40–49	0.0–2.0	0.0–2.5
50–59	0.0–4.0	0.0–3.5
60–69	0.0–4.5	0.0–3.5
70–79	0.0–5.5	0.0–3.5

Using PSA Density With Serum PSA by Age Category PSA Density = Serum PSA divided by prostate weight (calculated from measurements from a transrectal prostate ultrasound)	
40–49	0.0–0.10
50–59	0.0–0.12
60–69	0.0–0.14
70–79	0.0–0.16

Using PSA Velocity and Percent Free PSA to Aid Interpretation of PSA
An increase in PSA (PSA velocity) of >0.75 ng/mL/y is abnormal
If free PSA is <25% when PSA is between 4–10 ng/mL, recommend biopsy

TABLE 21.12
Prostatic Diseases

Condition	Symptoms	Examination	Lab Studies	Treatment
Benign hypertrophy	Nocturia, hesitancy, urge incontinence, dribbling, decreased urine flow, obstruction	Smooth, symmetrical enlargement	>150-mL postvoid residual, urinalysis, IVP, cystoscopy, urine flow studies, serum PSA	TURP, balloon dilation, α-blocker, finasteride
Acute bacterial prostatitis	Sudden onset of fever, chills, malaise, arthralgia, frequency, dysuria, pain in perineum	Tender and warm prostate, boggy enlargement (examine gingerly)	Urine culture, blood culture, avoid catheterization	IV antibiotics, analgesics, stool softeners, NSAIDs
Prostatic abscess	Acute bacterial prostatitis with spiking fevers and rectal pain, chills	Firm, tender, or fluctuant mass	Elevated blood glucose level, persistent leukocytosis despite antibiotics	Surgical drainage and antibiotics
Chronic bacterial prostatitis	Recurrent UTIs, irritative voiding symptoms, no systemic signs	Prostatic calculi, boggy enlargement	Persistent bacteria in prostatic fluid, hematospermia, split-voided urinalysis	4–6 weeks of antibiotic therapy, surgery if calculi

Condition	Symptoms	Examination	Lab Studies	Treatment
Nonbacterial prostatitis	Frequency, urgency, dysuria, testicular or penile pain, no systemic signs and no recurrent UTIs	Prostate may be normal on examination	$\leqslant$10 WBCs/HPF in prostatic secretions, no bacteria, lipid-laden prostatic macrophages, cystoscopy to rule out interstitial cystitis	Oxybutynin 5 mg po tid or propantheline 15 mg po tid or diazepam 2 mg po tid
Prostatodynia	Painful prostate, symptoms similar to chronic bacterial or nonbacterial prostatitis, history of sexual or marital difficulties	Normal prostate on examination, pelvic muscle tension	Prostatic secretions without WBCs	Prazosin 1 mg po bid or baclofen 5–10 mg po tid, warm sitz baths, psychosocial support

bid indicates twice daily; HPF, high-power field; IV; intravenously; IVP, intravenous pyelogram; NSAID, nonsteroidal anti-inflammatory drug; po, orally; PSA, prostate-specific antigen; tid, three times daily; UTI, urinary tract infection; WBC, white blood cell count.

TABLE 21.13

Prostatitis

Acute inflammation increases vascular permeability and antibiotics may gain easier access; chronic prostatic infection is " protected" from most antibiotics, which fail to diffuse into prostatic fluid.

Best antibiotics to use will:

- be lipophillic
- have a high ionization potential (pKa) ≥ 8.6
- have a gram-negative spectrum at pH of 6.6
- have a low degree of protein binding

Type	Organisms	Drug	Duration
Acute infection (associated with UTI and pyelonephritis)	*Escherichia coli, Klebsiella, Proteus, enterococci, Pseudomonas*	TMP-SMX Doxycycline 100 mg bid Ciprofloxacin 500 mg bid	3–4 weeks to prevent relapse
Chronic Infection (hemospermia present)	Gram-negative coliforms	TMP-SMX Norfloxacin (if TMP-SMX fails)	2–3 months
Chronic nonbacterial prostatitis (CNP)	Chlamydia, Ureaplasma, Mycoplasma	Doxycycline Minocin	2 weeks

TABLE 21.14

Benign Prostatic Hypertrophy Index

A. Symptom Index for Benign Prostatic Hyperplasia*							
	Over the past month or so, how often have you:	Never	Less than 1 time in 5	Less than ½ the time	About ½ the time	More than ½ the time	Almost always
1	had a sensation of not emptying your bladder completely after you finished urinating?	0	1	2	3	4	5
2	had to urinate again less than 2 hours after you finished urinating?	0	1	2	3	4	5
3	found you stopped and started again several times when you urinated?	0	1	2	3	4	5
4	found it difficult to postpone urination?	0	1	2	3	4	5
5	had a weak urinary stream?	0	1	2	3	4	5
6	had to push or strain to begin urination?	0	1	2	3	4	5
7	had to get up to urinate from the time you went to bed at night until the time you got up in the morning?	0 never	1 time	2 times	3 times	4 times	5 or more times

Symptom Score ________

*Adapted from the American Urological Association Symptom Index.

B. "Bother" Index for Benign Prostatic Hyperplasia				
Overall, how bothersome has any trouble with urination been during the past month?	Not at all	A little	Some	A lot

Scoring: A total score of 35 is possible. 0–7, "mild" symptoms; 8–18, "moderate" symptoms; 19–35, "severe" symptoms.

TABLE 21.15A

Balance Sheet for Benign Prostatic Hyperplasia Treatment Outcomes

	Surgical Options				Nonsurgical Options		
Direct Treatment Outcomes	**Balloon Dilation**	**TUIP**	**Open Surgery**	**TURP**	**Watchful Waiting**	**α-Blockers**	**Finasteride**
1. Change for improvement of symptoms (90% confidence interval)	37%–76%	78%–83%	94%–99.8%	75%–96%	31%–55%	59%–86%	54%–78%
2. Degree of symptom improvement (percent reduction in symptom score)	51%	73%	79%	85%	Unknown	51%	31%
3. Morbidity/ complications associated with surgical or medical treatment (90% confidence interval), about 20% of all complications assumed to be significant	1.78%–9.86%	2.2%–33.3%	6.98%–42.7%	5.2%–30.7%	1%–5% Complications from BPH progression	2.9%–43.3%	13.6%–18.8%
4. Chance of dying within 30–90 days of treatment (90% confidence interval)	0.72%–9.78% (high risk/elderly patients)	0.2%–1.5%	0.99%–4.56%	0.53%–3.31%	0.8% chance of death ≤90 days for 67-year-old man		
5. Risk of total urinary incontinence (90% confidence interval)	Unknown	0.06%–1.1%	0.34%–0.74%	0.68%–1.4%	Incontinence associated with aging		

Direct Treatment Outcomes	Surgical Options				Nonsurgical Options		
	Balloon Dilation	TUIP	Open Surgery	TURP	Watchful Waiting	α-Blockers	Finasteride
6. Need for operative treatment for surgical complications in future (90% confidence interval)	Unknown	1.34%–2.65%	0.6%–14.1%	0.65%–10.1%	0		
7. Risk of impotence (90% confidence interval)	No long-term follow-up available	3.9%–24.5%	4.7%–39.2%	3.3%–34.8%	About 2% of men aged 67 become impotent every year. Long-term data on α-blockers are not available		2.5%–5.3% (also decreased volume of ejaculate)
8. Risk of retrograde ejaculation (percent of patients)	Unknown	6%–55%	36%–95%	25%–99%	0	4%–1[illegible]%	0
9. Loss of work time (days)	4	7–21	21–28	7–21	1	3.5	1.5
10. Hospital stay (days)	1	1–3	5–10	3–5	0	0	0

Adapted from McConnell JD, et al. Benign prostatic hyperplasia: diagnosis and treatment. *Clinical Practice Guideline*, No. 8, AHCPR Publication 94-0582. Rockville, MD: Agency for Healthcare Policy and Research, Public Health Service, US Department of Health and Human Services; February 1994: 196–197.

Note: New minimally invasive therapies have been developed (eg, transurethral needle ablation [TUNA], transurethral microwave thermotherapy [TUMT], and interstitial laser coagulation [ILC]); however, there are no long-term data available to be able to include them in the decision balance sheet.

TABLE 21.15B

Assessment of Treatment Outcomes for Benign Hyperplasia Treatment

Explanation of Balance Sheet (Table 21.15A)	
Line 1	Likelihood that given patient will experience some symptom improvement; likelihood of improvement greater if pretreatment symptoms more severe
Line 2	Expected amount of improvement (for patients who improve)
Line 3	Likelihood that given patient will have treatment complications or adverse events
Line 4	Likelihood that given patient will die from any causes within 3 months of treatment
Line 5	Likelihood that a given patient will experience total incontinence caused by the treatment
Line 6	Likelihood that given patient will require surgical correction for a late complication of BPH treatment, such as bladder neck contracture or urethral stricture
Line 7	Likelihood that a patient who was potent before treatment will experience impotence following treatment
Line 8	Likelihood that a patient who was potent before treatment and still potent after treatment will experience retrograde ejaculation following treatment
Line 9	Estimated number of days a given patient may miss from work during first year of treatment
Line 10	Estimated number of days spent in the hospital

FIGURE 21.7

Evaluation and Management of Urinary Incontinence

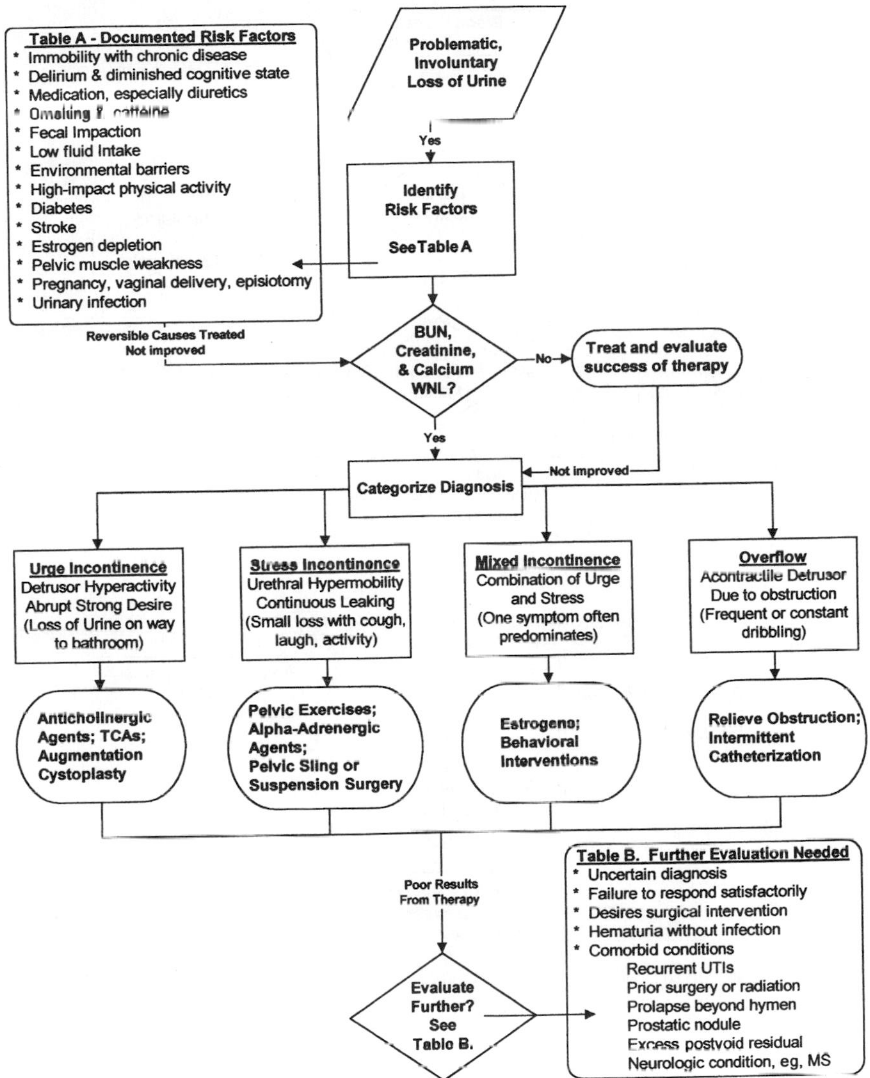

Reference: Bakris GL, Williams M, Dworkin L, et al. Preserving renal function in adults with hypertension and diabetes: a consensus approach. *Am J Kidney Dis.* 2000;36:646–661.

FIGURE 21.8

Blood Pressure Strategies for People With Renal Insufficiency and/or Diabetes

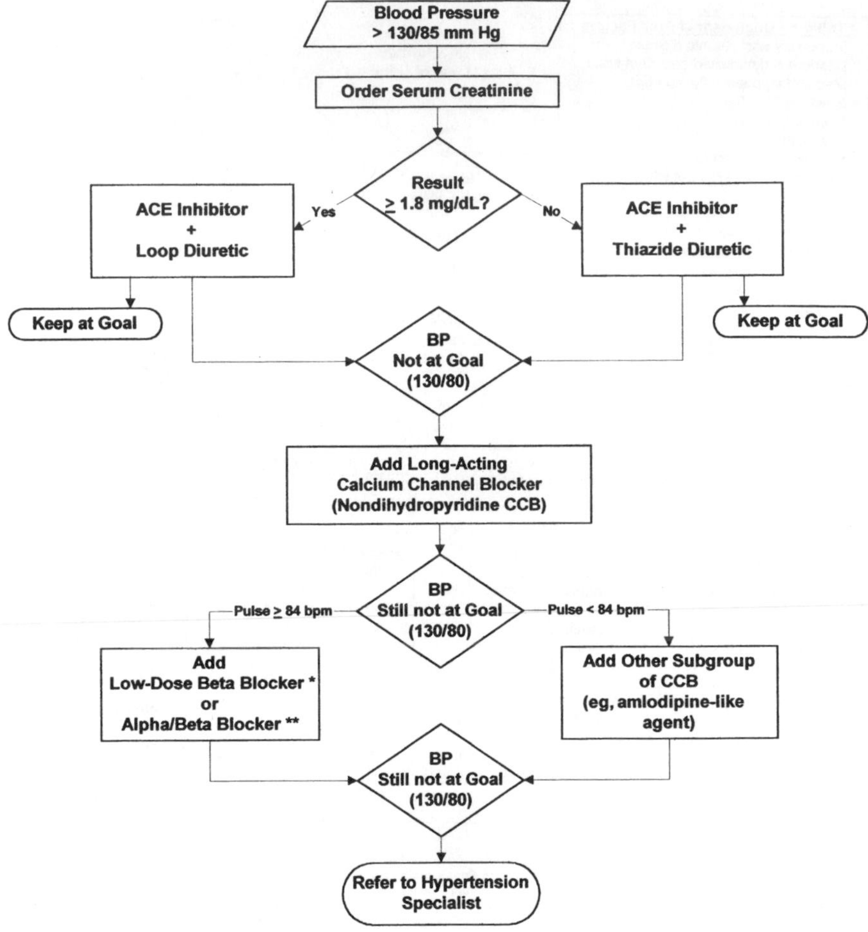

*Use of beta blocker in the presence of nondihydropyridine CCB should be avoided in the elderly and those with conduction abnormalities.

**Clonidine should not be used with beta blockers in order to avoid severe bradycardia.

TABLE 21.16

Asymptomatic Hematuria

Defined as abnormal presence of red blood cells in the urine, either gross or microscopic. Patients with ≥3 RBCs/hpf on two or more occasions have significant microscopic hematuria. Any episode of gross hematuria or microscopic hematuria of ≥100 RBCs/hpf requires attention to workup. The presence of red cell casts suggests glomerular bleeding; consult nephrologist. In men, distinguish between hematuria and hematospermia.

Age Group	Common Causes	Comment and Workup
Neonate/toddler	Nephroblastoma, renal vein thrombosis, polycystic kidney disease, obstructive uropathy, medullary sponge kidney, child abuse, infection, coagulopathy, ischemic injury	Usually presents as gross hematuria and is invariably serious; aggressive workup is indicated Renal sonogram
Children 5–19	Poststreptococcal glomerulonephritis, infection, sickle cell disease, drugs, hemorrhagic cystitis, trauma, orthostatic hematuria of heavy exercise, congenital renal abnormality, malignancy, menstruation, hypercalciuria	Usually benign with a good prognosis; workup needs to include an evaluation for reduced renal function Renal sonogram and possibly cystoscopy
Ages 20–40	Acute urinary tract infection, orthostatic hematuria of heavy exercise, "honeymoon" cystitis, urolithiasis, bladder tumors, inflammatory bladder conditions, essential or benign recurrent hematuria, urethritis	Rarely due to a life-threatening or surgical lesion; usual workup of IVP and cystoscopy Culture urine
Ages 41–60	Bladder tumor, urolithiasis, acute urinary tract infection, renal tumors, NSAID nephropathy, prostatic disease, interstitial cystitis, anticoagulants	Always suspect neoplasm until proven otherwise; IVP and cystoscopy are indicated Culture urine
Over 60 years	BPH, bladder tumor, acute urinary tract infection, renal tumors, medication-related, ischemic renal damage	Always suspect neoplasm until proven otherwise; IVP and cystoscopy are indicated Culture urine

BPH indicates benign prostatic hyperplasia; HPF, high-power field, IVP, Intravenous pyelogram; NSAID, nonsteroidal anti-inflammatory drug; RBC, red blood cell count.

FIGURE 21.9

Management Decisions for Patients With Hematuria

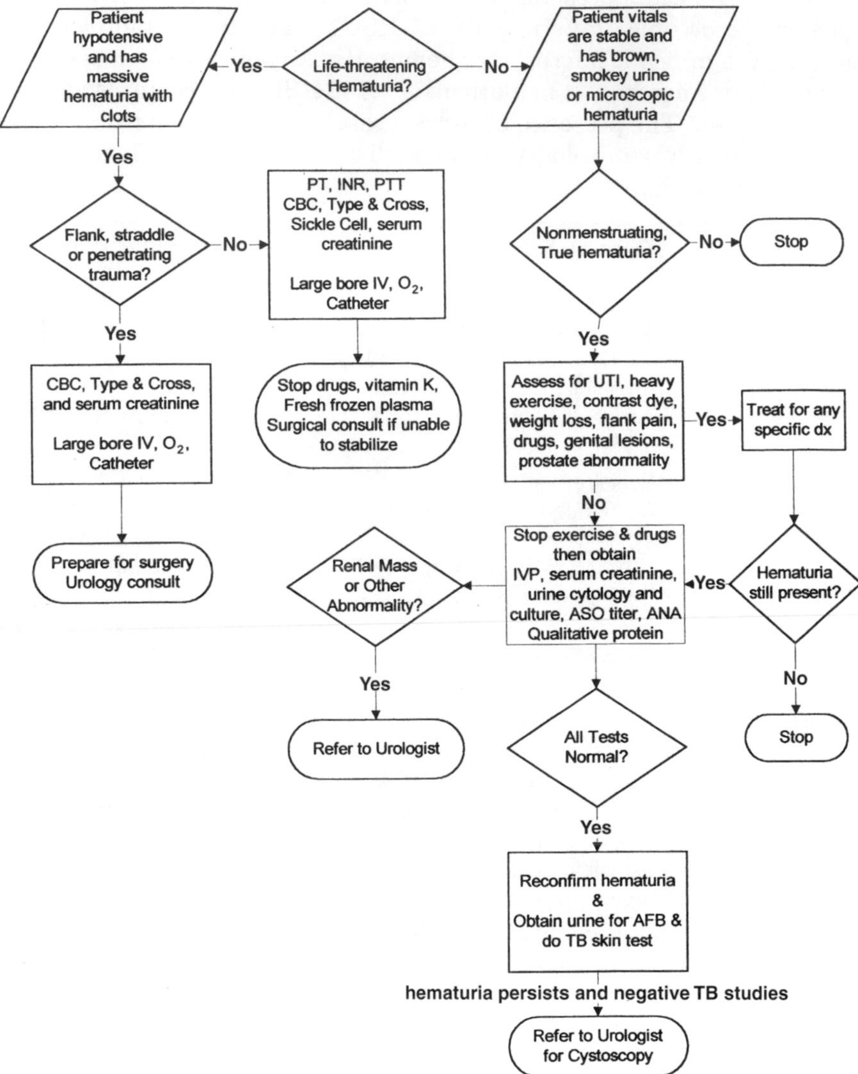

TABLE 21.17

Hematospermia

The problem of hematospermia is almost always benign and resolves spontaneously within several weeks.

Young Males

- Seminal vesicle inflammation or infection or trauma
- Not usually a cause for concern if a single episode

Males 20–40

- Acute prostatitis or seminal vesiculitis
- Effectively treated with tetracycline or erythromycin
- In the absence of other urological complaints, rarely caused by neoplasm in this age group

Males over 40

- Usually innocent cause
- Can be secondary to prostate cancer with extension to seminal vesicle
- Prostate-specific antigen and careful digital rectal exam before treatment
- Refer if persistent and unable to find cause

If spontaneous resolution is not observed, differential diagnoses are:

- Hemophilia or bleeding diathesis
- Tuberculosis
- Severe hypertension
- Urethral pathology
- Recent surgery on the prostate or vas deferens
- Schistosomiasis
- Cytomegalovirus
- Prostate or seminal vesicle carcinoma
- Prostatic, seminal vesicle, or ejaculatory duct calculi
- Prostatic, seminal vesicle, or ejaculatory duct cysts
- Masturbation

TABLE 21.18

Interstitial Cystitis

Definition
Chronic condition with irritative voiding symptoms and negative urine cultures Etiology is unknown Course marked by flare-ups and remissions
Epidemiology
■ 0.6 per 1000 ■ Women to men ratio is 9:1 ■ Nonulcerating type 90% of patients and severe form with Hunner ulcers 10% ■ Median age 45 (30–70 range)
Symptoms
■ Symptoms typically worsen the week prior to menses ■ Pelvic pain relieved by voiding small amounts ■ Urgency, frequency (17–40 times a day) ■ Dyspareunia
Clinical Evaluation
■ Usually a delay in diagnosis; must have a high index of suspicion ■ Urine culture to rule out infection and pelvic exam to rule out pelvic pathology ■ If urinalysis is positive for hematuria or sterile pyuria, culture for AFB ■ Refer for cystoscopy with hydrodistention under anesthesia
Diagnostic Findings
■ Pinpoint fissures or bleeding points called glomerulations ■ Small reddish-brown spots called Hunner ulcers ■ Drainage of bladder after hydrodistention reveals bloody-tinged fluid ■ Bladder biopsies reveal no evidence of neoplasm and indicate inflammation

Treatments
■ Hydrodistention of bladder may relieve symptoms for several months
■ Reduce foods that aggravate symptoms; caffeine, alcohol, spices, acidic foods
■ Tricyclic antidepressants, antihistamines, and pentosan polysulfate (Elmiron)
■ Systemic analgesics and NSAIDs may help by suppressing prostaglandins
■ Anticholinergics (oxybutynin), bladder analgesics (phenazopyridine), and calcium channel blockers (nifedipine)
■ Intravesicular treatments such as DMSO, BCG, heparin
■ Other therapies include TENS, pelvic floor exercises, and support groups

TABLE 21.19

General Management of Acute Renal Failure

Definition and Case Recognition
■ Occurs in 5% of hospitalized patients and is defined by an acute increase of the serum creatinine by 0.5 mg/dL over baseline
■ Complete renal shutdown is present when serum creatinine rises by 0.5 mg/dL per day and patient becomes oliguric (<400 mL/24 h)
General Emergent Management Steps
■ Correct fluid and electrolyte and acid-base balance
■ Resuscitate with normal saline for volume depletion
■ Furosemide 20–100 mg/d for volume overload
■ Temporary shift of K^+ into cells with glucose (25 g) and intravenous insulin (10 units), inhaled beta-agonist or Intravenous sodium bicarbonate (3 ampules in 1 L of 5% dextrose)
■ Short-term dialysis for BUN >100 mg/dL or creatinine >5 to 10 mg/dL
Mortality Rate
■ Averages 15% (range of 7%–80% dependent on severity)

BUN indicates blood urea nitrogen.

TABLE 21.20

Differentiating Types of Renal Failure

Definition
Urine volume <400 mL/24 hours
Serum BUN and creatinine elevation
BUN rises 10–20 mg/24 h and creatinine rises 0.5–1.0 mg/24 hours

Characteristics	Pre-renal	Renal	Postrenal
Urine osmolality	>500 mOsm/kg	<350 mOsm/kg	<350 mOsm/kg
Urine to serum osmolar ratio	>1.2	<1.1	<1.1
Urine sodium	<20 mEq/L	>40 mEq/L	Variable
Urine to serum urea ratio	>8	<3	<3
Urine to serum creatinine ratio	>40	<20	<20
Serum BUN to serum creatinine ratio	>20:1	<20:1	<20:1
Causes	Volume depletion, reduced cardiac output, reduced renal blood flow	Glomerular or renal tubular lesions Glomerular lesions nephritis, lupus, allergic angiitis, Wegener granulomatosis, polyarteritis nodosa, strep Tubular lesions ischemia, sepsis, eclampsia, drugs, contrast dyes, heavy metals, anesthetic gases, ethylene glycol, methanol, uricemia, carbon tetrachloride, hypercalcemia, myeloma	Urethral or ureteral obstruction

BUN indicates blood urea nitrogen.

TABLE 21.21

Clinical Management of Renal Failure

1. Establish a cause and treat those that are reversible
2. Stabilize and delay progression of the disease
3. Treat to prevent complications of chronic renal failure
4. Avoid further renal damage due to drugs or metabolic conditions
5. Assist patient and family to select options for ESRD (eg, dialysis, transplant)

Condition	Observation	Management
Hyperkalemia	Serum K^+, ECG	Kayexalate (oral or enema) 50 g in 200 mL of 70% sorbitol q 4 h; avoid ACE & β-blockers
Acidosis	Serum bicarbonate, serum pH	Oral bicarbonate tabs 650 1–3 times daily if serum HCO_3 <15 mEq/L; or sodium citrate 1 Tbsp 1–3 times daily
Malnutrition	Daily weights	Enteral hyperalimentation if gut works; restrict Na^+, K^+, and H_2O; give multivitamin
Hypermagnesemia	Serum magnesium	Avoid laxatives and antacids containing magnesium
Hyperphosphatemia	Serum phosphorus	Avoid aluminum-containing antacids; limit dietary phosphorus to ≤700 mg/d
Hypocalcemia	Serum calcium	Accompanies elevation of phosphorus. If Ca^{++} is <7.5 mg/dL give 2 g replacement/day and restrict dietary phosphate
Low vitamin D, hyperparathyroidism	1,25-Dihydroxyvitamin D and intact PTH level	If vitamin low and PTH high, give 1,25 dihydroxyvitamin D 25 μg daily; watch for elevated calcium
Anemia	CBC, serum iron	Recombinant erythropoietin 50–75 units subcutaneously twice weekly if Hct is <30%

Continued

TABLE 21.21

Clinical Management of Renal Failure, cont'd

Hypertension	Blood pressure	Control BP to ≤130/80 mm Hg
Fluid overload	Loss of thirst, serum sodium and osmolality, urine specific gravity	If hyponatremic, restrict water access and give loop diuretic
Azotemia rising	BUN, creatinine	Restrict protein to 0.6 g/kg/d, avoid NSAIDs, nephrotoxic drugs, hypotension, radiocontrast dyes

ACE indicates angiotensin-converting enzyme; BP, blood pressure; BUN, serum urea nitrogen; CBC, complete blood cell count; ECG, electrocardiogram; ESRD, end-stage renal disease; NSAID, nonsteroidal anti-inflammatory drug; q 4 h; every 4 hours.

TABLE 21.22

Indicatons for Renal Hemodialysis

- Volume expansion with life-threatening CHF and pulmonary edema
- Severe hypernatremia/hyperkalemia uncontrolled medically
- Metabolic acidosis (pH < 7.2) uncontrolled medically
- Refractory hypermagnesemia, hyperuricemia, hyperphosphatemia
- Serum calcium × serum phosphate product is ≥6
- Poisoning with salicylates, ethanol, methanol, barbiturates, or other drugs
- Chronic renal failure with acute decline
- Uremic syndrome with pericarditis
- Severe azotemia (serum BUN >100 mg/dL)
- Acute renal failure with creatinine >5.5 mg/dL

Usually performed for 4 hours three times in a week
Anticoagulation necessary
Risks: bleeding, hypotension, cardiac dysrhythmia, hypoxia, infection

BUN indicates serum urea nitrogen; CHF, congestive heart failure.

TABLE 21.23
Scrotal Problems

Condition	Clinical Differentiation	Diagnostic Studies	Treatment
Cryptorchidism	Nonexistent testicle, asymptomatic	Chromosome studies if bilateral	Surgical exploration
Epididymo-orchitis	Gradual onset (hours to days, worsening incrementally); males 12–20 y; sexually active, usually secondary to GC/*Chlamydia*, rarely from UTI/prostatitis—*Escherichia coli*; elevate scrotum decreases pain; cremasteric reflex present and fever/discharge present	WBCs in U/A, positive GC or *Chlamydia,* normal Doppler	GC:azithromycin 2 g or ceftriaxone IM Chlamydia: azithromycin or doxycycline
Fournier gangrene	History of trauma, UTI, rectal disease, diabetes, compromised immunity, explosive onset, edema, extreme pain, black necrotic skin, crepitance	Aspiration of skin yields purulent fluid with bacteria. Do sigmoidoscopy	Acute surgical emergency; debriding of necrotic tissue skin grafting. Broad-spectrum antibiotics
Hydrocele	Rule out hernia; irreducible painless mass, occurs in all age groups; may communicate intra-abdominally	No bowel sounds in scrotum on auscultation; transilluminates	Because of likelihood of associated hernia, surgical exploration and repair if persists after 1 year of age
Spermatocele	Painless lump in spermatic cord often following vasectomy	No transillumination	NSAIDs; surgical removal if large, tender, cosmetically undesirable
Testicular cancer	Painless firm enlarging mass; often ignored for months	Ultrasonography, biopsy of mass	Exploratory surgery, removal and lymph node dissection
Testicular torsion	Males 12–20 y; early morning or after trauma to area; pain gets worse on elevating scrotum; loss of cremasteric reflex; testes pulled up	Unequal Doppler flow or nuclear perfusion studies, but time is crucial	Surgery is standard within 6 h (if manual detorsion attempted, do enroute to OR or on OR table and from medial to lateral)

Continued

TABLE 21.23

Scrotal Problems, cont'd

Condition	Clinical Differentiation	Diagnostic Studies	Treatment
Torsion of appendix testes	Not as painful; most tender on top pole of testes; +blue dot sign	Ultrasonography or Doppler flow study	No medical/surgical treatment; pain resolves in time
Trauma	Painful trauma, gross swelling with ecchymosis	Urethrography, U/S	Exploratory surgery
Varicocele	"Bag of worms" or "spaghetti" of spermatic cord; usually on left	IVP or CT scan of retroperitoneal space if acute onset	Surgical removal if painful or infertility problem

CT indicates computed tomography; IM, intramuscularly; IVP, intravenous pyelogram; NSAID, nonsteroidal anti-inflammatory drug; OR, operating room; U/S; ultrasound; UTI, urinary tract infection; WBC, white blood cell count.

TABLE 21.24
Management of Paraphimosis

Retraction Techniques

Administer sedation; relieve pain
Lubricate the corona with K-Y jelly

then

Grasp the penis and apply firm pressure around the circumference of the swollen area. Maintain pressure for 5–10 minutes to reduce the swelling, then try to gently draw the incarcerated foreskin forward over the glans

or

Apply pressure as above, then place the index and third fingers behind the edematous mass with the thumb on the meatus. Then apply opposing pressure to retract the foreskin back over the glans

Dorsal Slit Surgery

- Prep with antibacterial soap such as povidine-iodine
- Identify the opening of the prepuce, which appears as a constricting band within the edematous mass
- Infiltrate the area with 1% lidocaine, used sparingly so as to not increase the edema
- With a No. 15 blade, incise through the constricting band, extending the incision as necessary
- Reduce the paraphimosis
- Hemostasis is usually accomplished by a few minutes of pressure
- Elective circumcision can be done when the dorsal slit is healed

TABLE 21.25

Emergency Management of Priapism

Since impotence is a known complication of priapism, this possibility should be explained to the patient early on; informed consent for an emergency procedure should be obtained.

Aspiration

Thoroughly cleanse penis with povidine-iodine to prep the skin.

Wearing sterile gloves, drape off surrounding area to create a sterile field.

Locate the 3 o'clock or 9 o'clock position on the shaft of the penis, approximately 1 inch proximal to the corona. Avoid the dorsal neurovascular bundle and the ventral urethral areas. Inject 0.5–1.0 mL of lidocaine to anesthetize skin over the aspiration site. Only one side of the penis needs to be aspirated because of the cross-flow of circulation.

Insert a 19-gauge butterfly needle into the corpora through the anesthetized skin and aspirate blood into a sterile 20-mL syringe. If blood gases on sludged penile blood are desired, use a 5-mL glass heparinized syringe to do the first aspiration, then change to the 20-mL syringe. If the condition has persisted for >36 hours and/or pH is <7.25, $Po_2 < 30$ and Pco_2 is >60 mm Hg, a significant ischemic condition exists, and the patient should be referred for surgical shunt procedure.

Continue aspiration until all possible blood is obtained and the penis loses its rigidity. Squeezing, or "milking," of blood from the penis may help in removing blood.

When aspiration is no longer productive, move to the irrigation stage of the procedure.

Irrigation

Add 1 mL of epinephrine 1:1000 to a 1-L bag of sterile saline. Attach an intravenous administration set, run some fluid through the tubing, and fill a clean sterile 20-mL syringe from it.

Slowly inject epinephrine/saline solution into cavernosa and aspirate back into syringe and discard.

Repeat the step above until satisfactory detumescence has occurred and blood returned from the penis is bright red instead of dark and viscous. Then withdraw the butterfly needle from the penis, and cover the aspiration site with a sterile dressing. If no satisfactory results are obtained after 200 mL of irrigation, abandon the procedure and plan for surgical shunting.

Hospitalize the patient for 24 hours of observation to ensure that priapism does not recur. Success should be anticipated in ≥75% of the cases regardless of cause.

TABLE 21.26

Evaluation of Adrenal Masses Discovered Incidentally

At autopsy, the incidence of masses >1 cm is approximately 3%.
Most are of little or no clinical significance. During workup of urological abnormalities or other abdominal symptoms, adrenal masses are incidentally discovered. Approximately 14% are hyperfunctioning.

Steps in evaluation:

1. Do a thorough history and physical exam focus on hyperfunction
   —"moon" facies, "buffalo" hump, striae, hypertension, glucose intolerance, menstrual abnormalities, deepening of voice, virilization, acne, baldness, hirsutism, clitoral hypertrophy
2. Twenty-four-hour urine for metanephrines and cortisol and 17 ketosteroids
3. If hypertensive, serum potassium and plasma aldosterone concentration, and plasma renin
4. If metanephrines are normal, mass can be biopsied if worrisome for metastatic disease

Nonfunctioning adrenal mass <4 cm	Repeat CT scan and function tests in 6–12 months; **no changes** noted	No treatment and no further follow-up
Nonfunctioning adrenal mass <4 cm	Repeat CT scan and function tests in 6–12 months; **functional** or **increase** in diameter >1 cm	Surgical resection
Hyperfunctioning or adrenal mass >4 cm		Surgical resection

5. Laparoscopic removal may be used for benign functional masses.
   If only biopsy is intended, metanephrines must be normal to avoid precipitating a life-threatening hypertensive crisis
6. If mass is suspected to be a malignancy, laparoscopic surgery is contraindicated. Laparotomy is recommended to avoid spillage of malignant cells and to facilitate wide margins of excision

CT indicates computed tomography.

TABLE 21.27

Nephrotic Syndrome

Diagnosis

>3.5 g/d of proteinuria
Hypoalbuminemia
Edema
Hyperlipidemia
Lipiduria

Classification

Primary (idiopathic): Minimal change or membranous glomerulonephritis; most common cause in adults is membranous glomerulonephritis

Secondary: Associated with diabetes, cancer, amyloidosis, lupus erythematosus, drug-induced and in preeclampsia

Thromboembolic Complications

Renal vein thrombosis
DVT
PE

People at Increased Risk

Serum albumin <25 g/L
Protein excretion >10 g/24 hrs
Increased fibrinogen level
Decreased antithrombin III levels

Treatment

For primary subtype:

Empiric trial of prednisone can be given starting with 2 mg/kg/d × 1 week, then q o d × 7 weeks. About 80% of adults respond and are believed to have minimal change disease.

If no response is evident, proceed to referral for renal biopsy.

Cyclophosphomide: 1–2 mg/kg/d, has side effects and monitoring of CBC, fluid intake, and contraception in females needed.

Cyclosporine: Can be used in both children and adults for those nonresponsive to steroids.

For secondary subtype:

Remove or treat the underlying cause.

Restrict sodium; judiciously use loop diuretics to reduce edema; and give a trial of bed rest.

A low dose of ACE inhibitor or calcium channel blocker (verapamil or diltiazem but not nifedipine or other dihydropyridine) is indicated for patients with diabetes.

Use lipid-lowering agents if needed.

FIGURE 21.10

Urologic Management of the Stroke Patient

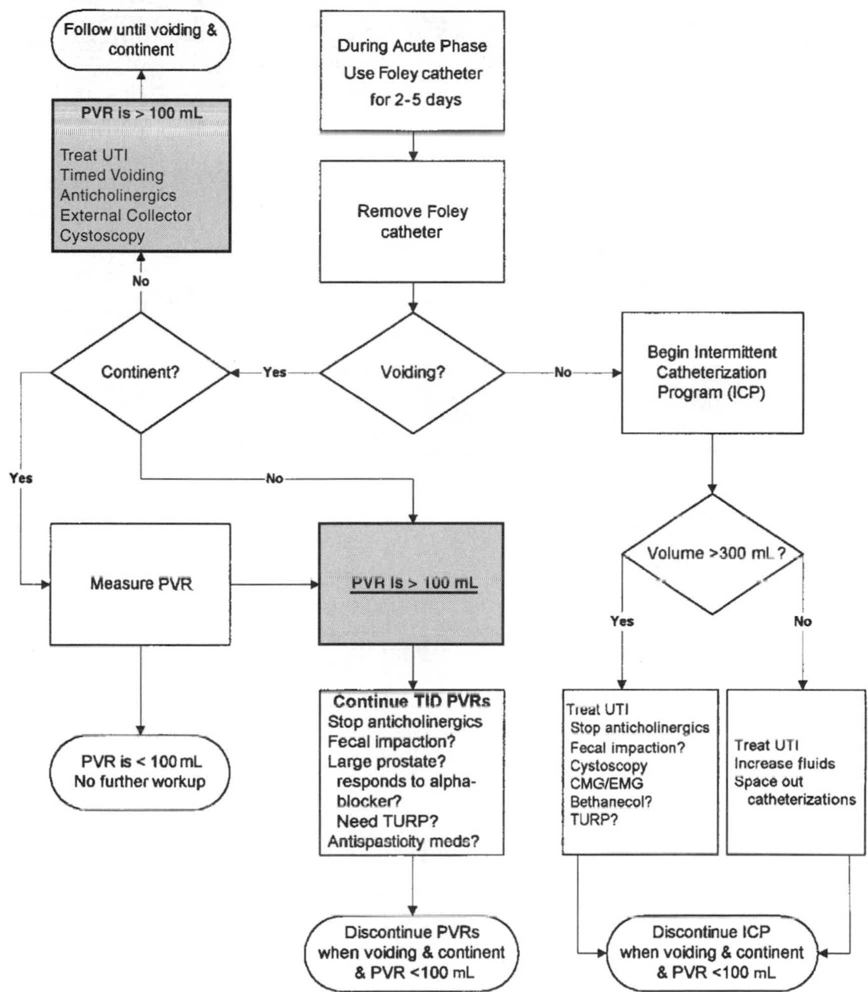

Adapted from *Stroke Clinical Updates*, "Urologic Problems After Stroke (Parts I and II)"; September 1993.

TABLE 21.28

Drugs Affecting Bladder Function

Muscle Affected	Action	
	Contraction	**Relaxation**
Detrusor/fundus (muscarinic receptors)	Bethanechol Neostigmine	Atropine Disopyramide Amantadine Imiprimine Antihistamines
Detrussor/fundus/sphincters (α- and β-receptors)	Ephedrine Pseudoephedrine Imipramine Propranolol Metoprolol	Prazosin Clonidine Terazosin α-Methyldopa
External sphincter (nicotinic receptors)		Diazepam Baclofen Dantrolene

Adapted from *Stroke Clinical Updates*, "Urologic Problems After Stroke (Parts I and II)," September 1993.

chapter 22

Emotional Illness and Adjustment

Ann M. Aring, MD

IN THIS CHAPTER

- Definitions of typical psychiatric signs and symptoms
- Psychiatric rating scales
- Child and adolescent developmental and psychological tests
- Childhood mood disorders
- Selective serotonin reuptake inhibitors to treat depression in children
- Attention deficit-hyperactivity disorder (ADHD)
- Evaluation and treatment for childhood attention deficit-hyperactivity disorder
- Adult mood disorders
- Laboratory monitoring for lithium, valproic acid, and carbamazepine
- Drug interactions with lithium
- Adult depressive disorders
- Treatment of depression: use of antidepressants
- Anxiety disorders
- Common peripheral manifestations of anxiety
- Organic differential diagnosis for anxiety disorders
- Benzodiazepines commonly prescribed for anxiety disorders
- Efficacy of pharmacologic agents for treatment of anxiety disorders
- Schizophrenia symptoms and treatment
- Properties of common antipsychotic agents
- Geriatric psychiatry: organic brain syndrome
- Borderline personality disorder: red flags
- Borderline personality disorder: diagnosis and treatment

- Substance abuse disorders
- Alcoholism screening tests
- Alcohol detoxification orders
- Psychiatric diagnoses to consider when physical symptoms are unexplained
- Relaxation therapy
- Counseling the family or individual
- Alternative medicine
- Risk factors associated with completed suicide
- Interviewing a patient with suicidal ideation
- Algorithm for the evaluation and treatment of suicidal patients
- Common psychiatric emergencies
- The hostile, agitated patient
- Medical reference software for handheld computers
- Internet references

BOOKSHELF RECOMMENDATIONS

- *Diagnostic and Statistical Manual of Mental Disorders*. 4th ed. Washington, DC: American Psychiatric Association; 2000.
- Barkley RA. *Attention Deficit Hyperactivity Disorder: A Handbook for Diagnosis and Treatment*. New York, NY: Guilford Press; 1990.

THE PSYCHIATRIC INTERVIEW

Family physicians play a key role in assessing and managing mental illness. Patients are more likely to consult a family doctor than a mental health specialist for depression and anxiety. In fact, primary care physicians write more prescriptions for antidepressants than do psychiatrists. In addition, patients with undiagnosed psychiatric disorders tend to be high utilizers of medical care. Family physicians have a unique opportunity to recognize and manage mental health problems as a result of the long-term relationship with the patient and the patient's family.

The psychiatric interview has two purposes: obtaining information to assess the patient's condition and establishing a doctor-patient relationship. In the psychiatric interview, patients may conceal feelings that they perceive to be shameful or threatening until they feel certain disclosing the information will not affect their doctor's respect. This illustrates an advantage family doctors have in the long doctor–patient relationships. The psychiatric interview may also be complicated by the fact that not all psychiatric patients have voluntarily sought medical help and may not be willing to cooperate for this reason. Initial consultations may be brief due to ill patients who find the interview stressful. Remember to position yourself between the patient and door in case the interview needs to be stopped abruptly.

TABLE 22.1

Definitions of Typical Psychiatric Signs and Symptoms

Disturbance of Consciousness

- Disorientation: disturbance of orientation in time, person, or place
- Delirium: confusion, restlessness, associated with fear and hallucinations
- Twilight state: disturbed consciousness with hallucinations
- Stupor: lack of reaction and unawareness of surroundings

Disturbance of Attention

- Hypervigilance: excessive attention and focus on all internal and external stimuli due to paranoid state
- Selective inattention: blocks out only those things that cause anxiety
- Distractibility: not able to concentrate; attention drawn by unimportant, irrelevant external stimuli

Disturbance of Affect (Expression of Emotion as Observed by Others)

- Appropriate affect: full range of emotions is appropriately expressed
- Inappropriate affect: emotional tone is not congruent with the patient's thoughts, ideas, and speech
- Flat affect: absence of any signs of affective expression
- Restricted affect: reduction in intensity of expressed feelings less severe than flat affect
- Blunted affect: disturbance in affect seen as a reduction in expression of emotions less severe than restricted affect
- Labile affect: abrupt and rapid change in emotions

Disturbance of Mood (Sustained Emotion, Subjectively Reported by the Patient and Observed by Others)

- Dysphoric mood: unpleasant mood
- Euthymic mood: normal range
- Irritable mood: easily annoyed and provoked to anger
- Labile mood: swings between depression or anxiety or elation
- Euphoric mood: elation with feelings of grandeur
- Depression: prolonged feeling of sadness
- Anhedonia: loss of interest and withdrawal from pleasurable activities
- Grief or mourning: appropriate sadness to a real loss

- Anxiety: feeling of apprehension caused by anticipating unpleasant event
- Agitation: severe anxiety associated with restlessness
- Panic: acute episodic attack of anxiety associated with overwhelming feelings of dread and autonomic symptoms
- Apathy: decreased emotional tone associated with indifference
- Ambivalence: coexistence of two opposing impulses toward the same thing at the same time

Disturbance in Motor Behavior

- Echopraxia: pathological imitation of movements of one person by another
- Catatonia: motor anomalies in nonorganic disorders
- Negativism: resistance to all attempts to instructions without a clear motive
- Cataplexy: temporary loss of muscle tone and weakness
- Psychomotor agitation: excessive motor and cognitive overactivity usually in response to inner tension
- Acting out: direct expression of an unconscious wish or impulse in action
- Tic: involuntary, spasmodic motor movement
- Akathesia: subjective feeling of muscular tension due to antipsychotic medication which can cause pacing and restlessness
- Compulsion: uncontrollable impulse to perform an act repetitively

Disturbance in Formation of Thought

- Neologism: new word created by the patient often formed by combining syllables of other words
- Word salad: incoherent mixture of words and phrases
- Circumstantiality: indirect speech that is delayed in reaching the point but eventually gets the message across
- Tangentiality: inability to have goal-directed thoughts
- Perseveration: persisting response to a prior stimulus after a new stimulus has been presented
- Echolalia: repeating of words or phrases, may be spoken with mocking or staccato intonation
- Loose associations: ideas shift from one subject to another in an unrelated way
- Flight of ideas: rapid continuous verbalizations of ideas that appear to be connected

Continued

TABLE 22.1

Definitions of Typical Psychiatric Signs and Symptoms, cont'd

- Blocking: abrupt interruptions in thinking before a thought is finished; after brief pause person indicates no recall of recent thought process

Specific Disturbances in Content of Thought

- Delusion: fixed, false belief based on incorrect interpretation of external stimuli that cannot be corrected by reasoning
- Obsession: persistence of an irresistable thought or feeling that will not go away despite logical effort
- Compulsion: need to act on an impulse that, if resisted, produces anxiety
- Phobia: persistent, irrational dread of some specific stimulus
- Dementia: deterioration of intellectual functioning without clouding of consciousness due to an organic cause
- Insight: ability of patient to understand cause of situation
- Judgment: ability to assess a situation correctly and act appropriately within that situation

Disturbance in Perception

- Hallucinations: false sensory perception not associated with real external stimuli; visual, olfactory, and gustatory most common in organic disorders
- Illusion: misinterpretation of real external sensory stimuli

TABLE 22.2

Psychiatric Rating Scales

Rating Scales Used for Mood Disorders	
Beck Depression Inventory	*Archives of General Psychiatry*, 1961;4:561
Standard Assessment of Depressive Disorders	*Psychological Medicine*, 1979;10:743
Zung Self-rating Scale for Depression	*Archives of General Psychiatry*, 1965;12:63
Mania Rating Scale	*Journal of Clinical Psychiatry*, 1983;44:98
Pediatric Symptom Checklist	*Journal of Pediatrics*, 1988;112:201–209
Rating Scales for Anxiety Disorders	
Anxiety States Inventory	*Psychosomatics*, 1971;12:371
Acute Panic Inventory	*Archives of General Psychiatry*, 1984;41:764
Leyton Obsessional Inventory	*Psychological Medicine*, 1970;1:48
Maudsley Obsessional-Compulsive Inventory	*Behavioral Research and Therapeutics*, 1977;15:389
Rating Scales for Schizophrenia and Psychosis	
Brief Psychiatric Rating Scale	*Psychological Reports*, 1962;10:799
Schedule for Affective Disorders and Schizophrenia	*Archives of General Psychiatry*, 1978;35:837
Scale for Assessment of Negative Symptoms	The University of Iowa Press, 1983
Thought Disorder Index	*Archives of General Psychiatry*, 1983;40:1281

TABLE 22.3

Selected Child and Adolescent Developmental and Psychological Tests

Test	Age Range	Test Description
Denver Developmental Screening Test	2 months–6 years	Developmental milestones
Stanford-Binet	2 years–24 years	Intelligence, IQ equivalent
Wechsler Intelligence Scale for Children-Revised	6 years–17 years	Full-scale IQ
Draw-a-Person	All ages	Perceptual ability
Test of Early Language Development	3 years–8 years	Speech and language
Rorschach test	3 years to adult	Personality
Peabody Individual Achievement Test	5 years–18 years	School grade skills level

CHILDHOOD MOOD DISORDERS

Mood disorders in childhood and adolescence are defined as a disturbance of mood such as depression or elation. Depression is more common. Mania or hypomania is very rare before the onset of puberty. Irritability is also a sign of mood disorders in children and adolescents. Suicide ideation, gestures, and attempts are associated with depression particularly in the adolescent population. The medical evaluation should include complete blood cell count, electrolytes, blood urea nitrogen, creatinine, liver function studies, thyearsoid function studies, and electrocardiogram as baseline, if considering a tricyclic antidepressant.

TABLE 22.4

Childhood Mood Disorders

Major Depressive Episode (296.2)

This is a very common disorder. There cannot be an organic factor as the etiology, nor is it a normal reaction to grief. There must be a depressive episode in which there is either a depressed mood or a loss of interest or pleasure in daily activities, or both. If both are present, there must be at least three of the following findings (four if only one is present):

1. Increase or decrease in weight or failure to make expected weight gains in children
2. Increase or decrease in sleep
3. Psychomotor agitation or retardation
4. Fatigue, feelings of worthlessness or guilt, cognitive changes, and recurrent thoughts of death.

According to the *Diagnostic and Statistical Manual of Mental Disorders*, fourth edition (DSM-IV), the core symptoms of a major depressive episode are the same for children and adolescents. Somatic complaints, irritability, and social withdrawal are common in children. In addition, excessive clinging to parents and school phobia may be symptoms of depression in children. Poor academic performance, drug abuse, antisocial behavior, and sexual promiscuity may be symptoms of depression in adolescence. Hypersomnia, psychomotor retardation, and delusions are more common in adolescence and young adulthood.

Dysthymia (300.4)

There are two significant differences in the diagnostic criteria for dysthymia in children and adolescents and those in adults. First, children and adolescents may have an irritable mood instead of the depressed mood required for adults. Second, the mood disturbance in children and adolescents must be present for only 1 year rather than 2 years for

Continued

TABLE 22.4

Childhood Mood Disorders, cont'd

adults. Patients with dysthymia have never had a manic episode. In addition, while feeling depressed, these patients must have at least two of the following three symptoms:

1. Increased or decreased appetite
2. Increased or decreased sleep
3. Fatigue, low self-esteem, poor concentration, difficulty making decisions, or feeling hopeless

Cyclothymia (301.13)

For child and adolescent cyclothymia, a period of 1 year of numerous mood swings between hypomania and depression is necessary for diagnosis instead of the adult criterion of 2 years. It is likely that most adolescents with cyclothymia will eventually develop bipolar disorder.

Bipolar Disorder (296)

Elevated, expansive, or irritable mood is the hallmark. Other signs include a disinhibited nature and impulsive behavior. Mania in adolescents may include severe, persistent symptoms of psychosis, alcohol or drug abuse, academic difficulties, multiple somatic complaints, antisocial behavior, or suicide attempts.

TABLE 22.5

Selective Serotonin Reuptake Inhibitors to Treat Depression in Children

Medication	Dosing Range	Available Formulations
Sertraline (Zoloft)	25–125 mg daily	50- and 100-mg tablets
Fluoxetine (Prozac)	5–40 mg daily	Suspension (20 mg/5 mL), 10- and 20-mg capsules
Paroxetine (Paxil)	5–40 mg daily	10-, 20-, 30- and 40-mg tablets
Fluvoxamine (Luvox)	25–125 mg twice daily	Suspension (10 mg/5 mL), 25-, 50- and 100-mg tablets

TABLE 22.6

Attention Deficit-Hyperactivity Disorder (314.9)

Attention deficit-hyperactivity disorder (ADHD) includes behavioral symptoms of short attention span, impulsivity, and hyperactivity. In order to diagnose ADHD, the symptoms must have started prior to age 7 years and be present for at least 6 months. The principal sign of hyperactivity should alert clinicians to the possibility of ADHD. Reports on the incidence of ADHD estimate 3% to 5% of prepubertal elementary school children have the disorder. Many rating scales exist for parents and teachers to assess for ADHD. For more information, see Barkley, RA. *Attention Deficit Hyperactivity Disorder: A Handbook for Diagnosis and Treatment*. New York, NY: Guilford, 1990. The family physician should also screen the child for other illnesses with a complete blood cell count, blood lead level, and thyearsoid function tests.

FIGURE 22.1

Evaluation for ADHD

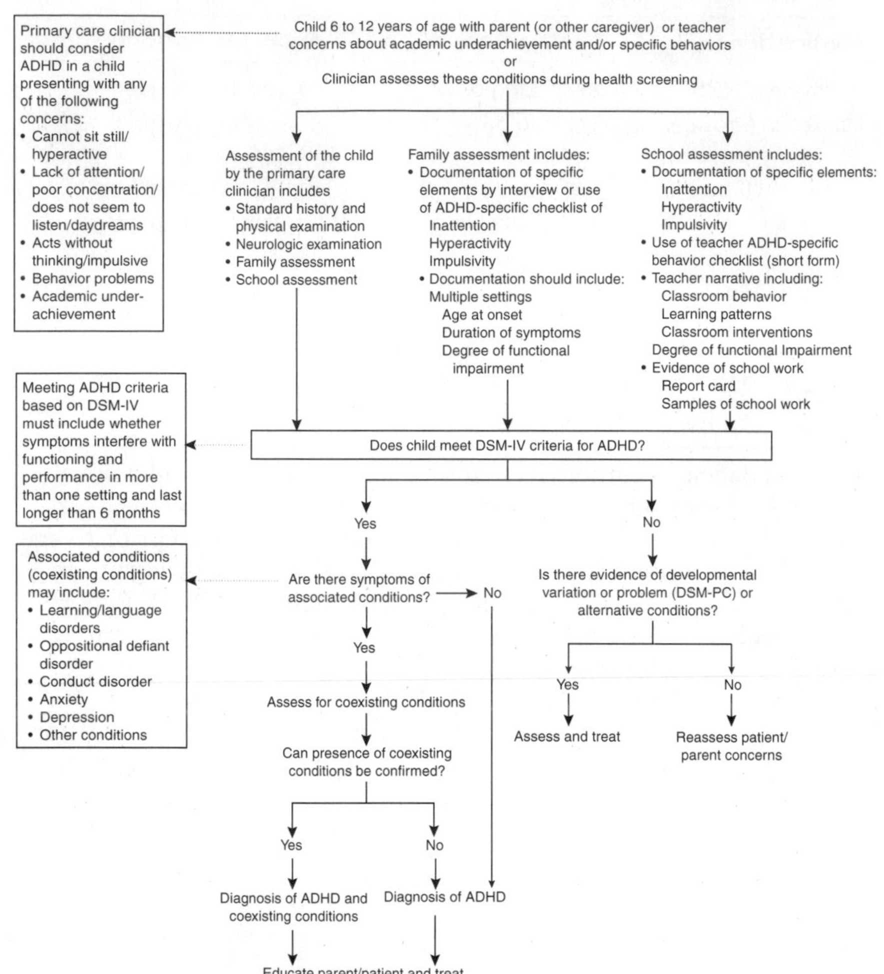

Reproduced with permission from the American Academy of Pediatrics. (Clinical Practice Guideline: diagnosis and evaluation of the child with ADHD. *Pediatrics.* 2000;105:1158–1170.)

ADHD indicates attention deficit-hyperactivity disorder; DSM-IV, *Diagnostic and Statistical Manual of Mental Disorders*, 4th edition; DSM-PC, *Diagnostic and Statistical Manual of Mental Disorders*, 4th edition, primary care version.

TABLE 22.7

Treatment for Childhood Attention Deficit-Hyperactivity Disorder

Medication	Dose	Side Effects	Monitoring
Methylphenidate (Ritalin) (5-, 10-, 20-mg tablets) Methylphenidate SR 20 mg	0.3–0.5 mg/kg/dose; initially, 5 mg q am and q noon; max dose 60 mg/d	Weight loss, high blood pressure, insomnia	CBC q 6 mo; weight, height, blood pressure each visit
Methylphenidate extended release (Concerta)	For Concerta, start at 18 mg q am with max dose 54 mg/d		
Dextroamphetamine (Dexadrine) Amphetamine mixtures (Adderall)	0.2–0.4 mg/kg/dose; usual starting dose 5 mg/d or bid; max dose 40 mg/d	Weight loss, high blood pressure, insomnia	Weight, height, blood pressure each visit
Pemoline (Cylert) (18.75, 37.5, 75 mg)	0.5–3 mg/kg/d; initial dose is 37.5 mg/d	Weight loss, high blood pressure, insomnia, hepatotoxicity	Baseline LFTs then 1 month later then q 6 mo; similar to Ritalin

ADULT MOOD DISORDERS

Mood disorders represent a disturbance of mood with a manic or depressive syndrome. Mood is a prolonged emotion and is usually depression or elation. The mood disorders are subdivided into bipolar disorders and depressive disorders. To qualify as a bipolar disorder, there must have been one or more manic or hypomanic episodes.

TABLE 22.8

Bipolar Disorders

Bipolar I Disorder (296.60)

There is a community prevalence of 0.5%. These patients have had one or more manic episodes and have often had previous major depressive episodes. The manic episode is not explained by schizoaffective disorder or is not superimposed on a psychotic disorder.

Bipolar II Disorder (296.60)

There is a community prevalence of 0.5%. These patients have recurrent major depressive episodes with one or more hypomanic episodes. Hypomanic episodes have the same characteristics as manic episodes but are not severe enough to impair the patient socially or occupationally or require hospitalization. If the hypomanic episode becomes manic, then the diagnosis becomes bipolar I.

Cyclothymia (301.13)

This disorder must have occurred for 2 years for adults or 1 year for children and involves numerous hypomanic episodes as well as recurrent periods of depressed mood not severe enough to be diagnosed as major depression. There is a prevalence of 0.4% to 1%.

TABLE 22.9

Treatment for Bipolar Disorder: Dosages of Lithium, Valpropic Acid, and Carbamazepine

Initial Starting Dose	Maintenance Dose	Side Effects
Lithium		
900 mg/d; increase 2 to 3 days by 300 to 600 mg as tolerated	900 to 1800 mg/d; therapeutic blood level 0.8 to 1.5 mEq/L	Thirst, polyuria, tremor, weight gain, nausea, hypothyroidism
Valproic acid (Depakene)		
20 mg/kg/d for mania; adjust dose in 3 to 5 days	1000 to 3000 mg/d; therapeutic blood level 50 to 125 μg/mL	Tremor, sedation, nausea, diarrhea, mild elevation of liver function tests
Carbamezepine (Tegretol)		
200 to 400 mg/d; increase by 200 mg daily every 2 to 4 days	400 to 1200 mg/d; therapeutic blood level 4–12 μg/mL	Headache, rash, leukopenia, mild elevation of liver function tests

TABLE 22.10

Laboratory Monitoring for Lithium, Valproic Acid, and Carbamazepine*

Lithium

- First 2 months of therapy: serum level every 1 to 2 weeks
- Long-term therapy: serum level every 3–6 months, yearly thyroid function tests, renal function every 6–12 months

Valproic Acid

- First 2 months of therapy: serum level every 1 to 2 weeks, CBC and LFTs monthly
- Long-term therapy: serum level every 3–6 months, CBC and LFTs every 6 to 12 months

Carbamezepine

- First 2 months of therapy: serum level every 1 to 2 weeks, CBC and LFTs monthly
- Long-term therapy: serum level every 1 to 2 weeks, CBC and LFTs monthly

*Serum levels of mood stabilizers should be checked whenever the clinical situation or dosage changes.

TABLE 22.11

Drug Interactions With Lithium

Drug	Effect on Lithium Level	Management
Nonsteroidal anti-inflammatory	Increased lithium level	Use lower dose of lithium; consider aspirin
Thiazide diuretics	Increased lithium level	Avoid combination or reduce doses
Loop diuretics	Increased or decreased lithium level	Avoid combination or reduce doses
Potassium-sparing diuretics	Decreased lithium level	Monitor lithium level; adjust prn
ACE inhibitors	Increased lithium level	Use lower dose of lithium; monitor

ACE indicates angiotensin converting enzyme; prn, when necessary.

TABLE 22.12
Adult Depressive Disorders

This is a very common disorder affecting mood. There cannot be an organic factor as the etiology, not is it a normal reaction to bereavement. Delusions or hallucination may occur but not in the absence of mood symptoms. Naturally, there must be a depressive episode in which there is either a depressed mood or a loss of interest or pleasure in daily activities, or both. If both are present, then there must be at least three of the following findings (four if only one is present):

1. Increase or decrease weight
2. Increase or decrease in sleep
3. Psychomotor agitation or retardation
4. Fatigue, feelings of worthlessness or guilt, cognitive changes, and recurrent thoughts of death

Major Depression (296.2)
The essentials of the diagnosis are a major depressive episode as described earlier without a history of a manic episode. Fifty percent of people who have major depression will have another episode. The range of incidence for females is 9% to 26% and for males the incidence is 5% to 12%. The disorder is 1.5 to 3 times more common in first-degree relatives. Up to 15% of individuals with major depression die of suicide during this episode.

Mnemonic for symptoms of major depression is **SIG E CAPS:**

S Sleep (insomnia or hypersomnia)
I Interest (loss of interest)
G Guilt
E Energy (feeling of fatigue)
C Concentration (inability to concentrate)
A Appetite (increase or decreased)
P Psychomotor (agitation or retardation)
S Suicidality (ideation, plan)

Dysthymia (300.4)
Individuals with dysthymia have never had a manic episode. Symptoms of depressed mood have existed for 2 years (1 year for children) without evidence of a major depressive episode as defined previously. While feeling depressed, these individuals must have at least two of the following three symptoms:

1. Increased or decreased appetite
2. Increase or decrease in sleep
3. Fatigue, low self-esteem, poor concentration or difficulty making decisions, and feeling of hopelessness.

Continued

TABLE 22.12

Adult Depressive Disorders, cont'd

Postpartum Depression (648.44)
Many women experience "postpartum blues" 3 to 7 days after the birth of a baby. These feelings include a state of sadness, dysphoria, frequent tearfulness, and clinging dependency. Postpartum blues have been attributed to the rapid change in hormone levels, stress of childbirth, and the increased responsibility of motherhood. Postpartum depression has an onset within 4 weeks of the postpartum period. Selective serotonin reuptake inhibitors are typical used for prolonged symptoms. In rare cases, a postpartum psychosis may develop, which is characterized by delusions, hallucinations, or severe anxiety.

TABLE 22.13

Treatment of Depression: Use of Antidepressants

Class	Drug	Dose*	NE	SER	Anticholinergic	Sedation	Ortho
Tertiary Amines	Amitriptyline (Elavil and generic)	50–150 mg hs	++	++++	++++	++++	++
	Imipramine (Tofranil and generic)	50–150 mg hs	++	++++	++	++	+++
	Doxepin (Sinequan and generic)	50–150 mg hs	+	++	++	+++	++
	Clomipramine (Anafranil)†	25–250 mg hs	++	+++++	+++	+++	++
	Trimipramine (Surmontil)	50–150 mg hs	+	+	++	+++	++
Secondary Amines	Desipramine (Norpramin and generic)	50–150 mg hs	++++	++	+	+	+
	Nortriptyline (Aventyl and generic)	25–100 mg hs	++	+++	++	++	+
	Protriptyline (Vivactil)	15–40 mg hs	++++	++	+++	+	+

Continued

TABLE 22.13

Treatment of Depression: Use of Antidepressants, cont'd

Class	Drug	Dose*	NE	SER	Anticholinergic	Sedation	Ortho
Tetracyclic	Maprotiline (Ludiomil and generic)	50–150 mg hs	+++	+	++	++	+
Bicyclic	Fluoxetine (Prozac)	20–60 mg in the morning	+	+++++	0	0	+
Triazolopyridine	Trazodone (Desyrel and generic)	150–400 mg hs or twice daily	0	+++	+	+++	+++
Aminoketone	Bupropion[‡] (Wellbutrin)	100 mg AM and PM for 3 days, then 100 mg tid	0/+	0/+	++	++	+
	Paroxetine (Paxil)	20–50 mg in the morning	0/+	+++++	0	0	0

Class	Drug	Dose*	NE	SER	Anticholinergic	Sedation	Ortho
New Agents	Sertraline (Zoloft)	50–200 mg in the morning	0/+	+++++	0	0	0
	Venlafaxine (Effexor)	75–150 mg in 2–3 daily doses	+++	+++	0	0	0
	Remeron (Mirtzaepine)	15–45 mg/d	++[1]	+++[2]	++	−++	++
	Serzone (Nefazadone)	200 mg/d in 2 individualized doses ↑ to 300–600 mg/d	0/+[3]	+++	+/0	−+	+

[1]Alpha 2 presynaptic antagonist.

[2]5++72 and SI + T3 antagonist.

[3]5++72 antagonist.

NE indicates Norepinephrine; SER, serotonin; Ortho, orthostatic; tid, three times daily; 0, none; +, slight; ++, moderate; +++, high; −+++, very high; +++++, extremely high.

*Doses listed are usual daily doses. Initiate the dosage at the low end of the range indicated and slowly titrate upward over several days or weeks. The dosage in elderly patients or children should be reduced (see product labeling).

†Clomipramine is only indicated for obsessive-compulsive disorder.

‡Also inhibits dopamine update. To avoid seizures, dosage increases of bupropion must not exceed 100 mg in a 3-day period, and no single dose should exceed 150 mg. The maximum dose is 450 mg daily (150 mg tid).

ANXIETY DISORDERS

Anxiety is a vague unpleasant feeling of apprehension accompanied by one or more somatic sensations. Pathologic anxiety can be a symptom of an organic anxiety disorder, an anxiety disorder, or an adjustment disorder with anxious mood. The lifelong prevalence of anxiety disorders is estimated between 10% and 15%. The hallmark symptoms of panic disorder are spontaneous, episodic, intense periods of anxiety, which last less than 1 hour. Panic attacks usually occur about two times a week but may occur more or less frequently.

TABLE 22.14

Anxiety Disorders

ICDA-9 Code	DSM-IV Classification	Definition: Excessive, Irrational, Worry Plus
300.22	Agoraphobia without panic disorder	Fear of being in a place where escape might be embarrassing
300.21	Panic disorder without agoraphobia	Fear of having a panic attack
309.21	Separation anxiety	Fear of separation from well-known people; onset before age 18
300.29	Specific phobia	Fear of an item
300.23	Social phobia	Fear of embarrassment or humiliation
300.3	Obsessive-compulsive disorder	Recurrent obsessions or compulsions
300.02	Generalized anxiety disorder	Non-stressor related, lasting ≥6 months
309.81	Posttraumatic stress disorder	Recurring thoughts of traumatic event
300.00	Anxiety disorder not otherwise specified	Do not meet other criteria
308.3	Acute stress disorder	Occurs within 4 weeks of a stressful event
293.89	Anxiety disorder resulting from a general medical condition	Physiologically linked to medical condition (eg, thyrotoxicosis)
—	Substance-induced anxiety	Related to chemical agent or withdrawal

TABLE 22.15

Common Peripheral Manifestations of Anxiety

- Diarrhea
- Dizziness
- Hyperhidrosis
- Palpitations
- Restlessness
- Syncope
- Tingling in the extremities
- Tremors
- Upset stomach
- Urinary frequency, hesitancy, urgency

TABLE 22.16

Organic Differential Diagnosis for Anxiety Disorders

Cardiovascular	**Drug Withdrawal**
Anemia	Alcohol
Angina	Antihypertensives
CHF	Opiates
HTN	Sedative hypnotics
Mitral valve prolapse	**Endocrine**
Pulmonary	Diabetes
Asthma	Hyperthyroid
Hyperventilation	Hypoglycemia
PE	Menopausal
Drug Intoxication	Neurological
Amphetamine	CVA
Cocaine	Epilepsy
Marijuana	Migraine headache
Theophylline	Multiple sclerosis
	Tumor

TABLE 22.17

Benzodiazepines Commonly Prescribed for Anxiety Disorders

Name	Half-life (h)	Dose/d*	Initial Dose
Oxazepam (Serax)	9	30 to 90 mg	15 to 30 mg tid
Lorazepam (Ativan)	14	1 to 6 mg	0.5 to 1 mg tid
Alprazolam (Xanax)	14	1 to 4 mg	0.25 to 0.5 mg qid
Chlordiazepoxide (Librium)	20	15 to 40 mg	5 to 10 mg tid
Diazepam (Valium)	40	6 to 40 mg	2 to 5 mg tid
Clonazepam (Klonopin)	50	0.5 to 4 mg	0.5 to 1 mg bid
Clorazepate (Tranxene)	60	15 to 60 mg	7.5 to 15 bid

*For geriatric patients, use half the daily dose listed.

bid indicates twice daily; qid, four times daily; tid, three times daily.

TABLE 22.18

Efficacy of Pharmacologic Agents for Treatment in Anxiety Disorder

Disorder	BZs	SSRIs	TCAs	Bu	ACs	ANs
Acute anxiety		++	–	–	–	–
Generalized anxiety disorder	++	+	++	++	+/–	–
Obsessive-compulsive disorder		++	+	+	–	+/–
Panic disorder		++	++	++	–	+
Posttraumatic stress disorder	+/–	+	+	+	+	+
Social phobia		+	++	+	+	–

Adapted from Longo LP, Johnson B. Addiction: Part I. Benzodiazepines—side effects, abuse risk and alternatives. *Am Fam Physician.* 2000;61:2121–2128.

BZs indicates benzodiazepines; SSRIs, selective serotonin reuptake inhibitors; TCAs, tricyclic antidepressants; Bu, buspar; ACVs, anticonvulsants; ANS, atypical neuroleptics.

TABLE 22.19

Schizophrenia: Symptoms and Treatment

Disorder	Major Symptoms	Treatment Plan
Schizophrenia	Delusions that may or may not have persecutory or jealousy content; auditory hallucinations; incoherence; decrease in level of functioning; symptoms present for 6 months at some time in life	See individual types
Catatonic	Mutism; negativism; rigid posture in inappropriate positions; may have motor excitement	Major tranquilizer; hospitalization; structured protective environment
Disorganized	Incoherent; delusions in fragments only; affect blunted, inappropriate, or silly	Major tranquilizer; structured environment
Paranoid	Delusions that are persecutory, grandiose, or jealous; hallucinations of same three types	Major tranquilizer; supportive but not overly friendly environment
Undifferentiated	Prominent delusions; incoherence; tangential thinking; hallucinations; grossly disorganized; other types excluded	Major tranquilizer; structured environment; routine medical follow-up; socialization groups
Residual	Emotional blunting; social withdrawal; eccentric behavior; illogical behavior; loose associations; past history of one of the above types	Major tranquilizer; routine medical care

TABLE 22.20

Properties of Common Antipsychotic Agents

Class	Drug	Dose*	EPS	Sedation	Anticholinergic	Ortho
Aliphatic	Chlorpromazine (Thorazine and generic)	50–1000 mg daily in three doses	++	+++	++	+++
	Promazine (Sparine and generic)	50–1000 mg in four doses	++	++	+++	++
	Triflupromazine (Vesprin)	60–150 mg IM daily	++	+++	+++	++
Piperidine	Mesoridazine (Serentil)	50–400 mg in three doses	+	+++	+++	++
	Thioridazine (Mellaril and generic)	150–800 mg in three doses	+	+++	+++	+++
Piperazine	Acetophenazine (Tindal)	40–80 mg daily in three doses	+++	++	+	+
	Fluphenazine (Prolixin and generic)	0.5–10 mg once or twice daily	+++	+	+	+

Class	Drug	Dose*	EPS	Sedation	Anticholinergic	Ortho
	Perphenazine (Trilafon and generic)	12–24 mg in three doses	+++	+	+	+
	Prochlorperazine (Compazine and generic)	25–150 mg in three doses	+++	++	+	+
	Trifluoperazine (Stelazine and generic)	4–30 mg in two doses	+++	+	+	+
Butyrophenone	Haloperidol (Haldol and generic)	1–15 mg in two or three doses	+++	+	+	+
Thioxanthene	Chlorprothixene (Taractan)	75–600 mg in three doses	++	+++	++	++
	Thiothixene (Navane and generic)	6–30 mg in three doses	+++	+	+	+

Continued

TABLE 22.20

Properties of Common Antipsychotic Agents, cont'd

Class	Drug	Dose*	EPS	Sedation	Anticholinergic	Ortho
Dibenzodiazepine	Clozapine (Clozaril)	300–900 mg daily in one or two daily doses†	+	+++	+++	+++
Benzisoxazole	Risperidone (Risperdal)	4–16 mg in two daily doses	0	+	+	+
Diphenylbutylpiperidine	Pimozide (Orap)	1–10 mg in two or three doses	+++	++	++	+
	Olanzapine (Zyprexa)	5–20 mg/d	+/0	++	+++	++
	Quetiapine (Seroquel)	300–400 mg/d; 2–3 ind doses start 25 mg bid	+/0	++/+++	0	++

bid indicates twice daily; EPS, extrapyramidal side effects; IM, intramuscularly; Ortho, orthostatic hypotension; 0, none; +, slight; ++, moderate; +++, high; ++++, very high.

*Doses listed are usual daily doses. Initiate the dosage at or below the low end of the range indicated and slowly titrate upward over several days or weeks. The dosage in elderly patients or children should be reduced (see product labeling).

†Initial dose should be 25 mg once or twice daily and should be titrated to the target range by 14 days. The use of clozapine must be accompanied by weekly blood tests to detect agranulocytosis.

TABLE 22.21

Geriatric Psychiatry: Organic Brain Syndrome

Disease	Major Symptoms	Etiology and Treatment Plan
Organic brain syndrome	Disturbance of attention, memory, intellect, and orientation; may have delusions or hallucinations	Systemic infections; metabolic disorders, including hypoxia; postoperative state; substance abuse
Delirium	Clouded state of consciousness; disorientation; memory deficit; misinterpretations; illusions or hallucinations; incoherent; increased or decreased psychomotor activity	Tranquilizers prn for agitation; structured environment
Dementia	Decrease intellectual ability leading to decrease in level of function; memory deficit; deficit in abstract thinking; impaired judgment; aphasia; agnosia; state of consciousness clear	Primary degenerative dementia (Alzheimer); CNS infection; brain trauma; toxic metabolic disturbances; vascular diseases; normal-pressure hydrocephalus; neurologic diseases
Amnestic syndrome	Long- and short-term memory deficit; clear state of consciousness; intellectual function intact	Head trauma; hypoxia; infarction; encephalitis; thiamine deficiency; alcohol abuse
Organic delusional syndrome	Delusions; intellect normal; state of consciousness clear; features resemble schizophrenia	Drug abuse; lesion in nondominant hemisphere
Organic hallucinosis	Persistent or recurrent hallucinations; intellect normal; state of consciousness clear; features resemble schizophrenia	Hallucinogen abuse; alcohol abuse; sensory deprivation structured, supportive, protective environment

CNS indicates central nervous system; prn, when necessary.

TABLE 22.22

Borderline Personality Disorder Red Flags

An important personality disorder to recognize is borderline personality disorder. Patients with this disorder cause hostility toward caregivers and have low rates of treatment compliance. In addition, patients with borderline personality disorder have high rates of suicidal ideation and a higher comorbidity of other psychiatric illness.

Red Flags for Borderline Personality Disorder

- History of doctor shopping
- History of legal suits against physicians or other professionals
- History of suicide attempts
- History of several brief marriages or relationships
- An immediate idealization of you as the "best doctor"

TABLE 22.23

Borderline Personality Disorder Diagnosis and Treatment

According to the criteria set forth by the American Psychiatric Association in the DSM-IV, the patient begins in early adulthood to show five of the following features as characteristics of her or his current and/or long-term functioning:

- Impulsivity or unpredictability in at least two areas that are potentially self-damaging: spending money, sex, gambling, substance abuse, overeating, inflicting self-harm
- A pattern of unstable and intense interpersonal relationships
- Inappropriate, intense anger or lack of control of anger (temper)
- Identity disturbance described many times by metaphors ("I feel like a robot") and that may involve poor self-image or gender identity confusion
- Marked shifts of mood lasting only a few hours and rarely a few days
- Chronic feelings of boredom, loneliness, and emptiness
- Concerned about real or imagined abandonment
- Transient stress-related paranoid ideation or dissociative symptoms

Treatment must be individualized, but the cornerstone is surely patience, support, and limits. Psychotherapy must be weekly for about 2 years; medications, though not useful for the long term, may be needed to control temporary crises.

State	Drug or Class
Emotional lability	Lithium carbonate
Anxiety states	Benzodiazepines
Psychotic episodes	Phenothiazines
	Atypical antipsychotics

TABLE 22.24

Substance Abuse Disorders

Scope of Problem

Alcoholism is one of the leading causes of death and disability. It is certainly the nation's number 1 drug problem. Early recognition and treatment are important.

Features That May Indicate an Alcohol Problem

Historical Features	Symptoms	Signs
■ GI bleeding	■ Abdominal pain	■ Decreased levels of consciousness
■ Recent auto accident or arrest record	■ Anxiety	■ Tremors
■ Unusual trauma or fracture	■ Depression	■ Spider nevus
■ Blackouts with drinking	■ Hallucinations	■ Abdominal tenderness
■ Hypertension	■ Insomnia	■ Hepatomegaly
■ Heart disease	■ Headache	■ Splenomegaly
■ Sexual dysfunction	■ Impotence	■ Testicular atrophy
■ Amenorrhea		■ Cigarette burns
■ Seizures		■ Parotid gland enlargement
■ Marital discord		■ Elevated BP
■ Legal or job problems		■ Gynecomastia
		■ Unexplained bruises

BP indicates blood pressure; GI, gastrointestinal.

TABLE 22.25A

Short Michigan Alcoholism Screening Test (SMAST)

	Yes	No
1. Do you feel you are a normal drinker? (By *normal* we mean do you drink less than or as much as most other people.)	______ (0 points)	______ (1 point)
2. Do others who are important to you ever worry or complain about your drinking?	______ (1 point)	______ (0 points)
3. Do you ever feel bad about your drinking?	______ (1 point)	______ (0 points)
4. Do friends or relatives think you are a normal drinker?	______ (0 points)	______ (1 point)
5. Are you always able to stop drinking when you want to?	______ (0 points)	______ (1 point)
6. Have you ever attended a meeting of Alcoholics Anonymous (AA) for yourself?	______ (3 points)	______ (0 points)
7. Has your drinking ever created problems between you and others who are important to you?	______ (1 point)	______ (0 points)
8. Have you ever gotten into trouble at work because of your drinking?	______ (1 point)	______ (0 points)
9. Have you ever neglected your obligations, your family, or your work for two or more days in a row because you were drinking?	______ (1 point)	______ (0 points)
10. Have you ever gone to anyone for help about your drinking?	______ (3 points)	______ (0 points)
11. Have you ever been in a hospital because of your drinking?	______ (3 points)	______ (0 points)

	Yes	No
12. Have you ever been arrested for drunken driving, driving while intoxicated, or driving while under the influence of alcoholic beverages?	______	______
	(1 point)	(0 points)
13. Have you ever been arrested, even for a few hours, because of other drunken behavior? (1 point) (0 points)	______	______

Scoring System
0–1 points: Normal
2 points: Possibly alcoholic
3 or more points: Probably alcoholic

TABLE 22.25B

CAGE Survey

Are you . . .

Cutting down or feel the need to?
Annoyed when people criticize your drinking?
Guilty about your drinking?
Eye-opening with a drink in the morning?

If you answered yes to any question, there is a high probability of alcoholism.

TABLE 22.26

Alcohol Detoxification Orders

- Obtain current drinking history with emphasis on prior withdrawal experience; inquire specifically about other drug use (tranquilizers, sedatives, cocaine, etc) in addition to alcohol
- Regular diet; between-meal feeding as needed
- Up ad lib, with help first 24 hours
- Take vital signs every 3 hours
- Pajamas or hospital gown first 72 hours
- Milk of magnesia 30 mL po prn
- Encourage po fluid intake
- Unless otherwise specified, the following medications:
  —Multivitamin tablets, 1 po bid
  —Thiamine HCl, 100 mg IM
  —Aspirin, 650 mg, or Tylenol, 650 mg
  —$MgSO_4$, if serum magnesium is low
- PPD and *Candida* control
- On admission, order the following lab tests: CBC with platelets, SMA 6/60 and 12/60, ALT, GGT, PT, PTT, serum magnesium, folic acid, RPR, urinalysis, blood alcohol, urine drug screen, consider HIV
- PA and lateral chest x-ray examination and ECG
- Detoxification regimen:
  —Phenobarbitol 60–90 mg every 6 hours po
  —Alternate with diazepam 10–20 mg every 6 hours prn
  —Decrease the regimen daily if vital signs remain stable
- Alternate regimen: choose one or more of the following to sedate patient, then wean over 2–3 days:
  —Chlordiazepoxide (Librium)
  —Diazepam (Valium)
  —Lorazepam (Ativan)
  —Phenobarbital
- Additional meds used as adjuncts:
  —Clonidine: to relieve autonomic hyperactivity
  —Beta-blockers: for persistent tachycardia
- For imminent delirium tremens, which usually occurs 48–72 hours after blood pressure, pulse, and respiration increase, use additional phenobarbital or diazepam

ALT indicates alanine aminotransferase; bid, twice daily; CBC, complete blood cell count; ECG, electrocardiogram; HIV, human immunodeficiency virus; IM, intramuscularly; PA, pulmonary artery; po, orally; PPD, purified protein derivative; prn, when necessary; PT, prothrombin time; PTT, partial thromboplastin time; RPR, rapid plasma reagin.

TABLE 22.27

Psychiatric Diagnoses to Consider When Physical Symptoms Are Unexplained

- Alcohol or drug dependence
- Anxiety disorders
  —Generalized anxiety disorder (300.02)
  —Panic disorder without agoraphobia (300.01)
  Factitious disorder with physical signs and symptoms (300.19)
- Mood disorders
  —Major depressive disorder (296.2)
  —Dysthymic disorder (300.4)
- Somatoform disorders
  —Somatization disorder (300.81)
  —Hypochondriasis (300.7)

TABLE 22.28

Relaxation Therapy

Relaxation therapy can be used to relieve stress and tension in some patients. It can be done in 5–10 minutes in the office and repeated by the patient several times a day. It is best introduced in a quiet, uninterrupted atmosphere with the patient in a comfortable position. The patient should understand that he or she is not being hypnotized and will remain in control of his or her body. You will need to speak in a soft, soothing, monotone and continue talking until the therapy ends. You can use your own script or this sample:

"You are going to relax to the best of your ability. Please close your eyes. As you relax you will feel tension leave your body, to be replaced by a calm, soothing sensation. I want you to think of a pleasant landscape scene and see yourself relaxing there. Already you can feel your tense muscles relax. You may feel sleepy as relaxation takes over your body. With each breath you become more relaxed. Breathe in relaxation and exhale tension. Breathe in relaxation and breathe out all tension. Feel your arms and legs relax as we count to ten. 1, 2, 3, 4, 5, 6, 7, 8, 9, 10. [You may ad lib here and discuss each area of the body.] Now feel how calm you are becoming and see yourself resting in that pleasant landscape scene. Every part of your body is relaxing now, your arms, your legs, your feet, your back, and your scalp. Breathe in relaxation and exhale tension. Now as we count backward from 10 to 1 you will become more alert and more rested. 10, 9, 8, 7, 6, 5 . . . Breathe in relaxation and exhale tension. At zero you will be more alert and well rested . . . 4, 3, 2, 1, 0. Open your eyes and feel how relaxed you are."

TABLE 22.29

Counseling the Family or Individual

Counseling Format

Outline of Counseling Session

Build a therapeutic relationship

Assess the Problem

Let each member describe the problem
Reflect the problem to make sure you understand it
Ask each member how it affects him or her
Allow ventilation and give support

Problem Solve

How has it been dealt with in the past?
What can be done to change the problem?

Form a Treatment Plan

Summarize the Session

First the patient, then the counselor

Counseling Techniques

Engaging the Family

The process of beginning a trusting relationship is more difficult with the family than with the individual. Some guidelines are to talk to all family members, beginning the session by addressing each member with polite social questions. It is usually best not to address the patient first, particularly if it is a child. Make an attempt to pull in the member who seems the most reserved. Recognize the member whose opinion is valued—there is probably one—and make a point to honor this authority. Adopt the family's style of conversation so that everyone is at ease.

Initiating Discussion of the Problem

Open the discussion by asking a family member (other than the patient) how it came about that you are meeting today. Another approach is to ask what it is like being in this family these days. You may want to address this question to the youngest member since he/she is likely to be totally honest. When dealing with a child problem, it is best to ask the parent what problems the family needs to work on. Even though one member may have already given you details of the problem, it is better to let someone repeat it in front of the whole group. In supportive counseling sessions, such as grief, you may be the one to summarize the situation.

Structuring the Session

The family or individual must perceive you as able to lead the session to feel secure enough to talk about painful material. There may be a struggle for control and leadership. You must win this struggle to be an effective counselor. Doherty and Baird suggest six core family counseling rules:

1. Each person has the right to speak without being interrupted.
2. When you have announced a procedure or plan of action, do not become sidetracked (eg, if you say you want to hear everyone's opinion, do not let an argument interrupt that plan).
3. Steer the family back to the issues at hand when they stray.
4. Resist requests for solutions if requests seem premature or inappropriate (eg, "I think the solution will come from you as a family. I will have ideas to help you").
5. Take charge of the physical arrangement of the session. Observe the seats they choose. Rearrange when needed. A circle is often good.
6. Take charge of who attends the session; make sure everyone knows who is expected to come to each meeting and insist that they be there.

Defining the Problem

You may wish to define the problem by asking each member how he/she would like to see this relationship change. "What changes would you like to see?"

You should encourage these to be specific, concrete, and positive.

History Taking

This should occupy less than a third of the initial interview. The two most basic pieces of information are the onset of the problem and how the family or person has attempted to cope with it.

Remaining Neutral

To avoid casting family members in roles, you must believe that there are not villains or victims. Your support must seem to be distributed equally among the group.

Encouraging a Collaborative Set

Encourage the family to work on the problem together. Explain that they got to the problem together and now must pull together to get out.

Facilitating Family Discussion

Encourage the family to talk directly to one another during the session. They may resist and say that they feel silly, etc. If you have asked them to speak directly to each other, insist on it and don't back down. There are three good opportunities for this direct communication:

1. When a joint decision is being reached.
2. When a positive comment about a member is made to you, respond with "Why don't you *ask/tell* her that now."
3. If a member says another member will not listen, ask him if he will listen.

Generally, communications must be practiced in the session before being used by the family. Give support when dealing with stress,

Continued

TABLE 22.29

Counseling the Family or Individual, cont'd

grief, or dislocation. To be an effective counselor you must provide support, and to do that you must genuinely want to support them. Here are five guidelines:

1. Listen; let people express their feelings.
2. Let them know that you are with them emotionally by reflecting the emotion you hear them expressing (eg, "You still miss him a lot").
3. Do not move ahead of the family emotionally by promising that they will feel better soon or that it may not be as bad as they think.
4. Mobilize support systems for the family or individual.
5. Teach when you can clarify a situation. The art is to teach when information is needed and back out when the family processes that information.

Challenging the Family

If is often best to let a member challenge the group. When a challenge is made a treatment plan should be in place.

Dealing With Resistance

The two most common primary care counseling forms of resistance are tardiness or absenteeism and arguing with you. Schedule problems should be addressed to see if there is a hidden meaning in the tardiness. If not, you may want to confront them by saying, "My time is important to me, and I would like you to respect it." If a member wants to argue with you, ask that he/she simply think about what you have said, or encourage him/her to describe how he/she sees the issues and how he/she would like to change things. You may gain valuable information by following his/her lead. Don't work hard to persuade the family that you are right; maybe you aren't.

Making Behavioral Contracts

You should encourage all members to identify clearly the specific, concrete changes they are willing to make. This must be done in a cooperative, nonhostile group mood. Members must be willing to make the changes in good faith so that the other will make their changes. The family should plan to evaluate the contract to see if it is working.

After-Session Assignments

It may be useful to follow through on some issues that arise during the session. For example, if sharing household tasks is an issue, you might help the family make specific assignments for the week. If the parents want to spend more time together, let them make specific plans for an event that week. Follow up on these assignments. Failure to follow through would be an important family dynamic to address.

Adapted from Guilford Publications Doherty WJ, Baird MA. *Family Therapy and Family Medicine*. New York, NY: Guilford Press; 1983.

TABLE 22.30

Alternative Medicine

Name	Use	Dose	Side Effects
St John's wort (*Hypericum perforatum*)	St John's wort is used for depressed mood and anxiety	900 mg/d, followed by 300–600 mg/d for maintenance therapy	Can cause gastro-intestinal symptoms and fatigue and can induce hypomania
Kava kava (*Piper methysticum*)	Kava kava is used to treat nervous anxiety, stress, and restlessness	60–120 mg/d. Usually 1 cup kava kava is consumed three times daily. Prepared by simmering 2–4 g of the root in 150 mL boiling water for 5–10 minutes. Should not be taken for more than 3 months without medical supervision	Can cause gastrointestinal upset, dizziness, headache, and enlarged pupils. Concomitant use of kava kava with alcohol can increase kava kava toxicity.

TABLE 22.31

Risk Factors Associated With Completed Suicide*

Epidemiological Factors	Psychiatric Disorders	Past History
White male, age greater than 65 years	Major depression	History of previous suicide attempt
Widowed or divorced	Substance abuse (especially alcohol)	Family history of suicide attempt
Living alone	Borderline personality disorder	Presence of family violence and disruption
Access to firearms	In adolescents:	
Stressful life events	impulsive, aggressive and antisocial behavior	

*Discussing suicidal ideation with patient does not increase the risk of a suicide attempt.

TABLE 22.32

Interviewing a Patient With Suicidal Ideation

1. When did you begin to have suicidal thoughts?
2. Was there a stressor that caused you to consider suicide?
3. Do you feel you are a burden or that life is not worth living?
4. Do you have a plan to end your life?
5. Do you have access to a gun or harmful medications?
6. Have you changed your life insurance policy or will or given away your possessions?
7. Can you call someone for help?

FIGURE 22.2

Algorithm for the Evaluation and Treatment of Suicidal Patients

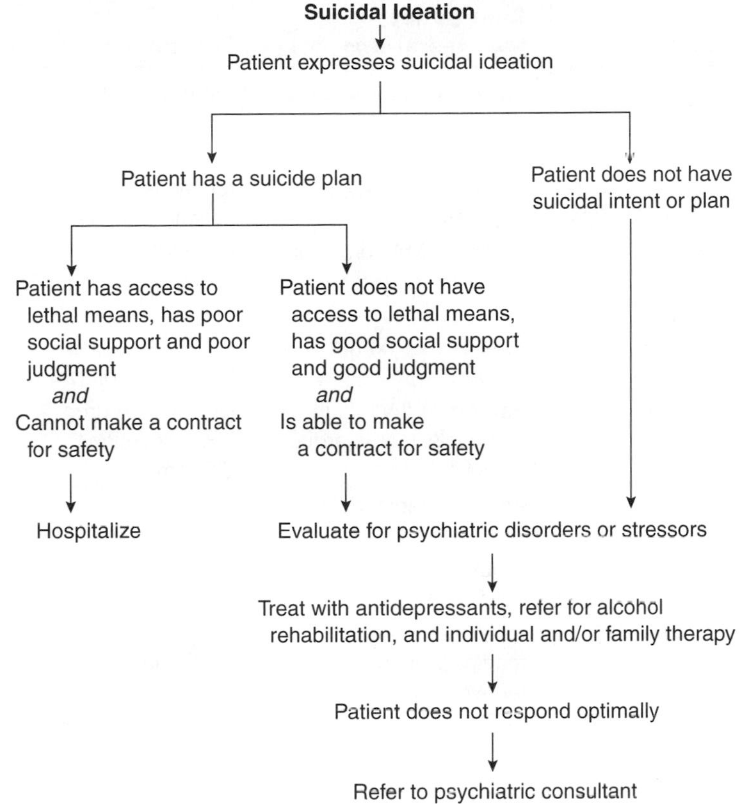

Reproduced with permission from Gliatto MF, Rai AK. Evaluation and treatment of patients with suicidal ideation. *Am Fam Physician.* 1999;59:1500–1506.

TABLE 22.33

Common Psychiatric Emergencies

Syndrome	Emergency Manifestations	Treatment
Agoraphobia	Panic and depression	Propranolol, SSRI, benzodiazepines
Amphetamine intoxication	Delusions, paranoia, violence, delirium, depression	Antipsychotics, restraints, hospitalization prn
Alcohol withdrawal	Autonomic hyperactivity, irritability, seizures	Benzodiazepines, thiamine 100 mg IM, monitor vital signs
Anorexia nervosa	Loss of 25% normal body weight	ECG, electrolytes, fluid, hospitalization prn
Anticholingeric intoxication	Psychotic, dry mouth, mydriasis, tachycardia, restless	Discontinue drug, physostigmine 0.5–2 mg
Caffeine intoxication	Anxiety, mania, delirium	Stop caffeine, benzodiazepines
Cannabis intoxication	Delusions, panic, dysphoria	Benzodiazepines prn; antipsychotics prn
Cocaine intoxication	Paranoia, anxiety, manic, delirium, violent, tachycardia	Antipsychotics, benzodiazepines, hospitalization, desipramine may decrease cravings
Depression	Suicidal ideation, self-neglect	Hospitalize if danger to self and others
Dystonia, acute	Involuntary spasm of neck, tongue, face, eyes, jaw, or trunk	Cogentin or Benadryl IM; decrease dose of antipsychotic
Grief and bereavement	Insomnia, somatic complaints	Benzodiazepines for sleep
Hyperventilation	Anxiety, terror, faintness	Breathe into paper bag, antianxiety medications
Mania	Impulsive, psychosis, substance abuse, indiscriminate sexual or spending behavior	Rapid tranquilization with antipsychotics, hospitalization if necessary
Neuroleptic malignant syndrome	Hyperthermia, muscle rigidity, autonomic instability, parkinsonian symptoms	Stop antipsychotic; bromocriptine po or dantroline IV; hydration and cooling, follow CPK levels

Syndrome	Emergency manifestations	Treatment
Opioid intoxication and withdrawal	Intoxication can lead to coma; withdrawal has abdominal cramps, HTN, diarrhea, nausea, sweating	IV naloxone for intoxication; use clonidine, Bentyl, Kaopectate, and/or methadone for withdrawal
Panic disorder	Acute onset of panic	Propranolol 10–30 mg, alprazolam 0.25–2 mg
Posttraumatic stress disorder	Flashbacks, terror, suicidal ideation	Monitor suicidal ideation, reassurance, hospitalization if needed
Schizophrenia	Command hallucinations, threat to others or themselves, self-neglect	Rapid tranquilization with Haldol, hospitalization, notify other people who are threatened
Tardive dyskinesia	Dyskinesias of mouth, tongue, face, neck, and trunk; appears after long-term antipsychotic use especially if dose is lowered	No effective treatment

CPK indicates creatine kinase; ECG, electrocardiogram; IM, intramuscularly; IV, intravenously; po, orally; prn, when necessary; SSRI, selective serotonin reuptake inhibitor.

FIGURE 22.3

The Hostile, Agitated Patient

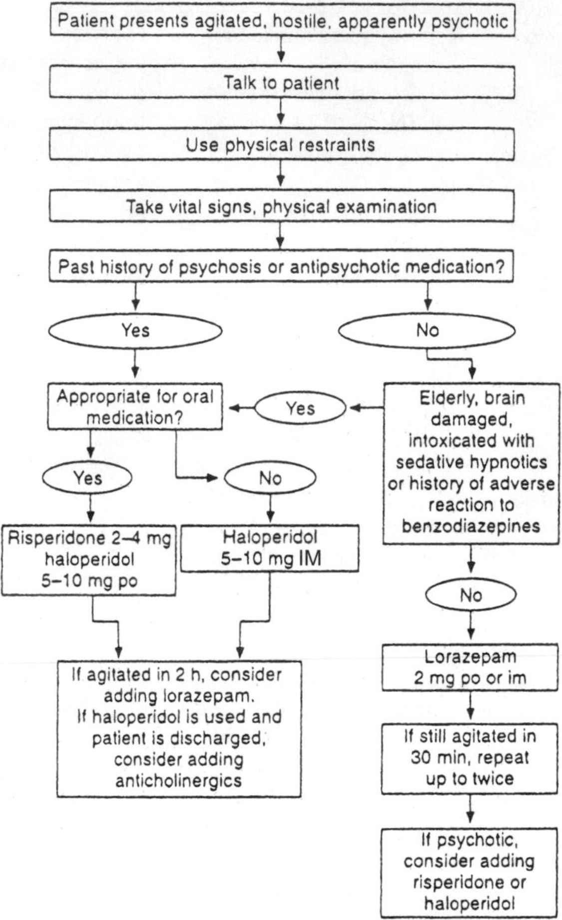

Reproduced with permission from Hillard JR. Emergency treatment of acute psychosis. *J Clin Psychiatry*. 1999;33:660–666.

IM indicates intramuscularly; po, orally.

TABLE 22.34
Internet References

American Psychiatric Association	www.psych.org
American Psychological Association	www.apaa.org
National Alliance for the Mentally Ill (NAMI)	www.nami.org
National Depressive and Manic-Depressive Association	www.ndmda.org
Obsessive-Compulsive Foundation	www.ocfoundation.org
Children and Adults with Attention-Deficit Hyperactivity Disorder	www.chadd.org
National Information Center for Children and Youth With Disabilities	www.nichcy.org
National Foundation for Depressive Illness	www.depresion.org
National Mental Health Association	www.nmha.org
Anxiety Disorders Education	http://nimh.nih.gov/anxiety

chapter 23

Surgical Care

Edward T. Bope, MD
Stephen A. Markovich, MD

IN THIS CHAPTER

- Suturing
- Facial skin lines
- Tetanus immunization schedule
- Breast mass evaluation
- Thyroid mass evaluation
- Hemorrhoid management
- Fluid management
- Prevention of deep venous thrombosis
- Pancreatitis
- Diverticulitis
- Cholecystitis/cholelithiasis
- Assessing surgical risk
- Indications for preoperative testing
- Obstruction and ileus
- The acute abdomen
- Decubitus ulcers

BOOKSHELF RECOMMENDATIONS

- Norton LW, Eiseman B, Steigmann G, eds. *Surgical Decision Making*. 4th ed. Philadelphia, PA: WB Saunders; 2000.
- Schwartz SI, Galloway AC, Shires GT, eds. *Principles of Surgery*. 7th ed. New York, NY: McGraw-Hill; 1998.
- Weinstock MB, Neides DM. *The Resident's Guide to Ambulatory Care*. 4th ed. Columbus, OH: Anadem Publishing; 2000.

TABLE 23.1

Absorbable Sutures

Suture Type	Frequent Uses	Maintains Strength	Tissue Reactivity
Surgical gut	Any short-term approximation/ligation Not for use in cardiovascular or neurological tissues	7–10 days	Some
Chromic gut	Any short-term approximation/ligation Not for use in cardiovascular or neurological tissues	10–14 days	Some
Uncoated Vicryl	Any short-term approximation/ligation	14–21 days	Minor
Coated Vicryl	Not for use in cardiovascular or neurological tissues	14–21 days	Minor
Polydioxanone	Any short-term approximation/ligation	14–30 days	Minimal
Monocryl	Any short-term approximation/ligation Not for use in cardiovascular, neurological, or ophthalmic procedures	7–14 days	Minimal

TABLE 23.2

Nonabsorbable Sutures

Suture Type	Frequent Uses	Maintains Strength	Tissue Reactivity
Silk	Any long-term approximation/ligation	Up to 1 year	Possible acute reaction
Nylon	Any long-term approximation/ligation	Decreases 15% per year	Minimal
Polyester	Any long-term approximation/ligation	Indefinitely	Minimal
Prolene	Any long-term approximation/ligation	Indefinitely	Minimal
Surgical steel	Abdominal wound closure, sternal closure, hernia repair, orthopedic procedures	Indefinitely	Minor

FIGURE 23.1

Wound Care: Laceration Repair

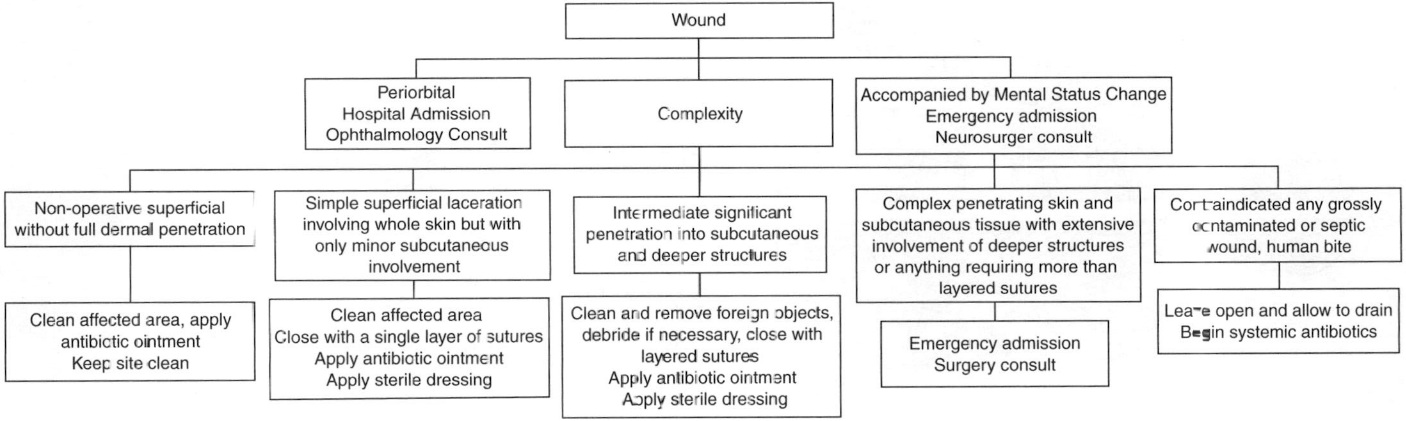

Wound

- Periorbital
  Hospital Admission
  Ophthalmology Consult
- Complexity
  - Non-operative superficial without full dermal penetration
    - Clean affected area, apply antibiotic ointment
      Keep site clean
  - Simple superficial laceration involving whole skin but with only minor subcutaneous involvement
    - Clean affected area
      Close with a single layer of sutures
      Apply antibiotic ointment
      Apply sterile dressing
  - Intermediate significant penetration into subcutaneous and deeper structures
    - Clean and remove foreign objects, debride if necessary, close with layered sutures
      Apply antibiotic ointment
      Apply sterile dressing
  - Complex penetrating skin and subcutaneous tissue with extensive involvement of deeper structures or anything requiring more than layered sutures
    - Emergency admission
      Surgery consult
  - Contraindicated any grossly contaminated or septic wound, human bite
    - Leave open and allow to drain
      Begin systemic antibiotics
- Accompanied by Mental Status Change
  Emergency admission
  Neurosurger consult

FIGURE 23.2

Wound Care: Skin Tension Lines

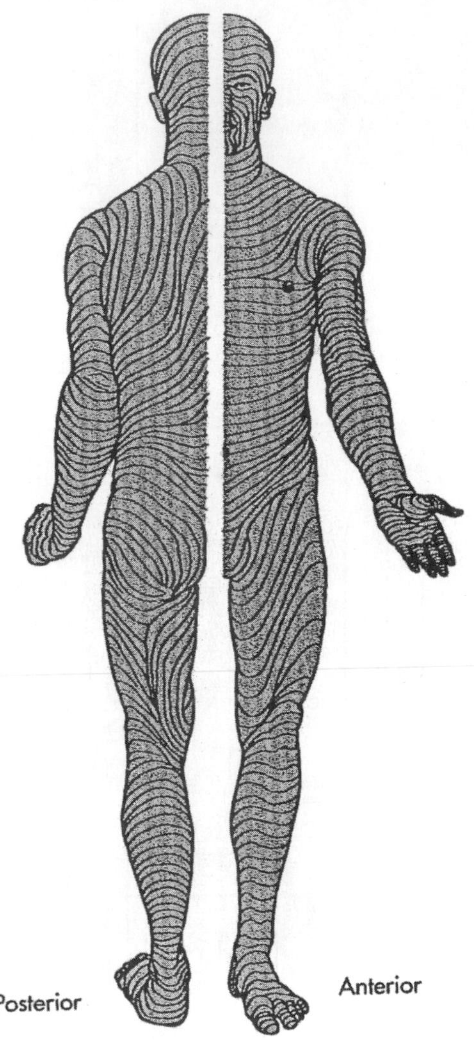

Adapted from Usatine RP, Moy RL, Tobinick EL. *Skin Surgery: A Practical Guide.* St Louis, MO: Mosby, Inc; 1998.

FIGURE 23.3

Facial Skin Lines

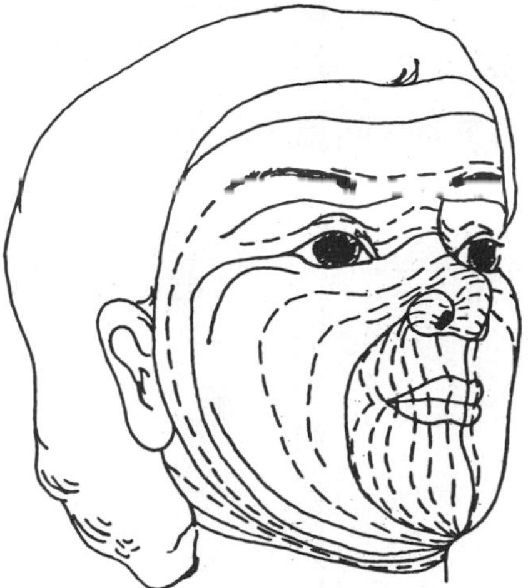

Adapted from Riley WB. Wound healing and problem scars. In: Barrett BM, ed. *Surgery*. Boston, MA: Little, Brown & Co; 1982:132.

FIGURE 23.4
Tetanus Prophylaxis Guideline

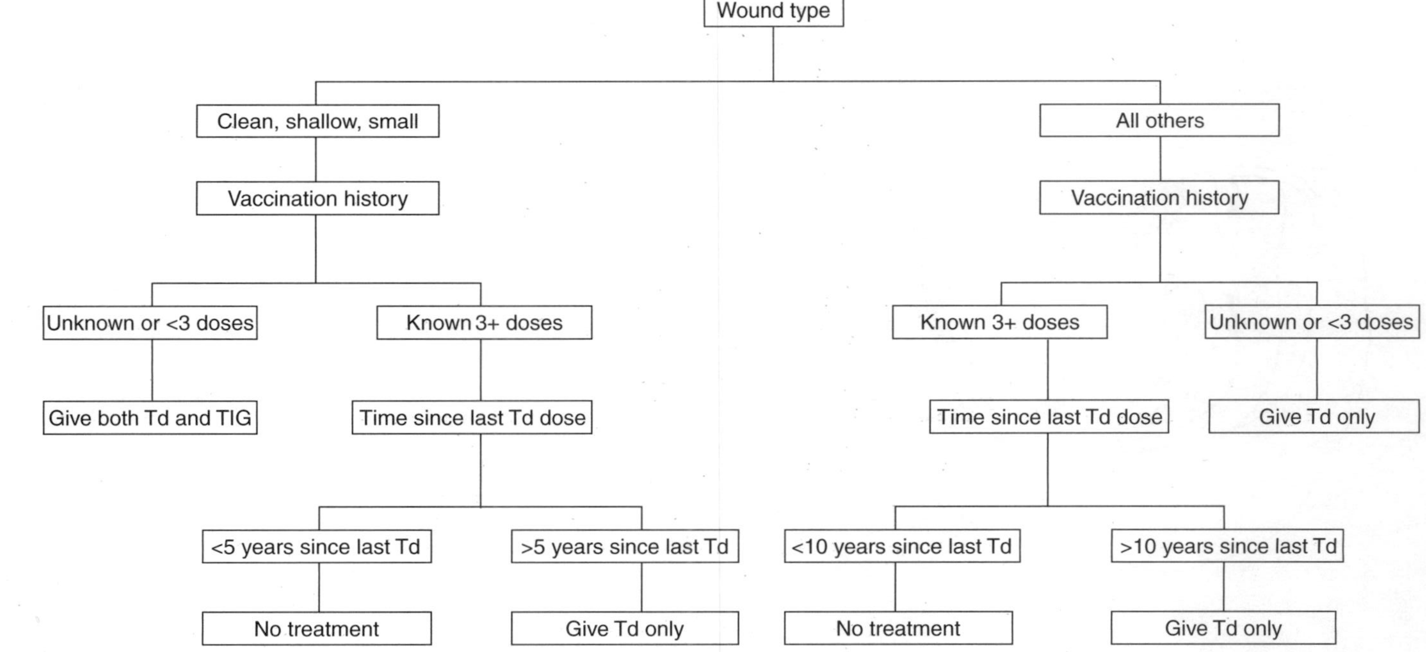

Courtesy Maciej Kedzierski, family practice medical student, Ohio State University College of Medicine and Public Health.

FIGURE 23.5

Evaluation of a Breast Mass

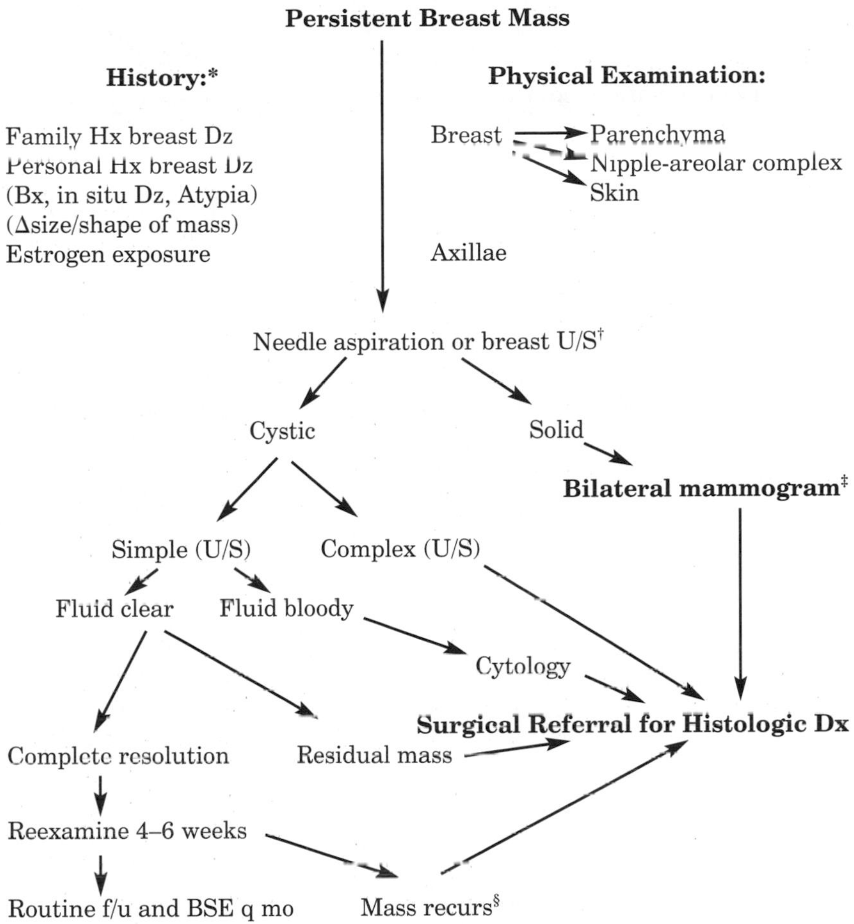

Courtesy Lance H. Shoemaker, MD, surgery resident, Riverside Methodist Hospital, Columbus, Ohio.

*Historical details modify physician's index of suspicion for malignancy. May hasten surgical referral.

†Ultrasound gives more detail as to character of lesion but is less widely available and more expensive.

‡Mammography to detect occult lesions in either breast. Not useful in patients under age 25 because of breast tissue density.

§Cysts may be aspirated one additional time. Recurrence requires histologic diagnosis.

TABLE 23.3

Risk Factors for Thyroid Cancer

- Age <20
- Age >45
- History of radiation exposure
- Family history

TABLE 23.4

Management of Thyroid Fine Needle Aspiration (FNA) Results

FNA Diagnosis	Malignant or "suspicious" FNA	Benign adenomas 1. Follicular adenomas 2. Colloid adenomas 3. Thyroiditis 4. Cyst	Cellular adenoma (all benign) 1. Follicular neoplasm 2. Hurthle cell adenoma 3. Microfollicular adenomas
Plan	Surgery plus lifelong thyroid replacement	Observe with serial ultrasounds Consider oral thyroid suppression Biopsy if change occurs	Thyroid scan: if "cold" nodule rebiopsy or do surgery Follow every 6 months with serial ultrasounds

TABLE 23.5

Workup of Patient with a Solitary Thyroid Nodule

TSH high	TSH normal	TSH low
■ Work up and treat hypothyroidism ■ If there is a solitary nodule, do FNA	■ Do FNA	■ Do a thyroid scan ■ If nodule is "cold," do FNA ■ If nodule is "hot," draw a free T_4 ■ For high free T_4 ablate or do surgery ■ For NL T_4 observe or consider ablation or surgery

TABLE 23.6

Classification and Management of Hemorrhoids

Staging Criteria for Hemorrhoids

Stage	Description
1	Bleeding only, no prolapse
2	Prolapse: reduces spontaneously
3	Prolapse: requires manual reduction
4	Irreducible prolapse, any producing anemia

Treatment of Hemorrhoids

<table>
<tr><th rowspan="2"></th><th colspan="4">Stage</th></tr>
<tr><th>1</th><th>2</th><th>3</th><th>4</th></tr>
<tr><td>Treatment</td><td colspan="2">■ Conservative management:
Topical therapy
Dietary modification
Stool softening
■ Any removal method if conservative therapy fails</td><td>■ Conservative management
■ Hemorrhoidal banding
■ Clot evaluation if thrombosed and painful</td><td>■ Laser hemorrhoidectomy
■ Anemic patient requires gastrointestinal bleed workup
■ Postoperative conservative management</td></tr>
<tr><td>Recurrence</td><td colspan="2">10%</td><td>30%</td><td>5%</td></tr>
</table>

TABLE 23.7

Fluid Maintenance for Adults

Cause of Fluid Loss	Approximated Fluid Replacement Required
Urine/insensible losses	2500 mL/d Sodium, 156 mEq; chloride, 190 mEq; potassium, 40 mEq
Emesis	Replace lost volume
Fever, 101–103° F	500 mL
Fever, 103° F or more	1000 mL
Hyperventilation	500 mL
Diarrhea	Replace lost volume Sodium, 60 mEq/L; chloride, 45 mEq/L; potassium, 30 mEq/L

TABLE 23.8

Deep Venous Thrombosis Prevention

Moderate Risk	High Risk	Highest Risk
■ Major surgery >45 minutes ■ Laparoscopic surgery >45 minutes ■ Confined to bed >72 hours ■ Immobilizing plaster cast ■ Central venous access	■ Major surgery plus any one of the risk factors below	■ Elective joint replacement ■ Hip, pelvis, or leg fracture ■ Stroke (new or old) ■ Multiple trauma ■ Acute spinal cord injury with paralysis

Medical Risk Factors:* MI, CHF, sepsis, immobility, malignancy, central venous access, varicose veins, obesity, inflammatory bowel disease, oral contraceptives or hormone replacement, age >60, pregnancy or post partum less than 1 month.

History of: Hypercoagulable state or DVT or PE moves the patient to the next higher risk category.

Treatment	Treatment	Treatment
■ Antiembolism stockings or ■ Heparin 5000 units SC q 8 h or ■ Sequential compression hose (knee high)	■ Heparin 5000 units SC q 8 h plus either: ■ Antiembolism stockings (TEDS) or ■ Knee-high sequential compression hose	■ Antiembolism stockings (TEDS) and knee sequential compression hose and one of the following: 1. Dalteparin 2500 units 6 hours after surgery then 5000 units SC q 24 h 2. Dalteparin 5000 units SC q 24 h 3. Warfarin 5 mg/d po and PT/INR daily 4. Heparin 5000 units SC q 8 h

*Patient with two or three risk factors is in the high-risk category. Patient with more than three is in the highest-risk category.

TABLE 23.9

Fluids in Surgery: Blood Products

Blood Products	Indication	Comments
Fresh whole blood	Massive hemorrhage; rarely used	Poor source of platelets, factor V, factor VIII
Packed red blood cells	Anemia, hemodynamic instability secondary to blood loss	Each unit raises hemoglobin 1 g/dL or hematocrit 3%; approximately 300 mL total volume
Leukocyte-poor washed cells	Hypersensitivity to leukocytes or platelets (buffy coat reaction)	White blood cells removed by washing or centrifugation
Platelets	Thrombocytopenia due to massive blood loss, decreased production, or increased destruction	One unit (35 mL) raises platelet count 10 K/mm^3; half-life is 6 days
Fresh frozen plasma	Bleeding and coagulation defects; rapid reversal of Coumadin	Stored at $-20^\circ C$ to preserve factor V, VIII; may also be used to supplement factor II, V, IX, XI; increases factors 2%
Cryoprecipitate	Consumption coagulopathy, hemophilia, and von Willebrand disease	Contains concentrated factor VIII and von Willebrand factor

TABLE 23.10

Fluids in Surgery: Crystalloids

	Crystalloids (mEq/L)						
	Na+	K+	Cl−	Lactate	Ca2+	Calories	Osmolarity
0.2NS	34	0	34	0	0	0	68
0.45NS	77	0	77	0	0	0	154
0.9NS	154	0	1540	0	0	0	308
Lactated Ringer	130	4	109	28	3	9	273
D_5W	0	0	0	0	0	0	170
$D_{10}W$	0	0	0	0	0	0	340

TABLE 23.11

Fluids in Surgery: Maintenance

Maintenance IV Fluid: D5.45 NS + 20 mEq K+ Maintenance IV Rate Calculation		
Patient Weight	**Fluid Rate per Day**	**Fluid Rate per Hour**
First 10 kg	100 mL/kg/d	4 mL/kg/h
Second 10 kg	1000 + 50 mL/kg/d	40 + 2 mL/kg/h
Over 20 kg	1500 + 20 mL/kg/d	60 + 1 mL/kg/h

IV Fluid Boluses	
Pediatrics	20 mL/kg isotonic solution (0.9NS or lactated Ringer)
Adults	500–1000 mL, titrate to maintain 30–50 mL/h urine output, adjust for CHF, electrolyte imbalance, renal failure

TABLE 23.12

Management of Acute Pancreatitis

Presentation

- Epigastric abdominal pain radiating through to the back
- Nausea
- Vomiting

History

- Alcohol use (40%)
- Gallstones (40%)
- Hypertriglyceridemia
- Prior pancreatitis
- Medication list

Physical Examination

- Epigastric tenderness without overt peritonitis
- Palpable mass or phlegmon may be present
- Fever, leukocytosis, tachycardia in 90%

Laboratory Evaluation

- Amylase, lipase, and glucose (lipase is specific to pancreas)
- Total bilirubin, AST, ALT, and alkaline phosphatase
- BUN, creatinine, hemoglobin, hematocrit, total calcium

Radiographic Evaluation

- RUQ ultrasound to evaluate for gallstones, required in most cases
- CT scan should be strongly considered in complicated pancreatitis
- MRI is rarely indicated

Treatment

- NPO
- IV fluid hydration with D5LR or D5 0.9NS
- Consider nasogastric tube if the patient is vomiting
- Recommend Foley catheter to monitor fluid status

Complications of Pancreatitis

- ARDS, acute renal failure, hypocalcemia, bleeding, pseudocyst, necrosis, infection of necrosis or pseudocyst
- Consider consulting surgery and critical care medicine in patients with complicated pancreatitis

Continued

TABLE 23.12

Management of Acute Pancreatitis, cont'd

Etiology

- Alcohol (refer for alcohol cessation)
- Gallstones (consult surgery)
- Hypertriglyceridemia
- Medications: Lasix, thiazide diuretics, sulfonamides, tetracycline, valproic acid, mercaptopurine
- Other: familial, postprocedural (ERCP), trauma, anatomic, scorpion sting

Diagnoses Often Confused With Pancreatitis

- Perforated duodenal ulcer will cause an isolated mild elevation of the amylase level, with or without identifiable free air on plain radiographs
- Ischemic bowel also causes elevation of the amylase, but late in the course of the disease. The abdominal examination is typically unremarkable despite the patient's complaints of excruciating pain
- Acute cholecystitis has a similar distribution of pain. The lab findings are normal in uncomplicated cholecystitis.

Courtesy Thomas Sonnanstine, MD, surgery resident, Riverside Methodist Hospital, Columbus, OH.

ALT indicates alanine aminotransferase; ARDs, acute respiratory distress syndrome; AST, aspartate aminotransferase; BUN, serum urea nitrogen; CT, computed tomography; ERCP, endoscopic retrograde cholangiopancreatography; IV, intravenous; MRI, magnetic resonance imaging.

TABLE 23.13

Risk Assessment in Pancreatitis (Ranson's Criteria)

Admission (1 Point Each)

- Age >55 years
- WBC >16 K/mm^3
- Blood glucose >200 mg/dL
- Serum LDH >350 IU/L
- AST >250 IU/dL

First 48 Hours (1 Point Each)

- Hematocrit fall >10%
- BUN rise >8 mg/dL
- Serum Ca^{++} <8 mg/dL
- Arterial PO_2 <60 mm Hg

Adapted from Ranson JH. Diagnositc standards for acute pancreatitis. *World J Surg.* 1997; 21(2):136–142.

AST indicates asparate aminotransferase; BUN, blood urea nitrogen; Po_2, arterial oxygen pressure; WBC, white blood cell count.

≤2 = 1% mortality

3–4 = 15% mortality

≥6 = 100% mortality

FIGURE 23.6

Tests for the Evaluation of a Patient With Suspected Diverticulitis

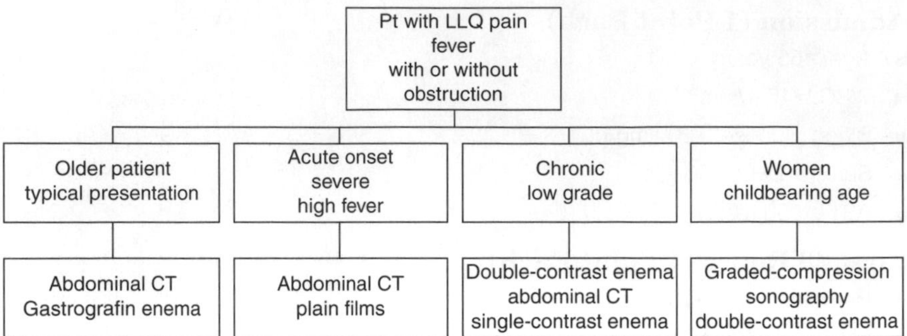

FIGURE 23.7

Management of Patient With Diverticulitis

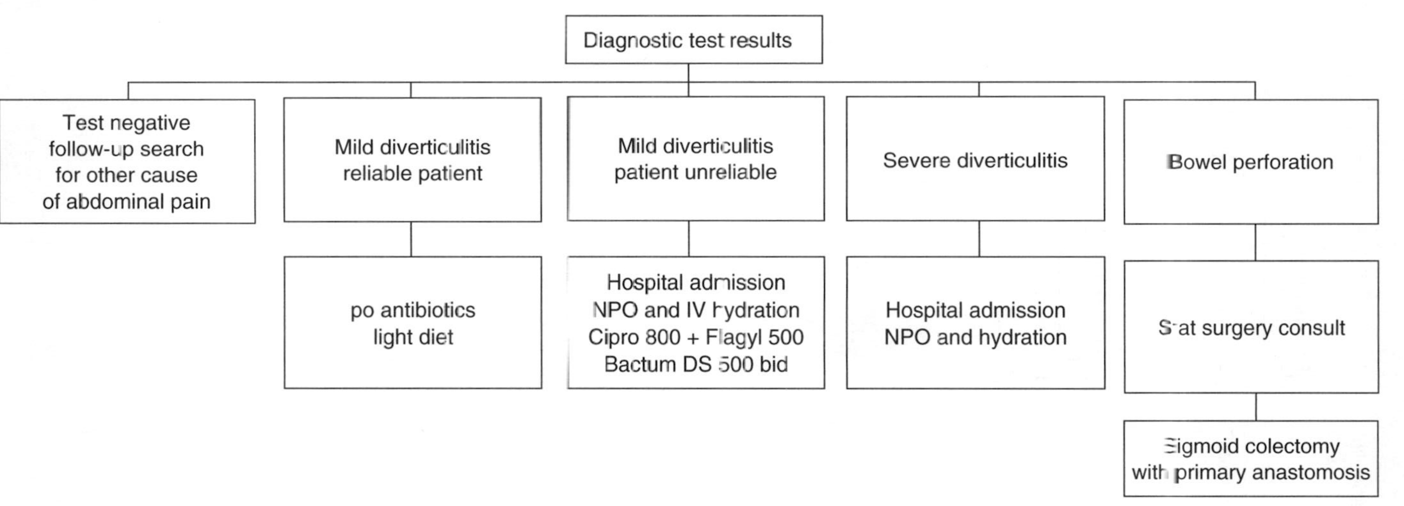

FIGURE 23.8

Follow-up of Patient With Diverticulitis

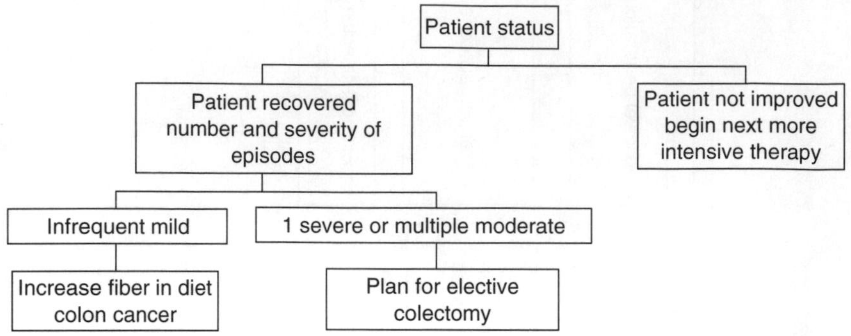

TABLE 23.14

Management of Cholecystitis and Cholelithiasis

Asymptomatic Cholelithiasis

- 15% of population have gallstones; usually found incidentally
- Over 50% of individuals with gallstones are asymptomatic and most will remain asymptomatic
- No proven role for prophylactic cholecystectomy in the asymptomatic patient

Symptomatic Cholelithiasis (Biliary Colic)

- Episodic in nature with recurrent episodes of constant postprandial RUQ abdominal pain
- Episodes usually occur 30 to 60 minutes after fatty or protein-rich meals and are always self-limited in lasting for several hours or less
- May have pain referred to right shoulder/scapula or midepigastrum
- Diagnosis is made by history, physical exam, and with abdominal ultrasonographic evidence of gallstones; laboratory evaluation is usually normal
- No evidence that dietary modification alters duration, intensity, or frequency of symptoms
- Recurrent biliary colic is an indication for surgical referral and elective cholecystectomy

Acute Cholecystitis

- Acute inflammation of the gallbladder with associated cystic duct obstruction
- Patients usually have a history of biliary colic
- Pain persists beyond the usual 4 to 6 hours common with biliary colic
- Localized RUQ abdominal pain (Murphy sign), leukocytosis (12,000 to 15,000/mm^3), low-grade fever, nausea and vomiting, liver function tests normal without involvement of the common bile duct (choledocholithiasis) or pancreas (gallstone pancreatitis)
- Differential diagnosis: acute appendicitis, perforated peptic ulcer, pancreatitis, pyelonephritis, RLL pneumonia, acute myocardial infarction, cholangitis
- Abdominal ultrasonography reveals gallstones, gallbladder wall thickening, pericholecystic fluid, sonographic Murphy sign; hepatobiliary scintigraphy for equivocal U/S in cases of acalculous acute cholecystitis

Continued

TABLE 23.14

Management of Cholecystitis and Cholelithiasis, cont'd

- Acute surgical consultation for cholecystectomy during hospitalization (for diagnosis within 48 hours of symptom onset) or interval cholecystectomy (delayed surgical treatment after course of IV or oral antibiotics) in cases of diagnosis after 3 to 4 day history of symptoms

Biliary Dyskinesia

- Functional disorder of the gallbladder in its ability to eject bile; also known as chronic acalculous cholecystitis
- Pain, often vague and RUQ/midepigastric, routinely after eating fatty foods or injection of CCK as part of hepatobiliary scintigraphy
- Diagnosis by clinical history and hepatobiliary scintigraphy with measured ejection fraction; abnormal ejection fraction defined as below 45% to 55% depending on the lab
- Treatment is elective cholecystectomy

Gallstone Pancreatitis

- See Acute Pancreatitis section

Courtesy Eric R. Dritsas, MD, surgery resident, Riverside Methodist Hospital, Columbus, OH.

FIGURE 23.9

Preoperative Cardiac Workup

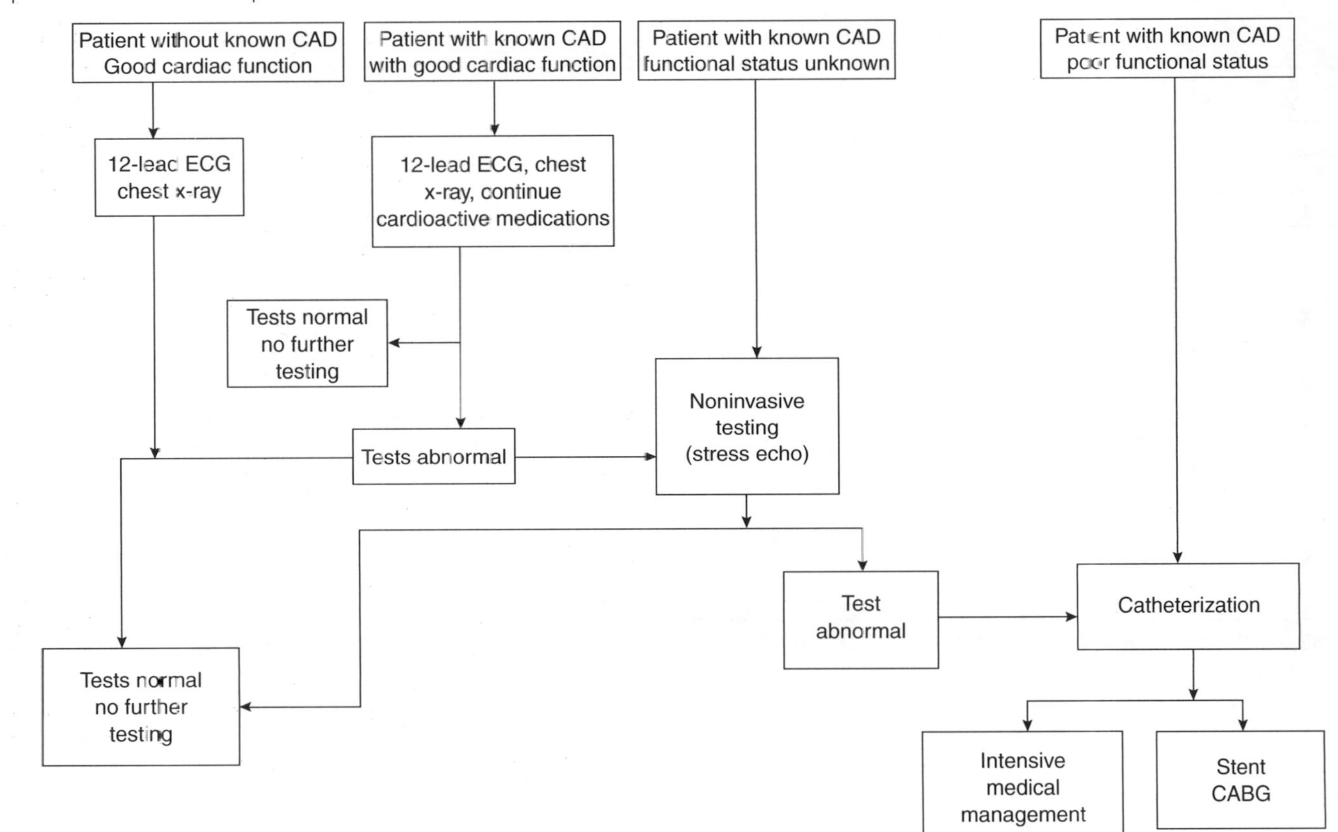

TABLE 23.15

Indications for Preoperative Testing

	Hb/Hct	PT/PTT	Type/Screen	Electrolytes	Creatinine/BUN	Glucose	CXR	ECG
1. Age <40 years	X							
Age 40 to 65 years	X				X	X		X
Age >65 years	X				X	X	X	X
2. All ages, major surgery*	X	X	X	X	X	X	X	X
3. Associated conditions:								
Cardiovascular pulmonary					X		X	X
Diabetes				X	X	X	X	X
Renal	X			X	X			
Hypertension					X			X
Smoking (>20 pack-years)	X				X		X	
Use of diuretics				X	X			
Use of digoxin				X	X			X
Use of anticoagulants	X	X						
Use of steroids				X		X		
Antiarrhythmics				X				X

Adapted from Weinstock MB, Neides DM. *The Resident's Guide to Ambulatory Care*. 4th ed. Columbus, OH: Anadem Publishing; 2000.

TABLE 23.16

Comparison of Paralytic Ileus, Intestinal Obstruction, and Diverticulitis

Aspect	Paralytic Ileus	Mechanical Obstruction	Diverticulitis
Symptoms			
Pain	Mild, diffuse aching; pain with a bloating sensation	Cramping, often severe in mid to low abdomen	Left lower quadrant with rebound
Vomiting	Mild if any	Bilious or feculent	Mild with anorexia
Physical Signs			
Distention	Persistent, early and marked	Moderate, worsens with time	Mild
Bowel sounds	Decreased or absent	Increased with rushes	Decreased
Tenderness	Mild and diffuse	Mild and diffuse	Mild to severe
Plain X-ray Signs			
Gas in stomach	Increased	Normal amount	Normal
Bowel gas	Marked throughout large and small	Proximal to the obstruction with rectum empty	Perforation may occur
Fluid in bowel	Minimal	Large amounts	With obstruction
Air/fluid levels	Same level across abdomen	Different levels with "J" loops seen	With obstruction

TABLE 23.17

Presentation of Common Conditions Leading to an Acute Abdomen

Diagnosis	Presentation	Evaluation
Peritonitis	Diffuse, severe tenderness; guarding or rigidity; absent bowel sounds; rebound	*Diagnosis is clinical*; upright chest film may show free intraperitoneal air
Appendicitis	Focal, lower right quadrant (McBurney point) tenderness, with rebound; anorexia	*Diagnosis is clinical*; ultrasound, CT, spiral CT, or barium enema may aid in diagnosis
Acute pancreatitis	Diffuse upper abdominal tenderness radiating to the back; mild rebound; ileus; Grey Turner sign (flank hematoma)	Serum amylase and lipase; ultrasound or CT
Acute cholecystitis	Right upper quadrant tenderness; muscle guarding; worse with inspiration	Ultrasound
Diverticulitis	Left lower quadrant tenderness; rebound; guarding; fever; quiet bowel sounds	CT; barium enema (Gastrografin should be used if a perforation is a possibility)
Small bowel obstruction: proximal	Nausea, vomiting; alkalosis; normal or quiet bowel sounds; no distention	Abdominal film; upper GI series; endoscopy
Small bowel obstruction: distal	Nausea, vomiting; tenderness, distention; hyperactive bowel sounds	Abdominal film; angiogram; serum amylase
Cholangitis	Fever, jaundice; right upper quadrant pain	Ultrasound; ERCP; cholangiogram
Ectopic pregnancy	Peritonitis, hypotension; anemia; shock	B-hCG; vaginal ultrasound; culdocentesis
Ruptured aortic aneurysm	Upper abdominal tenderness; back pain; pulsatile mass; hypovolemic shock	Angiogram; ultrasound, CT
Diseases related to AIDS:		
CMV	Peritonitis	CT; paracentesis
Opportunistic infections	Peritonitis	CT; paracentesis
Lymphoma	Distention; obstipation; GI bleeding	CT; upper GI series; endoscopy
Kaposi sarcoma of GI tract	Distention; obstipation; GI bleeding	Endoscopy

Adapted from Weinstock MB, Neides DM. *The Resident's Guide to Ambulatory Care.* 4th ed. Columbus, OH: Anadem Publishing; 2000.

AIDS indicates acquired immunodeficiency syndrome; CMV, cytomegalovirus; CT, computed tomography; ERCP, endoscopic retrograde cholangiopancreatography; GI, gastrointestinal.

TABLE 23.18

Classification and Treatment of Pressure Ulcers

Ulcer Classification	Description	Treatment
Stage 1	■ Nonblanchable erythema ■ Skin intact ■ Warmth over bony prominence	■ Relieve local pressure ■ Maximize mobility/activity ■ Assess support and ADLs ■ Assess nutritional adequacy
Stage 2	■ Partial-thickness skin loss ■ Ulcer is superficial ■ Appears like blister or abrasion	Stage 1 recommendations plus ■ Antibiotic ointment ■ Gentle cleansing ■ Exudate culture if present ■ Consider excision/primary closure
Stage 3	■ Full-thickness skin loss ■ Extends to subcutaneous tissue ■ Does not penetrate fascia	Stage 2 recommendations plus ■ Blood cultures ■ Debride in stages as needed ■ Consider operative debridement
Stage 4	■ Full-thickness skin loss ■ Lesion penetrates fascia ■ Any lesion with damage to underlying structures	Stage 3 recommendations plus ■ Hospitalization ■ Operative debridement with flap closure

ADLs indicates activities of daily living.

chapter 24

Emergencies, Poisoning, and Trauma

J. Dan Johnson, DO
Michael R. Cook, MD

IN THIS CHAPTER

- Management of poisoning
- General wound management
- Management of cat, dog, and human bites
- Emergencies involving the eye, ear, nose, and mouth
- Acute management of dental fractures
- Acute management of upper and lower airway emergencies
- Management of swallowed foreign bodies
- Management of acute allergic reactions
- Management of urologic emergencies
- Management of ectopic pregnancy
- Approach to the sexually assaulted patient
- Management of acute dystonic drug reaction
- Approach to the hyperventilating patient

BOOKSHELF RECOMMENDATIONS

- American College of Surgeons on Trauma. *Advanced Trauma Life Support Program for Surgeons*. 6th ed. Chicago, IL: American College of Surgeons on Trauma; 1997.
- Buttaravoli PM, Stair TO. *Minor Emergencies: Splinters to Fractures*. St Louis, MO: Mosby, Inc; 2000.
- Cline DM, Ma OJ. *Just the Facts in Emergency Medicine*. New York, NY: McGraw-Hill Professional Publishing; 2000.

TABLE 24.1

General Management of Systemic Poisoning*

Contact a Poison Control Center for emergent information in the management of all acute poisonings.

American Association of Poison Control Centers
3201 New Mexico Avenue NW
Suite 310
Washington, DC 20016
Internet address: www.aapcc.org
(800) 222-1222

Steps Before the Patient Is Seen by the Emergency Department

Ipecac

- There is a consensus that ipecac should *not* be used.
- It can be dangerous and should be avoided in certain poisonings including ingestion of calcium channel blockers, beta-blockers, digitalis, or when there has been an ingestion of a corrosive agent.
- Ipecac is contraindicated for ingestions that can produce changes in levels of alertness because of aspiration risks.
- Specific complications of ipecac may include aspiration, diarrhea, ileus, arrhythmia during vomiting, dystonia from treatment for vomiting, and hematemesis from vomiting.*

Activated Charcoal

- Treatment of choice for gastrointestinal decontamination
- There are concerns about correct dosing in the home and the difficulty in having children swallow it. However, can be administrated successfully in the home environment.
- Dosing of generic charcoal, activated (30 g/150 mL suspension)
  —Adults: 1 g/kg
  —Children <1 year old: 1 g/kg po q 4–6 h; do not use charcoal with sorbitol, as it may increase risk of dehydration
  —Children (1 to 12 years old): 1 g/kg po q 2–4 h; do not use charcoal with sorbitol for >1–2 doses/d

Steps to Be Taken in the Emergency Department

The general approach to the treatment of the acute ingestion includes:

- Decontamination
- ABCs of basic life support (assessment of airway, breathing, circulation)
- Toxic elimination

The treatment of an acute ingestion includes:

Stabilization

- Start the ABCs of basic life support if needed.

Protect the Airway

- If gastric lavage will be performed, secure the airway by intubation, especially in the obtunded patient.

Skin Decontamination

- Remove clothing and wash the skin copiously with water.

Gastric Decontamination

- Administer activated charcoal at dosage of 1 g/kg.

Continue Stabilization

- For the patient who presents with altered mental status, supplement with oxygen and consider the administration of glucose and thiamine.
- If narcotic use is suspected, naloxone should be administrated.

---

*For more information, see Pond SM, Lewis-Driver DJ, Williams GM, et al. Gastric emptying in acute overdose: a prospective randomized controlled trial. *Med J Aust.* 1995;163:345–349.

TABLE 24.2

Managing Acetaminophen Ingestion

Symptoms and Toxicity

Early Symptoms

- Within a few hours following ingestion, the only symptoms include anorexia, nausea, and vomiting. The patient may remain asymptomatic.

Late Symptoms

- Without treatment the patient may symptomatically improve over the next 24–48 hours; however, hepatic damage continues. This is reflected by a rise in bilirubin and liver enzymes. There is a prolongation of PT/INR. Jaundice, coagulation defects, and encephalopathy secondary to hepatic necrosis occur over the next 72–96 hours, ultimately progressing to death.

Estimating Risk of Hepatotoxicity

- Draw a serum acetaminophen level (mg/dL) 4 hours following ingestion.
- Levels drawn before 4 hours are not reliable when estimating risk.
- Serum levels in the *possible risk* or *probable risk* categories should receive acetylcysteine.

Hours After Acute Ingestion	No Risk	Possible Risk	Probable Risk
4	<150	150–200	>200
6	<100	100–150	>150
8	<75	75–100	>100
10	<50	50–75	>75
12	<40	40–50	>50
14	<22	22–40	>40
16	<18	18–22	>22
18	<12	12–18	>18
20	<8	8–12	>12
22	<5	5–8	>8
24	<4	4–5	>5

Note: With the marketing of slow-release, higher-dosage acetaminophen formulations, it may be necessary to continue assessing acetaminophen levels 12–24 hours after ingestion to ensure that levels are falling.

Treatment

- Administer activated charcoal within 1 to 2 hours after ingestion.
- Withhold acetylcysteine until the results of the 4-hour serum level are known. (See previous chart, estimating risk of hepatotoxicity.)
- If serum level is in the possible or probable risk category, initiate acetylcysteine.
- Acetylcysteine should be given as soon after the 4-hour window as possible, yet it remains effective when started within 8 hours of ingestion. While it is less effective when initiated up to 30 hours after ingestion, it is beneficial and should usually be given even late in the course of overdose.
- It is suggested that your local poison control center be contacted to assist in management of the acetaminophen ingestion.

Dosing of Oral Acetylcysteine (Mucomyst 20%)

- Acetylcysteine 20% should be diluted to a 5% concentration with cola, juice, or water
- Loading dose: 140 mg/kg po or NG
- Maintenance dose: 70 mg/kg po q 4 h for 17 doses
- The dose should be repeated if vomiting occurs within 1 hour of a given dose
- Monitor liver function tests, electrolytes, CBC, glucose, BUN, creatinine, prothrombin times in all patients

---

BUN indicates serum urea nitrogen; CBC, complete blood cell count; po, orally.

TABLE 24.3

Managing Salicylate Ingestion

Symptoms and Toxicity

- Acute ingestion results in nausea, vomiting, tinnitus, lethargy, hyperpnea, mixed respiratory alkalosis, and metabolic acidosis. Severe ingestions can progress to coma, seizures, pulmonary edema, hypoglycemia, hyperthermia, and death.
- Chronic ingestion can lead to confusion, dehydration, metabolic acidosis, cerebral edema, and pulmonary edema.

Severity

- Ingestions of >150 mg/kg are expected to cause toxicity, ingestions of 300–500 mg/kg are serious, and ingestions of >500 mg/kg are potentially lethal.

Estimating Risk

- Measure serum levels 6 hours or later after acute ingestion. Levels measured before 6 hours may indicate toxicity but not severity. Levels may continue to rise because of sustained-release products or large tablet mass.

Hours After Acute Ingestion	Potentially Mild (mg/dL)	Potentially Moderate (mg/dL)	Potentially Severe (mg/dL)
6	45–65	65–90	>90
12	35–52	52–72	>72
24	22–35	35–50	>50
30	20–30	30–40	>40
36	15–25	25–32	>32
42	12–20	20–28	>28
48	10–15	15–20	>20
60	<10	10–13	>13

Note: Serum levels must be interpreted in the content of signs and symptoms of toxicity; overreliance on serum levels can underestimate the severity of intoxication.

Therapy

- Begin treatment before serum levels are known—contact local poison control center.
- If the patient is alert, give activated charcoal, 1 g/kg.
- Maintain ABCs, administer oxygen, and obtain arterial blood gases.
- Activated charcoal and a cathartic should be given within 1–2 hours after ingestion.
  - —With very large ingestions (>30 g) doses of 300–600 g of charcoal may be necessary.
  - —25- to 50-g doses can be given at 3- to 5-hour intervals.
- Treat metabolic acidosis with IV sodium bicarbonate and do not allow serum pH to fall below 7.4.

Fluid Management

- Start with normal saline bolus for initial resuscitation if needed.
  —All additional fluids should contain a 5% dextrose solution.
  —A second IV line should be established to assist in alkalinization of the serum and urine.
- A bolus of 1 to 2 mEq/kg of sodium bicarbonate should be administered.
- Then 2 to 3 ampules of sodium bicarbonate should be added to 1 L of D5W and infused at 1.5 to 2 times the patient's maintenance IV rate.
  —Adjust the infusion to maintain a urine pH greater than 7.5.
- Monitor electrolytes; potassium will likely need to be added to IV fluids as alkalization decreases the serum potassium level. Carefully monitor volume status.

Hemodialysis

- Hemodialysis is indicated if continued clinical deterioration, including renal failure, severe acid-base disturbance, altered mental status, or ARDS develops.

Additional Therapy

- Correct prolonged PT with vitamin K and fresh frozen plasma.
- Psychiatric consultation and admission if appropriate.
- Arrange admission if large ingestions of enteric-coated or sustained-release tablets for continued observation and monitoring to ensure declining serum salicylate levels and improving clinical status.

ARDS indicates acute respiratory distress syndrome; IV, intravenous; PT, prothrombin time.

TABLE 24.4

Digitalis Glycoside Poisoning

Signs and Symptoms

Acute Ingestion

- The patient may experience nausea and vomiting.
- Serum chemistries will reveal hyperkalemia in acute poisoning with large ingestions.
- Arrhythmias occur based on digitalis effect. Digitalis increases vagal tone and decreases conduction though the atrioventricular node; therefore, a wide variety of arrhythmias can result.

Chronic Ingestion

- The patient may experience gastrointestinal disturbances including:
  —Nausea
  —Vomiting
- Central nervous system disturbances including:
  —Weakness
  —Seizures
  —Visualization of yellow-green halos around objects
  —Altered mental status
- Ventricular dysrhythmias

Therapy

- Immediately establish IV access, place the patient on a cardiac monitor, and administer activated charcoal.
- Hyperkalemia is treated with glucose followed by insulin, sodium bicarbonate, potassium-binding resin or hemodialysis.
- Calcium chloride should be avoided.
- The treatment for bradydysrhythmias with hypotension, ventricular dysrhythmias, and hyperkalemia ($K > 5.5$ mEq/L) is the administration of digoxin immune Fab (Digibind).
- Patients who are asymptomatic after 12 h of observation may be medically cleared.
- Patients with signs of toxicity or history of large overdose should be admitted to a monitored setting.
- Patients receiving Fab should be admitted to an intensive care unit.

Calculating Digoxin-Specific Fab Fragment Dosage

- 2–20 vials IV is the usual dose
- Number of vials = (serum digoxin level in ng/mL) × (kg)/100

TABLE 24.5

Hydrocarbon Ingestion

Symptoms and Toxicity

- Most morbidity and mortality involving hydrocarbon ingestion are from aspiration pneumonitis; however, ingestion can lead to systemic toxicity.
- Symptoms include:
  —Choking
  —Coughing
  —Tachypnea
  —Nausea
  —Vomiting
  —Fever
  —Irritability
  —Drowsiness
  —Lethargy
  —Seizures
  —Coma

Treatment

- **Do not induce emesis**, give activated charcoal immediately.
- Most accidental ingestions are less than 5-10 mL, and toxicity is rare.
- For suspected large ingestions:
  —Monitor vital signs and order electrolytes, in addition to glucose, BUN, creatinine, liver function studies, serum bilirubin, and serum haptoglobin.
  —Also order ABGs to include carboxyhemoglobin.
- Radiographic evidence of pulmonary toxicity is usually seen within 4–6 hours of exposure.
- Cardiac toxicity includes ventricular dysrhythmias, decreased cardiac contractility, bradycardia, and AV heart block.
- For suspected pneumonitis:
  —Observe for a minimum of 6 to 8 hours, monitoring for cardiac arrhythmias, serial chest x-rays, and ABGs.
- All symptomatic patients should be admitted.
- Avoid the use of steroids, epinephrine, and other catecholamines.
- Do not use prophylactic antibiotics unless the patient is debilitated or has preexisting respiratory disease.

TABLE 24.6

Tricyclic Ingestion

Products

- Amitriptyline, nortriptyline, imipramine, doxepin, trimipramine, amoxapine, desipramine, protriptyline, clomipramine, maprotiline

Symptoms and Toxicity

- Lethal dose is generally considered to be 1000 mg in an adult.
- Life-threatening ingestions usually require at least 10 mg/kg.
- Serum levels are not reliable in predicting severity.
- Signs of toxicity include hypotension, shock, arrhythmias, tachycardia, AV block, mydriasis, sedation, coma, seizures, irritability, restlessness, delirium, urinary retention, decreased bowel sounds, and fever.
- QRS prolongation to 0.1 second or longer suggest serious toxicity (except with amoxapine, which causes seizures and coma without changing the QRS).
- Hypotension is independent of QRS prolongation.

Therapy

- *Do not induce emesis*; immediately administer activated charcoal.
- Maintain airway and assist ventilation: be prepared for rapid development of respiratory arrest.
- If patient has central nervous system depression, give Narcan, dextrose, and thiamine.
- Give repeated doses of charcoal for intestinal dialysis.
- Sodium bicarbonate should be used to treat QRS widening > 100 ms, hypotension refractory to IV fluids, and ventricular dysrhythmias.
  —Sodium bicarbonate should be dosed at 1 to 2 mEq/kg IV followed by a continuous infusion of 2 to 3 ampules of sodium bicarbonate in 1 L of D5W at a rate of 3 mL/kg/h.
- Carefully monitor for electrolyte abnormality, especially potassium.
- Hypotension refractory to IV fluids and sodium bicarbonate therapy should be treated with norepinephrine infusion.
- Treat acute seizures with IV diazepam or lorazepam.

TABLE 24.7

Wound Management

- In the management of any open wound, the health care professional should understand and follow the universal precaution guidelines established by the Centers for Disease Control and Prevention.
- Perform a careful physical exam before repairing any wound, meticulously documenting any significant findings, including sensory and motor deficits, noting nerve, muscle, tendon, and vascular involvement distal to the wound.

Puncture Wounds

- Evaluate wounds for underlying structural damage including bone, tendon, nerve, and vascular injury.
- Consider the presence of a retained foreign body.
- Radiographs may be helpful.
  —Retained glass and metal splinters are often seen on plain radiographs.
  —Plastic, wood, and aluminum are more radiolucent.
- In such cases where a foreign body is highly suspected, consider ultrasound, CT scan, or MRI.
- Uncomplicated wounds can be managed with local cleaning and protective dressing.
- Tetanus prophylaxis is also recommended.
- Irrigation may be helpful, but the wound usually does not allow effective irrigation.
- Prophylactic antibiotics are usually not indicated in the otherwise healthy patient.
  —Aggressive antibiotic therapy is indicated if infection occurs.
  —If an infection occurs in a plantar puncture wound of the foot, an anti-pseudomonal antibiotic (a quinolone) is recommended.
- Outpatient antibiotic failure frequently occurs because of retained foreign body. In this setting, strong consideration must be given to careful surgical exploration.

Bites

- Bites, single or multiple, may cause various types of injuries, including injury to nerve, tendon, and bone.
- Be alert to vascular injury and occult fractures.
- A low threshold for radiographs will assist in diagnosing occult fractures.

Cat Bites

- Approximately 80% of cat bites become infected, with *Pasteurella multocida* being the most common pathogen.
- All wounds should be copiously irrigated with saline.
- Primary closure should be avoided if possible.
- Consider delayed primary closure or referral to plastic surgeon if extensive wound repair is necessary.

Continued

TABLE 24.7

Wound Management, cont'd

- Hand bites frequently result in tenosynovitis.
- Prophylactic antibiotics are frequently indicated.
  —*P multocida* is extremely sensitive to penicillin; however, amoxicillin/clavulanate is the drug of choice because of its effective coverage against additional pathogens including *Staphylococcus* and *Streptococcus*.*

Dog Bites

- Approximately 20% of dog bites become infected.
- Infections may be polymicrobial, including anaerobic and aerobic organisms.
  —Organisms include *Staphylococcus aureus, P multocida, Eikenella corrodens, Bacteroides*, and other zoonotic bacteria.
  —*Capnocytophaga canimorsus* has been associated with severe infections in immunocompromised patients.
- Prophylactic antibiotics are usually not indicated.
- Copiously irrigate wounds with NS or other irrigating solution.
- Use of a splash shield attached to an IV setup is very helpful in reducing the bacterial load within the wound.
- A low threshold for radiographs helps to avoid missing a fracture or retained foreign body.

Human Bites

- Radiographs are often helpful when evaluating for bony involvement as well as retained tooth fragments.
- Copious wound irrigation with saline or other irrigating solution will decrease the bacterial wound load.
- Lacerations are preferably not sutured closed, especially hand lacerations; however, lacerations may be closed with early follow-up.
- Prophylactic antibiotics should be initiated for bites involving the hand.
- Patients who are immunocompromised should also be started on antibiotics.

Clenched Fist Injuries

- An injury frequently occurring during a fistfight in which a clenched fist strikes against the teeth of another person, causing a hand laceration or puncture wound.
- A small laceration in the metacarpophalangeal joint region should increase clinical suspicion, as the patient will often deny the mechanism of injury.
- Antibiotic therapy and early follow-up are recommended because of potential serious infection to underlying tendon and bone.[†]
- Wounds that present already infected should be cleaned and cultured.
- With extensive wound involvement, surgical consultation and IV antibiotics are necessary.
- Suggested antibiotics include cefazolin, cefoxitin, or ampicillin/sulbactam.

Minor Wounds

- Consider tetanus immunization status.
- Gently irrigated with clean water once daily.
- For faster healing, apply topical antibiotic and occlusive bandages for 1 week.
- Change dressings and apply topical antibiotic once or twice daily.
- Close superficial wounds with suture or tissue adhesive.
  —Tissue adhesive may be used:
  - On cutaneous facial injuries excluding the lips and mucosa.
  - On the extremities and torso excluding joints.
  - On minor lacerations of the hands and feet.[‡]

  —Poor results can occur over areas of flexion.

  —Tissue adhesive has been proven to be as strong as sutures with similar cosmetic results if used appropriately.

---

*For more information, see Griego RD, Rosen T, Orengo IF, et al. Dog, cat, and human bites: a review. *J Am Acad Dermatol.* 1995;33:1010.

†For more information, see Zubowicz VN, Gravier M. Management of early human bites of the hand: a prospective randomized study. *Plast Reconstr Surg.* 1991;88:111.

‡For more information, see Quinn J, Wells G, Sutcliffe T, et al. Tissue adhesive versus tissue wound repair at 1 year: randomized clinical trial correlating early, 3 month, and 1 year cosmetic outcome. *Ann Emerg Med.* 1998;32:645–649.

TABLE 24.8

Eye Emergencies

Corneal Abrasions

- Patients present with severe pain, photophobia, tearing, and blepharospasm, which is relieved by a topical anesthetic.
- Topical-instilled fluorescein will reveal the site of defect.
- Simple abrasions should be irrigated with saline.
- Topical antibiotics are recommended if any defect is found.
- Patching is usually not effective and contraindicated in contaminated abrasions. Consider reevaluation in 24 hours or consider ophthalmology referral.
- This injury is frequently associated with traumatic iritis.

Corneal Foreign Bodies

- After applying a topical anesthetic gently remove the FB under magnification with cotton-tip applicator, fine needle, or ophthalmic burr, then treat as corneal abrasion discussed above.
- Remember to invert the eyelid with cotton-tip applicator looking for underlying foreign body.

Hyphema

- Traumatic injury to the eye can result in blood in the anterior chamber.
- Emergent care includes application of topical atropine 1% and topical steroid.
- A Fox shield should be applied for continued eye protection.
- The patient should be referred to ophthalmology.
- The patient should remain in the upright position.

Traumatic Iritis and Iridocyclitis

- Results from trauma to the eye causing inflammation of the iris and ciliary body.
- The patient presents with photophobia, ciliary flush, and consensual pain.
- Treatment includes a cycloplegic such as 5% homatropine.
- After consulting with ophthalmology, a topical steroid such as prednisone acetate may be prescribed.
- Ophthalmologist referral is suggested within 24 hours.

Orbital Fractures

- Occurs as a result of blunt trauma to orbit.
- This type of trauma often results in fractures to the inferior and medial wall of the orbit.
- Physical exam may include periorbital ecchymosis with diplopia on upward gaze.
- Plain film x-ray may reveal clouding of maxillary sinus with air-fluid levels.
- CT of orbits very helpful.
- All patients should be referred to facial surgeon or plastic surgeon.

Penetrating Globe Trauma

- This type of injury is often the result of a high-velocity small projectile striking and penetrating the globe.
- Teardrop-shaped pupil, shallow anterior chamber, and marked reduction in visual acuity are seen on physical examination.
- Orbital thin-sliced CT scanning vs orbital MRI is the test of choice for identifying penetrating foreign bodies.
- Avoid eye manipulation such as measuring intraocular pressures.
- Apply a protective eye shield, update tetanus, and consult ophthalmology immediately.

CT indicates computed tomography; MRI, magnetic resonance imaging.

TABLE 24.9

Ear Emergencies

Trauma to the External Ear

- Trauma to external ear may result in significant cosmetic deformity.
- Hematomas require immediate incision and drainage with the application of a compressive dressing.
- Failure to evacuate the hematoma may result in cartilage necrosis resulting in significant cosmetic "cauliflower" deformity.
- ENT consult is often helpful.

Tympanic Membrane Perforations

- Blunt trauma to the ear may result in tympanic membrane perforation with subsequent pain and hearing loss.
- If the patient also complains of deafness and vertigo, an emergent ENT consult is warranted, as these symptoms suggest injury to the ossicles and related anatomical structures.
- Most perforations heal spontaneously.
- Antibiotics are not necessary unless the perforation is associated with a coexistent otitis media.

ENT indicates ear, nose, and throat.

TABLE 24.10

Nasal Emergencies

Nasal Fracture

- Nasal bone fracture is often seen associated with facial trauma.
- Physical findings usually include periorbital ecchymosis, swelling, tenderness, epistaxis, and rhinorrhea; crepitance and deformity may also be present.
- Radiographs are usually not helpful.
- Nondisplaced fracture usually requires supportive therapy, including ice and analgesics.
- ENT referral is usually not needed.
- Refer to ENT if gross deformity is present after swelling subsides in 2 to 3 weeks.

Nasal Septal Hematoma

- Nasal septal hematoma may occur following facial trauma and present as a collection of blood along nasal septal wall.
- This hematoma requires immediate incision and drainage with anterior nasal packing.
- The patient should be referred to ENT for follow-up evaluation.

Nasal Foreign Bodies

- Always suspect a nasal foreign body in the presence of unilateral nasal obstruction accompanied with malodorous rhinorrhea.
- The foreign body can frequently be removed after the use of a vasoconstrictive agent such as nasal phenylephrine with suction, balloon-tipped catheter, or firm metal probe under direct visualization.
- In children successful removal has been well documented by occluding the unaffected nares and having the parent apply a puff of positive-pressure air to the patient's mouth.*

ENT indicates ear, nose, and throat.

*For more information, see Backlin SA. Positive pressure technique for nasal foreign body removal. *Ann Emerg Med.* 1995;25:554.

TABLE 24.11

Orofacial Injuries

- Patients with dentoalveolar injuries often have other injuries that may be more serious or even life threatening.
- All intraoral lacerations must be cleaned and explored, looking for additional evidence of trauma including retained foreign bodies such as fractured teeth.
- Careful examination of the mandible and maxilla must be included when looking for other evidence of trauma.*
- Malocclusion or pain on range of motion at temporomandibular joint is suggestive of fracture.

*For more information, see Dale RA. Dentoalveolar trauma. *Emerg Med Clin North Am.* 2000;18:521–538.

TABLE 24.12

Dental Fractures

Dental fractures are graded using the Ellis classification system.

Ellis Class 1 Fracture

- Involvement of the enamel of the tooth.
- Treatment includes analgesics and nonemergent referral to dentist for cosmetic repair.

Ellis Class 2 Fracture

- A fractured tooth that has exposed the yellow dentin.
- The patient complains of increased dental pain especially with air sensitivity.
- The exposed dentin must be dried and protected with dental cement and referred to dentist within 24 hours.

Ellis Class 3 Fracture

- The fracture is noted by blood or reddish-appearing dentin at fracture site.
- Treatment consists of analgesic medication.
- Avoid the use of topical anesthetics.
- Immediately refer the patient to a dentist or oral surgeon for further treatment.

Complete Tooth Avulsion

- The complete dislocation of a tooth requires immediate medical attention.
- Primary (deciduous) teeth should not be replaced.
- Permanent teeth should be gently cleaned in saline, Hanks solution, or saliva and reimplanted as soon as possible.
- A delay of more than 3 to 4 hours results in extremely poor prognosis for a successful reimplantation.

TABLE 24.13

Upper Airway Emergencies

Foreign Body Aspiration

- Most foreign body aspirations occur in children under the age of 4 years.
- Physical findings may include stridor, wheezing, tachypnea, cough, or apnea.
- Negative radiographs *do not* rule out FB aspiration if history suggests it.
- Air trapping may lead to hyperinflation.
- Treatment consists of airway support, O_2, direct laryngoscopy, or bronchoscopy in the operating room under anesthesia.

Epiglottitis

Overview

- The median age at presentation is 7 years.
- Most cases are due to gram-positive organisms.
  —There has been a marked reduction in the number of pediatric cases since the introduction of *Haemophilus influenzae* type B vaccine.*
- Patients may present with dysphagia, fever, drooling, and stridor that have developed over the past 24 hours.
- Diagnosis is confirmed by visualization of a swollen erythematous epiglottis. (*Only an experienced clinician skilled in the emergent management of the difficult airway should perform this procedure*).

Treatment

- Airway support, humidified O_2, and nebulized epinephrine.
- Vascular access is needed.
- Steroids are controversial but frequently used.
- Select antibiotics from third-generation cephalosporins, such as ceftriaxone 100 mg/kg q 24 h.
- Vancomycin should be considered in hospitals with increasing cephalosporin resistance.
- The classic approach to the child with epiglottis is described as follows:
  —Do not agitate the patient in any way.
  —Do not apply a face mask or attempt to start IV.
  —Do not attempt to visualize the epiglottis unless prepared to perform an emergent surgical airway.

Continued

TABLE 24.13

Upper Airway Emergencies, cont'd

Peritonsillar Abscess

- The patient usually presents with fever, sore throat, dysphagia, trismus, muffled voice, and occasionally drooling.
- Physical findings include unilaterally enlarged tonsillar swelling, loss of definition of the anterior tonsilar pillar, and contralateral deviation of the uvula.
- Palpation of the soft palate may reveal localized areas of fluctuance.
- CT scanning or ultrasound may be helpful in children.
- Treatment of the abscess by needle aspiration is diagnostic and therapeutic.
- If successful aspiration is accomplished the stable patient may be discharged home with broad-spectrum antibiotics and analgesics.
- Consider emergent ENT consult.

CT indicates computed tomography; ENT, ears, nose, and throat; IV, intravenous.

*For more information, see Gorelick MH, Baker MD. Epiglottis in children, 1979–1992: effects of *Haemophilus influenzae* type B immunization. *Arch Pediatr Adolesc Med.* 1994;148:47.

TABLE 24.14

Respiratory Distress, Pulmonary Emergencies

Overview

- The patient with acute dyspnea presenting with increasing shortness of breath, tachypnea, use of accessory respiratory muscles, and tachycardia will require emergent medical intervention.
- Initial assessment includes examination for assessment of the airway, breathing, and circulation (ABCs).
- Provide supplemental oxygen to maintain Pao_2 >60 mm Hg. (O_2 saturation >91%).
- If unable to provide adequate oxygenation, consider BiPAP or CPAP until underlying etiology is found; proceed to mechanical intubation if needed.

Tension Pneumothorax

- A tension pneumothorax is a medical emergency.
- It must be recognized by rapid assessment of clinical features, including hypoxia, hypotension, unilaterally decreased breath sounds, distended neck veins, and displaced trachea.
- A tension pneumothorax requires emergent medical treatment, including oxygen and needle thoracentesis, followed by chest tube insertion.
- A follow-up chest x-ray is always necessary following chest tube insertion.

Needle Thoracentesis Procedure

- After carefully evaluating the patient's respiratory status, administer high-flow oxygen and ventilate as necessary.
- Identify the second intercostal space, in the midclavicular line on the side of the tension pneumothorax.
- Prepare the chest with antiseptic scrub if time permits.
- Locally anesthetize the area if the patient is conscious or if time permits.
- Keeping the Luer-Lok in the distal end of the catheter, insert an over-the-needle catheter (2 inches or 5 cm long) into the skin and direct the needle just over (ie, superior to) the rib into the intercostal space.
- Puncture the parietal pleura.
- Remove the Luer-Lok from the catheter and listen for a sudden escape of air when the needle enters the parietal pleura, indicating that the tension pneumothorax has been relieved.
- Remove the needle and replace the Luer-Lok in the distal end of the catheter. Leave the plastic catheter in place and apply a bandage or small dressing over the insertion site.
- Prepare for a chest-tube insertion.

TABLE 24.15

Swallowed Foreign Bodies

The pediatric population accounts for approximately 80% of cases presenting to the emergency department.

Coin Ingestion

- The child usually presents with parents and appears comfortable without specific complaints.
- Radiographs should be performed on all patients.
- Coins lodged in esophagus require endoscopic removal; GI consult is necessary.
- Patients may occasionally be placed in radiology suite and the coin removed under fluoroscopy with balloon catheter technique.
- Balloon catheter removal of an esophageal foreign body is generally considered safe for an object that is smooth, radiopaque, and lodged for less than 72 hours. The child must be cooperative and not require sedation.
- The airway should not be compromised in any manner.
- Prior esophageal disease or surgery is a contraindication.
- This procedure is not without risks, such as aspiration, and must be performed by a skilled and experienced physician.
- Once the FB has passed the pylorus, it will usually pass the remainder of GI tract without problems.
- Some physicians recommend follow-up x-rays to verify that the FB has passed the entire GI tract.

Food Bolus Impaction

- This diagnosis is generally confirmed by the regurgitation of swallowed water and ruled out by the ability to swallow water without difficulty.
- Examine patient to be assured that patient is tolerating his or her own secretions.
- If patient cannot swallow liquids, a GI consult is necessary.
- Consider administration of glucagon 1 mg IV/IM (pediatric dose 0.025–0.1 mg/kg IV/IM/SC); avoid proteolytic enzymes as the risk of esophageal perforation is increased.
- Avoid contrast-enhanced swallowing studies as this may impair a needed endoscopic procedure.

Button Battery Ingestion

- Contacting a Poison Control Center at (800) 222-1222 is suggested.
- Endoscopic removal is suggested after radiographic documentation of battery lodged in the esophagus.
- Esophageal burns and perforation can occur as early as 4 hours after ingestion.

- If battery has passed the esophagus and the patient is asymptomatic, the battery most likely does not need to be retrieved; however, if the battery has not passed the pylorus within 48 hours then endoscopic retrieval is necessary.
- Ipecac is contraindicated.*

---

*For more information, see Litovitz T, Schmitz BF. Ingestion of cylindrical and button batteries. *Pediatrics*. 1992;89:727.

TABLE 24.16

Anaphylaxis and Acute Allergic Reactions

The patient with an acute allergic reaction may present with symptoms ranging from a cutaneous rash to severe life-threatening presentations including respiratory distress and cardiovascular collapse.

- Treatment includes a secure airway with anticipation of intubation.
- Administration of high-flow oxygen:
  —If bronchospasm is present, use nebulized epinephrine or albuterol.
- If hypotensive, rapidly administrator large volumes of crystalloid.
- Discontinue further antigen exposure by removal of the bee stinger, etc.
- Epinephrine (0.3 to 0.5 mL of 1:1000 q 5 to 10 min) may be administered IV, SC, or by nebulizer.
- Antihistamines are helpful, including H_1 blockers such as IV or IM diphenhydramine. H_2 blockers have also proved helpful such as the administration of famotidine 20 mg po or IV.
- Steroids are used to control persistent allergic reactions.
  —Methylprednisolone 125 mg IV is ordered for severe cases.
  —In less severe cases, prednisone 60 mg po, either in a pulse dose or tapering dose, is prescribed over several days.
- Patients with less severe reactions can be observed for several hours. Admit all patients with a severe reaction to an intensive care unit.
- Provide all patients with serious reactions with Epi-pens and Med-Alert bracelets. Consider referral to an allergist for further testing and desensitization therapy.

TABLE 24.17
Urologic Emergencies

Testicular Torsion

- Testicular torsion usually occurs in a young postpubertal male.
- The patient usually presents with acute severe pain in one testicle.
  —The involved testicle usually swells, with developing erythema in the skin overlying the testicle.
  —The patient complains of increasing abdominal pain, associated with nausea and vomiting.
  —The physician should be aware that the "shy" adolescent male might only report abdominal pain.
  —Urological exam should be performed on all patients presenting with abdominal pain.
- Physical examination reveals a swollen, tender, retracted testicle, that often lies in the horizontal plane (bell clapper deformity).
  —The cremasteric reflex is usually absent on the affected side.
  —In delayed presentations the entire hemiscrotum will appear swollen, tender, and tense.
  —The urine is generally clear with a normal microscopic urinalysis.
- Emergent urologic consultation is necessary with anticipation of operative intervention.
- Doppler ultrasound or technetium scan may prove helpful but should not be ordered if it will delay surgery.
- Detorsion may be attempted if the patient is seen within a few hours of onset.
  —If detorsion is attempted use the "opening a book technique."
  —When viewed from below, the right testicle is turned counterclockwise, and the left testicle turned clockwise.
- If successful detorsion, pain relief should be almost immediate.

Paraphimosis

- Paraphimosis is described as entrapment of the retracted foreskin behind the coronal sulcus that cannot be reduced.
- The constriction causes pain and severe swelling that can lead to arterial constriction and tissue necrosis.
- Squeezing the glans firmly for 5 minutes to reduce swelling may lead to successful reduction of foreskin.
- Use opiate analgesics to provide relief of significant pain for the patient.

Urethral Rupture

- Anterior urethral injuries are most often the result of a straddle-type injury.
- Posterior urethral injuries often occur as a result of motor vehicle and motorcycle accidents with resultant pelvic fracture.
- These patient's have blood in the urethral meatus, cannot void, and have perineal bruising.

- In males the prostate is often free-floating or may not be palpable at all if a rectoperitoneal hematoma has collected between the prostate and rectum.
- Urethral instrumentation should not occur prior to performing a retrograde urethrogram.
- If there is marked bladder distention, consider placement of a suprapubic catheter.
- Emergent urological consult should be considered.

Fracture of Penis

- Patients usually present complaining of trauma during sexual intercourse and may present with acute penile pain and deformity.
- The shaft of the penis is swollen and often angulated at the fracture site.
- If the patient is unable to void, a retrograde urethrogram may be required.
- Immediate urological consult is needed as the patient is often taken directly to the operating room for repair.

Blunt Scrotal Trauma

- This type of trauma usually results as a result of a straddle injury or as a result of a direct blow, such as being kicked or incurring a baseball injury to the groin.
- There is an associated high risk of urethral injury with straddle-type trauma.
- Look for bloody penile discharge or laceration, scrotal swelling, or dislocated testicle.
- Do a digital exam of the prostate looking for elevation of prostate, which implies injury to the membranous urethra.
- Consider pelvic x-rays if the injury is associated with significant trauma.
- An ultrasound study or testicular scan is necessary to diagnose disruption of intrascrotal anatomy.
- Be aware that testicular torsion can be associated with scrotal trauma.
- If the testicle cannot be palpated within scrotum, consider the diagnosis of a dislocated testicle with immediate urological consultation.

TABLE 24.18

Obstetric and Gynecologic Sexual Assault Emergencies

- One should think of pregnancy or a complication related to pregnancy in any female between menarche and menopause of reproductive age presenting with abdominal pain, vaginal hemorrhage, and/or vomiting.
- The words "I'm not sexually active" *should not reassure* the clinician that there is no chance for a pregnancy.
- A pregnancy test is always indicated in such patients regardless of last menses or method of contraception.

Sexual Assault

- The evaluation and treatment of the sexual assault victim requires a multidisciplinary team approach.
- This includes a careful medical evaluation, a psychological assessment with appropriate counseling, forensic evidence gathering, and appropriate authority contacts.
- All efforts should be directed toward ensuring patient comfort and confidentiality.
- A thorough physical examination should be performed looking for abrasions, contusions, and other soft tissue injury.
- A careful examination of the perineum, vagina, vaginal fornices, cervix, and rectum is required to identify injuries and potential mechanisms of trauma.
- Because the evaluation of the rape victim is technically a legal assessment, meticulous attention to documentation is an absolute necessity.
- Forensic evidence gathering includes a Wood lamp examination to identify semen for collection, pubic hair sampling, vagina and cervical smears, vaginal wet preparation to identify sperm, vaginal aspirate to test for acid phosphatase, and rectal and buccal swabs for sperm.
- Many localities have found forensic nursing programs to be of great benefit.
- Cervical cultures for *Chlamydia* and gonorrhea should be obtained in addition to obtaining serum testing for syphilis, hepatitis, and HIV.
- Also offer empiric antibiotic coverage against sexually transmitted diseases.
- After confirming that the patient is not pregnant, an oral contraceptive (morning-after pill) may be offered to prevent an unwanted pregnancy.

TABLE 24.19

Obstetric and Gynecologic Emergencies: Ectopic Pregnancy

Ectopic Pregnancy

- Ectopic pregnancy occurs in as many as 2% of all pregnancies.
- It is the leading cause of maternal obstetric morbidity in the first trimester of pregnancy.

Signs and Symptoms

- Consider ectopic pregnancy in any female of reproductive age presenting with syncope.
- Ectopic pregnancy usually presents as the triad of lower abdominal pain, mild vaginal bleeding, and a positive pregnancy test.
- Patients can present in shock secondary to massive bleeding.
- The patient may complain of pain in the upper abdomen and shoulder secondary to bleeding into the peritoneum.

Physical Findings

- Findings vary from stable vital signs and normal pelvic exam to unstable with massive vaginal bleeding.
- A urine pregnancy test should be immediately ordered; if positive, an emergent pelvic ultrasound is ordered to identify an ectopic pregnancy.
- If the pelvic ultrasound establishes an intrauterine pregnancy, an ectopic pregnancy is extremely unlikely; however, there is a chance of a coexisting ectopic pregnancy, especially in women on fertility drugs.
- Pelvic ultrasound findings of an "empty uterus" with an adnexal mass suggest a diagnosis of ectopic pregnancy.*
- Serum quantitative β-HCG levels greater than 6000 IU/L accompanied by sonographic findings of an "empty uterus" are highly suggestive of an ectopic pregnancy.[†]
- A quantitative β-HCG level less that 1500 IU/L indicates that the pregnancy is too early to be appreciated on sonography and that the pregnancy may be intrauterine or ectopic.
- A repeat β-HCG is usually ordered in 48 hours.
- In a normal intrauterine pregnancy the rate of rise of the β-HCG should be greater than 66% at 48 hours.[‡]
- Serum β-HCG between 1500 and 6000 IU/L with a nondiagnositic sonogram strongly suggests ectopic pregnancy

Treatment

- For the unstable patient:
  —Immediate IV access with two large-bore needles.
  —The rapid administration of crystalloid.
  —Packed RBCs transfused.
  —Emergent laparotomy.

Continued

TABLE 24.19

Obstetric and Gynecologic Emergencies: Ectopic Pregnancy, cont'd

- For the stable patient:
  —If the patient has a low quantitative HCG level and a sonogram that is nondiagnostic, patient may be sent home with careful instructions to return to the ED if there is vaginal bleeding and/or abdominal pain.
  —These discharge instructions must be given to a reliable patient as she must be expected to follow up for a reevaluation and repeat quantitative HCG in 2 days.
  —Further treatment may require obstetric/gynecologic consultation and may include the use of abortifacient agents (methotrexate) vs laparoscopy.

ED indicates emergency department; IV, intravenous; RBC; red blood cell count.

*For more information, see Brown DL, Doubilet PM. Transvaginal sonography for the diagnosis of ectopic pregnancy: positivity and performance characteristics. *J Ultrasound Med.* 1994;13:259.

†For more information, see Zinn HL, Cohen HL, Zinn DL. Ultrasonographic diagnosis of ectopic pregnancy: importance of transabdominal imaging. *J Ultrasound Med.* 1997;16:603.

‡For more information, see Barnhart K, Mennuti MT, Benjamin I, et al. Prompt diagnosis of ectopic pregnancy in an emergency department setting. *Obstet Gynecol.* 1994;81:1010.

TABLE 24.20

Neuropsychiatric Emergencies

Dystonic Drug Reactions

- The patient often presents to the office or emergency department anxious with peculiar posturing and/or difficulty speaking.
- Check history for the recent use of phenothiazines or butyrophenones.
- Even a single dose of an antiemetic agent such as prochlorperazine (Compazine) may induce dystonic reaction.
- Treatment includes the IV administration of benztropine (Cogentin) or diphenhydramine (Benadryl).
- If this is a true dystonic reaction, dramatic improvement should be appreciated within 5 minutes.
- Discontinue the use of the offending drug.
- If the offending agent has a prolonged half-life, prescribe benztropine 2 mg or diphenhydramine 25 mg po q 6 h for 24 hours to prevent a relapse.

Hyperventilation

Signs and Symptoms

- The patient presents with extreme anxiousness with increasing complaints of shortness of breath, chest pain, palpitations, and numbness of the hands, fingers, and perioral area.
- The physical examination is normal, with the occasional exception of flexor spasm of the hands and feet.
- A careful physical examination is required to exclude serious medical emergencies such as pneumothorax, acute pulmonary embolus, myocardial infarction, reactive airway disease, foreign body ingestion, DKA, and salicylate overdose.
- Pulse oximetry should reveal an O_2 saturation approaching 97% to 100%.

Treatment

- Use of the traditional paper bag rebreathing is generally discouraged, due to hypoxic events.*
- Pharmacological therapy should be reserved as a last resort.
- If the patient fails to improve despite continued observation, the administration of hydroxyzine (Vistaril) 50 to 100 mg IM, diphenhydramine (Benadryl) 25 to 50 mg IM, or lorazepam (Ativan) 1 to 2 mg IM may calm the anxious patient.
- If symptoms are not reversed within 20 minutes, reconsider diagnosis.
- ABGs should be consistent with an acute respiratory alkalosis.
- Frequently "benign neglect" of the patient allows for spontaneous resolution of symptoms.
- This should then be followed by a thorough interview, with emphasis on management of social stressors.

---

*For more information, see Callaham M. Hypoxic hazards of traditional paper bag rebreathing in hyperventilating patients. *Ann Emerg Med.* 1989;18:622–628.

chapter 25

Practice Management and Enhancement

Alex Wilgus, MD

IN THIS CHAPTER

- Internet-based reference tools
- Handheld computers/personal digital assistants (PDAs)
- Electronic medical record primer
- Internet-based practice enhancement tools
- Documentation guidelines
- Health Insurance Portability and Accountability Act (HIPAA)

BOOKSHELF RECOMMENDATIONS

- Due to the rapidly changing nature of this field, any printed book will unlikely be able to provide current information, especially with regard to electronic medical records and other computer resources, and HIPAA. Thus, I recommend the American Academy of Family Physicians Family Practice Management Web site as an unparalleled, frequently updated resource, located on the World Wide Web at www.aafp.org.

INTERNET-BASED REFERENCE TOOLS

There are a large number of Internet-based reference tools that can be of great assistance to the clinician of all disciplines. There is perhaps a greater variety of resources for primary care providers. It must be emphasized that Web sites are under no obligation to ensure the accuracy of the information they offer: many use the World Wide Web (WWW) as a forum to promote personal opinions and viewpoints. You are best served by using information from reputable sources and sites. Many of the "old standards" of medical reference are available on the Internet. US government agencies maintain many sites that are highly useful.

- For those who are new to the Internet as a tool for finding medical information, a primer is available on the WWW at www.physiciansguide.com/newbies.html.
- An excellent site that contains regularly updated links to various sites of interest to family physicians is maintained by the American Academy of Family Physicians at www.aafp.org/x7684.xml.

TABLE 25.1

Web Sites of Interest to Primary Care Providers

Any listing of medical Web sites is destined to be incomplete. Table 25.1 is intended only as a sampling of some of the more common Web sites of general interest to family physicians. It is best to explore the Internet periodically to determine what has become available. It is also wise to "bookmark" sites (Netscape) or place them in the "favorites" heading (Internet Explorer) in an organized fashion to be able to retrieve Web site addresses easily.

Category	Name	Web Site Address (URL)	Comments
General Reference	Merck Medicus	www.merckmedicus.com	Free to holders of a valid state medical license. Includes several reference texts and MD Consult
	MD Consult	www.mdconsult.com	Medical texts, patient education, medical headlines
	Family Doctor	www.familydoctor.org	Done by AAFP, many patient-oriented information links
	Centers for Disease Control	www.cdc.gov	Centers for Disease Control and Prevention—MMWR, etc
Medical Literature	PubMed	www.ncbi.nlm.nih.gov/entrez/query.fcgi?db=PubMed	User-friendly free MEDLINE searches—includes a way to have your local medical library forward articles to you
	Cochrane abstracts	www.update-software.com/Cochrane/default.HTM	Allows free searching of the abstracts of evidence-based reviews of the medical literature
	JFP POEMS	www.medicalinforetriever.com/poems/poemsearch.cfm	Free searching of a subset of the "patient-oriented evidence that matters" reviews published in the *Journal of Family Practice*
	National Guideline Clearinghouse	www.guideline.gov	Searchable database of various practice guidelines from many different organizations

Continued

TABLE 25.1

Web Sites of Interest to Primary Care Providers, cont'd

Category	Name	Web Site Address (URL)	Comments
Primary Care Index Sites	Primary Care Network	www.primarycarenetwork.com	Site with many categories of links of interest to primary care physicians
	American Academy of Family Physicians	www.aafp.org	AAFP's wide-ranging site with volumes of information: CME reporting, access to *American Family Physician*, etc
	Medscape	www.medscape.com/familymedicinehome	Commercial site with many links of interest
Online Journals	Various	www.ncbi.nlm.nih.gov/entrez/journals/loftext_noprov.html (list of over 2000 journals available online, maintained by the National Library of Medicine)	Many medical journals are available online free of charge, or free to current subscribers. Many of these allow downloading, viewing, and printing of high-quality reproductions of articles in Adobe PDF format*

AAFP indicates American Academy of Family Physicians; CME, continuing medical education.

*The Adobe Acrobat Reader is available for free download at www.adobe.com/products/acrobat/readstep.html.

HANDHELD COMPUTERS/PERSONAL DIGITAL ASSISTANTS (PDAS)

The emergence of handheld computers has been one of the most notable recent technological advances in medicine. These small computers have many times the computing and storage power of their "mainframe" forebears. They can be used for many different medical applications as well as more general business applications, such as word processing.

TABLE 25.2

Reasons to Consider Clinical PDA Use

- Organize and rapidly access personal information, like phone numbers, calendar items, and to-do lists
- Access medical information at the "point of care" in the exam room
- Choose from thousands of medical applications on the Web and download those you want
- Synchronize your information on your home or clinic PC
- Share information quickly with others who have PDAs by infrared "beaming"
- Write prescriptions electronically
- Interface directly with some EMR (Electronic Medical Records) Systems

Adapted with permission from www.aafp.org/fpnet.xml.

There are two types of handheld computers readily available: those that use the Palm OS (operating system), and those that use the Windows CE OS (Pocket PC). (Other systems, such as EPOC, are not widely available.) The former is an operating system that was created de novo for Palm handheld devices, while the latter is an adaptation of the familiar Microsoft Windows operating system. Presently, the Palm devices are in wider use, but each camp has its strong proponents. Differences are summarized in Table 25.3. There are many software resources available on the Internet for these devices, many free. There are likewise many sites that serve as clearinghouses for actual product sites.

TABLE 25.3

Differences Between Palm and Pocket PC Personal Digital Assistants

	Palm OS Devices	Pocket PC
Operating system	Palm OS	Windows CE (3.0)
Major brands	Palm, Handspring, HandEra, Sony, IBM, Symbol, Kyocera, Samsung	Compaq, Casio, HP
Least expensive model (8MB+)	\$169 (Palm m105 and Visor Neo) (prices dropping)	\$499 (iPAQ H3650 from Compaq) (prices dropping)
Smallest size	11.4 × 7.9 × 1.0 cm (Palm VX and IBM Workpad)	13.0 × 7.8 × 1.6 cm (HP Jornada 548)
Lowest weight	113 g (Palm VX and IBM Workpad)	179 g (Compaq iPAQ H3650
Display	160 × 160 pixels monochrome (most) to 65 K colors	240 × 320 pixels 4096 (most) to 65 K colors
Software available	++	+
Expandability	+/− (depends on model)	+
Pros	Simple, lower cost, energy efficient	Versatile, powerful, voice recorder, pocket Word/Excel
Cons	Less versatile	Higher cost, energy-consuming

Adapted from www.aafp.org/fpnet.

TABLE 25.4

Internet Sites for Personal Digital Assistant Software

Clearinghouse Sites	
Family Physician's Guide to Handheld Computers	www.fphandheld.com
Peripheral Brain	http://pbrain.hypermart.net
PdaMD	www.pdamd.com
Healthy Palm Pilot	www.healthypalmpilot.com
Handheld Med	www.handheldmed.com
Collective Med	www.collectivemed.com
Medical Pocket PC	www.medicalpocketpc.com

Adapted with permission from www.aafp.org/fpnet.

TABLE 25.5

Personal Digital Assistant Software Categories

Medical Applications	Medical References	Utility
Billing and coding	General medicine	Database
Prescribing	EBM/guidelines	Document readers
Medical calculators	Pharmacological	Document converter
Patient tracking/EMR	Specialty medicine	Security
OB calculators		Synch/scheduling
Procedure logging		

Adapted with permission from www.aafp.org/fpnet.

ELECTRONIC MEDICAL RECORDS

There has been an explosion of development in electronic medical record (EMR) systems. The intent is to provide a technological solution to the disorganized, illegible traditional medical record many of us have come to know, thus markedly improving patient care.

There two basic formats available: those that are provided as an application accessed through the Internet (known as application service providers or ASPs), as well as stand-alone systems that run on computers in or near your office.

There are more ideas about the features that should be included in an EMR than there are companies making them. There is a wide variety available, some of which cater particularly to large or small office practices. Others still concentrate on hospital information systems.

EMR systems typically consist of three modules:

- Patient management and scheduling
- Clinical records
- Practice management and billing

Some vendors offer only one or two of these modules, while a few offer a fully integrated system that is meant to handle a patient encounter from scheduling through billing. Several companies cooperate in ensuring their modules are compatible.

A checklist of features one may want in an EMR system is available on the Internet at www.aafp.org/fpnet/x3701.xml.

An EMR vendor survey has been published in *Family Practice Management* (www.aafp.org/fpm/20010100/45elec.html). This survey is a useful tabulation of the different features that EMRs may contain; however, it should be noted that this is not a *user* survey, and thus contains claims of included features that may be incompletely or imperfectly implemented.

It is a generally recognized principle that an EMR system should be seen in use in a genuine clinical setting before decisions about its usefulness are made.

TABLE 25.6

Partial Listing of Leading EMR Vendors

Vendor	Web Site Address (URL)	Product
A4 Health Systems (919) 851-6177	www.a4healthsystems.com	HealthMatics
Care Is #1 (949) 753-1900	www.careis1.com	Medinformatix
Cerner (816) 201-2722	www.cerner.com	Power Chart
Chart Ware (800) 642-4278	www.chartware.com	Chart Ware
DOCS, Inc (800) 455-7627	www.docs.com	SOAPware
e-MDs (512) 257-5200	www.e-mds.com	TOPS
Epic Systems (608) 271-9000	www.epicsystems.com	Epic Care
HBOC (404) 338-6000	www.hboc.com	Pathways
Healthcare Data, Inc (765) 342-9947	www.healthprobe.com	Health Probe
IMcKesson (612) 814-7160	http://imckesson.com	iMcKesson Clinical Suite
Infor*Mod, Inc.	www.infor-med.com	Praxis
JMJ Technologies (800) 677-5653	www.jmjtech.com	Enounter PRO
Medic (800) 334-8534	www.medcmp.com	Auto Chart
Medical Manager (650) 969-7047	www.medicalmanager.com	Omni Docs
MEDCOM Information Systems (800) 213-2161	www.idt.net	Dr. Welford's Chart Notes
MedicWare (626) 303-4000	www.medicware.com	MedicWare EMR
MedInformatix (310) 348-7367	www.medrecords.com	MedInformatix
Medscape (503) 466-3628	www.medicalogic.com	Logician
Micromed-Clinitec (215) 657-7010	www.micromed.com	Next Gen
Pen Chart (860) 537-1823	www.penchart.com	Pen Chart

Continued

TABLE 25.6

Partial Listing of Leading EMR Vendors, cont'd

Vendor	Web Site Address (URL)	Product
Physician Micro Systems, Inc. (206) 441-8490	www.pmsi.com	Practice Partner
Pocket Chart (425) 482-7000	www.datacritical.com	Data Critical
STAT! Systems (510) 705-8700	www.statsystems.com	Q.D. Clinical
STI Computer Systems (610) 768-9030	www.chartmaker.com	ChartMaker

Adapted with permission from www.aafp.org/x477.xml.

INTERNET-BASED PRACTICE ENHANCEMENT TOOLS

Once again, the Family Practice Management Web site (www.aafp.org/fpm/) has a number of forms and flow sheets that can be used in traditional paper charts to organize and to standardize care. These are best browsed periodically on the Internet at www.aafp.org/fpm/toolbox/index.html. This is the main site for the Family Practice Management "Toolbox," which is frequently updated with resources that have been published in the journal.

A practice quality enhancement project proposed by the AAFP called Practice 2010 seeks to redefine medical office practice as usual by implementing several technology, office efficiency, and patient care enhancements. This is an ongoing project, and modules for the Practice 2010 initiative will be added to the Web site at www.aafp.org/quality/index.html as they are developed.

TABLE 25.7

Components of the Practice 2010 Initiative

Technology Enhancements	Office Efficiency and Patient Care Enhancements
Clinic Web site for patient access/info	Open access office scheduling
Patient e-mail communication	Group medical visits
Electronic medical record	Clinic productivity planning (demand/supply for encounters)
Internet use for timely data access for patients and providers	Practice measurement of outcomes and employee satisfaction
Palmtop computer use	Patient satisfaction

Adapted with permission from www.aafp.org/x3847.xml.

Documentation Requirements

Current Procedural Terminology (CPT) codes (which include Evaluation and Management codes) are owned, written, and maintained by the American Medical Association. Documentation guidelines (DGs) are maintained by HCFA (now known as CMS—Centers for Medicare and Medicaid Services) and are intended to provide guidance on the required documentation to appropriately submit a given E/M CPT code. There are currently two sets of guidelines in effect, 1995 (15 pages) and 1997 (51 pages), with a third set still in process. These DGs can be downloaded and printed out from the HCFA Web site at www.hcfa.gov/medlearn/emdoc.htm.

The 1999/2000 guidelines are a work-in-progress in response to complaints by many physicians about the crushing documentation requirements of the 1997 DGs in particular. An optimistic estimate is that the new guidelines will be rolled out sometime in 2002. Pending the release/rollout of the 2000 DGs, HCFA has stated that physicians may employ either of the existing DGs, whichever is more "beneficial" for the physician. There are significant discrepancies between how physicians code their visits and how experts feel they should be coded, based on written chart documentation, as evidenced in Table 25.8. At press time, a CMS advisory committee has recently voted to abolish the current system of DGs, in favor of more self-explanatory E/M code.

TABLE 25.8

Number and Percentage of Family Physician CPT Coding of Six Hypothetical Cases Compared With Expert Consensus, by CPT Coding Level*

Case	No (%)	No (%)	No (%)	No (%)	No (%)
Coding level, established patient	*99211*	*99212*	*99213*	*9921*	*99215*
1. Pneumonia	2 (1)	13 (6)	132 (64)	**55 (27)**	3 (1.4)
2. Cramps, hypertension	2 (1)	41 (20)	**137 (66)**	25 (12)	0 (0)
3. Deep vein thrombosis follow-up	11 (5)	**125 (60)**	65 (31)	3 (1.4)	0 (0)
Coding level, new patient	*99201*	*99202*	*99203*	*99204*	*99204*
4. Asthma	3 (1.4)	**39 (19)**	114 (55)	143 (21)	6 (3)
5. Gastroenteritis	**18 (9)**	128 (62)	53 (26)	5 (2)	0 (0)
6. Sinusitis, hypertension	4 (2)	**49 (24)**	119 (58)	30 (15)	0 (0)

Used with permission from King MS, Sharp L, Lipsky MS. Accuracy of CPT evaluation and management coding by family physicians. *J Am Board Fam Pract.* 2001;14(3):184–192.

CPT indicates Current Procedural Terminology.

*Responses in boldface indicate the number and percentage of physicians agreeing with the experts' consensus coding.

The task of assigning Evaluation and Management (E/M) codes to accurately reflect the work performed in the course of a patient encounter is daunting. There are many publications aimed at demystifying the process. Tables 25.9 through 25.16 break down the different elements of history, exam, decision-making, and time investment that must be satisfied for a given type of patient encounter. This is an incomplete listing, but includes the most commonly used E/M codes. The examination requirement in the tables assumes a "General Multisystem" examination.

TABLE 25.9

Documentation Requirements for New Patient Office Visits*

	99201	99202	99203	99204	99205
HISTORY					
CC	Required	Required	Required	Required	Required
HPI	1–3 elements	1–3 elements	4+ elements (or 3+ chronic diseases)	4+ elements (or 3+ chronic diseases)	4+ elements (or 3+ chronic diseases)
ROS	N/A	Pertinent	2-9 systems	10+ systems	10+ systems
PFSH	N/A	N/A	1 element from any 1 area	1 element from each of 3 areas	1 element from each of 3 areas
EXAMINATION					
1997 documentation guidelines	1–5 elements	6–11 elements	12 or more elements	Comprehensive	Comprehensive
1995 documentation guidelines	System of complaint	2–4 systems	5–7 systems	8+ systems	8+ systems
MEDICAL DECISION MAKING					
	Straight-forward	Straight-forward	Low	Moderate	High
TIME					
Half the total must involve counseling or coordination of care.					
	10 minutes	20 minutes	30 minutes	45 minutes	60 minutes

*Three of the three key components—history, exam, and medical decision-making—are required.

TABLE 25.10

Documentation Requirements for Established Patient Office Visits*

	99211	99212	99213	99214	99215
HISTORY					
CC	N/A	Required	Required	Required	Required
HPI	N/A	1–3 elements	1–3 elements	4+ elements (or 3+ chronic diseases)	4+ elements (or 3+ chronic diseases)
ROS	N/A	N/A	Pertinent	2–9 systems	10+ systems
PFSH	N/A	N/A	N/A	1 element from any 1 area	1 element from each of 2 areas
EXAMINATION					
1997 documentation guidelines	N/A	1–5 elements	6–11 elements	12 or more elements	Comprehensive
1995 documentation guidelines	N/A	System of complaint	2–4 systems	5–7 systems	8+ systems
MEDICAL DECISION MAKING					
	N/A	Straight-forward	Low	Moderate	High
TIME					
Half the total must involve counseling or coordination of care.					
	5 minutes	10 minutes	15 minutes	25 minutes	40 minutes

Adapted with permission from Hill E. How to get all the 99214s you deserve. *Fam Pract Manag.* 2001;8:43–47

*Two of the three key components—history, exam, and medical decision-making—are required.

TABLE 25.11

Documentation Requirements for Initial Hospital Patient Visits*

	99221	99222	99223
HISTORY			
CC	Required	Required	Required
HPI	4+ elements (or 3+ chronic diseases)	4+ elements (or 3+ chronic diseases)	4+ elements (or 3+ chronic diseases)
ROS	2+ systems	10+ systems	10+ systems
PFSH	1 element from each of 1+ area	1 element from each of 3 areas	1 element from each of 3 areas
EXAMINATION			
1997 documentation guidelines	12 or more elements	Comprehensive	Comprehensive
1995 documentation guidelines	5–7 systems	8+ systems	8+ systems
MEDICAL DECISION MAKING			
	Straightforward or Low	Moderate	High
TIME			
Half the total must involve counseling or coordination of care.			
	30 minutes	50 minutes	70 minutes

*Three of the three key components—history, exam, and medical decision-making—are required.

TABLE 25.12

Documentation Requirements for Subsequent Hospital Patient Visits*

	99231	99232	99233
HISTORY			
CC	Required	Required	Required
HPI	1–3 elements	1–3 elements	4+ elements (or 3+ chronic diseases)
ROS	N/A	Problem pertinent	2–9 systems
PFSH	N/A	N/A	1 element from any 1 area
EXAMINATION			
1997 documentation guidelines	1–5 elements	6–11 elements	12 or more elements
1995 documentation guidelines	System of complaint	2–4 systems	5–7 systems
MEDICAL DECISION MAKING			
	Straightforward or Low	Moderate	High
TIME			
Half the total must involve counseling or coordination of care.	15 minutes	25 minutes	35 minutes

*Two of the three key components—history, exam, and medical decision-making—are required.

TABLE 25.13

Documentation Requirements for Same-Day Observation Patient Visits*

	99234	99235	99236
HISTORY			
CC	Required	Required	Required
HPI	4+ elements (or 3+ chronic diseases)	4+ elements (or 3+ chronic diseases)	4+ elements (or 3+ chronic diseases)
ROS	2+ systems	10+ systems	10+ systems
PFSH	1 element from each of 1+ area	1 element from each of 3 areas	1 element from each of 3 areas
EXAMINATION			
1997 documentation guidelines	12 or more elements	Comprehensive	Comprehensive
1995 documentation guidelines	5-7 systems	8+ systems	8+ systems
MEDICAL DECISION MAKING			
	Straightforward or Low	Moderate	High

*Three of the three key components—history, exam, and medical decision-making—are required. Also, contact time may not be used as a criterion for E/M coding for same-day discharge observation patients.

TABLE 25.14

Documentation Requirements for Emergency Department Patient Visits*

	99281	99282	99283	99284	99285
HISTORY					
CC	Required	Required	Required	Required	Required
HPI	1–3 elements	1–3 elements	1–3 elements	4+ elements (or 3+ chronic diseases)	4+ elements (or 3+ chronic diseases)
ROS	N/A	Pertinent	Pertinent	2–9 systems	10+ systems
PFSH	N/A	N/A	N/A	1 element from any 1 area	1 element from each of 2 areas
EXAMINATION					
1997 documentation guidelines	1–5 elements elements	6–11 elements	6–11 elements	12 or more	Comprehensive
1995 documentation guidelines	System of complaint	2–4 systems	2–4 systems	5–7 systems	8+ systems
MEDICAL DECISION MAKING					
	Straight-forward	Low	Moderate	Moderate	High

*Three of the three key components—history, exam, and medical decision-making—are required. Also, contact time may not be used as a criterion for E/M coding in the ED.

TABLE 25.15

Documentation Requirements for New Patient Home Visits*

	99341	99342	99343	99344	99345
HISTORY					
CC	Required	Required	Required	Required	Required
HPI	1–3 elements	1–3 elements	4+ elements (or 3+ chronic diseases)	4+ elements (or 3+ chronic diseases)	4+ elements (or 3+ chronic diseases)
ROS	N/A	Pertinent	2–9 systems	10+ systems	10+ systems
PFSH	N/A	N/A	1 element from any 1 area	1 element from each of 3 areas	1 element from each of 3 areas
EXAMINATION					
1997 documentation guidelines	1–5 elements	6–11 elements	12 or more elements	Comprehensive	Comprehensive
1995 documentation guidelines	System of complaint	2–4 systems	5–7 systems	8+ systems	8+ systems
MEDICAL DECISION MAKING					
	Straight-forward	Low	Moderate	Moderate	High
TIME					
Half the total must involve counseling or coordination of care.	20 minutes	30 minutes	45 minutes	60 minutes	75 minutes

*Three of the three key components—history, exam, and medical decision-making—are required.

TABLE 25.16

Documentation Requirements for Established Patient Home Visits*

	99347	99348	99349	99350
HISTORY				
CC	Required	Required	Required	Required
HPI	1–3 elements	1–3 elements	4+ elements (or 3+ chronic diseases)	4+ elements (or 3+ chronic diseases)
ROS	N/A	Pertinent	2–9 systems	10+ systems
PFSH	N/A	N/A	1 element from any 1 area	1 element from each of 2 areas
EXAMINATION				
1997 documentation guidelines	1–5 elements	6–11 elements	12 or more	Comprehensive
1995 documentation guidelines	System of complaint	2–4 systems	5–7 systems	8+ systems
MEDICAL DECISION MAKING				
	Straight-forward	Low	Moderate	Moderate to high
TIME				
Half the total must involve counseling or coordination of care.	15 minutes	25 minutes	40 minutes	60 minutes

*Two of the three key components—history, exam, and medical decision-making—are required.

TABLE 25.17

The Elements of HPI

- Location
- Quality
- Severity
- Duration
- Timing
- Context
- Modifying factors
- Associated signs and symptoms

TABLE 25.18

The "System" of the ROS

- Constitutional symptoms (eg, fever, weight loss)
- Eyes
- Ears, nose, mouth, throat
- Cardiovascular
- Respiratory
- Gastrointestinal
- Genitourinary
- Musculoskeletal
- Integumentary (skin and/or breast)
- Neurological
- Psychiatric
- Endocrine
- Hematologic/lymphatic
- Allergic/immunologic

TABLE 25.19

Elements of the General Multisystem Exam

The "elements" of the general multisystem physical exam referenced to 1997 guidelines in Tables 25.9 through 25.16 are defined as follows. Note that there are specific body system exams that have their own criteria for "completeness".

"12 or more elements" (detailed examination)	At least two elements identified by a bullet from each of six areas/systems OR at least twelve elements identified by a bullet in two or more areas/systems, as listed in Table 25.20.
"Comprehensive"	*Perform* all elements identified by a bullet in at least nine organ systems or body areas and *document* at least two elements identified by a bullet from each of nine areas/systems as listed in Table 25.20. Note the distinction made between "perform" and "document."

TABLE 25.20

General Multisystem Exam

System/ Body Area	Elements of Examination
Constitutional	■ Measurement of **any three of the following seven** vital signs: (1) sitting or standing blood pressure, (2) supine blood pressure, (3) pulse rate and regularity, (4) respiration, (5) temperature, (6) height, (7) weight (May be measured and recorded by ancillary staff) ■ General appearance of patient (eg, development, nutrition, body habitus, deformities, attention to grooming)
Eyes	■ Inspection of conjunctivae and lids ■ Examination of pupils and irises (eg, reaction to light and accommodation, size and symmetry) ■ Ophthalmoscopic examination of optic discs (eg, size, C/D ratio, appearance) and posterior segments (eg, vessel changes, exudates, hemorrhages)
Ears, Nose, Mouth and Throat	■ External inspection of ears and nose (eg, overall appearance, scars, lesions, masses) ■ Otoscopic examination of external auditory canals and tympanic membranes ■ Assessment of hearing (eg, whispered voice, finger rub, tuning fork) ■ Inspection of nasal mucosa, septum and turbinates ■ Inspection of lips, teeth and gums ■ Examination of oropharynx: oral mucosa, salivary glands, hard and soft palates, tongue, tonsils and posterior pharynx
Neck	■ Examination of neck (eg, masses, overall appearance, symmetry, tracheal position, crepitus) ■ Examination of thyroid (eg, enlargement, tenderness, mass)
Respiratory	■ Assessment of respiratory effort (eg, intercostal retractions, use of accessory muscles, diaphragmatic movement) ■ Percussion of chest (eg, dullness, flatness, hyperresonance) ■ Palpation of chest (eg, tactile fremitus) ■ Auscultation of lungs (eg, breath sounds, adventitious sounds, rubs)
Cardiovascular	■ Palpation of heart (eg, location, size, thrills) ■ Auscultation of heart with notation of abnormal sounds and murmurs

System/ Body Area	Elements of Examination
	■ Examination of: 1. carotid arteries (eg, pulse amplitude, bruits) 2. abdominal aorta (eg, size, bruits) 3. femoral arteries (eg, pulse amplitude, bruits) 4. pedal pulses (eg, pulse amplitude) 5. extremities for edema and/or varicosities
Chest (Breasts)	■ Inspection of breasts (eg, symmetry, nipple discharge) ■ Palpation of breasts and axillae (eg, masses or lumps, tenderness)
Gastrointestinal (Abdomen)	■ Examination of abdomen with notation of presence of masses or tenderness ■ Examination of liver and spleen ■ Examination for presence or absence of hernia ■ Examination (when indicated) of anus, perineum and rectum, including sphincter tone, presence of hemorrhoids, rectal masses ■ Obtain stool sample for occult blood test when indicated
Genitourinary	**MALE** ■ Examination of the scrotal contents (eg, hydrocele, spermatocele, tenderness of cord, testicular mass) ■ Examination of the penis ■ Digital rectal examination of prostate gland (eg, size, symmetry, nodularity, tenderness) **FEMALE** ■ Pelvic examination (with or without specimen collection for smears and cultures), including 1. Examination of external genitalia (eg, general appearance, hair distribution, lesions) and vagina (eg, general appearance, estrogen effect, discharge, lesions, pelvic support, cystocele, rectocele) 2. Examination of urethra (eg, masses, tenderness, scarring) 3. Examination of bladder (eg, fullness, masses, tenderness) 4. Cervix (eg, general appearance, lesions, discharge) 5. Uterus (eg, size, contour, position, mobility, tenderness, consistency, descent or support) 6. Adnexa/parametria (eg, masses, tenderness, organomegaly, nodularity)

Continued

TABLE 25.20

General Multisystem Exam, cont'd

System/ Body Area	Elements of Examination
Lymphatic	Palpation of lymph nodes in **two or more** areas: ■ Neck ■ Axillae ■ Groin ■ Other
Musculoskeletal	■ Examination of gait and station ■ Inspection and/or palpation of digits and nails (eg, clubbing, cyanosis, inflammatory conditions, petechiae, ischemia, infections, nodes) Examination of joints, bones and muscles of **one or more of the following six** areas: (1) head and neck; (2) spine, ribs and pelvis; (3) right upper extremity; (4) left upper extremity; (5) right lower extremity; and (6) left lower extremity. The examination of a given area includes: ■ Inspection and/or palpation with notation of presence of any misalignment, asymmetry, crepitation, defects, tenderness, masses, effusions ■ Assessment of range of motion with notation of any pain, crepitation or contracture ■ Assessment of stability with notation of any dislocation (luxation), subluxation or laxity ■ Assessment of muscle strength and tone (eg, flaccid, cog wheel, spastic) with notation of any atrophy or abnormal movements
Skin	■ Inspection of skin and subcutaneous tissue (eg, rashes, lesions, ulcers) ■ Palpation of skin and subcutaneous tissue (eg, induration, subcutaneous nodules, tightening)
Neurologic	■ Test cranial nerves with notation of any deficits ■ Examination of deep tendon reflexes with notation of pathological reflexes (eg, Babinski) ■ Examination of sensation (eg, by touch, pin, vibration, proprioception)
Psychiatric	■ Description of patient's judgment and insight ■ Brief assessment of mental status including: 1. Orientation to time, place and person 2. Recent and remote memory 3. Mood and affect (eg, depression, anxiety, agitation)

TABLE 25.21

Table of Risk*

Level of Risk	Presenting Problem(s)	Diagnostic Procedure(s) Ordered	Management Options Selected
Minimal	■ One self-limited or minor problem, eg, cold, insect bite, tinea corporis	■ Laboratory tests requiring venipuncture ■ Chest x-rays ■ EKG/EEG ■ Urinalysis ■ Ultrasound, eg, echocardiography ■ KOH prep	■ Rest ■ Gargles ■ Elastic bandages ■ Superficial dressings
Low	■ Two or more self-limited or minor problems ■ One stable chronic illness, eg, well controlled hypertension, non-insulin dependent diabetes, cataract, BPH ■ Acute uncomplicated illness or injury, eg, cystitis, allergic rhinitis, simple sprain	■ Physiologic tests not under stress, eg, pulmonary function tests ■ Non-cardiovascular imaging studies with contrast, eg, barium enema ■ Superficial needle biopsies ■ Clinical laboratory tests requiring arterial puncture ■ Skin biopsies	■ Over-the-counter drugs ■ Minor surgery with no identified risk factors ■ Physical therapy ■ Occupational therapy ■ IV fluids without additives
Moderate	■ One or more chronic illnesses with mild exacerbation, progression, or side effects of treatment ■ Two or more stable chronic illnesses ■ Undiagnosed new problem with uncertain prognosis, eg, lump in breast	■ Physiologic tests under stress, eg, cardiac stress test, fetal contraction stress test ■ Diagnostic endoscopies with no identified risk factors ■ Deep needle or incisional biopsy ■ Cardiovascular imaging studies with contrast and no identified risk factors, eg, arteriogram, cardiac catheterization	■ Minor surgery with identified risk factors ■ Elective major surgery (open, percutaneous or endoscopic) with no identified risk factors ■ Prescription drug management ■ Therapeutic nuclear medicine ■ IV fluids with additives

Continued

TABLE 25.21

Table of Risk, cont'd*

Level of Risk	Presenting Problem(s)	Diagnostic Procedure(s) Ordered	Management Options Selected
	■ Acute illness with systemic symptoms, eg, pyelonephritis, pneumonitis, colitis ■ Acute complicated injury, eg, head injury with brief loss of consciousness	■ Obtain fluid from body cavity, eg lumbar puncture, thoracentesis, culdocentesis	■ Closed treatment of fracture or dislocation without manipulation
High	■ One or more chronic illnesses with severe exacerbation, progression, or side effects of treatment ■ Acute or chronic illnesses or injuries that pose a threat to life or bodily function, eg, multiple trauma, acute MI, pulmonary embolus, severe respiratory distress, progressive severe rheumatoid arthritis, psychiatric illness with potential threat to self or others, peritonitis, acute renal failure ■ An abrupt change in neurologic status, eg, seizure, TIA, weakness, sensory loss	■ Cardiovascular imaging studies with contrast with identified risk factors ■ Cardiac electrophysiological tests ■ Diagnostic Endoscopies with identified risk factors ■ Discography	■ Elective major surgery (open, percutaneous or endoscopic) with identified risk factors ■ Emergency major surgery (open, percutaneous or endoscopic) ■ Parenteral controlled substances ■ Drug therapy requiring intensive monitoring for toxicity ■ Decision not to resuscitate or to de-escalate care because of poor prognosis

*The "level" of Medical Decision Making (MDM) is a very complex determination. It is important to note that the highest level of risk in any one category (presenting problem(s), diagnostic procedure(s), or management options) determines the overall risk; thus, "prescription drug management" alone during an encounter would assume "moderate" risk.

FIGURE 25.1

E/M Coding Assistants

Given the obvious complexity of the foregoing documentation guidelines, an automated system to ease and improve compliance is useful. One Palm OS compatible coding assistant is presently available for handheld computers in the form of STAT E&M Coder, available on the Internet at www.statcoder.com. Screen shots from this program are shown below.

St. Anthony Publishing compiles perhaps the best-known published E/M coding resources. Their current offerings can be found on the Internet at www.st-anthony.com/Modules/default/default.asp.

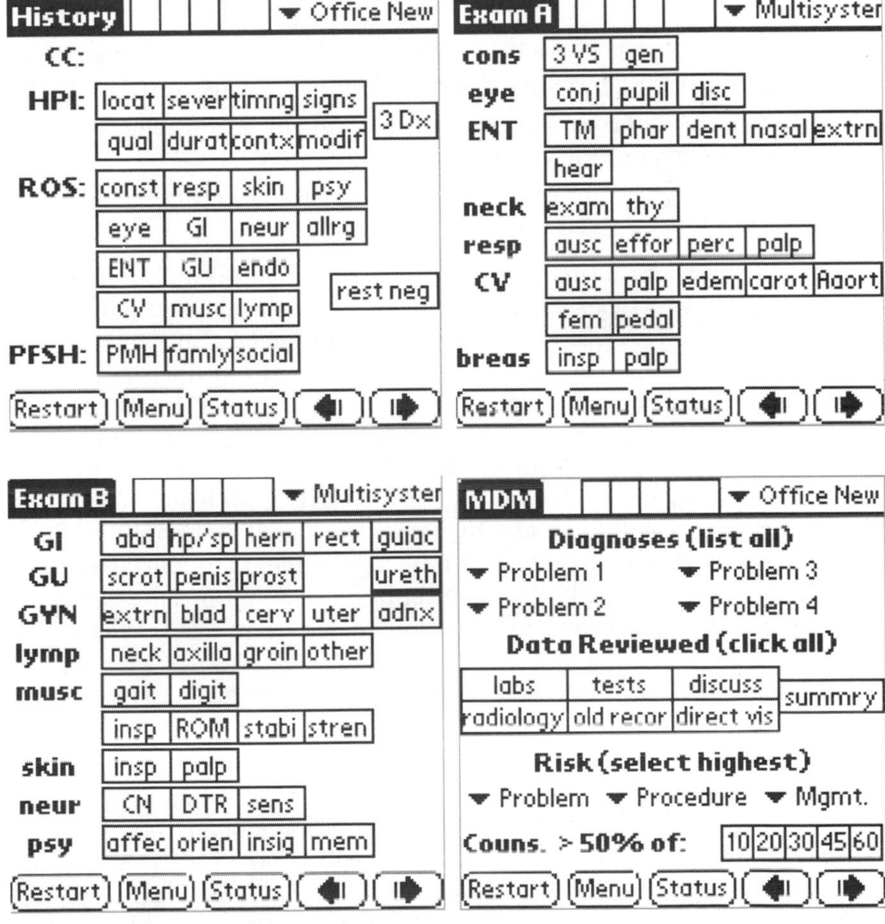

THE HEALTH INSURANCE PORTABILITY AND ACCOUNTABILITY ACT (HIPAA)

The Health Insurance Portability and Accountability Act (HIPAA) is a wide-ranging governmental regulatory effort that will alter fundamentally day-to-day business in physician offices. The Act includes regulations for electronic data transfer, patient rights over personal health information, and stringent security protections to ensure the confidentiality of a patient's medical information, among other issues.

The Department of Health and Human Services maintains a HIPAA Web site at http://aspe.hhs.gov/admnsimp/index.htm that addresses many questions physicians and administrators may have about implementing HIPAA. Also, the AAFP maintains a site with recent HIPAA articles on the Web at www.aafp.org/fpm/hipaa.html.

There are three aspects to the HIPAA regulations:

- Privacy (for confidentiality of patient health information)
- Transactions and code sets (for streamlining electronic claims and eliminating paper forms)
- Security measures (for protecting patient records from improper access or loss)

The final regulations for transactions have been issued, with compliance required by October 2002. This deadline has been extended to October 2003; however, the extension is not automatic, and must be pre-approved. The final rules for privacy were issued in April 2001, with compliance required by April 2003. The final rules for security have not yet been finalized as of press time. This schedule is subject to change, and more current sources should be sought for more up-to-date information on compliance, such as the DHHS Web site.

Noncompliance will come at a high cost, with civil and criminal penalties: fines of up to $25,000 for multiple-incident standard violations, and fines and/or jail time for intentionally inappropriate violation of the "protected health information" rules, up to $250,000 and 10 years in jail.

The final rules as published thus far are voluminous, but some summary sheets are available on the DHHS Web site. A good brief overview can be found on the Internet at www.hhs.gov/news/press/2001pres/01fshippa.html.

TABLE 25.22

Key HIPAA Terms

Understanding the HIPAA regulations will be a lot easier if you familiarize yourself with the following five terms:

Protected Health Information (PHI): HIPAA regulations apply to "protected health information," that is, medical information that contains any of a number of patient identifiers including name, Social Security number, telephone number, medical record number, or zip code. The regulations protect all individually identifiable health information in *any* form (electronic, paper-based, oral) that is stored or transmitted by a covered entity.

Covered Entities: Any health care providers, health plans, or clearinghouses that electronically transmit medical information such as billing, claims, enrollment, or eligibility verification must meet HIPAA regulations. Covered entities also include medical practices (including solo practices), employers, rehabilitation centers, nursing homes, public health authorities, life insurance agencies, billing agencies and some vendors, service organizations, and universities.

Business Associates: Covered entities cannot circumvent HIPAA regulations by using a "business associate," such as a billing service or other agency, to handle their electronic transactions. HIPAA requires covered entities to guarantee that their business associates and partners have security measures in place and technology sufficient to avoid accidental disclosure or mishandling of individually identifiable health information. This is known as a "chain of trust" relationship. Business associates must also abide by HIPAA regulations, for example, by ensuring that the individuals who are the subject of the information have access to it.

Privacy: HIPAA regulations protect an individual's right to the privacy of his or her medical information, that is, to keep it from falling into the hands of people who would use it for commercial advantage, personal gain, or malicious harm. The HIPAA privacy regulations require providers to obtain a signed consent form in order to use and disclose PHI for activities related to treatment, payment, and health care operations and to obtain a separate authorization to use or disclose PHI for any other purposes (eg, marketing).

Security: Security refers to a covered entity's specific efforts to protect the integrity of the health information it holds and *prevent unauthorized breaches of privacy* such as might occur if data are lost or destroyed by accident, stolen by intent, or sent to the wrong person in error. Security measures can be physical (eg, locking rooms and storage facilities), administrative (eg, policies and procedures covering access to information, user IDs and passwords, or punishments for violations of these), or technological (eg, encryption of electronic data and use of digital signatures to authenticate users logging into a computer system).

Adapted from Kibbe DC. What you need to know about HIPAA now. *Fam Pract Manag.* 2001;8(3):43–47.

HIPAA indicates Health Insurance Portability and Accountability Act.

INDEX

J

K

M

S

U